microbiology

and infection control for health professionals

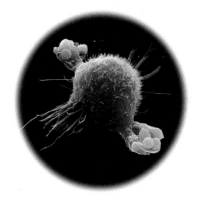

I dedicate this book to my wife Cathie, and my parents Phillip and Phyllis,
for their support and encouragement

Gary Lee

For my daughters, Karin, Christine and Genevieve

Penny Bishop

microbiology

and infection control for health professionals

GARY LEE & PENNY BISHOP [3RD EDITION]

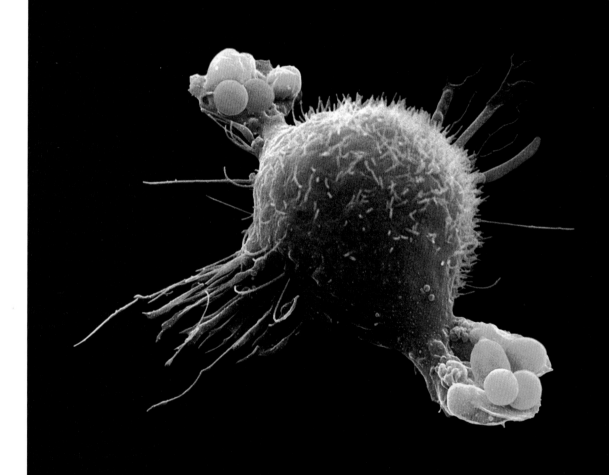

PEARSON

Prentice
Hall

Pearson Education Australia
Unit 4, Level 3
14 Aquatic Drive
Frenchs Forest NSW 2086
www.pearsoned.com.au

Acquisitions Editor: Michelle Aarons
Project Manager: Loretta Barnard
Senior Project Editor: Carolyn Robson
Copy Editor: Jo Rudd
Senior Permissions Coordinator: Louise Burke
Proofreader: Loretta Barnard
Indexer: Russell Brooks
Editorial Coordinators: Natalie Crouch, Maria Lynch
Cover and text design: Liz Nicholson, designBITE
Illustrations: Nives Porcellato and Andy Craig; Lorenzo Lucia
Typeset by Midland Typesetters, Maryborough, Victoria
Printed in China (GCC)

4 5 10 09 08 07 06

National Library of Australia
Cataloguing-in-Publication Data

Lee, Gary Mark.
Microbiology and infection control for health professionals.

3rd ed.
Includes index.
For tertiary students.
ISBN 0 7339 7344 2.

1. Medical microbiology. I. Bishop, Penny. II. Title.

616.9041

Cover
The cover shows a coloured scanning electron micrograph of a macrophage engulfing rod shaped bacteria. Macrophages are one of the first lines of defence in the body's immune system.

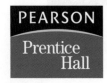

An imprint of Pearson Education Australia (a division of Pearson Australia Group Pty Ltd)

Contents in brief

Contents

Preface

Microbiology and Infection Control for Health Professionals was written in response to a perceived need for a text suitable for use in degree programs in nursing and the health sciences. The text has been widely adopted in universities throughout Australia and has also made its way into many clinical and professional libraries. The first edition of the book received an award for Excellence in Educational Publishing in 1997 as the best Australian tertiary text book and the second edition received the same award in 2002. The authors were also the recipients of the 1998 Excellence in Teaching Award from the Australian Society for Microbiology. The response of students and our colleagues in academic and clinical areas of microbiology has been very rewarding and we are pleased to be able to present a revised and updated text for this third edition.

The role of the health professional in today's society is complex, and the level of knowledge and skill required to work effectively is very high. Changing patterns of health care, new technologies, the emergence of new pathogens and increasing concerns about the incidence of hospital-acquired infections, all highlight the need for health professionals to have a thorough understanding of the microorganisms responsible for infectious diseases, a knowledge of the way they are spread, and the current research regarding methods for the prevention and control of infection.

The incidence and spread of infectious diseases in different parts of Australia are affected by socioeconomic conditions as well as geographical considerations. There is a wide variation in climatic conditions, in the distribution of insect vectors and also in people's access to health services. Because Australia is geographically isolated from the rest of the world, it is free of some of the diseases that are prevalent in other countries. However, increasing world travel creates opportunities for these diseases to spread to Australia. There is thus a risk of the global spread of new and recurrent diseases, such as occurred with the SARS epidemic.

In this edition, we maintain our approach of presenting a comprehensive text on the subject of microbiology and infection control, and as before, there is an emphasis on Australian data throughout the book. We have updated the book throughout, reflecting the important new discoveries and changes to clinical practice recommended in the 2004 CDNA *Infection Control Guidelines for the prevention of transmission of infectious diseases in the health care setting*.

Microbiology is a field that is continually and rapidly changing as a result of new research, the discovery of new diseases and pathogens, and changes in clinical practice. This edition again represents a comprehensive analysis of the current literature in the fields of medical microbiology and infection control. Topics that have been added or substantially revised include diagnostic molecular biology, the pathogenic mechanisms of microorganisms, the importance of the increase in antibiotic resistant organisms, the worldwide impact of HIV infection and AIDS, systemic fungal infections in immunocompromised patients, hepatitis, measures to prevent the spread of prion diseases (including variant Creutzfeldt-Jakob disease).

The occurrence of the SARS epidemic is used as an example of a successful epidemiological investigation and the implications of the outbreak for the development of better infection control procedures is discussed.

The sections on epidemiology have been expanded and there is increased emphasis on public health issues and the impact of globalisation on the spread of disease. The incidence rates, methods of diagnosis, treatment and prevention of specific diseases reflect current research and clinical practices. Health professionals need a thorough understanding of microbiology in order to provide safe, effective health care and this book provides current information with applications to clinical situations wherever possible. The central theme throughout the book is the relevance of microbiology to patient care.

The book is designed to enable information to be accessed in a number of ways. For students, it can be used at different levels depending on their science background and the number of hours of microbiology in their course. The content has been arranged so that educators can use the book according to the way they prefer to teach the course. For example, the major groups of microorganisms could be covered, followed by applications to transmission and control. Alternatively, the nature of infectious diseases could be covered using the 'body systems' approach and then relating it to transmission and prevention. The content of the book is selected specifically for health professionals and many of the chapters can be used for self-directed learning activities.

There are 21 chapters, divided into four units. The first unit contains basic information about the different types of microorganisms (bacteria, viruses, fungi and parasites) and the types of diseases they cause. The introduction highlights the importance of microbiology and presents an overview of the issues confronting the health professional. It contains the historical background to our current knowledge of medical microbiology, an overview of microbial metabolism and a description of the techniques of microscopy.

The second unit deals with general host-microbe relationships. A description of types of infection and disease is followed by a discussion of the ways in which microbes gain access to, and exit from, the human body. General principles of epidemiology and the value of epidemiological studies are presented with an increased emphasis on the value of surveillance and the need for evidence-based practice. The balance between pathogenic mechanisms and host defence mechanisms is discussed. This unit also includes a description of the non-specific and specific immune defences of the human body. Special emphasis is placed on the increasing occurrence of opportunistic infections in immunodeficient patients and the roles of the immune system in both preventing infection and contributing to certain disease conditions.

The third unit addresses the methods of disease prevention and control, with a special emphasis on guidelines recommended for use in Australia and New Zealand. It covers principles of sterilisation and disinfection and provides information on current recommended procedures. Antimicrobial agents and their use are described and the problems associated with the development of resistant organisms are discussed. The chapter on health care associated infections details the incidence of infection in Australian hospitals, describes methods of infection control and refers to the 2004 CDNA guidelines for the control of transmission of infectious diseases.

A unique feature of this unit is Chapter 14, 'Issues in Public Health', which addresses topics of particular interest to Australian students in the health professions. These include notifiable diseases, community health services, primary health care, Australian immunisation schedules, infection control in child-care centres, Aboriginal health and infectious diseases in remote areas of Australia. There is also a description of the health scene in New Zealand, including a comparison of the health of different ethnic groups.

The fourth unit is intended as a reference section for students and scholars of medical microbiology and uses the 'body systems' approach to give a detailed description of individual diseases. It includes a chapter on methods of specimen collection and techniques for identification of particular pathogens. The major diseases that affect each body system are described, together with relevant data, where appropriate, on their incidence in the world and Australia, diagnosis, treatment and prevention.

The third edition of *Microbiology and Infection Control for Health Professionals* is intended to provide a comprehensive guide to microbiology, infectious diseases and infection control, suitable for students in health professions, clinicians, educators and scholars of microbiology. Wherever appropriate, the emphasis is placed on Australian data, the incidence of diseases in Australia, and CDNA guidelines for infection control practices.

Features

The major pedagogical features of the book have been retained. The Spotlight boxes found throughout the text deal with incidents or events that are of general interest. They have been increased and updated.

Case study boxes are also included in the text to highlight clinical issues and to provide a focus for questions designed to test student understanding. They too have been updated.

Each chapter has an introductory list of focus questions, a chapter summary and questions at two levels: revision and 'test your understanding'. Each chapter ends with a list of material for further reading.

Where relevant website addresses have been included to enable students to access the latest information for themselves.

The book contains a comprehensive glossary and is fully indexed. Extensive use is made of diagrams and colour figures to illustrate the text.

We hope that students and clinicians will continue to find this book a valuable addition to their professional libraries.

Penny Bishop
Gary Lee

Acknowledgments

The authors would like to thank their many colleagues who convinced them of the need for the original text and have willingly offered advice and encouragement during the preparation of subsequent editions. Many of them have also generously provided us with their colour photographs to enhance the new edition (see Credits at the end of the book).

Our thanks also go to Michelle Aarons and Loretta Barnard and the other members of the editorial and production team at Pearson Education Australia.

We are grateful to our colleagues who have carefully reviewed various sections of the manuscript: Dr Richard Benn, Dr Ross Bradbury, Dr C Shu Chan, Professor Yvonne Cossart, Ms Ilze Dalins, Dr Ian Denham, Dr Sharyn Errington, Mr Glen Funnell, Dr Edward Hettiaratchi, Dr Bernie Hudson, Dr Tom Jeavons, Dr Vicki Krause, Professor Adrian Lee, Mr David Muir, Ms Virginia Jacques, Professor Margaret Burgess, Associate Professor Margaret Deighton, Associate Professor William Rawlinson, Associate Professor David Ellis, Ms Terry McAuley, Dr Joan Faoagali, Ms Irene Wilkinson, Dr Bart Currie, Dr Richard Hillman, Dr Catherine Willis.

About the Authors

Penny Bishop M Sc, Ph D, MASM

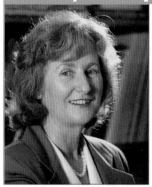

Dr Penny Bishop has recently retired from her position as a Senior Lecturer in the Department of Clinical Nursing in the Faculty of Nursing at the University of Sydney, where she was responsible for the development and integration of science courses into the nursing curriculum. Her main area of teaching was microbiology and infection control in the pre- and post-registration program for nursing students, and also in the Master of Nursing program.

Penny Bishop graduated with Honours in Biochemistry from the University of Sydney and then worked in research at the Children's Medical Research Foundation, Sydney, and overseas, in the Department of Bacteriology and Immunology at Harvard Medical School, and at the Karolinska Institute in Stockholm.

She was awarded her Ph D from the University of Sydney for studies on the biochemical properties of bacterial cell membranes. She has a number of research publications in microbiology and molecular biology to her credit, and she has taught across a wide range of courses in the faculties of Science and Medicine at the University of Sydney and the University of New South Wales.

Penny Bishop is a member of the Australian Society for Microbiology (MASM), the Australian Society for Biochemistry and Molecular Biology (ASBMB) and the Australian Infection Control Association (AICA). Her interests include the use of techniques of molecular biology to study the epidemiology of hospital-acquired infections. In 1998 she was the recipient of the Excellence in Teaching Award from the Australian Society for Microbiology (ASM) with Dr Gary Lee.

She is currently an Honorary Senior Lecturer in the Faculty of Health Sciences at the University of Sydney and for the last three years has been editor of *Microbiology Australia* – the journal of the Australian Society for Microbiology.

Gary Lee B Sc, Ph D, MBA, MASM

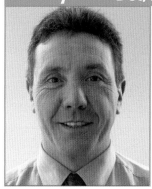

Dr Gary Lee is a Senior Lecturer in the School of Biomedical Sciences, Faculty of Health Sciences, University of Sydney. Since 1980 he has been teaching microbiology, immunology, physiology and pathophysiology at tertiary level in a broad range of health professional courses including nursing, medical radiation technology, occupational therapy and physiotherapy. He has also had several years experience in diagnostic pathology laboratories, particularly those specialising in microbiology, haematology, blood banking and serology.

Gary Lee received his BSc in microbiology and immunology from the University of New South Wales, and obtained his Ph D for his work on infection and immunity to *Salmonella typhimurium*. He completed an MBA at the University of Central Queensland.

Gary Lee is a member of the Australian Society for Microbiology and an Associate Member of the Australian Institute of Project Management. His research interests focus on infection control and antibiotic usage in hospitals, vaccination uptake by the community, evidence-based education, and the relationships between learning styles, approaches to study, student pedagogical preferences and performance. Dr Lee had a principal role in a major, innovative reform of all Faculty of Health Sciences undergraduate programs in 2001–2002. He also led the development of a generic Health Sciences degree program that was first offered in 2002, and he is currently leading its further development to establish it as a foundation program for graduate entry courses in health sciences. From 1995–1997, Dr Lee was Associate Dean and Chair of the Faculty of Health Sciences Undergraduate Studies Committee, and was Head of the School of Biomedical Sciences from 1998 to 2001. In 1998 he received, in conjunction with Dr Penny Bishop, the Australian Society for Microbiology Excellence in Teaching Award.

Fundamental Microbiology

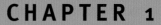

CHAPTER 1

Microbiology:
Past, Present, Future

[CHAPTER FOCUS]

- *Why is the study of microbiology essential for the health professional?*

- *What have been the major discoveries in microbiology in the last 100 years?*

- *How have these discoveries contributed to the prevention and treatment of infectious diseases?*

- *What are the major challenges posed by infectious diseases in the world today?*

- *How will infectious diseases impact on our health in the future?*

Why study microbiology?

In recent years a number of new infectious diseases have emerged, some of which have had serious implications for human health as well as significant economic impact. The most recent of these was the outbreak of severe acute respiratory syndrome, SARS, in March 2003 (see page 11 and Chapter 8, page 162). These new diseases have focused world attention on the global spread of disease and the need to identify, control and treat the agents responsible for these new infections.

One hundred years ago more than 60% of all deaths were attributed to infectious diseases. In Western countries that figure is now less than 5%, but in developing countries millions of people still die from infections that could be prevented or treated. Modern medicine has been able to identify the cause of most infectious diseases and devise strategies for their control. However, the ability to reduce mortality from infections is jeopardised by the appearance of new diseases such as AIDS and SARS, and the increasing resistance of many microorganisms to antimicrobial drugs. The purpose of this text is to introduce health professionals to the microorganisms that cause infection (**pathogens**) and the methods used to prevent or control the spread of infection.

Microorganisms (microbes) are organisms too small to be seen with the naked eye. The science of microbiology is the study of microorganisms, their properties, classification, growth requirements, method of reproduction and distribution in nature. These organisms range in size from tiny viruses to the larger organisms – bacteria, protozoa, algae, fungi and some of the microscopic stages in the life cycles of worms (helminths). They are present everywhere in our environment, in our homes, on our bodies, on the things we touch and on the food we eat. They are important for human survival on Earth, playing an essential role in many processes that maintain life.

In nature, microorganisms carry out a number of important functions. They are responsible for the decomposition of organic matter and the recycling of nutrients that help to maintain the balance of chemicals in the soil. Special nitrogen-fixing bacteria live symbiotically with certain plants, absorbing nitrogen from the air and converting it into compounds that can be used by the plant for growth. Some algae carry out photosynthesis, using energy from the sun to convert carbon dioxide in the air into carbohydrates. Marine microorganisms form the basis of the food chain in lakes, rivers and oceans. One of the most important groups of microorganisms are the **normal flora**, the microbes that reside on the human body.

As well as their role in nature, microorganisms are of benefit to humans in many other ways. Certain microorganisms are used in the manufacture of food and various pharmaceuticals and drugs, and in other industrial processes (see Chapter 3, page 46). They are a valuable tool for scientific research, and their use in laboratory experiments has been fundamental to many of the breakthrough discoveries made in biochemistry and molecular biology, including the understanding of metabolic pathways and the discovery of the genetic code.

The science of microbiology includes the study of the relationship between microorganisms and their environment (which includes the human host). In many circumstances this interaction is beneficial but, if the balance between microbe and nature is disturbed, a situation can arise where microbial growth becomes uncontrolled and the microorganisms cause disease. Some microorganisms cause disease in plants, while others infect animals and/or humans. Very few of the thousands of different microorganisms in our environment actually cause disease although, up until the last 50 years, infectious diseases were a major cause of illness and death throughout the world.

The main focus of this book is on medical microbiology, the study of the microbes that are responsible for infectious diseases, the nature of the diseases they produce in humans and the way in which they are spread. Infectious diseases have a great impact on human lives and a knowledge of this topic is essential for all health professionals.

The Past: discovery of the causes of infectious diseases

Our understanding of the relationship between microorganisms and infectious diseases dates back only to the late 19th century. Before that time, people viewed infectious diseases and epidemics with fear and superstition. Voyages of exploration throughout the world in the 16th and 17th centuries led to the development of trade routes that were responsible for carrying, not only goods, but also diseases from one part of the world to another. Travellers from the East brought diseases such as plague and cholera to Europe, where they were easily spread in the crowded, unsanitary and unhygienic conditions that existed in many cities. People thought that infections were spread in 'miasmas', or bad air, and blamed travellers for bringing disease. In Italy, travellers were isolated for 40 days to prevent the spread of plague – the Italian word for 40 is the origin of our word 'quarantine'.

Although various practices were followed to prevent the spread of diseases, they were not particularly effective because people had no real knowledge of the cause of the infection. Our current understanding of the nature of infection and transmission of infectious diseases is the outcome of the painstaking work of a number of scientists and doctors, which led to significant discoveries. Some of these are listed in Table 1.1.

'SEEING IS BELIEVING'

Until the 17th century there were no instruments that could magnify sufficiently to make microorganisms visible to the human eye. The first person to use lenses for magnification was a Dutchman, ANTON VAN LEEUWENHOEK, who observed microorganisms (or 'animalcules', as he called them) suspended in a drop of pond water in front of

Table 1.1
Scientific discoveries

YEAR	SCIENTIST	DISCOVERY
1665	Robert Hooke	Light microscope
1673	Anton van Leeuwenhoek	Lens-observed microbes
1796	Edward Jenner	Smallpox vaccine
1840	Ignaz Semmelweis	Childbirth fever
1854	John Snow	Epidemiology of cholera
1857	Louis Pasteur	Fermentation
1861	Louis Pasteur	Disproved spontaneous generation
1864	Louis Pasteur	Pasteurisation
1867	Joseph Lister	Use of disinfectants in surgery
1876	Robert Koch	Discovery of anthrax; germ theory of disease
1880	Louis Pasteur	Immunisation for cholera
1884	Elie Metchnikoff	Phagocytosis
1884	Hans Christian Gram	Gram staining method
1888–1910	Various scientists	Bacteria responsible for most diseases isolated and characterised
1898	Ross, Grassi	Malaria: mosquitoes
1900	Walter Reed	Yellow fever: mosquitoes
1910	Paul Ehrlich	Sulpha drugs
1928	Fleming, Chain, Florey	Penicillin
1953	Watson and Crick	Structure of DNA

the presence of microorganisms in air and in liquids. Figure 1.1 describes Pasteur's experiment.

Pasteur demonstrated that microorganisms are present in and on all kinds of non-living matter – solids, liquids and air. He went on to show that organisms can be destroyed by heat and that methods can be developed to prevent microbes from gaining access to solutions that have been heat-treated. The knowledge that there are microorganisms everywhere in the environment and that, given the right conditions of temperature, water and nutrients, they can reproduce and multiply is of great significance medically, scientifically and in everyday life.

During the second half of the 19th century, a number of scientists and doctors were working on a variety of medical and scientific problems in different parts of Europe. They each contributed ideas and observations which together formed a picture of how microorganisms survive, reproduce and cause disease. Some of the discoveries they made were in response to economic pressures and had a commercial basis. For example, in France, wine merchants were concerned because the wine they made sometimes turned sour when stored or shipped. Pasteur, from his work on the growth of microorganisms in liquid cultures, showed that the conversion of sugar to alcohol in the absence of air (a process called **fermentation**) was due to the activity of small organisms called yeasts. The presence of other organisms (bacteria) caused further reactions and led to souring of the wine. He showed that the troublesome organisms could be destroyed by heating the wine to 56°C for 30 minutes (a procedure now called **pasteurisation**), thus preventing the souring of the wine while still retaining

a carefully ground hand lens. His paper to the Royal Society in 1673 showed pictures of small creatures which look very like the familiar bacteria observed in laboratories today. In 1665 ROBERT HOOKE built a simple compound microscope and was able to observe the structure of a thin layer of cork. He used the term 'cells' to describe the orderly arrangement of units that he saw. However, their observations were largely forgotten for almost 200 years.

SPONTANEOUS GENERATION VERSUS BIOGENESIS

In the second half of the 19th century there was considerable discussion among scientists as to the origin of living matter. One theory was that living cells could arise from non-living matter, the theory of **spontaneous generation**. This theory arose from the observation that food left out in the air was soon found to contain millions of microscopic organisms. Other scientists contended that life could only arise from pre-existing living cells, the theory of **biogenesis**.

The arguments for each point of view became quite heated but the debate was finally settled by LOUIS PASTEUR who, with a series of ingenious experiments, demonstrated

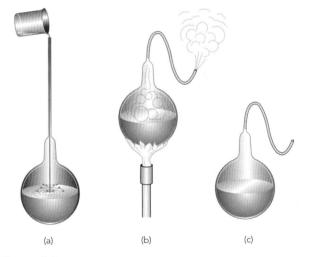

(a)   (b)   (c)

Figure 1.1

Pasteur's experiment
In order to disprove the theory of spontaneous generation, Pasteur devised the following experiment. He poured nutrient broth into a flask with a long thin neck, then heated the neck and bent it into an S-curve, a 'swan-necked' flask. He then boiled the broth in the flask, thus killing all the bacteria present in the flask, and expelling all the air. On cooling, air re-entered the flask, but the bacteria were trapped in the S-bend in the tube. Even after a long period of time, no growth of microorganisms occurred in the flask, showing that new cells could only arise from pre-existing living cells.

its quality. This method was later extended to treat milk in order to remove undesirable organisms, some of which caused souring of the milk and others that were the cause of diseases such as tuberculosis. Pasteurisation is still widely used to preserve milk products and destroy any pathogens that may be present.

The observation that microorganisms were linked to food spoilage provided a basis for the concept that they might also be responsible for infectious diseases.

TRANSMISSION OF INFECTION

In the 19th century people had little, if any, knowledge about the cause of infections or how they were spread. In Europe, the Hungarian physician IGNAZ SEMMELWEIS was concerned at the high incidence of **puerperal** (childbirth) **fever**. He thought it might be due to the transfer of an 'infectious agent' from one patient to the next by the midwives. He also observed that many doctors were in the habit of going from patient to patient, or from an autopsy to a delivery, without washing their hands. He instituted methods of handwashing in chlorinated solutions for all physicians and nurses. Although there was a significant reduction in infections, his ideas were largely ridiculed by his colleagues. His abrasive personality led to his dismissal, he spent some time in an asylum and, ironically, is said to have died from a streptococcal infection.

At about the same time, an American, OLIVER WENDELL HOLMES, also noticed that women suffered fewer infections when they gave birth at home rather than in hospital, and concluded that the infection was carried from person to person on the hands of midwives and doctors.

Other ways in which infections could be transmitted were still not well understood. JOHN SNOW, an English physician who worked in London in the 1850s, was intrigued by the fact that some of his patients contracted cholera while others did not. Although the causative agent of cholera was not known at that time, he suspected that it was being transmitted in water. He surmised that the agent responsible for cholera was being excreted by people suffering from the disease into the sewage which was dumped in the river, contaminating the water used by other inhabitants. His work was confirmed by ROBERT KOCH in Germany. The work of these two scientists laid the basis for our modern epidemiological ideas of common vehicle transmission and water purification (see Chapter 8).

In England, a surgeon named JOSEPH LISTER had heard of Pasteur's work on bacterial fermentation. He wondered if the incidence of infections, such as gangrene, in surgical wounds might be reduced if microbes were prevented from gaining access to the wounds. He knew that phenol (carbolic acid) could kill bacteria so he began to treat surgical wounds with carbolic acid and developed procedures for surgery that were quickly adopted by other surgeons. These included boiling the instruments, soaking linen and bandages in carbolic acid, and spraying a fine mist of the disinfectant into the air during surgery. Carbolic acid is quite corrosive and its use must have caused severe pain

and discomfort, but the incidence of post-surgical infections (and deaths) was dramatically reduced.

THE GERM THEORY OF DISEASE

The stage was set for the next important discovery – that bacteria are the cause of many of the known infectious diseases. In the middle of the 19th century, in Europe, the disease anthrax was killing large numbers of cattle. Both Pasteur and the German microbiologist, ROBERT KOCH, were trying to find the cause of the disease. Koch examined a sample of blood from an animal that had died from anthrax and observed rod-shaped cells (bacilli) under the microscope. He transferred a drop of blood to a flask of nutrient broth in the laboratory, allowed the bacteria to multiply, and then injected the bacteria into otherwise healthy animals. The animals developed anthrax and died (see Figure 1.2). Koch then isolated the same bacteria from the blood of the dead animals. Based on these results, Koch proposed the **germ theory of disease**, which states that each infectious disease is caused by a particular microorganism.

The experimental procedure he developed was referred to as **Koch's Postulates**, and formed the basis of a set of principles to be followed in order to determine whether an organism was the causative agent of a particular disease. The organism had to be isolated from the diseased patient, grown in culture away from the patient, and then produce the same disease when introduced into a susceptible host. It was further required that the same organism could then be isolated from the new host (see Figure 1.2). These principles were eagerly adopted by other scientists and during the next 30 years were used successfully to isolate and identify the causative organisms of most of the then known diseases of bacterial origin (see Table 1.2). To a large extent these principles are still valid today, although they require some modification in light of our current understanding of the nature of infections. They are discussed further in Chapter 7.

The methods developed by Koch were applicable only to diseases caused by bacteria. Viruses, which can replicate only inside living cells and cannot be seen under a light microscope, could not be isolated and identified in this way, so the viral nature of some diseases was not established until much later.

Another important contribution made by Koch was the development of a technique for growing bacteria on plates of nutrient medium, solidified with agar. This technique is still the basis for the isolation and identification of bacteria in diagnostic microbiology laboratories (see Chapter 15).

INSECTS AS CARRIERS OF DISEASE

A further important discovery that occurred about this time was that diseases could be spread by insects. Two diseases that were shown to be carried by mosquitoes were malaria and yellow fever. Scientists in several countries had been studying malaria, which was originally thought to be acquired by drinking contaminated water. By 1895, due mainly to the work of the French doctor CHARLES

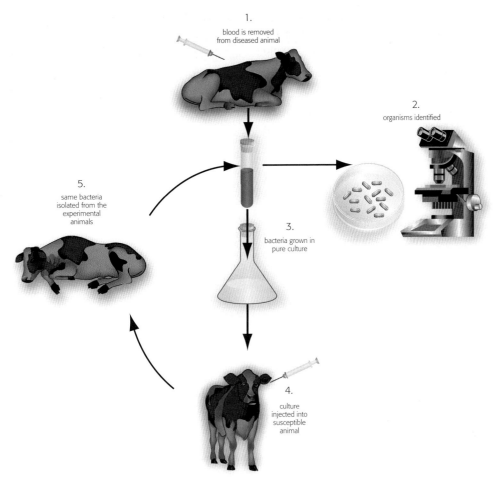

Figure 1.2

Koch's experiment showing that anthrax is caused by a particular bacterium

Table 1.2

Identification of bacteria responsible for disease

DATE	DISEASE	ORGANISM	SCIENTIST
1876	Anthrax	*Bacillus anthracis*	Koch
1878	Skin infection	*Staphylococcus*	Koch
1879	Leprosy	*Mycobacterium leprae*	Hansen
1880	Gonorrhoea	*Neisseria gonorrhoeae*	Neisser
1880	Typhoid	*Salmonella typhi*	Eberth
1880	Pneumonia	*Pneumococcus*	Pasteur, Sternberg
1882	Tuberculosis	*Mycobacterium tuberculosis*	Koch
1883	Cholera	*Vibrio cholerae*	Koch
1883	Diphtheria	*Corynebacterium diphtheriae*	Klebs
1885	Cystitis	*Escherichia coli*	Escherich
1885	Tetanus	*Clostridium tetani*	Nicolaier
1886	Pneumonia	*Streptococcus pneumoniae*	Fraenkel
1887	Meningitis	*Neisseria meningitidis*	Weichselbaum
1887	Brucellosis	*Brucella melitensis*	Bruce
1889	Tetanus	*Clostridium tetani*	Kitasato
1892	Gangrene	*Clostridium perfringens*	Welch, Nutall
1894	Plague	*Yersinia pestis*	Roux, Kitasato
1897	Botulism	*Clostridium botulinum*	van Ermengem
1898	Dysentery	*Shigella dysenteriae*	Shiga
1905	Syphilis	*Treponema pallidum*	Schaudinn, Hofmann
1906	Whooping cough	*Bordetella pertussis*	Bordet, Gengou

LAVERAN, the protozoan that causes malaria had been identified and the different forms of the parasite in the human body had been described. However, there was no agreement on how the infection was acquired or transmitted from person to person.

In 1898 the work of the English army physician RONALD ROSS in India, and GIOVANNI GRASSI in Italy, finally demonstrated that the malaria parasite was spread by a particular type of insect, the Anopheles mosquito. There were many arguments about these findings and it was not until many years later that it was accepted that control of mosquitoes was the most effective way to limit the spread of malaria. However, the implementation of mosquito eradication programs has not been successful and malaria, which is endemic in many parts of the world, is still responsible for between one and two million deaths each year.

In 1900, during the building of the Panama Canal, many workers died from the haemorrhagic disease, yellow fever. It was shown by the US army surgeon, WALTER REED, that this disease is also transmitted by mosquitoes. Although the viral nature of the disease was not known at the time, the discovery was important as it was the first time that the transmission of a viral disease by an insect was recorded. Drainage of the swamps and a spraying program successfully eliminated mosquitoes from the area, dramatically reducing the incidence of the disease and allowing the completion of the canal.

TREATMENT AND PREVENTION

By the early part of the 20th century the causative organisms of many diseases had been identified, and in many cases it was known how they were spread from person to person. The work of Semmelweis and Lister had introduced the concept of transmission by human hands or contaminated instruments. Insects had also been implicated as carriers (vectors) of disease. However, effective methods for the treatment and prevention of infectious diseases had not yet been developed. To a large extent, treatment for infectious diseases was merely supportive, using procedures that relieved the symptoms but did not cure the disease or prevent its transmission.

The worldwide influenza epidemic of 1917–18 killed 21 million people, more than three times the number of deaths that occurred during World War I. Scientists such as PAUL EHRLICH began the search for a drug, 'a magic bullet', that could destroy pathogens in the human body without harming the patient. This resulted in the discovery of the first chemotherapeutic agent, salvarsan, which was active against *Treponema pallidum*, the bacterium responsible for syphilis. The discovery of sulpha drugs followed and then the discovery of penicillin by ALEXANDER FLEMING in 1928. Penicillin was developed as a therapeutic agent during World War II by HOWARD FLOREY and ERNST CHAIN. Since then, many other antimicrobial drugs have been isolated and synthesised (see Chapter 12).

IMMUNOLOGY

The work of other scientists expanded our knowledge of the disease process and the way in which the body responds to invasion by foreign organisms. As far back as 1796, EDWARD JENNER observed that milkmaids who suffered from cowpox, a relatively mild disease that produced pustular lesions similar to smallpox, appeared to be immune to smallpox. He tested his theory by inoculating a child with material taken from a cowpox lesion and subsequently exposing him to smallpox (see Figure 1.3). The child appeared to be immune. This procedure laid the basis for our modern methods of vaccination (named after the pox virus *Vaccinia*). At that time, the viral nature of the disease was not known.

Almost 100 years later, Pasteur was experimenting with chicken cholera and accidentally used an old culture of the bacteria to inject some chickens. They did not become sick and were subsequently shown to be immune when exposed to a fresh culture. Pasteur realised that he had found an 'attenuated' or weakened strain of the pathogen which was able to protect the chickens against the virulent (disease-causing) strain in the same way as Jenner's cowpox had protected against smallpox. This concept was carried further by Pasteur when he developed a weakened strain of anthrax which provided protection against that disease.

A number of scientists attempted to produce effective vaccines by treating infectious organisms in various ways. Some of these were successful, but others – such as the tuberculin preparation against *Mycobacterium tuberculosis* developed by Koch – had disastrous consequences. Several of Koch's patients developed tuberculosis and the vaccine was discredited. Many modern vaccines consist of attenuated strains of viruses and are particularly effective because they mimic the disease, producing an immune response without any symptoms of the disease. Others consist of killed microorganisms or fragments of bacteria or viruses which are able to provoke an immune response

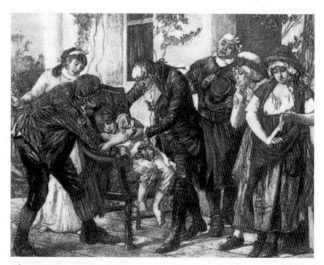

Figure 1.3

Jenner inoculating a child
Source: The Granger Collection

without producing symptoms of disease (see Chapter 9). Vaccination is the main method of protection against viral diseases as there are few effective antiviral drugs that do not also damage the host cells (see Chapters 5, 12).

Although these early scientists had some success in producing vaccines, they had little understanding of how the immune system functions. In the late 19th century many scientists believed that immunity was due to the presence of special components in the blood. The Russian zoologist ELIE METCHNIKOFF discovered that certain blood cells could ingest microbes. He called these cells **phagocytes**, meaning 'cell-eating'. We now know that phagocytes play an important role in the non-specific defences of the body. However, an understanding of the specific immune response whereby the body produces antibodies to specifically inactivate the invading organism, and memory cells to maintain immunity, did not come until late in the 20th century. The discovery in the 1980s of the AIDS virus, which attacks the T lymphocytes of the immune system, has generated a huge amount of research and contributed significantly to our knowledge of the functioning of the cell-mediated immune system.

THE AUSTRALIAN CONTRIBUTION

Although Australia has a relatively small population, the standard of scientific and medical knowledge has always been in the forefront of world achievement. A number of Australian scientists have made major discoveries in microbiology and related disciplines, working alone or in groups, or collaborating with researchers in other countries. Some of the more important are mentioned here. For a more complete description the reader is referred to Fenner 1999.

Perhaps the most famous is HOWARD FLOREY who was educated in Adelaide but worked mainly in England. Based on Alexander Fleming's earlier observations, Florey and Ernst Chain developed penicillin as a therapeutic agent. The three scientists shared the Nobel Prize in 1945.

One of the most significant discoveries was the recognition in the early 1940s by NORMAN GREGG, a paediatrician at the Royal Alexandra Hospital for Children in Sydney, that rubella infection in the first trimester of pregnancy was the cause of congenital defects, including deafness, heart and brain lesions and cataracts. The successful development of a vaccine for rubella has greatly reduced the incidence of congenital rubella syndrome.

Australians have been world leaders in the fields of immunology and viral research. Another Nobel Prize winner in 1960 was F. MACFARLANE BURNET. His early work was in the fields of viral, rickettsial and bacterial infections, but he gained most recognition in the field of immunology for his work on immunological tolerance, the biology of self-recognition, and his development of the theory of clonal selection and antibody response.

Throughout his lifetime, FRANK FENNER has also made major contributions to an understanding of the nature of viral infections and played a major role in the World

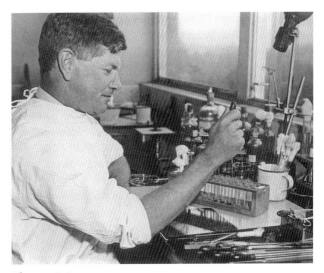

Figure 1.4
Nobel laureate Sir Frank MacFarlane Burnet

Health Organization's successful campaign to eradicate smallpox.

In 1996 PETER DOHERTY (together with the American Rolf Zinkernagel) received the Nobel Prize for his work on the role of the major histocompatibility complex (MHC) antigens in T cell recognition of virus-infected cells. The work was first published in 1972, but the significance of the observations became more apparent as knowledge of the nature of viral infection and the immune response increased.

A number of disease-causing microorganisms were first identified in Australia and found to have worldwide significance. In 1973 RUTH BISHOP and IAN HOLMES described a virus responsible for severe gastroenteritis in children. It was later named *rotavirus* and found to be a major cause of infant diarrhoea and mortality throughout

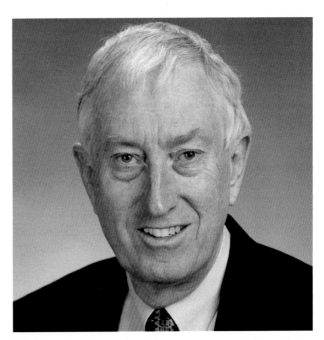

Figure 1.5
Nobel laureate Professor Peter Doherty

the world. YVONNE COSSART demonstrated the presence of human parvovirus in blood donors and IAN GUST worked on the classification of hepatitis A. Another important organism first described by Australians is the rickettsia responsible for Q fever, *Coxiella burnetii*, (MACFARLANE BURNET and EDWARD DERRICK).

The bacterium *Mycobacterium ulcerans* which causes necrotising ulcers (Bairnsdale ulcers) was identified by JEAN TOLHURST and GLENN BUCKLE. Although not common in Australia (see page 372), these ulcers are a major problem in Africa where they are called Buruli ulcers. The agent that has been implicated as a cause of gastric ulcers, *Helicobacter pylori*, was first identified by Perth doctors ROBIN WARREN and BARRY MARSHALL (see page 431). Antibiotic treatment of this condition gives dramatic results (see page 431).

A number of viral pathogens that are found mainly in Australia and New Guinea have been identified by other Australian groups. They include many of the arboviruses transmitted by mosquitoes, such as Ross River virus (RALPH DOHERTY), Murray Valley encephalitis virus (ERIC FRENCH) and Barmah Forest virus. In 1994 a new virus was discovered which could cross the species barrier and infect animals as well as humans – the equine morbil-livirus – now renamed Hendra virus. This was followed soon after by the discovery of the rabies-like bat lyssavirus and the Menangle virus. These are discussed further in Chapter 5 on page 89 and Spotlight box Chapter 8, page 157.

The Present: achievements in the control of infectious diseases

PUBLIC HEALTH

During the last hundred years, there has been a dramatic increase in our understanding of the microbial causes of infection and with it has come an improvement in our ability to deal with outbreaks of disease.

We now know the cause and method of transmission of many diseases and can implement strategies to deal with outbreaks when they occur. Improvements in hygiene and sanitation in the developed world have significantly reduced the mortality rates from infectious diseases. The area of disease prevention and health maintenance is called Public Health and is of vital importance when developing strategies to deal with major global events such as the Olympic Games, mass gatherings for sporting events and pilgrimages such as the Haj. Electronic communication between health authorities around the world enables rapid dissemination of information about an outbreak, the reporting of cases and sharing of experience for treatment and control.

Today, when people can travel from one side of the world to the other in less than 24 hours, the possibility of an infectious agent being introduced into an unsuspecting population is very high. Any major international event involving thousands of travellers from all parts of the world, often crowded into a relatively closed environment,

creates a situation where infections can spread very easily. Increased medical services are required for the large number of people who attend, the environment must be continuously monitored and the provision of safe food and water is essential.

An important aspect of the organisation of any major event involves the public health strategies put in place to monitor and protect the health of residents and visitors, and the coordination of health services so that swift action can be taken in the event of an outbreak of disease, or a natural or man-made disaster. If a serious outbreak of infection occurs among athletes or visitors to a city, it can spell disaster for an event that has taken years to plan and organise.

Prevention: the Olympic Games

An example of the use of public health measures was the Olympic Health Surveillance System which was set up by the New South Wales Department of Health and played a coordinating role in protecting the health of the visitors and residents of Sydney during the Olympic Games in 2000 (see Figure 1.6).

The procedures put in place included:

- The Notifiable Diseases computerised database was used to detect outbreaks of communicable disease, and reporting was made on a twice daily rather than weekly basis. The emergency departments at several large hospitals were designated sentinel sites to detect whether an unusually high incidence of certain conditions or symptoms of infection occurred.

- Monitoring of food safety was of the utmost importance. About 1.8 million meals were prepared and served at the Olympic village. An outbreak of food-

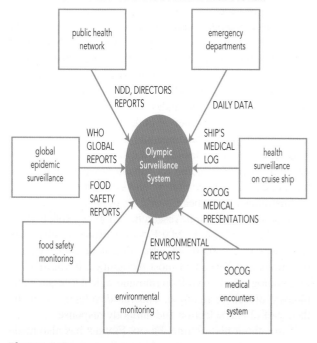

Figure 1.6

New South Wales Olympic surveillance system

borne illness in the village would have been disastrous for the athletes.

- Health surveillance was carried out on the cruise ships in the harbour which acted as floating hotels and provided beds for over 6000 people at a time, with a total of many thousands of people using their facilities. Outbreaks of diseases such as gastroenteritis, influenza, Legionnaires' disease and tuberculosis have all been reported from cruise ships where people are in a confined space and air conditioning facilitates the spread of respiratory diseases.
- Environmental monitoring of air and water quality was carried out and reported each day. In particular, steps were taken to prevent an outbreak of Legionnaires' disease by treatment and inspection of all water cooling towers at Olympic venues.
- Global outbreaks of infectious diseases were monitored so as to identify travellers arriving from high-risk areas.

The Health Surveillance System involved cooperation between local government and health care agencies in a way that would never have been imagined a hundred years ago, when our knowledge of the transmission of infection was very limited.

Dealing with an outbreak: SARS

The recent outbreak of SARS (Severe Acute Respiratory Syndrome), which originated in China and spread via Hong Kong to other parts of the world, is a striking example of the way in which a network of doctors, scientists and public health experts from all parts of the world worked together to identify the causative organism and contain the disease. World attention was focused on this new disease which could spread rapidly and was potentially fatal. A single person carrying the virus travelled from China to Hong Kong and stayed in a hotel where the infection was spread to other guests and subsequently carried to almost 30 other countries (see Spotlight box, page 162).

There were over 8000 cases of the disease and 774 deaths, a large number of them health care workers and their families who were exposed to infected patients before the disease was diagnosed (51% in Toronto and 33% in Hong Kong). The virus is highly infectious and transmitted mainly by contact and in aerosol droplets.

The speed with which the world community reacted prevented the occurrence of a potentially serious pandemic. Experts in infection control from many countries (including Australia) travelled to Hong Kong, Singapore and other affected countries to advise on containment of the disease. Meanwhile, scientists worked on the isolation and identification of the new virus. Only two months after the index case arrived in Hong Kong, the virus responsible for SARS had been isolated and its genome sequenced; it was identified as a new corona virus, SARS-CoV. The outbreak was brought under control in just a few months.

The World Health Organization (WHO), the Centers for Disease Control (CDC) and infectious diseases experts collaborated on guidelines for case definition and infection control protocols which effectively broke the chain of transmission. However, the virus is still endemic in the community and the potential exists for it to resurface at any time. The only real control for the future lies in the development of a vaccine.

The economic cost of the outbreak was huge – in terms of losses in trade, travel and tourism. In Hong Kong alone, the SARS outbreak is estimated to have cost the country 4% of its gross domestic product (GDP).

ANTIBIOTICS

Since the first antibiotic, penicillin, was discovered and developed in the 1940s, a number of other antimicrobial drugs have been produced to treat or cure disease. These have had a significant impact on the level of morbidity and mortality due to infectious diseases. Antibiotics have been used successfully to treat community-acquired infections as well as more serious life-threatening infections in hospital patients. However, there are increasing numbers of organisms that are resistant to antibiotics. Antibiotic therapy is described in detail in Chapter 12.

VACCINATION

Many infections can now be prevented by the administration of a vaccine. The World Health Organization's vaccination campaign against smallpox led to the worldwide eradication of this disease in 1977. Polio, which once crippled thousands of people annually, has almost been eradicated from Western countries including Australia, which was declared free of polio in 2000. The incidence of congenital rubella syndrome, which causes serious birth defects in babies whose mothers are infected in the first trimester of pregnancy, has been dramatically reduced by the development of a vaccine.

As well as vaccines to prevent the childhood diseases of diphtheria, whooping cough, measles and mumps, new vaccines have been developed for chickenpox, meningococcal disease and pneumococcal disease. A vaccine is available to protect against hepatitis A and B. Vaccines against influenza are developed each year to combat new strains of the virus. However, it is essential that a high level of vaccine coverage is maintained in the community to prevent the recurrence of vaccine-preventable diseases (see Chapter 14).

DIAGNOSTIC TECHNIQUES

In the last 50 years there has been a rapid expansion of knowledge in the fields of virology, immunology and molecular biology. Specialised techniques using sophisticated equipment have enabled scientists to carry out research in these areas. We now understand the basis of inheritance at a molecular level – how information can be carried from one generation to the next and translated into functional cell components. Techniques developed for use in molecular biology have enabled the production of genetically engineered compounds such as hormones and vaccines that are of benefit to humans (see Chapter 4).

Microorganisms can now be identified by their genetic

material, the DNA or RNA, using specific techniques to distinguish between closely related strains. This testing is often quicker than conventional techniques and enables 'real time' testing by diagnostic laboratories to identify microbial pathogens and follow their transmission in the clinical environment (see Chapter 15).

The Future: challenges for the health professional

In the 21st century there are new challenges for the health professional. They include new and re-emerging diseases, increased susceptibility of patients, changes in lifestyle, globalisation and opportunities for travel. Advances in medicine mean that many more patients survive, but they are also sicker and more susceptible to infection. The overuse or misuse of antibiotics has led to the emergence of antibiotic-resistant strains of bacteria, especially in hospitals. This poses special problems in the treatment of hospital-acquired infections (see Chapters 12, 13). The ability of viruses and bacteria to change their genetic properties means that preventative strategies (vaccines) and treatments (antimicrobial drugs) are not as effective as before.

The advances achieved in Western countries have not occurred in developing nations, where millions still die each year from infectious diseases. It is sobering to compare the challenges facing health care workers in different parts of the world (see Table 1.3).

MAJOR CHALLENGES

Throughout the world, earlier successes are now being clouded by the emergence of new diseases and drug-resistant microorganisms. Diseases that had almost been eradicated, such as tuberculosis, have re-emerged, often in a form exhibiting multi-resistance to existing antimicrobial drugs. Tuberculosis is now the greatest single cause of death throughout the world with an estimated four million deaths each year.

In some tropical areas, strains of malaria have appeared that are resistant to the usual antimalarial compounds, chloroquine and primaquine. Malaria poses a significant threat to residents, tourists and aid workers in these areas There are about three million new cases of malaria each year with between one and two million deaths.

AIDS

The world is now faced with a new kind of epidemic. AIDS (acquired immune deficiency syndrome), caused by the human immunodeficiency virus (HIV), appeared in the 1980s, attacking the immune system, destroying T cells and leaving the patient susceptible to opportunistic infections. Although the number of new cases in Australia has been contained, due largely to a public education campaign and needle exchange program, this is not the case in other parts of the world, especially the developing nations (see Figure 1.7).

In parts of sub-Saharan Africa, AIDS has gained a hold in the heterosexual population and there is a lack of gov-

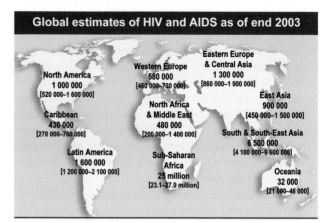

| Global estimates of HIV and AIDS as of end 2003 |

Total number of adults and children living with HIV: 38 million [35-42 million]

Number of people living with HIV	Total	37.8 million	[34.6–42.3 million]
	Adults	35.7 million	[32.7–39.8 million]
	Women	17 million	[15.8–18.8 million]
	Children <15 years	2.1 million	[1.9–2.5 million]
People newly infected with HIV in 2003	Total	4.8 million	[4.2–6.3 million]
	Adults	4.1 million	[3.6–5.6 million]
	Children <15 years	630 000	[570 000–740 000]
AIDS deaths in 2003	Total	2.9 million	[2.6–3.3 million]
	Adults	2.4 million	[2.2–2.7 million]
	Children <15 years	490 000	[440 000–580 000]

Figure 1.7

Adults and children estimated to be living with HIV/AIDS at the end of 2003

ernment support for education to prevent transmission, and no money to provide drugs for treatment. In these areas, it is estimated there are 25 million people living with HIV. In 2003 3 million people became newly infected. The Caribbean is the second-worst affected area.

The steepest increases in HIV infections are occurring in Southeast Asia, Eastern Europe and Central Asia, with injecting drug use contributing to a large share of infections. In Europe, heterosexual transmission is increasing and women account for an increasing proportion of new HIV-positive diagnoses. Although there have been advances in the development of antiviral drugs, there is still no cure for AIDS and no immediate prospect of a vaccine. Some 40 million people are estimated to be infected worldwide, of whom nearly 50% are women. There have been more than 20 million deaths since the beginning of the epidemic – 3 million of them in 2003.

VIRAL DISEASES

The last few years of the 20th century and the start of the 21st century were marked by reports of an increase in the number of 'new' viral diseases. Australia, because of its isolation, used to be relatively free of many of these diseases, but with the increase in speed and frequency of air travel it is possible for new diseases to be introduced. The introduction of multiple strains of dengue fever by travellers can give rise to cases of the haemorrhagic form of dengue fever (see page 467).

Japanese encephalitis, a mosquito-borne viral

Table 1.3

The global scene: major issues affecting health

DEVELOPED NATIONS	DEVELOPING COUNTRIES
• Improvement in patient survival due to advances in treatment and medical interventions	• Famine, lack of clean water, poor sanitation
• Increased susceptibility of patients to infection	• Poverty, malnutrition, high susceptibility to infection
• Increased resistance of hospital strains of bacteria to antibiotics	• Lack of drugs
• Changes in lifestyle, air conditioning	• Gastrointestinal diseases
• Travel – globalisation	• Parasitic diseases – helminth infestations
• Non-compliance with vaccination	• Vaccines not available due to expense or lack of transport
• Emerging viral infections – SARS	• HIV/AIDS
• Viral mutation – influenza A	• Blood-borne and haemorraghic diseases
• Arboviruses	• Malaria
• Multi-drug-resistant TB (MDRTB)	• TB
• Bioterrorism	• Civil war

encephalitis, is common throughout Asia and some cases have been reported in the Northern Territory and Torres Strait Islands. Given the right conditions this disease could spread to the southern, more populous states of Australia. Viruses transmitted by insect vectors are of increasing importance in Australia (see Chapter 5, page 100, and Chapter 8, page 169).

Ebola fever is caused by a deadly haemorrhagic virus that attacks every tissue and organ in the body, causing death in most patients within a few days. The patient is highly infectious and the virus is spread by contact with infected blood or other body fluids. Since the patient is bleeding from the skin and body orifices, it is very easy for the virus to spread, especially in the unhygienic conditions that prevail in developing countries. Ebola virus belongs to a group known as filo viruses. They are the causative agents of haemorrhagic fevers in humans, with mortality ranging from 20% to 80%. Another virus in this group is the Marburg virus. The natural reservoir for the filo viruses is unknown.

These viruses are not currently present in Australia and are unlikely to become established because of the short incubation time, easily identifiable symptoms and Australia's isolation.

Hantaviruses form another group of viruses which can produce haemorrhagic symptoms. An outbreak of disease with influenza-like symptoms, in which the lungs filled with fluid, leading to death by respiratory failure, occurred on an Indian reservation in New Mexico in 1993. It was found to be caused by a hantavirus and epidemiologists linked the outbreak to a recent plague of deer mice. Many of these viruses are maintained in nature in a rodent reservoir. Humans acquire the diseases by direct contact with the animals or with virus shed in urine or saliva. As yet there have been no reports of hantavirus infections in Australia.

In September 1994, in Queensland, there was an outbreak of a pneumonia-like disease among racehorses in a Brisbane stable. Fourteen horses died and their trainer also

contracted the disease and died. A previously unknown virus, initially called equine morbillivirus, now renamed Hendra virus, was isolated from both trainer and horses, and antibodies to the virus were found in the blood of a strapper who had cared for the sick horses. In October 1995 there was a report of the death of another person who had assisted at the autopsy of a horse that had died in Mackay in August 1994. He also had antibodies to Hendra virus.

Flying foxes (fruit bats) have been implicated as the reservoir for Hendra virus and also for the recently discovered rabies-like bat lyssavirus and the Menangle virus which affects pigs and humans. Nipah virus, which caused an outbreak of encephalitis among pig farmers in Malaysia, also has flying foxes as its natural reservoir. These are all examples of new viruses which appear to be able to cross the species barrier (see Spotlight box, page 157).

The avian flu virus, which has affected millions of birds and chickens in all parts of Asia, has now been classed as endemic in the bird population. The strain H5N1 has been responsible for a number of infections in humans, causing illness and sometimes death.

West Nile virus, which originated in North Africa, can also infect humans. It is carried by migratory birds and is now classified as endemic in North America. As yet there have been no reports of the virus in Australia.

It is probable that many more viruses will emerge or be identified in the future. There are a number of reasons for this.

- An increase in tourism and world travel allows viruses to spread around the globe at frightening speed (e.g. SARS).
- Building and development in previously unsettled areas brings humans into contact with hitherto unknown viruses.
- New molecular techniques allow identification of viruses without the need for culture. For example,

molecular techniques have identified TTV (transfusion transmissible virus) in blood – but as yet there is no obvious disease caused by the virus. It is possible there may be other unidentified viruses which can be transmitted in body substances (see Chapters 5 and 15).

Viral mutation

An important factor in the occurrence of epidemics of 'new' viral diseases is the ability of viruses to mutate and change their outer structure so that existing vaccines are no longer effective. This is best illustrated by the influenza A virus, which has undergone repeated changes to its outer envelope during the last century. It is thought that the virus is able to infect domestic animals, particularly pigs and ducks, where it undergoes genetic recombination and acquires new genetic characteristics, giving rise to a new and more virulent strain of the virus.

This passage of a human virus through an animal is also thought to account for the emergence of the virus responsible for SARS, a virulent **coronavirus**, related to the human cold virus.

Reactivation of viral infections

Several viruses have been identified that persist in the human body in a latent form, able to be reactivated if the immune system is depressed (see Chapter 5, page 95). Others, such as hepatitis B, hepatitis C and human papilloma virus (HPV), persist in a chronic, infective carrier state that can lead to cancer. It is thought that other viruses may play a part in the development of cancer but the link is not yet proven. Some viruses that persist in the body have been linked to diseases like chronic fatigue syndrome (CFS). A large number of CFS sufferers show evidence of previous exposure to viruses such as Epstein-Barr (EB), cytomegalovirus (CMV), coxsackie B virus, human herpes virus 6 (HHV6) and human T cell lymphotrophic virus 1 (HTLV1).

There is still very little understanding of how persistent viral infections affect the immune system, but there is some evidence that viruses play a part in autoimmune diseases.

VACCINES

Although vaccines are available for many infectious diseases, there is widespread complacency in developed countries and many people do not have their children immunised. As a result, epidemics of diseases such as measles, diphtheria and whooping cough still occur, even in Australia, where all these vaccines are freely available. If the level of vaccine coverage falls below a critical value the protective effect of 'herd immunity' is lost and there is a real risk of a recurrence of epidemics of diseases such as measles (see Chapter 14).

In developing countries, people are still suffering and dying from infectious diseases such as gastroenteritis, measles and polio, which would not occur if better hygiene, vaccines and medical treatment were available. Poverty, lack of education and lack of government finance for effective medical programs are largely to blame.

SUSCEPTIBILITY OF PATIENTS

Advances in medical treatments mean that there are increasing numbers of people whose immune system is compromised to some extent – from their illness, the medical treatment they have received, diseases such as cancer, the use of immunosuppressive drugs after transplant operations, or a disease such as AIDS. They are particularly vulnerable to a range of otherwise harmless microorganisms. They also act as reservoirs for some of the more serious pathogens (e.g. multi-drug-resistant tuberculosis in AIDS patients). In particular, susceptible patients are at risk from opportunistic pathogens (microorganisms that would not cause disease in healthy individuals).

The hospital environment may contain antibiotic-resistant microorganisms and other opportunistic pathogens. Fungal infections in immunocompromised patients are becoming more common. Building works that disturb the environment, create air currents and release fungal spores can also pose a significant risk to susceptible patients in a health care facility, see Chapter 7.

GLOBAL ISSUES

As humans penetrate into unsettled areas and disturb the natural environment, they are at risk of exposure to previously unrecognised microbes. Sometimes, these are organisms that would not otherwise come into contact with humans. Often, the changes that humans make to the environment create more favourable conditions for the animal reservoir or insect vector of the organism. For example, the planting of grain crops can encourage the rodents that carry some of the viruses described above (e.g. hantavirus in deer mice). Irrigation may establish breeding grounds for mosquitoes or sandflies that transmit diseases.

In Australia there has been an increase in reports of infections with mosquito-borne viruses such as Ross River and Barmah Forest virus. These are often related to rainfall and climatic conditions. Global warming and changes in climate also affect the environments where microorganisms can thrive.

In some cases, our modern lifestyle facilitates the spread of an organism. For example, in tropical regions, strains of cholera can be found in coastal waters. When this water is used as ballast for shipping, it is sometimes discharged into harbours or rivers in other parts of the world. The cholera bacteria are thus spread, contaminating the water and entering the food chain.

Another example is the widespread use of air-conditioning systems, which have been blamed for spreading organisms around a building. They have been linked to the occurrence of pneumonia caused by the organism *Legionella pneumophila*, which is spread in the fine aerosol vapour associated with water-cooled air-conditioning units.

The history of infectious diseases is also the history of exploration and the spread of disease by travellers carrying organisms around the world. In the early days of white settlement in Australia, infections such as influenza, measles and smallpox had a devastating effect on the Aboriginal population, which had never been exposed to these diseases before and therefore had no immunity.

As an island continent, Australia has been for many years free of diseases that are endemic in other parts of the world (e.g. plague, rabies). Our isolation and stringent quarantine regulations combined to prevent these diseases from entering the country or becoming established in animal reservoirs. However, travel, complacency, lack of compliance with health regulations and the emergence of resistant strains of organisms are rapidly creating a situation where no area can be considered free of a particular infectious disease.

This is illustrated by the devastating effects of the tsunami which hit Southeast Asia on Boxing day 2004. Outbreaks of disease resulted in many injured tourists returning home carrying unusual tropical infections. Flooding caused an increase in vector-borne diseases, malaria and dengue fever.

PRION DISEASES

Prions are unusual infective particles consisting only of protein. They are responsible for a group of fatal neurological disorders called **transmissible spongiform encephalopathies** (TSEs). See Chapter 20 and Spotlight box, Chapter 13. The appearance in England of cases of variant Creutzfeldt-Jakob disease (vCJD), a new prion disease with evidence of a link to mad cow disease (BSE), raised concerns about the number of people who may have been infected by eating contaminated beef. Although the number of cases of vCJD seems to have peaked, there is still little information about the risks of transmission in blood or body products or by medical procedures.

Because of the long incubation time for the disease, Australia, which is currently free of BSE, has banned blood and organ donations from any person who lived in England between 1980 and 1996 (see Spotlight box, page 240). The importation of beef and beef products has also been banned.

BIOTERRORISM

Since 11 September 2001 the threat of bioterrorism has been discussed constantly in the newspapers.

Bioterrorism is the fear created by the threat of biological warfare. Biological weapons (microorganisms) are popular with terrorists because they are easy to obtain, easy to produce in large quantities and easy to disseminate.

The damage that can be done by microorganisms, although real, is limited by the nature of the organisms, their stability, the way they are transmitted and environmental conditions. The Centers for Disease Control in the United States has ranked the most dangerous microorganisms. In the highest category are anthrax, smallpox, plague, botulism, tularaemia and the haemorrhagic fevers.

Among these, the smallpox virus is one of the most important because there is no treatment for it. Since it was eradicated globally (the last natural case occurred in 1977), most of the world's population are no longer immune. Stocks of the virus are supposed to be held only in Russia and the United States, but it is possible that during the dissolution of the Soviet Union stocks of the virus could have fallen into the hands of terrorists. It is a serious life-threatening disease and easily transmissible. However, there is a vaccine available which could be used if an outbreak occurs.

Anthrax spores are very stable and can be easily disseminated as fine powder or aerosol. Anthrax is treatable with antibiotics unless resistant strains are used, and a vaccine is also available. It does not spread easily from person to person. In the United States, the anthrax powder that was sent by mail after 11 September 2001 infected 22 people, of whom five died.

The food supply is a major area where bioterrorism is effective. **Food biosecurity** is the prevention of the intentional contamination of food and water with hazardous agents, including pathogens and toxins. The main risks are incurred during production and processing, and controls are needed over the importation and transportation of food. The main agents are *Salmonella*, toxigenic strains of *E. coli*, which cause haemolytic uremic syndrome, *Listeria* and botulinum toxin.

In agriculture, infectious diseases can have devastating economic effects; for example, the naturally occurring outbreaks of foot and mouth disease and avian flu have cost farmers all over the world billions of dollars and made a significant impact on the economies of affected countries.

Australia is very vulnerable to the importation of these diseases and this could be exploited by terrorists. Bioterrorists can cause physical, economic, social and political damage with minimal effort. The actual loss of life may not be great: the main aim of bioterrorism is to create panic and cause civil disorder, and it can have a major impact on the economy and political stability of a country.

The chapters in this book cover basic information about the microorganisms that can adversely affect humans. In this chapter we attempt to describe the current state of knowledge about infectious diseases and to show why an understanding of the properties of microorganisms, a knowledge of their transmission and control, as well as methods for the prevention and treatment of infection, are essential for the health professional.

SUMMARY

- Microorganisms are present everywhere and play an essential role in many processes that maintain life. Very few microorganisms actually cause disease.
- In the past, explorers spread diseases from the East to Europe.
- During the last 100 years, there has been a dramatic increase in knowledge and understanding of the microbial causes of infection.
- The development of suitable magnifying instruments was necessary in order to see microorganisms.
- Pasteur disproved the theory of spontaneous generation and showed that microorganisms were responsible for food spoilage.
- Scientists such as Semmelweis and Lister showed how transmission of infection could be prevented.
- In the 19th century Robert Koch proposed the germ theory of disease; he and other scientists isolated and identified the causative organisms of most of the then known diseases of bacterial origin.
- Work on malaria and yellow fever showed that some diseases are transmitted by mosquitoes.
- The search for drugs to treat infectious diseases led to the synthesis of sulpha drugs and the discovery of antibiotics.
- Edward Jenner used cowpox to prevent infection by smallpox; this laid the basis for modern vaccination programs.
- Some diseases have been eradicated (smallpox), are preventable (polio) or are controllable (plague).
- Research in immunology and molecular biology has increased our understanding of how infectious diseases affect the body and can be treated.
- A number of Australian scientists have made significant discoveries in microbiology.
- Improvements in public health have contributed to successful control of outbreaks of disease.
- The discovery of antibiotics and the introduction of vaccines have reduced mortality from infectious diseases.
- New diagnostic techniques help to quickly identify and track the organisms responsible for an outbreak of disease.
- The successful treatment of infectious diseases in the future is threatened by the emergence of new and resistant organisms.
- HIV/AIDS is the 'plague' of the new millenium.
- Bioterrorism using biological (microbial) weapons is a new threat.

STUDY QUESTIONS

1. Why is the study of microbiology important for the health professional?
2. Name the scientist responsible for proposing the germ theory of disease.
3. Describe some of the contributions made to microbiology by Louis Pasteur.
4. What is meant by the theory of spontaneous generation?
5. What contribution did Semmelweis make to our understanding of disease transmission?
6. How are malaria and yellow fever transmitted?
7. Who discovered penicillin?
8. What is the origin of the word 'vaccination'?
9. Which infectious diseases are responsible for most deaths in the world today?

TEST YOUR UNDERSTANDING

1. What are the major scientific achievements that have contributed to a reduction in deaths from infectious diseases?
2. Why is tuberculosis still a worldwide problem?
3. How has our modern lifestyle contributed to the spread of infectious diseases?
4. What are some of the major successes in the treatment and control of infectious diseases?

5. What are the major problems in infectious diseases confronting medicine today?
6. How can bioterrorists achieve their goals?

Further reading

Cumpston JHL 1989, *Health and Disease in Australia. A History*, Canberra: Australian Government Publishing Service.

Fenner F (ed.) 1990, *History of Microbiology in Australia*, Curtin ACT: Australian Society for Microbiology.

Fenner F, Some Notable Discoveries in Microbiology Made by Australians: The Discoveries and the Scientists. In Asche V (ed.) 1999, *Recent Advances in Microbiology* Vol 7: Melbourne, Australian Society for Microbiology Inc; 1–62.

Halstead SB 2001, Emerging and endangered infections. *Current Opinion in Infectious Diseases* 14(5): 503–506.

Mackenzie JS et al. 2001, Emerging Viral Diseases of Southeast Asia and the Western Pacific. *Emerging Infectious Diseases* 7(3) Supplement pp. 497–504.

Thackway SV, Delpech VC, Jorm LR, McAnulty JM, Visotina M, 2000, Monitoring acute diseases during the Sydney 2000 Olympic and Paralympic Games. *MJA*; 173: 318–321.

World Health Organization, Global Tuberculosis Control: WHO Report 2000 Geneva: World Health Organization.

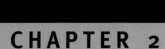

CHAPTER 2

Overview of the Microbial World

[CHAPTER FOCUS]

- *How are microorganisms classified?*

- *What are the major groups of microorganisms that cause disease in humans?*

- *What is the value of microscopy in medical microbiology?*

- *What types of microscopes and microscopic techniques are commonly used in medical microbiology?*

- *What is the value of the Gram stain in microbiology?*

Introduction

As scientists began to study the complex world of living organisms, the need arose to develop a system of classification. The earliest classification scheme put all living organisms into two groups: plants and animals. With the development of the microscope the world of cells and cell structure was revealed, and it became accepted that all living matter is made up of cells. It also became clear that some organisms consist of only one cell, whereas others are made up of many cells. Complex, higher organisms are made up of many parts, or organs, which are differentiated into various types of cells according to the function they perform. Improvements in microscopes enabled scientists to study the 'invisible' organisms – that is, those too small to be seen with the naked eye – and to show that some of these microscopic creatures were responsible for the infectious diseases of higher organisms.

Classification of living organisms

The classification of living organisms is a kind of short-hand used to describe groups of organisms which:

- have a similar genetic composition,
- have characteristics in common,
- have developed in similar ways,
- have certain growth requirements, or
- are found in certain locations.

CLASSIFICATION INTO DOMAINS AND KINGDOMS

Early scientific observations of living organisms were confined to a description of their **morphology** (external appearance). In 1866 the German scientist ERNST HAECKEL extended the classification of living organisms from two to three groups – animals, plants and **Protista**, which consisted of single-celled organisms such as bacteria and protozoa, together with some fungi and algae.

In the 20th century, new techniques and instruments enabled scientists to study the different life forms in more detail. As more microorganisms were discovered, and more was learnt about their structure, habitats and nutritional requirements, further refinements in classification were made. In 1969, R.H. WHITTAKER proposed a **five-kingdom classification** which placed all known organisms in five groups, or kingdoms – based on microscopic observations of morphology and methods of reproduction.

1. **Monera**, or **Procaryota** – single-celled organisms comprising the **eubacteria**, or **true bacteria**, and the **archaebacteria**, or ancient bacteria such as thermophiles and halophiles
2. **Protista** – including slime moulds, protozoa and some algae
3. **Fungi** – single-celled yeasts, multicellular moulds and mushrooms

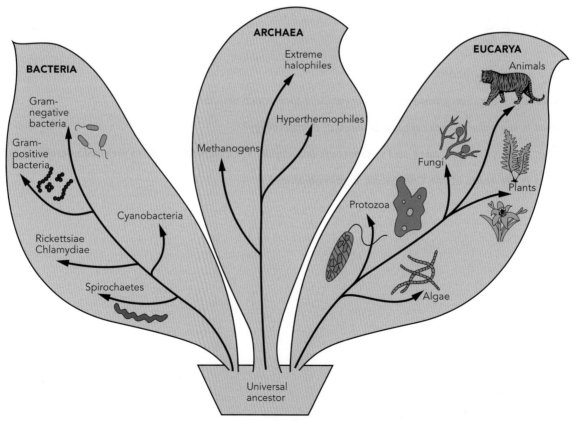

4. **Plants**
5. **Animals**.

The three domains

Recent developments in molecular biology have allowed scientists to compare the DNA and RNA from different organisms. In 1978, based on ribosomal RNA studies, CARL WOESE proposed that all organisms should be grouped in one of three domains. The domain, Archaea, contained the archaebacteria, the most primitive of all organisms. A second domain, the **Bacteria**, contained the eubacteria (true bacteria). All organisms in the other four kingdoms – protista, fungi, plants and animals – were grouped in a third domain, the Eucarya (see Figure 2.1). It may be that, in the future, further revisions of the system of classification will be required.

NAMING OF MICROORGANISMS

The Swedish botanist CARL LINNAEUS devised a careful naming system for each species within the kingdoms, a system still widely used today. Linnaeus proposed that each group of organisms should be placed into a **genus** (plural: genera), the name of which is always spelt with a capital letter. Within the genera there are different species which have discrete but related characteristics. A species can be further divided into different **strains** that exhibit specific properties. For example, under the Linnaean system a bacterium would be named *Escherichia* (genus) *coli* (species), O157 (strain).

The names assigned to organisms may reflect the place where the organism is commonly found (e.g. coli = of the colon), the name of the researcher who first described the organism (e.g. Escherich) or sometimes the disease the bacterium causes (e.g. tetani) or its shape (e.g. bacillus, meaning rod-shaped).

A further refinement in the classification of microorganisms has come with the development of serological techniques that enable the differentiation between strains of organisms on the basis of their antigenic properties or **serotypes** (i.e. the unique structure of the chemical molecules on the outside of the cell). The development of nucleic acid probes has enabled some organisms (viruses in particular) to be classified and named according to their type of RNA or DNA.

In the higher kingdoms of plants and animals, the genera are grouped into families, orders, classes and phyla. These are required to classify the huge diversity of plants and animals, but are of less importance in the microbial world.

Procaryotic and eucaryotic cells

The basic structural and functional unit of life is the cell. All cells contain a complex mixture of chemicals, consisting of proteins, lipids, nucleic acids and carbohydrates suspended in a watery fluid called **cytoplasm**, which is enclosed by the cell membrane and, in some cells, by a cell wall as well. The development of the electron microscope enabled the fine structure of cells to be examined in detail and revealed two distinct types of cells – **procaryotic** and **eucaryotic** – which can be distinguished on the basis of their subcellular structures. This is a useful distinction for the medical microbiologist and, for the purposes of this text, we shall continue to refer to them in this way.

Bacteria are procaryotes and all other living organisms are eucaryotes. Eucaryotic cells have structures that are quite distinct from procaryotes and these differences can be exploited in the development of drugs to treat microbial infections (see Chapter 12). All bacteria of medical importance are classified as true bacteria. The eucaryotic microorganisms of medical significance include some of the protozoa, fungi and helminths. Viruses are not capable of independent reproduction so are not included in this system of classification.

Table 2.1 summarises the principal characteristics of procaryotic and eucaryotic cells.

PROCARYOTES

Procaryotic organisms are unicellular and under the microscope appear to have a very simple structure usually bounded by a cell wall. The nuclear material is not contained within a membrane and there are no other discrete **organelles** visible in the cytoplasm. Although all bacteria are procaryotic, they are a very large heterogeneous group. The thousands of species of bacteria are differentiated by many factors, including appearance (morphology), chemical composition, nutritional requirements and biochemical properties. Procaryotic cells mainly reproduce by *binary fission*, a process in which the cell splits into two daughter cells with properties identical to the original cell. The classification and identification of bacteria is described in more detail in Chapter 4.

Structure of procaryotic cells

Figure 2.2 is a schematic diagram of a typical procaryotic (bacterial) cell. Almost all procaryotic cells are bounded by a **cell wall**, a complex semi-rigid structure that is responsible for the shape of the cell. The cell wall is located outside the plasma membrane and protects the membrane and the internal parts of the cell from changes in the external environment, such as a change in osmotic pressure.

The **plasma membrane** (or **cytoplasmic membrane**) is a semi-permeable membrane that lies underneath the cell wall and controls the passage of chemicals in and out of the cell. When examined by electron microscopy, the **cytoplasm** of procaryotic cells appears as a granular mass with no clearly defined regions. The cytoplasm is mainly water and contains enzymes, nutrients and chemicals.

The nuclear area of the cell contains its genetic information, **DNA**, which in most bacteria consists of a single circular chromosome. **Ribosomes**, which are the site of protein synthesis, appear as round particles in the cytoplasm. In the cytoplasm there are also various '**inclusions**', which are deposits of reserve nutrients such as starch. Some bacteria have **flagella** for motility (movement). **Pili**

Table 2.1

Characteristics of procaryotic and eucaryotic cells

CHARACTERISTIC	PROCARYOTIC	EUCARYOTIC
Size	0.4 to 2.0 μm diameter	5 to 100 μm diameter
Cell wall	Always present	Bounded by wall or membrane
Nucleus	No defined region	Contains DNA, bounded by double membrane
Genetic material	One circular chromosome of double-stranded DNA; plasmids in some cells	Double strand of DNA associated with proteins (histones) to form pairs (of chromosomes); DNA also present in mitochondria and chloroplasts
Membrane-bound subcellular organelles	Absent	Present – include mitochondria, chloroplasts, Golgi apparatus, lysosomes, endoplasmic reticulum
Motility	Some are motile, use flagella	Some are motile, e.g. protozoa; most are non-motile
Plasma membrane	Present – selectively permeable	Present – contains sterols; selectively permeable
Cytoplasm	Contains all enzymes and chemicals; no defined structures	Has cytoskeleton, exhibits streaming (moving of cytoplasmic fluid)
Endoplasmic reticulum	Absent	Present
Ribosomes	Present, smaller 70S	Present, larger 80S
Reproduction	Mainly asexual binary fission	Sexual or asexual

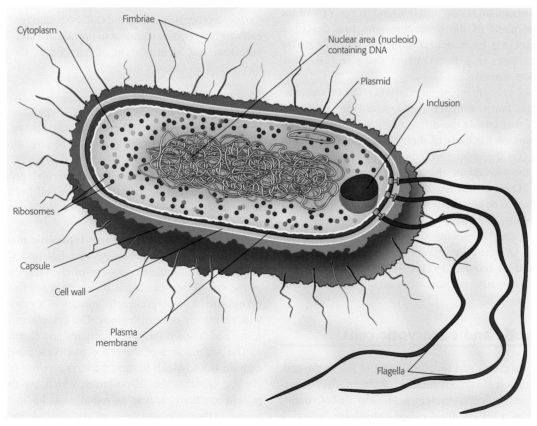

Figure 2.2
Schematic diagram of a procaryotic cell

and **fimbriae** are appendages for attachment of the cell to surfaces or to other cells. Many bacteria have a layer external to the cell wall which may be called a **capsule**, a **slime layer** or a **glycocalyx**, depending on its structure and function.

EUCARYOTES

Eucaryotic organisms include all organisms other than the bacteria. They comprise single-celled organisms (protozoa, yeasts and unicellular algae), multicellular organisms (some algae and fungi) and the much more complex higher plants and animals. Microscopic examination reveals that eucaryotic cells are larger and structurally more complex than procaryotic cells. They contain a defined nucleus enclosed by a membrane, as well as other **organelles** that are specialised structures responsible for carrying out specific functions.

Structure of eucaryotic cells

Figure 2.3 is a schematic diagram of a eucaryotic cell.

Not all cells contain all types of organelles. For example, only plant cells capable of photosynthetic activity contain chloroplasts. The most characteristic eucaryotic organelle is the **nucleus**. This is frequently the largest organelle in the cell and is easily visible under the light microscope. It contains most of the cellular DNA (some DNA is also found in the mitochondria and chloroplasts). The nucleus is surrounded by a double membrane, called the **nuclear membrane** or envelope. Pores in the membrane allow the passage of substances in and out of the nucleus. Within the nucleus are found one or more spherical bodies called **nucleoli** (singular: nucleolus) which are the sites of synthesis of ribosomal RNA.

The DNA in the nucleus is combined with proteins called **histones** to form **chromosomes**. **Centrioles** are located in the cytoplasm near the nucleus and are important in eucaryotic cell division.

The **endoplasmic reticulum** is a system of membranes located within the cytoplasm and connected to both the plasma membrane and the nuclear membranes. It forms a network of tubes on which are located the ribosomes – the sites of protein synthesis. The endoplasmic reticulum provides a surface area for chemical reactions and the membranes control transport of molecules within the cell.

The **ribosomes** of eucaryotic cells are larger and slightly more dense than the ribosomes of procaryotic cells. In both procaryotic and eucaryotic cells, ribosomes are the sites of protein synthesis. Messenger RNA attaches to ribosomes to provide a structure where amino acids can be incorporated and joined to form proteins (see Chapter 4).

The **Golgi complex** is another membranous structure found in the cytoplasm. It consists of a series of flattened sacs or vesicles and is responsible for the secretion of certain proteins, such as enzymes and hormones.

Mitochondria (singular: mitochondrion) are found in

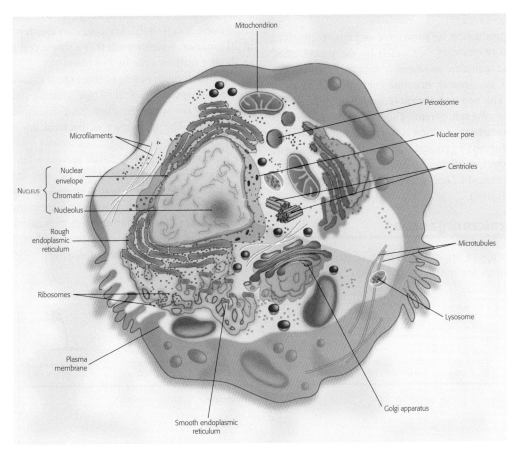

Figure 2.3

Schematic diagram of a eucaryotic cell

the cytoplasm of eucaryotic cells. They consist of a double membrane structure, the inner one arranged in a series of folds called **cristae**. The structure of the mitochondria makes it possible for enzyme reactions that are closely linked to be carried out in sequence. These include the energy-producing reactions involved in the metabolism of glucose and the production of ATP via the electron transport chain. Mitochondria are often called the 'powerhouses' of the cell as they are the main site of ATP production (see Chapter 3).

Chloroplasts are complex structures consisting of stacks of membranes and are found in photosynthetic algae and green plants. The chloroplast contains the pigment **chlorophyll** and the enzymes necessary to trap light energy and use it for synthesis of glucose during **photosynthesis**.

Lysosomes are small organelles, bounded by a single membrane and found mainly in animal cells. They consist of a sac containing digestive enzymes and are important in breaking down foreign material and microorganisms that have been ingested by the cell. Human white blood cells (phagocytes) contain large numbers of lysosomes.

Reproduction in eucaryotic cells can be sexual or asexual. **Asexual reproduction** occurs in protozoa and some algae and fungi and in normal cell division during growth of higher organisms. In this process, termed **mitosis**, the chromosomes replicate and two daughter nuclei are formed in a complex but organised process. The new nuclei move to opposite ends of the cell and the cell then splits into two identical daughter cells with identical sets of chromosomes.

Sexual reproduction in eucaryotic organisms involves the formation of gametes (sex cells) by the parent cells. Fusion of the gametes produces a new cell which has received half its genetic material (chromosomes) from each parent. The new cell therefore has some, but not all, characteristics of each parent. The cell division process involved in gamete production is termed **meiosis**. Meiotic division and fusion of gametes is then followed by mitosis. Sexual reproduction allows for mixing of genetic material (i.e. characteristics) to occur and produces genetic diversity in the offspring.

Types of microorganisms

The major groups of organisms that are of medical importance in humans are the bacteria, viruses, protozoa and fungi, and some multicellular parasites. These organisms vary in size from the viruses (the smallest of which are about 20 nm or 0.02 μm) to the macroscopic stages of some of the helminths, some of which are up to 35 cm in length and obviously visible to the naked eye.

Figure 2.4 illustrates the relative sizes of some of these organisms. The distinctive properties of each group of organisms are discussed in later chapters, together with descriptions of the types of diseases they cause. A brief overview of the various groups of organisms is presented here.

BACTERIA

There are many thousands of different species of bacteria, but relatively few of them actually cause disease in humans. Because bacteria are free-living and can be seen under an ordinary light microscope, they have been extensively studied. All bacteria are procaryotic; that is, they are simple, unicellular organisms with no defined nucleus or membrane-bound organelles in the cytoplasm. They absorb nutrients from their environment and are capable of carrying out all the metabolic reactions necessary for growth and reproduction.

Bacteria are remarkably adaptable and can grow in a variety of environmental conditions. While some are very fastidious (i.e. particular about their nutrient requirements), many bacteria can use a wide range of nutrients and adapt to growth at different temperatures and oxygen levels. Bacteria can multiply very rapidly. Under optimum conditions, a cell of *Escherichia coli* can reproduce itself in 20 minutes, which means that a single cell can give rise to about 1 million cells in 7–8 hours.

Most bacteria have one of three common shapes: spherical, rod-shaped or spiral. Their characteristic shape is important for classification and identification (see Figure 2.5). The properties of bacteria are described in detail in Chapter 4.

Chlamydiae and **rickettsiae** are classified as bacteria even though they do not have all the characteristics described above. They usually reproduce inside a living cell and cannot be grown on an agar plate in the laboratory. However, they can be stained with conventional bacterial stains and are sensitive to antibacterial drugs. They are the cause of a number of important diseases.

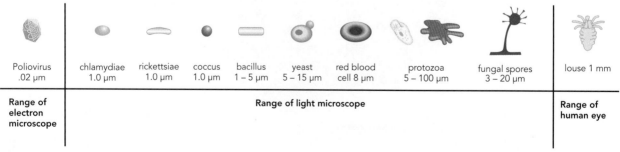

| Poliovirus .02 μm | chlamydiae 1.0 μm | rickettsiae 1.0 μm | coccus 1.0 μm | bacillus 1 – 5 μm | yeast 5 – 15 μm | red blood cell 8 μm | protozoa 5 – 100 μm | fungal spores 3 – 20 μm | louse 1 mm |

| Range of electron microscope | Range of light microscope | Range of human eye |

Figure 2.4
Relative size of microorganisms

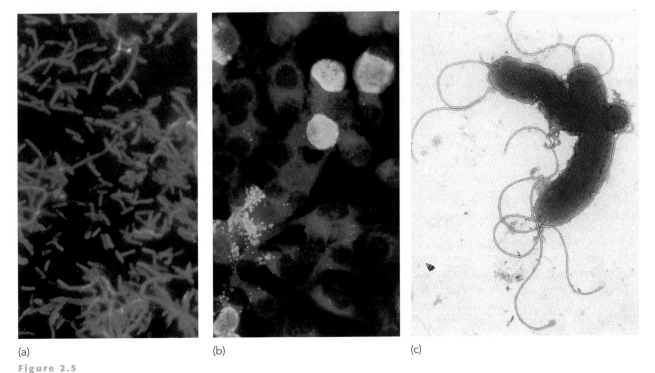

(a)   (b)   (c)

Figure 2.5

Diversity of bacterial morphology

Fluorescent antibody labelling reveals (a) large rod-shaped cells of *Legionella pneumophila*; (b) tiny cells of *Chlamydia trachomatis* shown as intracellular clusters and as free particles released when the host cell ruptures; (c) negative stain of *Helicobacter pylori*.

VIRUSES

According to the classification systems described earlier in this chapter, viruses are not considered to be living cells because they are unable to reproduce or carry out any metabolic reactions on their own. However, viruses are very important pathogens and, together with bacteria, are the cause of many infectious diseases.

Viruses are able to cause infection in many types of cells, including animal, plant and bacterial cells, but each virus is quite specific for the cell type(s) it attacks. In order to reproduce, a virus must take over the metabolic machinery of the host cell. This usually results in alteration, damage or destruction of the host cell. Viruses are often described as *obligate intracellular parasites*, because they can only reproduce inside the cells they have infected.

Viruses are very small and are not visible with the light microscope. It is only since the development of the electron microscope that much has been learnt about the structure of virus particles. Electron microscopy has revealed that viruses exist in a large range of shapes and sizes. They vary in size from the tiny polio virus which is only 20 nm (0.02 μm) to the large vaccinia (e.g. smallpox) virus which is 300 nm (0.3 μm). However, the largest viruses are still considerably smaller than even the smallest bacteria, which are about 1 μm in length or diameter.

ALGAE

Algae (singular: alga) are mainly aquatic eucaryotic organisms, occurring in freshwater ponds and streams, and some in salt water. Algae do not usually cause infections

in humans so are not discussed further in other chapters. However, some species of dinoflagellates (unicellular plankton), such as *Gonyaulax*, produce **neurotoxins**. When these algae are eaten by shellfish, the toxin is concentrated in the fish and can cause poisoning if the shellfish is eaten by humans. These dinoflagellates are red in colour and when in high concentration in the sea produce a 'red tide'. Health authorities usually prohibit the harvesting of shellfish for human consumption during a red tide.

Food poisoning associated with toxic shellfish occurs frequently along the coast of the North Island of New Zealand. Another alga, *Gambierdiscus toxicus*, is responsible for the production of a similar toxin, **ciguatera**, which may be found in fish in the South Pacific Ocean and the Caribbean.

Algae play an important role as part of the food chain, and seaweeds are a source of food in some countries. The gelling agent agar, used to prepare bacterial culture plates, is extracted from the red alga *Gelidium*. Algae carry out photosynthesis, converting atmospheric carbon dioxide into carbohydrate with the release of oxygen (see Chapter 3). Algae thrive in the upper layers of water where there is plenty of light, and when in large numbers may cause a green 'scum' to form on the surface. Heavy growth of algae (**algal bloom**) often indicates sewage pollution in rivers and waterways as algae thrive on the high concentrations of organic material and phosphates that exist in sewage or waste. When these blooms die and decompose, they severely deplete the water of oxygen and this can result in the death of the fish population.

True algae should be distinguished from **blue-green algae**, which can pollute inland waterways and produce a toxin that can affect animals that drink the water. Blue-green algae are really bacteria and are more correctly called **cyanobacteria**.

Some algae live in a symbiotic association with other organisms, the photosynthetic activity of the algae providing carbohydrate nutrients for the host. For example, algae are responsible for the bright blue/green colour of the 'lip' of the giant clam found on coral reefs. Lichens seen on rocks and decaying wood are combinations of algae and fungi.

PROTOZOA

Protozoa (singular: protozoan) are unicellular eucaryotic organisms that lack a cell wall (see Figure 2.6). They are much larger than bacteria and have visible organelles. Most of them are found in aquatic environments. They are usually colourless and are distinguished from algae because they do not contain chlorophyll. Protozoa ingest their food, either by surrounding the food with a portion of their cell membrane and engulfing it, or by swallowing it through a specialised structure or 'mouth'. Only a few protozoa cause human disease (see Chapter 6).

FUNGI

Fungi are a large, diverse group of eucaryotic organisms, ranging from microscopic yeast cells to large complex structures such as mushrooms. They are unicellular or multicellular and have a thick cell wall. Many fungi are beneficial to humans. They play an important role in the decomposition of organic matter and some species are a source of antibiotics. Yeasts are important in the food industry for making bread, wine and beer. Although many fungi are responsible for infections of plants, very few are pathogenic to humans. The fungi that cause human disease belong to two main groups: (1) the **yeasts** and (2) the **filamentous fungi**. Most fungal infections are cutaneous, affecting only the upper layers of the skin or mucosa, and do not cause severe illness. However, some fungal infections can become systemic, spreading throughout the body and causing life-threatening conditions. Fungi and fungal infections (**mycoses**) are discussed further in Chapter 6.

MICROSCOPIC PARASITES

Some worms have a microscopic stage in their life cycle, so infections caused by these parasites are usually classed as microbial diseases. Parasitic worms belong to the group called **helminths**. They include the **flatworms** (**tapeworms** and **flukes**) and roundworms. Infection of humans may occur in a number of ways – ingestion of the larvae or eggs, injection of the parasite by a blood-sucking insect, or the direct penetration of the skin by the larval stage of the parasite.

Helminth infections are most common in developing countries and transmission is influenced by socio-economic conditions, general hygiene and other lifestyle factors (see Chapter 6).

Microscopes

One of the major discoveries that gave birth to the field of microbiology was the development of instruments that enabled the observation of objects too small to be seen with the naked eye. Robert Hooke in the 1660s, using an instrument with two sets of lenses (a crude microscope), was the first person to describe cells as life's smallest structural units. In the early 1670s Anton van Leeuwenhoek used a simple but powerful magnifying lens to observe microbes he called 'animalcules' in rainwater. He was probably the first person to observe the individual cells of microorganisms. Since then, lenses and lens systems have been so extensively developed that we now have microscopes that can achieve magnifications hundreds of times greater than that of van Leeuwenhoek. The development of electron microscopes in the 1930s enabled magnifications of a further hundred times greater to be achieved.

Another major advance in microbiology was the development of stains that colour the normally colourless microbial cells, or specific structures in them, and enable them to be seen more readily under a microscope.

Three types of microscopes are used for the visualisation and examination of microorganisms. The **compound light microscope** uses visible light to illuminate the specimen and multiple lenses to magnify it. This is the most common type of microscope used in diagnostic microbiology laboratories because it is powerful enough to enable the observation of all types of microbes, except viruses. For the observation of viruses and small structures within microbes, much greater magnification is needed, requiring the use of a **transmission electron microscope**.

A special type of electron microscope, called a **scan-**

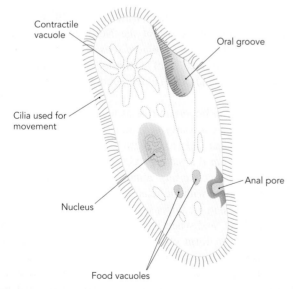

Figure 2.6

Schematic protozoan
Diagram showing cellular organelles of a typical ciliated protozoan (e.g. *Paramecium*).

Labels in figure:
- Contractile vacuole
- Oral groove
- Cilia used for movement
- Nucleus
- Anal pore
- Food vacuoles

ning electron microscope, provides a dramatic three-dimensional image of a specimen at very high magnifications. Electron microscopes are highly specialised, expensive pieces of equipment and are, therefore, found in research institutes and some virus laboratories but not in routine diagnostic laboratories.

THE COMPOUND LIGHT MICROSCOPE

The light microscope consists of a series of lenses (see Figure 2.7(a)). The condenser lens focuses the rays of light from the lamp onto the specimen. The light passes through the specimen and is directed by the condenser into the objective lens, which is the first of the magnifying lenses. A number of objective lenses are mounted on a revolving nosepiece that allows the desired lens to be selected and clicked into place. The objectives offer different magnifications – the usual combination is a $10 \times$ (10 times), $40 \times$ (40 times) and $100 \times$ (100 times). They are referred to,

respectively, as the low power, high power, and oil immersion objectives. The oil immersion objective is specially designed to be used with oil (actually immersed in a drop of it) to prevent excessive dispersion of the light and maximal collection by the objective lens. From the objective, the light passes through a tube containing a series of prisms to the eyepiece (ocular) lens, which magnifies the image a further 10 or 20 times. The operator observes the specimen by looking into the eyepiece. The total magnification achievable in a standard compound light microscope is the product of the magnifications of the objective and eyepiece lenses, and is therefore $100 \times$, $400 \times$ or $1000 \times$ (with a $10 \times$ eyepiece), depending on which objective lens is used.

The specimen for observation is usually mounted on a glass slide which is placed on the stage of the microscope. The use of coarse and fine focusing brings the specimen into focus for the eye. The condenser focusing knob is used to ensure proper focusing of the light onto the specimen. The amount of light (brightness) can be controlled by diaphragms, usually on the condenser lens and lamp.

Apart from magnification, the other main requirement of a high-performance microscope is *resolution* (or resolving power). This is the ability of the microscope to distinguish, as separate, two objects that are close together – that is, to distinguish fine detail – and provide a sharp, clear image. Resolution is related to the wavelength of light, and the maximum resolution of a microscope using white light is about 0.2 μm. That is, any objects that are closer to each other than 0.2 μm will appear to be joined. The highest useful magnification achievable with a light microscope is limited by this resolution, and is therefore about 2000 times. In contrast, the resolving power of the human eye is about 100 μm.

The use of a direct light source to illuminate the specimen fully is called **bright-field microscopy**. It is also possible to use the compound light microscope in other ways, such as in dark-field microscopy, fluorescence microscopy, phase microscopy and differential interference contrast microscopy. These techniques allow microorganisms to be observed in different ways, and provide a means of observing the special properties of some organisms. The first two of these techniques are described below to illustrate their different uses.

Dark-field microscopy

Dark-field microscopy involves the use of a special condenser that blocks light from entering the objective lens unless it is reflected from objects in the specimen. In this form of microscopy, objects in the specimen appear bright against a dark background. It is particularly useful for the visualisation of bacteria that are not readily seen or identified by conventional staining and microscopic methods. For example, *Treponema pallidum*, the causative agent of syphilis, can be seen by this method as a spiral-shaped organism that moves with a corkscrew-type action (see Figure 2.8). This organism is too thin to be readily seen using standard microscope methods. Since staining is not

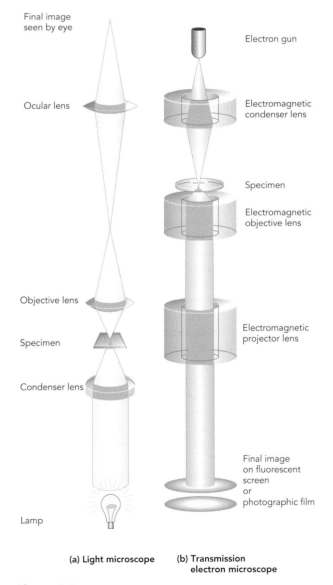

Figure 2.7

A comparison of the lens systems of (a) a compound light microscope and (b) an electron microscope

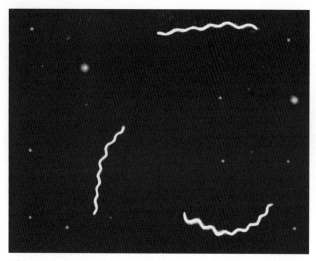

Figure 2.8
Dark-field micrograph of *Treponema pallidum*

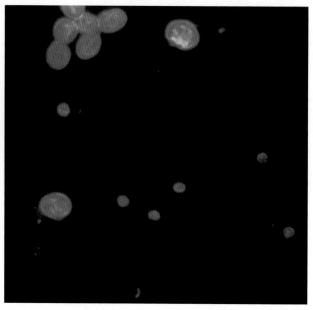

Figure 2.9
Fluorescent antibody stain
Showing different morphologies of *Giardia* (larger) and *Cryptosporidium*.

required, living organisms can be observed using this method.

Fluorescence microscopy

Fluorescence microscopy is based on the principle that certain compounds absorb invisible light of short wavelengths and give off visible light of longer wavelengths. Brilliant shades of yellow, orange or green are seen against a dark background. Ultraviolet light has a short wavelength and is used as the light source instead of white light. Some microorganisms naturally fluoresce, but most have to be coated with fluorescent dyes (e.g. fluorescein, rhodamine, acridine) in order to be seen in a fluorescence microscope.

The major application of this method is the fluorescent antibody (or immunofluorescence) technique. **Antibodies** are protein molecules present in serum, produced by the body to defend itself against foreign microorganisms (see Chapter 9). Antibodies react specifically with the microbes against which they are produced. In the fluorescent antibody technique, antibodies to a particular organism are collected and purified, and then a fluorescent dye is attached to them. If a patient is suspected of suffering from disease caused by that particular organism, the diagnosis can be confirmed by collecting an appropriate specimen, treating it with fluorescent antibodies and examining it microscopically. If the suspected organism is present, it will readily be seen as a brightly fluorescing object when observed microscopically (see Figure 2.9).

This technique is particularly useful for the visualisation and rapid identification of organisms that are otherwise difficult to detect in clinical specimens, such as *Legionella pneumophila* (Legionnaires' disease), *Treponema pallidum* (syphilis) and some viruses.

THE TRANSMISSION ELECTRON MICROSCOPE

The electron microscope is able to achieve much greater resolution (and magnification) than light microscopes because it uses rays of electrons to visualise the specimen.

These have a much shorter wavelength than white light (about 100 000 times shorter). Because the wavelength is so short, magnifications of more than 100 000 times can be achieved that will resolve minute structures as small as 0.001 μm (1 nm), the size of some viral structures.

Instead of a light source, the transmission electron microscope has an electron gun that emits a finely focused beam of electrons. The electrons are directed at the specimen, which is an ultra-thin section of the material fixed to a grid. The specimen has to be thin enough (20–100 nm) to allow the electrons to pass through it, and it must be specially treated with stains, usually salts of heavy metals such as lead, osmium, tungsten or uranium. These stains scatter electrons well and increase the contrast between structures. The electrons pass through the specimen and then through electromagnetic lenses (see Figure 2.7(b)) which magnify the degree of scatter of the electrons. Finally, the electrons are focused by another electromagnetic lens onto a fluorescent screen. An image of the specimen is then visible on this screen. For a permanent record of the observation, or for prolonged examination, the electrons can be directed onto a photographic plate to produce a photograph called an **electron micrograph** (see Figure 2.10).

Note that there is no natural colour in a specimen examined by an electron microscope, but sometimes micrographs are artificially coloured. The colour in an electron micrograph does not necessarily bear any relationship to the real colour of the object in the specimen.

The components of the electron microscope are contained within a sealed vacuum chamber (see Figure 2.11), to prevent the scattering of electrons by dust and other particles in air, which can cause distortion of the image. The basic principles of electron microscopy are similar to

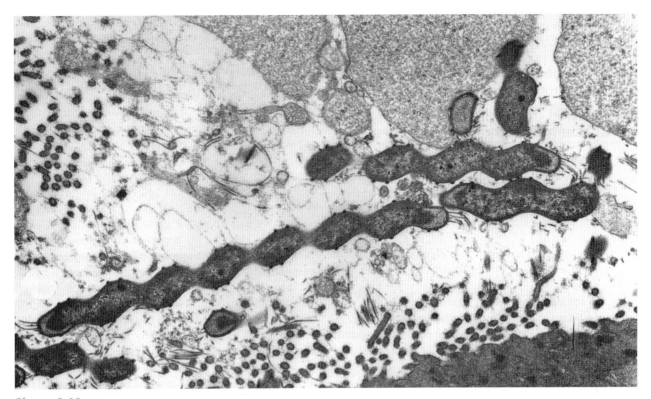

Figure 2.10
Electron micrograph
A photograph taken from an image produced in an electron microscope. This micrograph shows *Helicobacter* (spiral-shaped organism) in a gastric crypt.

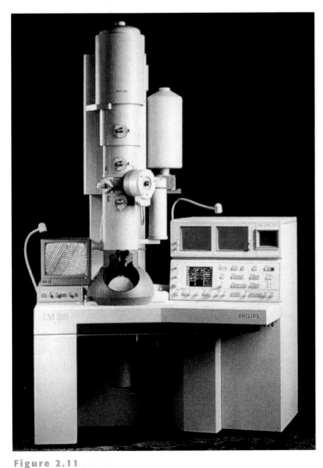

Figure 2.11
An electron microscope

those of light microscopy, except that the former utilises electrons, and electromagnets to focus them, where the latter uses white light and glass lenses.

The main advantage of transmission electron microscopy is the high resolution and magnification that can be achieved, allowing observation of the internal structure of microbial cells. However, it also has distinct disadvantages resulting from the severe treatments (fixing, dehydrating and staining) that the specimen must be subjected to when it is being prepared for electron microscopy. These treatments mean that living cells cannot be examined, and that alteration or distortion of cell structures may occur. Sometimes, new structures may even be created and these artefacts (not real cell structures) are an ever-present concern in the interpretation of electron micrographs.

THE SCANNING ELECTRON MICROSCOPE

The scanning electron microscope is a development of the electron microscope that produces three-dimensional images of objects with high resolution and magnification. In the scanning electron microscope the beam of electrons is directed at the specimen which has first been coated with a thin film of a heavy metal, such as platinum. The whole specimen is showered with electrons, which are deflected from the specimen at different angles and collected by a sophisticated detector that scans back and forth. As for the transmission microscope, the image is produced on a viewing screen or photographic plate.

The scanning electron microscope enables the three-dimensional structure and the surface of objects to be visualised and examined, as shown in Figure 2.12. Magnifications of up to 10 000 × can be achieved with this microscope.

Preparation of specimens for light microscopy

Two preparation methods are generally used for the observation of microorganisms with the light microscope: wet preparations and fixed, stained preparations. Living bacteria, yeasts and protozoa can be observed directly in a light microscope by suspending the organisms in a drop of fluid. This is called a **wet preparation**. However, most microorganisms are colourless, so they are usually stained (coloured) prior to microscopic examination. **Staining** provides a greater contrast between the microorganisms and the background.

WET PREPARATIONS

Microorganisms can be observed in the living state when suspended in fluid, placed on a microscope slide and observed with the light microscope. Using a wet preparation, certain characteristics of microorganisms such as their ability to move or their cellular arrangements (e.g. clusters or chains of bacteria) can be observed. Better contrast can be obtained in some situations with the use of weak stains, such as dilute methylene blue. Wet preparations are generally used for the examination of fungi and protozoa.

The India ink stain, a black suspension of carbon particles, is used specifically to examine and identify cells of the pathogenic yeast *Cryptococcus neoformans*. These cells have a thick capsule which excludes the stain and shows up in this procedure as a clear structure around the cell against a black background (see Figure 2.13). Wet preparations are also useful for the direct observation of urine and cerebrospinal fluid specimens, in which the presence of host cells, especially red and white cells, can be readily determined.

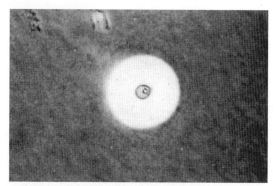

Figure 2.13

India ink stain of *Cryptococcus neoformans*

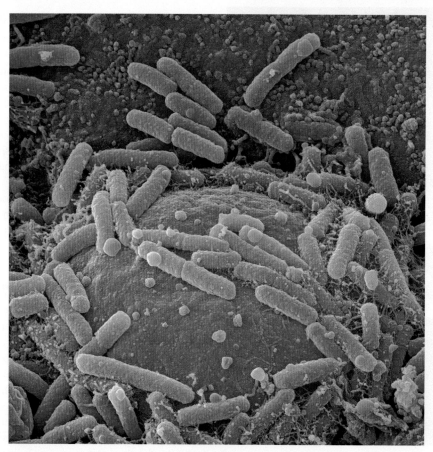

Figure 2.12

Coloured scanning electron micrograph of *Escherichia coli* in the gastrointestinal tract

FIXED AND STAINED PREPARATIONS

Generally, bacteria can be better visualised and examined in a light microscope when they are stained. Staining can also help to visualise some internal structures (e.g. spores) and to identify and separate different bacteria. Before staining, the bacteria must be fixed (or attached) to a microscope slide to prevent them being washed away by the liquid stains. To fix a specimen to a glass slide, a thin film of the material is spread over a portion of a glass slide. The film can be made in a number of ways: for example, by suspending a colony of bacterial growth from a culture plate in a small drop of tap water; or by wiping a swab, taken from a patient, over the surface of a slide. This smear of material is allowed to air dry completely. It is then fixed to the slide by gently heating the underside of the slide by passing it several times through the flame of a Bunsen burner. The stain(s) are then applied and after an appropriate time washed off with water.

Various stains are used in the microbiology laboratory to examine bacteria, or certain structures within them, but the **Gram stain** is undoubtedly the most useful and important staining procedure used. Developed in 1884 by the Danish bacteriologist Hans Christian Gram, it has become the standard procedure for staining bacteria because it divides almost all bacteria into two groups, and serves as the first step in classifying and identifying bacteria. Bacteria stain as Gram-positive or Gram-negative, depending on the composition of their cell wall (see Chapter 4). The Gram staining reaction is characteristic for each species.

The Gram staining procedure involves the application of several solutions to a fixed smear of bacteria (see Figure 2.14).

1. The slide is first covered with a solution of a purple dye, usually crystal violet. After a short time (approximately 30 seconds) the dye is washed off with water, leaving the bacterial cells purple-coloured.
2. The smear is next treated with an iodine solution, which fixes the purple dye firmly in the cells. After the iodine is washed off all cells are still coloured a dark purple.
3. The smear is then treated briefly (a few seconds) with an alcohol or alcohol-acetone solution, followed quickly by a water rinse. This decolourises some cells by removing the purple dye from them. In this critical stage, Gram-positive bacteria retain the purple dye, but Gram-negative bacteria lose it, becoming colourless.
4. The final treatment (or counterstain) is with a red/pink dye, usually safranin or neutral red. This is necessary because the Gram-negative bacteria, which have lost their purple colour, would not be visible under the microscope. The cells that retained the purple dye in step 3 remain purple because it is a darker colour. The safranin is washed off after a short time (approximately 30 seconds) and the slide is then gently blotted dry and is ready for microscopic examination.

As shown in Figure 2.14, after Gram staining bacterial cells are either a dark violet or purple colour (Gram-positive) or a pink/red or orange colour (Gram-negative) and can be readily seen in the light microscope. The Gram stain is thus termed a *differential stain*. In Gram-stained smears of clinical specimens (e.g. swabs, cerebrospinal fluid), bacteria as well as host cells, especially polymorphonuclear leucocytes (white cells or pus cells), can be observed if present. A direct Gram stain of a clinical specimen can be performed within minutes of receiving

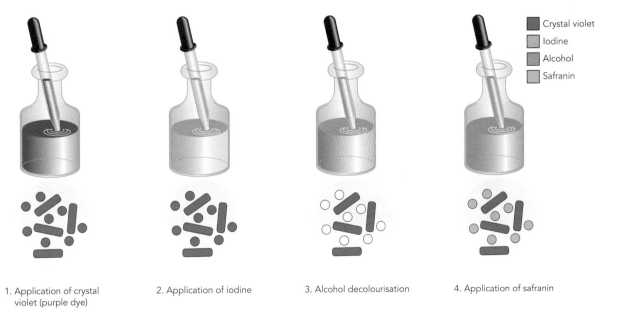

Crystal violet
Iodine
Alcohol
Safranin

1. Application of crystal violet (purple dye)
2. Application of iodine
3. Alcohol decolourisation
4. Application of safranin

Figure 2.14

The Gram stain procedure
(1) A heat-fixed smear of bacteria on a glass microscope slide is treated with crystal violet, then rinsed in water. (2) The smear is treated with iodine and then rinsed with water. (3) The smear is then briefly treated with ethanol or acetone and rinsed with water. (4) The smear is finally treated with safranin, rinsed with water and dried. Gram-positive bacteria are purple-coloured. Gram-negative bacteria have a pink/red or orange colour.

the specimen in the laboratory. After microscopic examination of the stained smear, a presumptive diagnosis can be made in some circumstances. For example, in bacterial meningitis, the observation of bacterial cells and pus cells in a Gram stain of cerebrospinal fluid can sometimes give a good indication of the possible causative agent.

Figure 2.15 shows a Gram stain of a mixture of organisms.

Several other stains are used by microbiologists for specific purposes. The **Ziehl-Neelsen**, or **acid-fast stain**, is an important one because it is used to identify bacteria belonging to the genus *Mycobacterium*, such as *M. tuberculosis* and *M. leprae*, the causative agents of tuberculosis and leprosy, respectively.

Mycobacteria have a waxy substance in their cell wall which prevents them from being stained using Gram's method. The acid-fast stain is a multi-step procedure that stains the mycobacteria a red colour, and all other bacteria and material another colour, usually blue (see Figure 2.16). It is useful for the detection of mycobacteria in sputum specimens from patients with pulmonary tuberculosis.

Other bacterial stains include the spore stain (see Figure 2.17) and flagella stain, used to highlight spores and flagella for easier recognition.

Stains are one of the more important techniques used by microbiologists to aid in the visualisation, classification and identification of bacteria. The Gram stain is particularly important because it is usually the first step in the identification of bacteria. Preliminary microbiology laboratory report forms often provide the results of Gram stains performed directly on clinical specimens. Although other more intricate and sensitive techniques are being developed for the detection of microorganisms in clinical specimens (e.g. the polymerase chain reaction and DNA probes – see Chapter 15), the ability to visualise the Gram reaction, shape and arrangement of bacterial cells is still very important in diagnostic medical microbiology.

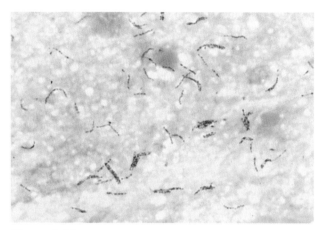

Figure 2.16
A Ziehl-Neelsen stain
The mycobacteria are stained a red colour against a blue background.

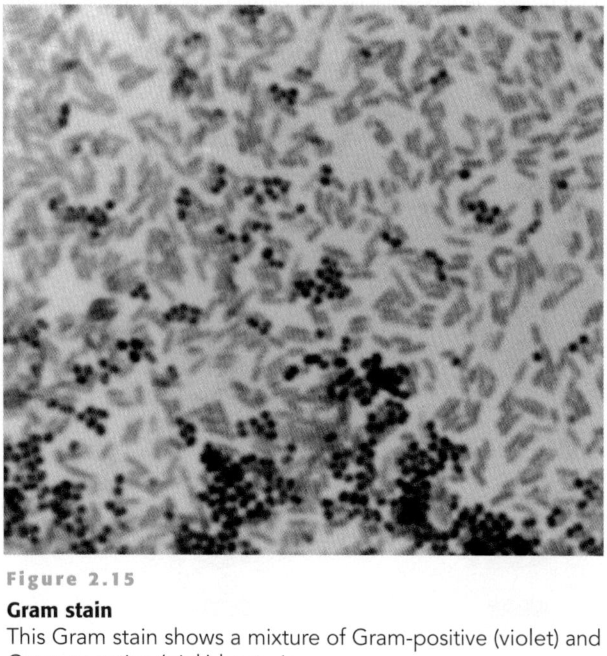

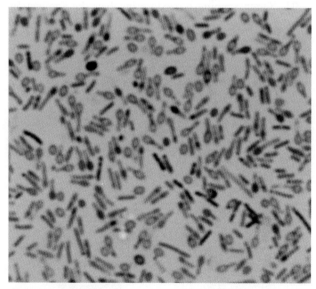

Figure 2.15
Gram stain
This Gram stain shows a mixture of Gram-positive (violet) and Gram-negative (pink) bacteria.

Figure 2.17
Spore stain
The spores are the clear structures surrounded by a red wall.

CLASSIFICATION AND NAMING OF LIVING ORGANISMS

- Classification is the grouping together of organisms that have characteristics in common.
- Carl Woese proposed a three-domain system of classification, consisting of the archaebacteria, and the Eucarya, which contains the kingdoms of Protista, Fungi, Animals and Plants.
- Microorganisms are named according to their genus, species and strain; they can also be classified according to their serological properties or DNA type.

PROCARYOTIC AND EUCARYOTIC CELLS

- All cells can be described as either procaryotic or eucaryotic.
- Procaryotic organisms are unicellular with a simple structure consisting of a cell wall located outside the plasma membrane. The cytoplasm contains enzymes, nutrients, chemicals, ribosomes and a nuclear area containing a single circular chromosome.
- All bacteria are procaryotic.
- Procaryotic cells reproduce asexually by binary fission.
- Eucaryotic organisms comprise all organisms other than the bacteria.
- Eucaryotic cells have a nucleus surrounded by the nuclear membrane. Other structures in the cytoplasm include the endoplasmic reticulum, ribosomes, the Golgi complex, mitochondria, lysosomes in animal cells, and chloroplasts in plant cells.
- Sexual reproduction in eucaryotic organisms involves the formation of gametes by meiosis.

TYPES OF MICROORGANISMS

- The major groups of organisms of medical importance are viruses, bacteria, protozoa and fungi, and some multicellular parasites.

Viruses

- Viruses cause infection in animal, plant and bacterial cells and are quite specific for the cell type they attack.
- Viruses consist of a core of RNA or DNA surrounded by protein and sometimes an envelope of glycoprotein.
- Viruses are very small and can only reproduce inside a cell they have infected.

Bacteria

- All bacteria are procaryotic and live freely in the environment.
- They occur in one of three common shapes: spherical, rod-shaped or spiral.
- Bacteria multiply very rapidly, a single cell giving rise to about 1 million cells in 7–8 hours.

Algae

- Algae are mainly aquatic organisms occurring in both fresh and salt water.

- All algae contain chlorophyll and can carry out photosynthesis.
- Algae do not usually cause infections in humans, but some species produce neurotoxins which can concentrate in fish or shellfish and cause poisoning when eaten by humans.

Protozoa

- Protozoa are unicellular eucaryotic organisms, enclosed in a membrane, and contain visible organelles.
- They live mainly in water and some species of protozoa are the cause of serious diseases.

Fungi

- Fungi are unicellular or multicellular and have a thick cell wall.
- They are important in the decomposition of organic matter and in the food industry; some species are a source of antibiotics.
- Very few fungi are pathogenic to humans.

Microscopic parasites

- Some worms (tapeworms, flukes and roundworms) have a microscopic stage in their life cycle, so infections with these parasites are usually classed as microbial diseases.

MICROSCOPY

- One of the main discoveries that gave birth to the field of microbiology was the development of magnifying instruments.
- Another major advance in microbiology was the development of stains to colour the normally colourless microbial cells.

MICROSCOPES

The compound light microscope

- The compound light microscope consists of a series of lenses.
- The maximum magnification achievable in a standard compound light microscope is 1000–2000 times.
- The specimen for observation is usually mounted on a glass slide and placed on the stage of the microscope.
- Apart from magnification, the other major requirement of a microscope is resolution – the ability of the microscope to separate two objects that are close together (i.e. to distinguish fine detail).

The transmission electron microscope

- The electron microscope is able to achieve much greater resolution (and magnification) than light microscopes because it uses rays of electrons, which have a much shorter wavelength than white light.
- Magnifications of more than 100 000 times can be achieved.
- Electrons can be directed onto a photographic plate to produce a photograph called an electron micrograph.
- The major disadvantages of transmission electron microscopy are: living cells cannot be examined; alteration or distortion of cell structures may occur.

The scanning electron microscope

- The scanning electron microscope is a development of the electron microscope. It produces three-dimensional images of objects at magnifications of up to 10 000 times.

PREPARATION OF SPECIMENS FOR LIGHT MICROSCOPY

- Living bacteria, yeasts and protozoa can be observed directly in a light microscope by suspending the organisms in a drop of fluid. This is called a wet preparation.

- Most microorganisms are colourless, so they are usually stained prior to microscopic examination.
- The Gram stain is the most useful and important staining procedure used in the microbiology laboratory because it divides almost all bacteria into two groups, thus serving as the first step in classifying and identifying bacteria.
- In the Gram staining procedure, bacteria stain as Gram-positive (purple) or Gram-negative (pink/red or orange), depending on the composition of their cell wall.

STUDY QUESTIONS

1. What are the major differences between a eucaryotic and a procaryotic cell?
2. Which organisms belong to the procaryotic kingdom?
3. In eucaryotic cells, what is the function of the mitochondria?
4. Describe the basic structure of a virus.
5. What are the three basic shapes of bacterial cells?
6. How do algae differ from protozoa and fungi?
7. What are fungal infections called?
8. Why are microscopes required for the study of micro-organisms?
9. What is meant by the term 'resolution' in microscopy?
10. What is the maximum useful magnification achievable with a light microscope?
11. What is fluorescence microscopy?
12. Why is an electron microscope able to achieve much greater magnifications than a light microscope?
13. What is an electron micrograph?
14. What are the main disadvantages of electron microscopy?
15. What is the main feature of a scanning electron microscope?
16. Why are preparations of microorganisms usually stained before they are examined with a light microscope?
17. Why is the Gram stain so important in microbiology?
18. What is the acid-fast stain and what is it used for?

TEST YOUR UNDERSTANDING

1. What methods are used to assign an organism to a particular classification?
2. How do viruses differ from other microorganisms?
3. Compare the resolving power of the human eye with that of a compound light microscope.
4. Describe the essential differences between a light microscope and an electron microscope.
5. Describe the essential differences between the images obtained with a transmission electron microscope and those obtained with a scanning electron microscope.
6. Explain how the different Gram-staining reactions relate to differences in the cell wall structure of bacteria.
7. Explain how the Gram stain can be used to achieve a rapid presumptive diagnosis of some infectious diseases.

Further reading

Murray PR, EJ Baron, MA Pfaller, FC Tenover & RH Yolken (eds) 2003, *Manual of Clinical Microbiology*, 8th edn, Washington DC: American Society of Microbiology. (Has chapters on microscopy and staining techniques.)

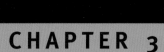

CHAPTER 3

Metabolic Processes in Microbial Cells

[CHAPTER FOCUS]

- **Why is an understanding of metabolic processes of relevance to the health professional?**

- **In what ways are the structures of biological compounds related to their function?**

- **What is the role of enzymes in biological processes?**

- **What are the principal pathways of energy production in microorganisms?**

- **What is the relationship between the breakdown and synthesis of different classes of biological molecules?**

- **What metabolic processes carried out by microorganisms are of use to humans?**

Introduction

All living cells, from the smallest microorganisms to the most complex animal cells, undergo continual processes of breakdown, synthesis, replication and repair. The overall term used to describe these processes is **metabolism** and it refers to all the different reactions that must occur in a cell in order for it to grow and reproduce. The pathways of metabolism are remarkably similar in all living cells. The differences that do occur usually reflect the availability of nutrients or the need for a cell to carry out a specialised function – which may be secretion, storage, structural support, energy for movement, or reproduction. Much of our knowledge of the processes that occur in human cells has been derived from research on the major metabolic pathways that occur in microbial cells.

Catabolism is the process of breakdown of complex molecules, usually with the release of energy. **Anabolism** refers to the synthesis of new or replacement molecules. This is an energy-requiring process. A **metabolic pathway** is a series of reactions in the process of metabolism.

Although metabolic processes are complex, consisting of thousands of chemical reactions, an understanding of the basic concepts of metabolism does not require an extensive knowledge of chemistry. The reactions are logical and can be understood in a simplified descriptive form. Many students are unnecessarily deterred from attempting to study the biochemistry of cells as they do not see its relevance to their work as health professionals. However, a knowledge of the processes that occur in all living cells will enable students to understand the chemistry underlying many of the phenomena they observe every day. For example:

- how pathogens invade, replicate and cause disease in a host
- why adequate nutrients are needed to provide energy for cellular activity, growth and repair
- why some microorganisms need a particular environment to survive
- how cells replicate and repair themselves
- the nature of the immune response
- the therapeutic use of drugs
- why some infections can be treated with antibiotics and others cannot
- how microorganisms are identified by biochemical tests
- how microbial reactions are used to produce compounds of use to humans.

This chapter assumes a basic knowledge of atoms and molecules, of ionic and covalent bonds and some carbon chemistry. The metabolic pathways are described using diagrams, words and simple chemical formulae. Students can therefore study the reactions at a level suitable to their chemistry background.

Structure of biological molecules

All living matter is made up of a number of complex molecules containing the elements carbon, hydrogen, oxygen, nitrogen, phosphorus and sulphur, with lesser (trace) amounts of other elements. The way in which the atoms of these elements are arranged determines the structure and unique function of each molecule. The most important element is carbon, a small atom with four electrons in its outer shell, capable of forming four covalent bonds. Compounds containing carbon are called **organic compounds**. When carbon combines with other atoms it forms a molecule with a particular shape (**stereospecificity**) (see Figure 3.1). The configuration of atoms in the molecules of carbon-containing compounds gives rise to the enormous diversity we observe in biological molecules; it is also responsible for the specific shape and function of these molecules.

FUNCTIONAL GROUPS

A number of specific structures are found joined to carbon in various organic compounds and are essential for the activity of these compounds. They are called 'active', or 'functional', groups. They include:

- Carboxylic acid – COOH in fatty acids (lipids), acetic acid (vinegar), amino acids (proteins)
- Amino – NH_2 in amino acids (proteins)
- Hydroxyl – OH in alcohols and glycerol (carbohydrates)
- Sulfhydryl – SH in proteins
- Organic phosphate – R CH_2 OPO_4 in phospholipids and nucleic acids
- Ester linkage – RC= OO R in triglycerides.

Another property conferred on biological molecules containing carbon is **stereoisomerism**. Because the carbon atom is linked to four other atoms, it often forms compounds which, although they have the same formula (composition), do not have the same structural configuration; they are mirror images and cannot be superimposed on each other (see Figure 3.2). This can be likened to a

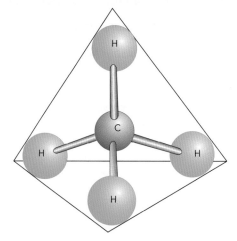

Figure 3.1

Structure of carbon-containing compounds
A carbon atom with four single bonds has this shape because of the direction of the bonds. The tetrahedral molecule of methane, CH_4, shown here, contains carbon bonded to four hydrogen atoms.

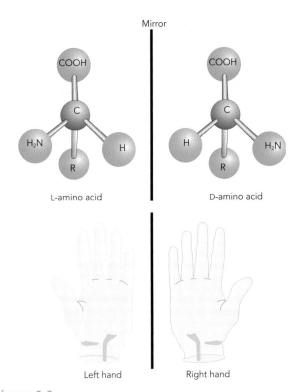

Mirror

L-amino acid   D-amino acid

Left hand   Right hand

Figure 3.2
Stereoisomerism
Models of the L- and D- forms of an amino acid are mirror images and cannot be superimposed, just like the right- and left-hand gloves illustrated.

pair of gloves, where the right-hand glove cannot be substituted for the left because it has a different configuration.

SPECIFICITY

One of the most fascinating things about biological molecules is their *specificity* – that is, the ability of a particular structure in a molecule to recognise and fit together with a complementary structure in another molecule. You may have experienced the frustration of having different pieces of electrical equipment that do not fit together – for example, having the wrong lead for a machine, or a plug and socket that do not 'match'. A similar situation occurs in living cells. Biological molecules contain particular chemical groups in unique structures that confer certain properties on the molecules. The way in which these molecules interact forms the basis for the regulation of all life processes. If the structures of two molecules are compatible, then those molecules can combine and interact in the same way that an electric plug will fit into a compatible socket (see Figure 3.3). To take this analogy further, sometimes an 'adaptor' is needed to join two pieces of equipment together. In biochemical terms, this adaptor molecule is called a **cofactor** or **coenzyme**.

The specific interaction between two compatible biological molecules determines which reactions can take place. It explains the unique mechanism of many important processes such as DNA replication, enzyme reactions, antigen–antibody interactions and the specificity of viral attack.

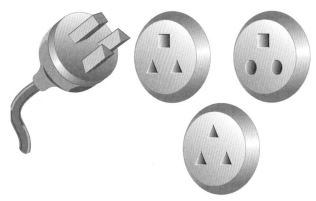

Figure 3.3
Specificity
The need for biological molecules to be the right shape in order to interact with each other is illustrated by this electrical plug and three different sockets.

Enzymes and chemical reactions

Metabolic processes involve thousands of chemical reactions. But what makes these reactions occur? A **catalyst** is defined as a substance that speeds up a chemical reaction by lowering the activation energy required for the reaction to take place. It takes part in the reaction but is itself unchanged.

What is **activation energy**?

The simplest definition is that it is the amount of energy required to make a reaction occur. For example, if two substances such as hydrogen and oxygen are mixed, a reaction will not occur at a measurable rate. However, if some energy is applied (in the form of a spark or heat), the reaction occurs very rapidly. The necessary input of energy is called the activation energy. In industry, the amount of energy in the form of heat that needs to be added is often very great, but the addition of a catalyst (e.g. a metal) will allow the reaction to occur with a much lower energy input. In other words, *the catalyst lowers the activation energy*.

In biological systems the addition of large amounts of heat would destroy the cellular proteins so an alternative way of providing the necessary energy has to be found. Cells use **enzymes** which act as biological catalysts and lower the amount of energy (activation energy) required to get a reaction started. This is why enzymes are sometimes described as 'speeding up a chemical reaction' (see Figure 3.4).

Enzymes enable reactions to occur that might not otherwise happen; they give the reaction a 'push' so that it acquires a momentum of its own. They do this by providing a surface or site on which the reaction can take place, thereby allowing the reactant molecules to be held in close proximity to each other and increasing the efficiency of their interaction. All this is done at a temperature compatible with the normal activities of the cell.

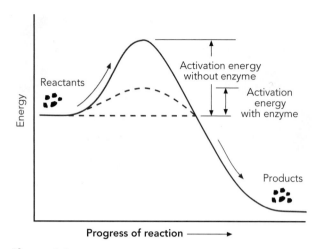

Figure 3.4

Activation energy

A chemical reaction cannot take place unless a certain amount of activation energy is available to start it. Enzymes lower the amount of activation energy needed to initiate a reaction. They thus make it possible for biologically important reactions to occur at the relatively low temperatures that living organisms can tolerate.

STRUCTURE OF ENZYMES

Enzymes are produced in cells in response to the metabolic requirements of the cell. The genetic information needed for the synthesis of each particular enzyme is coded for in the DNA of the cell, together with information that enables the cell to synthesise all its other protein requirements (see Chapter 4). The name of the enzyme is usually derived from the **substrate** it uses and the type of reaction that occurs. Most enzyme names end in *-ase*. For example, lactic dehydrogenase is an enzyme that removes hydrogen from its substrate, lactic acid.

Enzymes are proteins and are therefore made up of chains of amino acids. Each enzyme has its own unique sequence of amino acids and is folded in a certain way to give it a specific shape. Within this shape there is a particular location or area on the molecule called the **active site**. This site is rather like an electrical socket. It allows the attachment of a correspondingly shaped molecule or **substrate**. Once attached, this substrate can be modified or split; that is, it undergoes a metabolic reaction. It is then released and another substrate molecule takes its place and the reaction continues (see Figure 3.5).

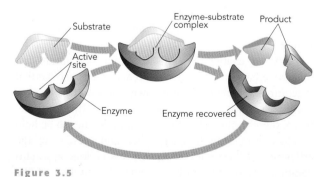

Figure 3.5

Enzyme-substrate complex

There are hundreds of different enzymes in each cell. Every reaction that occurs in a living cell is controlled by a specific enzyme. Each enzyme has an active site specific for the shape of a particular substrate. Some enzymes contain both a protein and a non-protein component. The non-protein part, called a **cofactor** or **prosthetic group**, is necessary for enzyme activity. If the cofactor is an organic molecule, it is called a **coenzyme**. These coenzymes fit into the active site like an adaptor (see Figure 3.6). Some coenzymes can be synthesised by the cell. Others must be obtained from the food supply and are considered **essential nutrients**. Some enzymes require the presence of divalent metal ions as cofactors for activity, such as magnesium Mg^{++}, calcium Ca^{++}, manganese Mn^{++} and zinc Zn^{++}.

Bacteria are usually able to synthesise all the coenzymes they require, whereas most animals need to receive them in their diet. They are called essential nutrients or **vitamins** (e.g. folic acid). These metabolic differences can be exploited when developing drugs to selectively inhibit the bacteria causing an infection without harming the host (human) cells. This topic is discussed further in Chapter 12.

FACTORS INFLUENCING ENZYME ACTIVITY

As mentioned before, enzymes usually react preferentially with a particular substrate. Sometimes, however, they may bind to a closely related compound, or **analogue**. When a compound with a structure similar to the substrate binds reversibly or irreversibly to the active site and prevents the real substrate reaching the enzyme, the activity of the enzyme is inhibited, or an inactive product is formed. This property has been used to design nucleotide analogues which are effective as antiviral drugs (see Chapter 12).

Enzymes have been found to function optimally at certain pH values and salt (ionic) concentrations. This is

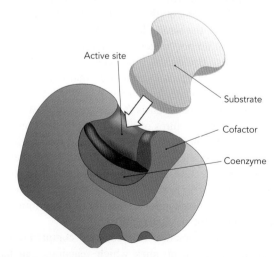

Figure 3.6

Components of an enzyme

Many enzymes require the protein portion of the enzyme as well as a cofactor (non-protein) portion for activity. Cofactors may be metal ions or organic molecules called coenzymes.

because a change in pH or ionic concentration may alter the charge on the protein molecule and therefore its shape. If the shape of the active site is altered, the substrate may not be able to attach. Temperature also affects the rate at which enzyme reactions take place. Bacteria therefore reproduce fastest at their optimum temperature.

It is important to remember all these factors when considering the metabolic reactions described below. Environmental factors can also exert some influence but, in general, microorganisms have shown themselves to be particularly adaptable to changes in their environment and can utilise a range of nutrients depending on what is available.

Energy production in biological systems

The basic metabolic process of life is the production of energy for use in other cellular processes. Initially, all energy comes from the sun, the radiant energy being trapped by the chlorophyll in green plants. In a process known as **photosynthesis**, the basic molecules of carbon dioxide (from the air) and water are converted to a simple carbohydrate molecule, glucose (containing six carbon atoms). In the process, oxygen is released. The removal of carbon dioxide from the atmosphere and the release of oxygen enables the survival of oxygen-requiring organisms such as humans, other animals and many microorganisms. This can be written as:

Photosynthesis

$$6\ CO_2 + 6\ H_2O + \Delta E \longrightarrow C_6H_{12}O_6 + 6\ O_2$$

carbon + water + energy $\longrightarrow$ glucose +
dioxide   (from sun)   oxygen

The same energy from the sun that is trapped and used to produce glucose is released when a molecule of glucose is broken down during metabolism. This complex process is called **oxidation**, or **respiration**, and consists of a number of interrelated biochemical pathways, including those of **glycolysis**, **fermentation** and **aerobic respiration**. Reactions that occur in the presence of oxygen are termed **aerobic**. Glycolysis and fermentation, which can occur in the absence of oxygen, are called **anaerobic**. Many of these reactions require the involvement of various cofactors as well as enzymes, and result in the production of energy which is trapped in a small molecule called **adenosine triphosphate (ATP)**. ATP is termed an 'energy-rich storage molecule' because the subsequent breakdown of ATP releases energy for use in other reactions in the cell.

In aerobic respiration (e.g. in muscle cells), glucose is completely broken down in a series of steps to form carbon dioxide and water, with the release of considerable amounts of energy. The reaction can be written as:

Respiration

$$C_6H_{12}O_6 + 6\ O_2 \longrightarrow 6\ CO_2 + 6H_2O + ATP$$

glucose + oxygen $\longrightarrow$ carbon dioxide +
water + energy

It is obvious that this is the reverse process to photosynthesis.

There are many other reactions that take place, depending on the needs of the cell and the availability of oxygen. The reactions described in this chapter are of importance in microbial cells.

The energy released during the breakdown of the glucose molecule in living cells is used to form ATP. ATP is a small, soluble, biological energy-storage molecule which can diffuse around the cell and provide energy for other reactions in the cell. ATP consists of a molecule of the purine base, adenine, joined to the pentose sugar, ribose, and then to three phosphate groups (see Figure 3.7). Each of these phosphate groups has a different 'bond energy' – that is, the amount of energy required to form or break the bond. The third phosphate bond, the 'triphosphate', is very labile; that is, it is readily broken with the release of a large amount of energy. It also requires a large amount of energy to form it. The triphosphate bond is therefore referred to as a 'high-energy bond'. The base-ribose unit is called a **nucleoside**, and the base-ribose-phosphate is a **nucleotide**. ATP is also one of the building blocks of the nucleic acids, RNA and DNA.

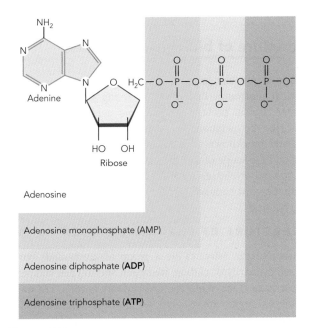

Figure 3.7

Structure of ATP
ATP is composed of the purine base, adenine, joined to the sugar, ribose, and three phosphate groups. The addition of the third phosphate group to ADP requires a large amount of energy which is released when the bond is broken.

For a molecule of glucose to be metabolised, it must first acquire some energy, or be 'activated'. This occurs through the removal of one phosphate group from ATP – that is, the conversion of ATP to ADP (adenosine diphosphate) and the transfer of the phosphate group to glucose.

$$glucose + ATP \rightarrow glucose\text{-}6\text{-}phosphate + ADP$$

The 'activated' glucose molecule (glucose-6-phosphate) is now ready to participate in other cellular reactions.

The processes that occur in living cells can be likened to those in a complex piece of machinery. Fuel (in the form of nutrients) is broken down (oxidised, metabolised) to provide energy to carry out the functions of the machine. Manufactured engines, however, waste a lot of energy as heat, whereas living cells are highly efficient and use sophisticated energy-capturing systems such as ATP and other complex molecules to conserve energy.

ENERGY REQUIREMENTS OF MICROBIAL CELLS

Microbial cells require energy to carry out a range of activities necessary for their growth and reproduction. These activities include:

- the synthesis of lipids, carbohydrates, enzymes and other types of proteins
- the formation of the various structural components of the cell
- the repair and maintenance of the cellular environment
- the accumulation and storage of nutrients and the disposal of waste products
- the active transport of substances into and out of the cell
- the movement of flagella and cilia.

Structure of biological molecules

We now consider in more detail the structure of the biological molecules that make up living cells – carbohydrates, lipids, proteins and nucleic acids – and briefly describe the metabolic pathways involved in their synthesis and breakdown. The details of all these pathways is beyond the scope of this text. However, a brief description of the major classes of molecules is given here together with the most common pathways of energy production and biosynthesis.

STRUCTURE OF CARBOHYDRATES

Carbohydrates (sugars) are a group of compounds composed primarily of carbon, hydrogen and oxygen and their breakdown is the major source of energy in cells. The most common sugar unit is glucose. Glucose is a **hexose**, a 6-carbon compound containing six hydroxyl (OH) groups. Because of the stereoisomerism of the carbon atom, these hydroxyl groups can be arranged in different ways, giving rise to different **isomers** of glucose. In the cell, glucose exists in a ring form with a three-dimensional shape (see Figure 3.8).

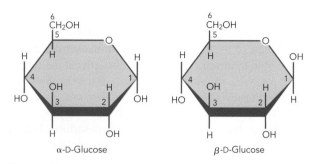

α-D-Glucose   β-D-Glucose

Figure 3.8

Ring structure of glucose
Sugars exist in biological molecules in a three-dimensional ring form.

The most abundant sugars are the 6-carbon sugars but another important group – the **pentoses** – contain five carbon atoms. The most important sugars in this group are **ribose** and **deoxyribose**, which occur in nucleic acids.

Monosaccharides, disaccharides and polysaccharides

Sugars are found in nature as single units (**monosaccharides**), double units (**disaccharides**) or polymers (**polysaccharides**). The monosaccharides include the hexoses and pentoses described above. Disaccharides and polysaccharides are made up of basic hexose units joined together. The way in which they are linked (i.e. the direction of the bond) is referred to as an α-linkage or a β-linkage and determines the shape of the molecule (see Figure 3.9).

STRUCTURE OF LIPIDS

Fats, or triglycerides, are lipids consisting of glycerol and long-chain fatty acids. **Glycerol** is a 3-carbon compound containing three hydroxyl (OH) groups. **Fatty acids** are long chains of carbon and hydrogen (usually 16 or 18 carbon atoms in length) with a single carboxyl (COOH) group at one end. Triglycerides consist of a glycerol molecule combined with three long-chain fatty acids joined by ester linkages (see Figure 3.10).

Another important group of lipid molecules are the **phospholipids**. These consist of glycerol esterified with two long-chain fatty acids. The third position is occupied by a phosphate group which can also be joined to another organic molecule such as choline. Phospholipids are an integral component of all cell membranes (see Chapter 4).

STRUCTURE OF PROTEINS

Proteins consist of chains of amino acids arranged in a specific sequence. There are 20 different naturally occurring amino acids which serve as the building blocks of proteins. Amino acids are a group of organic molecules which all contain an amino ($-NH_2$) group and a carboxyl (–COOH) group attached to various side chain groups (usually designated R). The differences in the side-chain groups confer different properties on the amino acids. For example, glutamic acid has a carboxyl group in its side chain, so is quite acidic; lysine has an amino group, so is

(a) Formation of sucrose

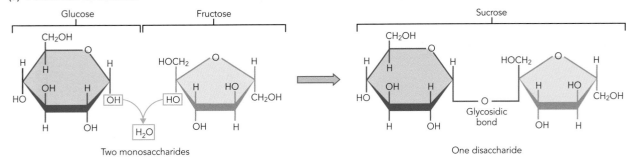

Figure 3.9
Structure of carbohydrates
(a) Two monosaccharides are joined to form a disaccharide by the removal of water and the formation of a glycosidic bond; (b) Polysaccharides such as starch are formed by the linking of many monosaccharides in long chains; (c) Structure of cellulose, β1–4 linkage, gives rise to a straight-chain polymer which cannot be broken down by human enzymes.

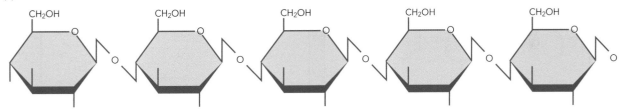

Figure 3.10
Structure of a triglyceride

basic; cysteine has a sulphydryl (SH) group, so is capable of forming disulphide bridges (S-S) within the protein molecule. The structures of the 20 naturally occurring amino acids are shown in Figure 3.11.

When two amino acids join together, they do so by the removal of a molecule of water from the amino and carboxyl groups of adjacent acids, forming a peptide bond (Figure 3.12). Short sequences of amino acids joined together are

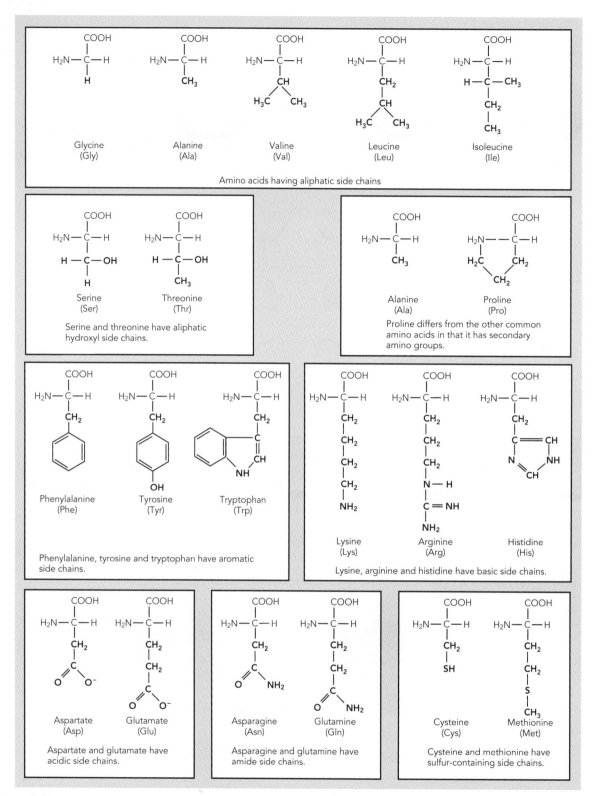

Figure 3.11

Structures of the 20 naturally occurring amino acids
The nature of the R side chain confers special properties on the amino acid molecule.

called **peptides**; longer ones are called **polypeptides**. Proteins are long polypeptide chains, folded and cross-linked to form compounds with a specific molecular structure.

The nature of the side chains of the amino acids affects the overall structure of the protein. The size, shape and charge of each amino acid determine the ability of the protein to fold and assume a particular conformation and activity (Figure 3.13). When this conformation is disrupted, the proteins are said to be 'denatured' and their function, or enzyme activity, may be lost.

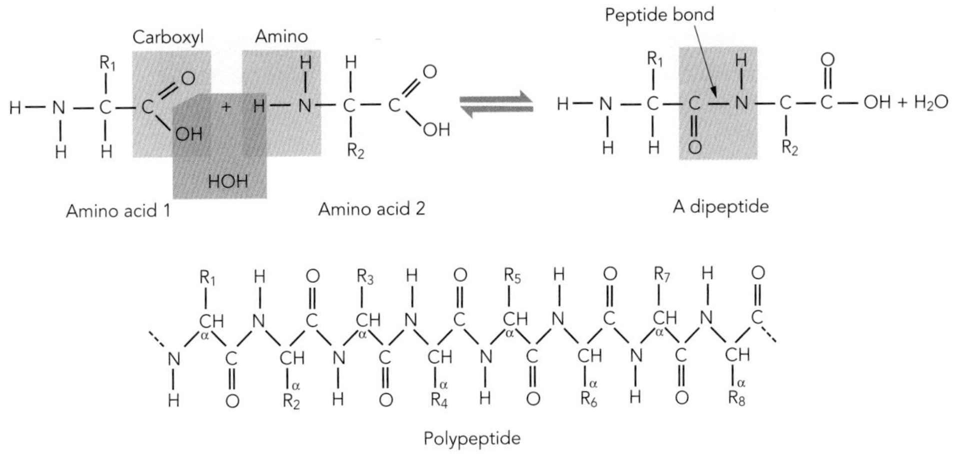

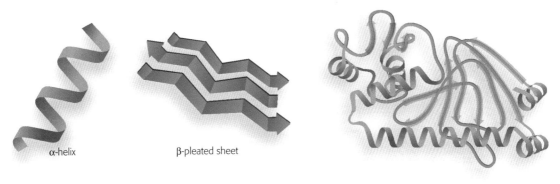

Figure 3.12

Synthesis of a peptide bond
Two amino acids join together to form a dipeptide. Water is eliminated from adjacent molecules to form the peptide bond.

α-helix   β-pleated sheet

(a) Secondary structure:
α-helix or β-pleated sheets held
together by hydrogen bonds.

(b)Tertiary structure:
3-dimensional shape of proteins involves
hydrogen bonds and covalent bonds.

Figure 3.13

Structure of proteins

Biochemical pathways of energy production

BREAKDOWN OF POLYSACCHARIDES

The ability of an organism to utilise different carbohydrates as an energy source depends on its ability to synthesise the appropriate enzymes. For example, human saliva contains the enzyme, amylase, which can break the α-linkages found between the glucose units in starch (Figure 3.9(b)). However, humans cannot synthesise the enzyme which breaks the β1–4 linkage that occurs between the glucose molecules in cellulose (Figure 3.9(c)), and so they are unable to metabolise cellulose. Cellulose therefore acts as fibre, or roughage, in the human diet and aids in digestion and formation of faeces without providing any energy.

Many microorganisms, however, produce an enzyme which can break this bond and release single glucose units. Ruminant animals such as cows rely on the bacteria present in their stomachs to break down cellulose, which is the primary polysaccharide in grass and other fibrous plants. The ability of soil microorganisms to break down cellulose is important for the decomposition of plant organic matter.

Starch, with its branched structure, is mainly a storage carbohydrate. It can be utilised by many organisms, including humans, as a source of energy. Enzymes in the mouth (salivary amylase) and small intestine (pancreatic amylase) break it down to the disaccharide, maltose, for digestion and absorption. Most microorganisms use carbohydrates as their primary source of energy. They are broken down by various reactions to single glucose units, which then enter the pathways described below.

BREAKDOWN OF GLUCOSE

This is a brief overview of the principal pathways of glucose catabolism in microorganisms. The first stage is called **glycolysis**, or the **Embden-Meyerhof pathway** (see Figure 3.14(a)). It consists of ten reactions, each catalysed by a different enzyme, and is essentially the same in all living cells, plant, animal or microbial. It does not require the presence of oxygen. During this process, each molecule of glucose (six carbon atoms) is broken down to form two molecules of **pyruvic acid** (three

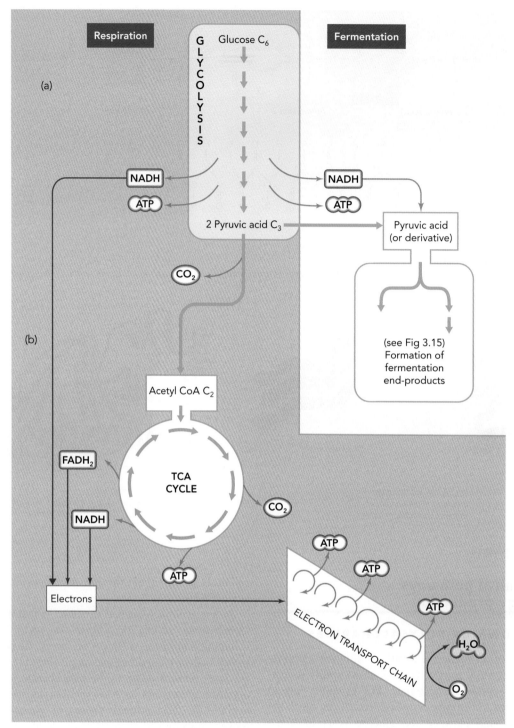

Figure 3.14

Overview of glucose metabolism

(a) Embden-Meyerhof pathway of glycolysis

One molecule of glucose gives rise to two molecules of pyruvic acid with the overall yield of two molecules of ATP.

(b) The reactions of the TCA cycle

Pyruvic acid from glycolysis is converted to the 2-carbon intermediate acetyl CoA which enters the cycle. Each turn of the cycle results in the release of two molecules of CO_2. ATP is produced by substrate-level phosphorylation and by oxidative phosphorylation via the electron transport chain.

carbon atoms), yielding only a small amount of energy. A number of other sugars, including fructose, can enter the glycolytic pathway and be converted to pyruvic acid but the pathways involved are not described here.

Pyruvic acid is an important intermediate that can be further metabolised, either aerobically (respiration) or anaerobically (fermentation). Under aerobic conditions, **respiration** occurs, in which pyruvic acid is first converted to **acetyl CoA**, which then undergoes a series of reactions known as the **Krebs cycle**, or **tricarboxylic acid**

(TCA) cycle. This cycle leads to the formation of carbon dioxide and water, and large amounts of energy are released and stored as ATP. Acetyl CoA is a central intermediate that also occurs in the metabolism of lipids and proteins.

Respiration

Organisms that are capable of respiration oxidise pyruvic acid (three carbon atoms) to acetyl CoA (two carbon atoms), which then enters the Krebs, or tricarboxylic acid (TCA), cycle (Figure 3.14(b)). The TCA cycle provides a mechanism whereby molecules of acetyl CoA continuously enter the cycle and are broken down to carbon dioxide (CO_2) and water with the release of large amounts of energy in the form of ATP. A supply of inorganic phosphate (Pi) is necessary for these reactions to occur.

The intermediate steps require the transfer of electrons to the coenzyme, nicotinamide adenine dinucleotide (NAD), which is part of the **electron transport chain** used to convert the energy from these reactions into ATP. The TCA cycle also provides intermediate compounds that link into pathways involved in the synthesis of lipids, proteins and nucleic acids (see Figure 3.16 on page 45).

Oxidative phosphorylation and the electron transport chain

In the presence of oxygen, pyruvic acid is oxidised via the TCA cycle with the release of large amounts of energy. The cell uses a process called **oxidative phosphorylation** to capture this energy in the storage molecule, ATP. The process involves the transfer of electrons from the reduced coenzyme, NADH, along a series of specialised carrier molecules located in the cell membranes to the final electron acceptor, molecular oxygen. This is known as the **electron transport chain**. It is a complex system comprising a series of steps in which each oxidation reaction is linked to a reduction reaction – that is, the energy released from one reaction is immediately used to carry out another reaction and to synthesise ATP.

Summary of glucose oxidation

The overall process of the aerobic oxidation of one molecule of glucose can be written:

$$C_6H_{12}O_6 \ + \ 6\,O_2 \ \rightarrow \ 6\,CO_2 \ + \ 6\,H_2O$$
glucose + oxygen → carbon dioxide + water

Each molecule of glucose produces 38 molecules of ATP.
The energy equation can be written:

$$38\,ADP \ + \ 38\,Pi \ \rightarrow \ 38\,ATP$$
adenosine + inorganic → adenosine triphosphate
diphosphate phosphate

Fermentation of pyruvic acid

Under anaerobic conditions pyruvic acid undergoes **fermentation**, which is the term used to describe catabolic reactions that occur in the absence of oxygen. The energy yield is low compared to respiration. In microorganisms a number of different fermentative pathways may be followed, some of which give rise to useful products (see Figure 3.15).

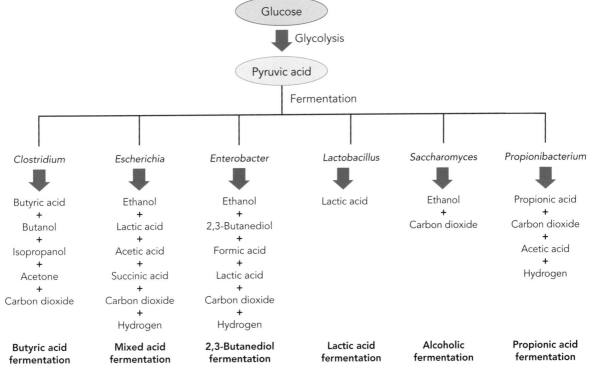

Figure 3.15

Major pathways of fermentation
Different microorganisms use characteristic fermentative pathways. The products of fermentation can be used to aid in identification of the microorganisms.

No single organism has all the enzymes required for all these pathways. In fact, most organisms use only one pathway. This is a useful property for microbiologists, since organisms can often be characterised by the end products they release into the environment from fermentation reactions. Conversely, pure cultures of specific microorganisms can be added to a particular substrate to produce a desired product. Many of the products of microbial fermentation are of great use to humans. For example, yeast (*Saccharomyces*) is added to grape juice to produce alcohol in winemaking; yeast is also added to bread to produce carbon dioxide which causes the bread to rise; lactobacilli are added to various milk products to induce 'souring' during the production of cheese and yoghurt. These processes are described in more detail later in this chapter (see Table 3.1, page 48).

Anaerobic respiration

Some microorganisms use inorganic substances as the final electron acceptor instead of oxygen. For example, some species of *Pseudomonas* and *Bacillus* can use the nitrate ion (NO_3^-) as the acceptor, forming nitrite (NO_2), nitric oxide (NO) or nitrogen gas. Others use sulphate or carbonate. The amount of ATP formed is not usually as great as that produced when molecular oxygen is the final electron acceptor, but is quite significant.

The metabolic reactions described above are for glucose, which is the primary source of energy in most cells. However, lipids and proteins are also broken down with the release of energy and the formation of small molecules (building blocks) that can be used in other cellular processes.

BREAKDOWN OF LIPIDS

Triglycerides are readily broken down by enzymes called **lipases** which split the fatty acids from the glycerol molecule. The glycerol is then converted to dihydroxyacetone phosphate, an intermediate in glycolysis (see step 5, Figure 3.14(a)). The fatty acids are broken down by β-oxidation into 2-carbon units of acetyl CoA which enter the TCA cycle. The metabolism of fats therefore yields large amounts of energy.

BREAKDOWN OF PROTEINS

Proteins are broken down in most bacterial cells by proteolytic enzymes (called proteases or peptidases) to form smaller peptide fragments or single amino acids. The amino acids are reused for protein synthesis or are metabolised further. The removal of the amino group gives rise to compounds that can enter the TCA cycle and be broken down, producing energy in the form of ATP.

Anabolism – biosynthesis of cellular components

The energy released in the reactions described above is used by the cell in a number of different ways. ATP is needed for the synthesis of the chemical components of the cell: carbohydrates, lipopolysaccharides, RNA and DNA, structural proteins and enzymes, the cell wall and the phospholipids of the cell membrane. The small building blocks of these complex macromolecules are activated by combining with ATP so that they have sufficient energy to enter their respective biosynthetic pathways.

Energy is also used for active transport of substances into and out of the cell and for the movement of flagella and cilia.

BIOSYNTHESIS OF CARBOHYDRATES

Microorganisms utilise different pathways for the synthesis of carbohydrates depending on the availability of nutrients and the particular needs of the organism.

Autotrophs are organisms that can use carbon dioxide as their primary source of carbon; that is, they can live without access to complex molecules. They are able to use energy from the sun during photosynthesis to synthesise glucose from carbon dioxide with the release of oxygen. These organisms include photosynthetic bacteria (cyanobacteria, green sulphur and purple sulphur bacteria), algae and green plants.

Heterotrophs, which include most bacteria, fungi and protozoa, must be provided with a source of organic carbon in their environment in order to synthesise glucose and larger polysaccharides. The intermediates in the TCA cycle, or other breakdown products from lipid or protein metabolism, can be a suitable source. Depending on the needs of the cell and the availability of energy in the form of ATP, various biosynthetic pathways are utilised which are the reverse of (or parallel to) those described for the breakdown of carbohydrates. However, some microorganisms have strict nutritional requirements; these are described in Chapter 4.

One important complex polysaccharide molecule that is synthesised only by procaryotic cells is **peptidoglycan**, a compound that provides strength and rigidity to bacterial cell walls. Peptidoglycan is a complex molecule composed of sugar molecules cross-linked by peptide bridges (see Chapter 4).

BIOSYNTHESIS OF LIPIDS

Bacterial lipids are usually formed by the condensation of long-chain fatty acids with a molecule of glycerol to form triglycerides. The fatty acids are synthesised from units of acetyl CoA which occur as a breakdown product of carbohydrate metabolism.

BIOSYNTHESIS OF AMINO ACIDS

Amino acids are required for the synthesis of proteins and also serve as precursors for the purine and pyrimidine bases which are the building blocks of the nucleic acids RNA and DNA. Amino acids are synthesised in microbial cells by the addition of an amino group ($-NH_2$) to various intermediates in the TCA cycle. The nitrogen may be derived from ammonium salts (NH_4^+) or nitrates (NO_3^-), or nitrogen in the atmosphere. Some bacteria are capable of using atmospheric nitrogen to form nitrogenous compounds in a process called **nitrogen fixation**.

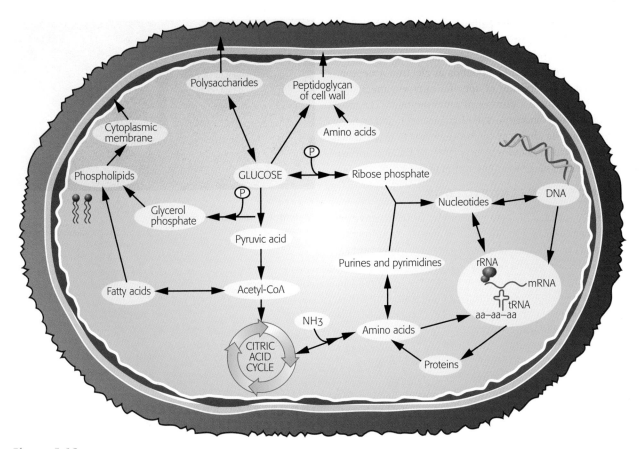

Figure 3.16

Interrelationship of metabolic pathways
Bacteria are able to synthesise all their cellular requirements when supplied with a simple carbon source, nitrogen (ammonia) and inorganic salts.

BIOSYNTHESIS OF PROTEINS

The biosynthesis of proteins occurs under the direction of the genetic material of the cell, the DNA. It requires the participation of RNA and other nucleotides and is described in detail in Chapter 4.

Interrelationship of metabolic pathways

Microorganisms show great diversity in their nutritional requirements (see Chapter 4). These differences reflect their biosynthetic abilities. For example, some microorganisms can synthesise all their cellular requirements from simple organic or inorganic compounds. Others require more complex molecules such as sugars, amino acids, and vitamins or cofactors. Some mutant strains may have an absolute requirement for a particular compound (e.g. a fatty acid or amino acid). Figure 3.16 illustrates the interrelationship between the pathways of bacterial metabolism. It is beyond the scope of this text to examine all these pathways in detail, but it is important to remember that most microorganisms of medical importance are **heterotrophic** – that is, they use complex carbon-containing molecules as their primary nutritional source. This property is useful for the identification and control of potential pathogens.

Practical applications of microbial processes

The metabolic pathways described in this chapter represent only a small fraction of the reactions carried out by living cells. These reactions are controlled by specific enzymes produced by cells according to the information contained in their genes. In animal cells, the production of a set of enzymes by a cell is usually fixed, and reflects the function of that cell. If the required enzymes are not produced or are produced in the wrong amount, the workings of the cell are greatly affected. The measurement of the amount of enzyme produced by a cell can be used to diagnose whether a cell is functioning normally. For example, in humans, liver function tests measure the levels of different liver enzymes in blood to determine whether the liver is damaged by diseases such as hepatitis or cirrhosis.

In the microbial world, bacteria are able to adapt the metabolic pathways they use to the nutrients available. Because the bacterial cell is so small, it only synthesises enzymes for its immediate need, even though it may carry the genetic information for other enzymes. When provided with alternative carbon sources it is often able to synthesise the enzymes necessary for metabolism of that compound. The metabolic pathways employed, therefore, reflect the environment in which the organism is generally found – for example, the sulphur bacteria occur in hot springs and use sulphur compounds as electron acceptors.

The metabolic abilities of specific microorganisms are used by scientists in a number of areas including diagnostic microbiology, industry, scientific research and genetic engineering. The ability of microorganisms to break down large biological molecules is important for the decomposition of waste matter in the environment.

DIAGNOSTIC MICROBIOLOGY

The ability (or lack of it) to grow under different environmental conditions is used by microbiologists to differentiate between species of organisms that may appear morphologically identical. This is the principle behind the selective and differential media used in a diagnostic microbiology laboratory. A brief introduction is appropriate here to show how an understanding of metabolic pathways helps to identify different pathogens.

A **selective medium** is one to which chemical compounds have been added to prevent the growth of certain microorganisms, but not others. The 'compound' is often something as simple as a high salt concentration. A **differential medium** is one to which some sort of indicator, usually a dye, has been added. This allows the clinical microbiologist to differentiate between various bacteria on the basis of chemical reactions that occur during growth.

Sometimes the medium is both differential and selective at the same time. For example, mannitol salt agar (MS agar) is used in the identification of a mixture of streptococci and different species of staphylococci. Staphylococci grow readily in the high salt concentration whereas the growth of streptococci is inhibited. *Staphylococcus aureus* produces enzymes which utilise mannitol (a sugar alcohol) and convert it to an acid that turns the pink indicator dye in the medium to yellow. *Staphylococcus epidermidis*, which appears similar under the microscope to *Staphylococcus aureus*, does not metabolise mannitol, so there is no acid production and no colour change in the medium (see Figure 3.17).

A battery of different tests is used in the microbiology laboratory to assist in the identification of a particular microorganism and many of these involve the measurement of an enzyme reaction. In effect, these tests detect the presence or absence of the enzyme required for a reaction similar to the ones described above, thus indicating the kind of organism that is present. The change in dye colour measures pH changes occurring as a result of the ability of the organism to produce the enzyme which can ferment mannitol. Enzyme reactions that produce gases such as carbon dioxide or hydrogen can also be seen by the appearance of bubbles in the culture medium. Enzymic breakdown of sulphur compounds with the release of hydrogen sulphide is detected by reacting the gas with iron (ferric) compounds – as well as by its offensive smell!

Many commercial companies market diagnostic kits for the identification of microorganisms. These kits test

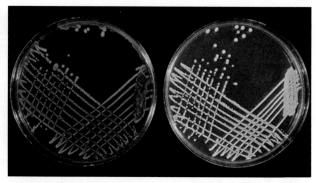

Figure 3.17

Mannitol-fermentation test
Growth on mannitol salt agar distinguishes different species of staphylococci. *Staphylococcus aureus* ferments mannitol, producing acid which turns the indicator in the medium to yellow. *Staphylococcus epidermidis* does not produce a colour change.

for the presence of several different enzymes in a single specimen. Some of these reagents are very sensitive and can give a positive diagnosis when only a small amount of specimen is available. This topic is discussed further in Chapter 15.

INDUSTRIAL APPLICATIONS OF MICROBIAL METABOLISM

Microorganisms are used in industry in a number of different ways, for example:

- as living cell cultures in the production of food
- in the preparation of purified enzymes
- as a source of primary or secondary metabolites.

Live microbial cells

Live cell preparations, such as yeasts, and lactic acid bacteria are widely used in the food industry. Fermentation of sugar by yeast cells under anaerobic conditions produces alcohol and carbon dioxide. For example:

- Wine is made from fermented grape juice. Wild yeast cells are found on grapes in nature. In practice, the wine they produce is of variable quality, so most winemakers add a pure culture of the yeast, *Saccharomyces ellipsoideus*, and control the fermentation by the amount of oxygen present. An understanding of metabolism can be used to achieve the desired product. When oxygen is low or absent, yeast fermentation produces mainly alcohol. When oxygen is available, carbon dioxide is also formed. When the alcohol concentration reaches 12–14% the yeast cells die. Champagne is made by a secondary fermentation in which fresh yeast cells and sugar are added to still wine in a sealed bottle. The carbon dioxide produced cannot escape and remains as bubbles in the champagne.
- Beer is also a product of yeast fermentation. An extract of grains such as barley is used to make a sugar substrate or 'malt'. Hops are added for flavour. Special strains of yeast, *Saccharomyces carlsbergensis* or *Saccharomyces cerevisiae*, are used.

- The leavening of bread also relies on the properties of the yeast cell. When added to the dough, yeast produces alcohol and carbon dioxide gas. The carbon dioxide causes the bread to rise. When the bread is baked, the alcohol and carbon dioxide are driven off, leaving the distinctive holes in the bread. Sour dough bread is made by adding cultures of lactic acid bacteria to the dough to produce the distinctive 'sour' taste.
- Lactic acid bacteria produce lactic acid by fermentation of glucose and are responsible for the 'souring' of milk to produce cheese, yoghurt, buttermilk and other products. Various other bacteria and some fungi are added to produce intermediate compounds which impart a distinctive appearance and flavour to cheeses (e.g. different strains of the mould, *Penicillium*, are used for blue cheeses and camembert).
- Cultures of the nitrogen-fixing bacterium, *Rhizobium*, are frequently inoculated onto leguminous plant seeds to encourage the formation of root nodules where nitrogen fixation can take place.
- Mushrooms are cultivated for food.

Microbial enzymes

Microorganisms are also used as a source of enzymes that are used industrially. Some chemical reactions are difficult to carry out by non-enzymic means. As explained earlier in this chapter, enzymes are biological catalysts that allow chemical reactions to occur more efficiently by lowering the activation energy – often giving a much higher yield of product for a lower cost. Specific enzyme proteins can be extracted from large-scale preparations of microorganisms, purified and used in the commercial production of a particular compound. Examples are protein-digesting enzymes (proteases in laundry detergents) and glucose isomerase, which converts glucose to fructose for use in the confectionery industry. Another useful enzyme is penicillin acylase, used in the manufacture of semi-synthetic antimicrobial drugs.

Primary metabolites

Many different organic compounds are produced by microorganisms in the metabolic reactions outlined in this chapter. **Primary metabolites** are products formed in the major pathways of fermentation. These compounds can often be obtained in sufficient yields to be of use commercially. Some of the more important metabolites are described below.

- Citric acid, an intermediate in the TCA cycle, is widely used as a flavouring in foods and beverages.
- Sorbose, produced when the bacterium *Acetobacter* oxidises sorbitol, is used to make ascorbic acid (vitamin C).
- Acetic acid (vinegar) is a product of the oxidation of alcohol (one of the products of fermentation) by members of the genera *Acetobacter* and *Gluconobacter*. Sometimes the *Acetobacter* are an accidental contaminant of food and cause acid production or 'souring'. Vinegar can be produced commercially from the alcohol present in wine or any other product of alcoholic fermentation. Vinegar is used to preserve (pickle) food because most harmful bacteria cannot tolerate acid conditions.
- Vitamins and growth factors are used as food supplements for humans and in animal feeds. Most vitamins are made commercially by chemical synthesis, but a few are too complex and so are produced by microbial fermentation. These include vitamin B12 and riboflavin.
- Some amino acids are produced by microbial means. Chemical synthesis of amino acids usually results in the formation of a mixture of the D- and L- stereoisomers. Naturally occurring amino acids are in only the L-form. Using microorganisms to produce the L-amino acid means that a pure product can be obtained. Some useful amino acids are:
  – the salt of glutamic acid, monosodium glutamate (MSG), used as a flavour enhancer
  – phenylalanine and aspartic acid, which are components of the sweetener, aspartame
  – lysine, an essential amino acid for humans, produced as a food supplement.

Some uses for products of microbial fermentation are listed in Table 3.1.

Secondary metabolites

Secondary metabolites are an interesting group of organic compounds, usually produced by microorganisms when nutrients have been depleted and the number of cells is no longer increasing rapidly. These compounds do not appear to be essential for growth or reproduction. The formation of these metabolites is limited to certain kinds of organisms and is very dependent on growth conditions. It is possible to select for specific strains of an organism in order to enhance the yield of the desired metabolite.

Antibiotics form one of the most important groups and their discovery has had an enormous impact on the practice of medicine since the first commercial development of penicillin in the 1940s. More than 5000 antibiotic substances have been described, but most of them are too toxic for human use. Most commercially useful antibiotics are produced by filamentous fungi and bacteria of the actinomyces group (see Table 3.2).

MICROORGANISMS AS TOOLS IN SCIENTIFIC RESEARCH

The metabolic processes that occur in microorganisms are very similar to those occurring in the cells of higher organisms. In fact, much of the scientific knowledge about cellular metabolism was derived from laboratory research using bacteria. Bacteria are easy to grow in large numbers on a defined medium (i.e. controlled nutrients and growth conditions). They provide the research worker with a uniform population of cells, making it easier to interpret results. The simple genetic material (the DNA is all on one circular chromosome) provided the ideal system for early genetic mapping experiments. The techniques and

Table 3.1

Some useful fermentation reactions

PRODUCT	USES	SUBSTRATE	MICROORGANISM
Lactic acid	Cheese, yoghurt	Milk	*Lactobacillus* spp.
	Sauerkraut	Cabbage	
Propionic acid and carbon dioxide	Swiss cheese	Milk	*Propionibacterium*
Ethanol	Beer	Malt extract	*Saccharomyces cerevisiae* (yeast)
	Wine	Grape juice	*Saccharomyces ellipsoideus* (yeast)
	Fuel	Agricultural waste	*Saccharomyces cerevisiae*
Acetic acid	Vinegar	Ethanol	*Acetobacter* (bacterium)
Glycerol	Industry/Food Pharmaceutical	Molasses	*Saccharomyces cerevisiae*
Citric acid	Flavouring	Molasses	*Aspergillus* (fungus)
Sorbose	Vitamin C	Sorbitol	*Acetobacter*

Table 3.2

Commercial production of antibiotics

ANTIBIOTIC	MICROORGANISM	TYPE
Penicillin	*Penicillium chrysogenum*	Fungus
Cephalosporin	*Cephalosporium* spp.	Fungus
Bacitracin	*Bacillus subtilis*	Bacterium
Polymixin B	*Bacillus polymyxa*	Bacterium
Cycloheximide	*Streptomyces griseus*	Actinomycete
Streptomycin	*Streptomyces griseus*	Actinomycete
Erythromycin	*Streptomyces erythreus*	Actinomycete
Aminoglycosides	*Streptomyces* spp.	Actinomycete
Tetracycline	*Streptomyces rimosus*	Actinomycete

knowledge obtained from this 'simple' system have now been adapted for use in more ambitious projects such as mapping of the DNA of the human genome. A knowledge of the processes of DNA replication in bacteria provided the scientist with a tool for manipulating the genetic information in cells – **genetic engineering**.

GENETIC ENGINEERING

A very important use for microorganisms in recent years has been the production of specific compounds for medical use by the process of genetic engineering. Scientists have developed methods of inserting genetic information into microbial cells in such a way as to direct the microbe to synthesise large amounts of a desired compound. Examples of genetic engineering include the production of human insulin, human growth hormone and some vaccines. Genetic engineering is described in more detail in Chapter 4.

ENVIRONMENTAL USES FOR MICROORGANISMS

Microorganisms play an essential role in the environment in decomposition and recycling of nutrients.

Decomposition

The catabolic reactions carried out by many microorganisms are essential for the decomposition of organic matter such as plant material and sewage. The enzymes produced by microorganisms break down complex carbohydrates and other biological compounds using the pathways described above, releasing small organic molecules into the soil. These molecules are a source of nutrients for growing plants.

Hydrocarbon metabolism

Hydrocarbons are organic compounds containing only hydrogen and carbon, and are usually insoluble in water. Two examples are oil and petroleum. The chemical breakdown of hydrocarbons is a slow process, requiring oxygen. Very few microorganisms can utilise hydrocarbons for growth. The exceptions are some strains of *Pseudomonas*, *Nocardia* and *Mycobacterium*, and some yeasts and moulds. Cultures of *Pseudomonas* have been used to help disperse oil spills. Usually, the hydrocarbon metabolism would proceed too slowly to be of use, but the addition of other nutritional requirements, nitrogen and phosphate, speed up metabolism and growth of the bacteria so that the oil is broken down and dispersed.

Microorganisms have been used in bioremediation projects such as those undertaken at the Sydney Olympic site (see Spotlight box on the next page).

SPOTLIGHT ON
Bioremediation – environmental uses for bacteria

When the Homebush site was chosen for the 2000 Olympic Games, one of the problems confronting the organisers was the fact that for many years the area had been used to dump Sydney's waste. Wilson Park is a 12-hectare portion of Crown Land adjacent to the Olympic site. It was used for the production of town gas for Sydney between 1953 and 1974 and approximately 230 000 tonnes of hydrocarbon (tar) waste remained buried on site (Figure 3.18(a)).

A feature of the Sydney 2000 bid had been the guarantee of a 'green games' so the main task was to clean up the site to a level where the risks to humans and the ecology of the area could be contained.

A number of toxic volatile organic compounds such as benzene, toluene, ethyl benzene and xylene were emanating from the buried tar and were found in the groundwater on site. The challenge was to remove these compounds and make the area safe.

Three Sydney scientists were commissioned by the Olympic Coordination Authority to undertake the project.

They found that there were high numbers of hydrocarbon-degrading bacteria present in the topsoil of the site. In the laboratory these bacteria were capable of completely metabolising benzene to carbon dioxide and water if simple plant fertilisers containing nitrogen and phosphorus were added to the cultures. The isolated bacteria included species of *Pseudomonas*, *Bacillus*, *Microbacterium*, *Actinomyces* and *Gordonia*. Some of these bacteria were similar to those used to clean up oil spills overseas.

The remediation project consisted of providing a healthy vegetated topsoil cover to act as a microbial biofilter. The enhanced bacterial activity in the soil was responsible for degrading the hydrocarbon gas pollutants and stopping their reaching the surface. In this way the park was made safe for human use once more (see Figure 3.18(b)).

Source: Sheumack D, M Howe, B Bicknell, M Muir, J Pym, E Ling & K Hughes 2000, Contamination Assessment and Bioremediation at Wilson Park, *Proceedings of the 15th International Clean Air and Environment Conference*, Sydney, November. Clean Air Society of Australia and New Zealand Inc., Vol. 1, pp. 191–98.

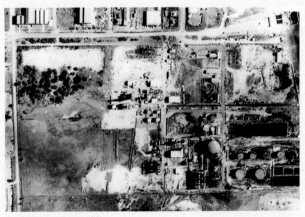

Figure 3.18(a)
Aerial view of gasworks at Wilson Park, Silverwater, in 1962

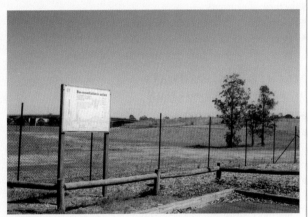

Figure 3.18(b)
Wilson Park 2000, prior to Sydney Olympic Games

SUMMARY

- Metabolism is the overall term used to describe the chemical reactions of breakdown (catabolism), synthesis (anabolism) and repair that occur in living cells.

STRUCTURE OF BIOLOGICAL MOLECULES

- Living matter is made up of complex molecules containing the elements carbon, hydrogen, oxygen, nitrogen, phosphorus and sulphur and other, trace elements.
- Organic compounds are compounds containing carbon; they exhibit stereoisomerism by forming four covalent bonds with other atoms.

- The arrangement of atoms within a molecule determines its shape and function.
- The particular structure of biological molecules enables them to combine with complementary molecules. This is termed 'specificity'.

ENZYMES AND CHEMICAL REACTIONS

- Enzymes are proteins that act as biological catalysts to lower the activation energy of a reaction.
- The production of enzymes is under the control of the DNA of the cell.

- Enzymes have a particular shape, containing an active site that is specific for the substrate; some require a cofactor for activity.

ENERGY PRODUCTION IN BIOLOGICAL SYSTEMS

- Photosynthesis uses energy from the sun to convert carbon dioxide and water to glucose.
- Cells break down glucose and release energy by the processes of glycolysis, fermentation and respiration.
- ATP is a small, biological, energy-rich storage molecule.
- Breaking the bond of the terminal phosphate group of ATP releases large amounts of energy, used by the cell for essential processes.

STRUCTURE OF BIOLOGICAL MOLECULES

Structure of carbohydrates

- Carbohydrates (sugars) are organic compounds made up of carbon, hydrogen and oxygen.
- The most common sugars are hexoses and pentoses; they may exist as monosaccharides, disaccharides or polysaccharides.

Structure of lipids

- Fats, or triglycerides, are composed of glycerol and long-chain fatty acids.

Structure of proteins

- There are 20 different naturally occurring amino acids.
- Proteins consist of chains of amino acids joined by peptide bonds in a specific sequence and folded into a particular shape.

BIOCHEMICAL PATHWAYS OF ENERGY PRODUCTION

Breakdown of carbohydrates

- Energy is produced from the oxidation of carbohydrates by a process of glycolysis, followed by either fermentation or respiration.
- Fermentation occurs anaerobically and results in the formation of a number of useful products, depending on the microorganism.

- Respiration via the Krebs (TCA) cycle occurs in the presence of oxygen with the formation of carbon dioxide, water and large amounts of energy, which is stored as ATP.
- Proteins are broken down by proteolytic enzymes into amino acids which can take part in other reactions or in the synthesis of new proteins.

ANABOLISM – BIOSYNTHESIS OF CELLULAR COMPONENTS

- Autotrophs are organisms that use carbon dioxide to synthesise glucose.
- Heterotrophs require a source of organic carbon to synthesise cellular components.
- Bacteria synthesise lipids from acetyl CoA and glycerol.
- Amino acids are synthesised by incorporation of nitrogen from nitrates or ammonia into the intermediates of the TCA cycle.
- Some bacteria can use atmospheric nitrogen to synthesise nitrates and ammonia.
- Proteins are formed in a complex series of reactions, directed by the nucleic acids, DNA and RNA.

INTERRELATIONSHIP OF METABOLIC PATHWAYS

- Microorganisms can use many different interrelated metabolic pathways to synthesise cellular requirements.

PRACTICAL APPLICATIONS OF MICROBIAL PROCESSES

- Many of the reactions carried out by microorganisms are of benefit to humans.
- Biochemical reactions are used to identify bacteria.
- Microorganisms and their products are used in the food industry.
- Genetic engineering involves the use of microorganisms to produce compounds for human use.
- Microbial metabolism is important for the decomposition of sewage and other organic matter.

STUDY QUESTIONS

1. What is meant by metabolism?
2. Which elements make up biological molecules?
3. What name is given to compounds containing carbon?
4. (a) What name is given to the process in which carbon dioxide from the air is converted to glucose?
   (b) What type of microorganisms can carry out this process?
5. How do microbial cells obtain energy for their synthetic reactions?
6. What is meant by a 'biological catalyst'?
7. What is meant by the 'active site' of an enzyme?
8. Give two examples of naturally occurring monosaccharides, disaccharides and polysaccharides.
9. What is the final product in glycolysis?
10. Which compound is the key intermediate that links different metabolic pathways?
11. Give three examples of fermentative processes that are of use to humans.
12. How do microorganisms contribute to the recycling of nutrients to the environment?

TEST YOUR UNDERSTANDING

1. Give three examples of specificity in biological systems.
2. Explain how the properties of the carbon atom contribute to the shape and function of biological molecules.
3. Explain how the energy released in the oxidation of glucose via the TCA cycle is converted into ATP.
4. How can the biochemical properties of microorganisms be used to aid in their indentification?

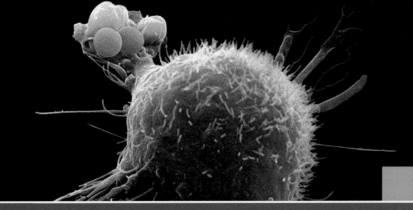

CHAPTER 4

Bacteria

[CHAPTER FOCUS]

- ■ *What are the major properties of bacterial cells?*

- ■ *What are the growth requirements of bacteria?*

- ■ *How are bacteria classified?*

- ■ *What are the major groups of medically important bacteria?*

- ■ *How does the genetic material determine the properties of a cell?*

- ■ *How has the discovery of the process of DNA recombination contributed to advances in biotechnology?*

Introduction

The largest group of microorganisms of medical significance are the **bacteria**. Most bacteria are able to survive and reproduce independently under a wide range of environmental conditions. There are thousands of species of bacteria which can be differentiated on the basis of size, shape, morphology, staining characteristics, nutritional requirements, biochemical activities, cell wall structure and the composition of their RNA and DNA. They are responsible for many skin and wound infections, and are the causative agents of various defined diseases. However, most bacteria are not pathogenic and, in fact, many are beneficial to humans. In this chapter we examine in detail the properties of bacteria, describe the way they are classified and introduce the reader to the way in which bacterial genetics has contributed to the science of molecular biology.

Bacteria are classified as procaryotes because they are single-celled organisms characterised by the lack of a membrane-bound nucleus or other defined organelles. According to the classification developed by CARL WOESE, they are grouped into two domains:

1. The domain **Bacteria** forms the largest group and includes the **eubacteria**, or true bacteria, and a small subgroup of bacteria capable of photosynthesis, the **cyanobacteria** (formerly called blue-green algae).
2. The domain **Archaea** contains the **archaebacteria**. These bacteria are thought to be of ancient origin and are able to live in extreme conditions of temperature and osmotic pressure. The features that distinguish the archaea from eubacteria include the lack of peptidoglycan in the cell wall, the presence of branched-chain fatty acids in their cell membranes and their unique ribosomal RNA. They are not known to cause disease in humans so are not discussed further in this text.

Nomenclature

All bacteria are given two names: the **genus**, which is usually signified by a capital letter, followed by the **species**. For example, *Staphylococcus aureus* and *Staphylococcus epidermidis* are the names of two different species within the same genus. A species may consist of a collection of similar **strains** that differ slightly from each other. The strain is usually designated by a letter or number after the species – for example, *Escherichia* (genus) *coli* (species) 0157 (strain). There are no rules about how bacteria get their names. The name may reflect the characteristic shape of the organism (Bacillus), where it is found (coli = colon), the name of the scientist who identified it (Neisseria) or the disease it causes (tetani = tetanus). Names are always written in *italics*.

Size, shape and appearance of bacterial cells

Bacteria vary significantly in their **morphology**, that is, their size and shape. They range in size from 0.2 μm to 1 μm in diameter and 1 μm to 10 μm in length. There are three basic shapes of cells: spherical, rod-shaped and spiral (see Figures 4.1, 4.2, 4.3). Sometimes, groups of cells remain together after cell division to form clusters or chains. Some bacteria are motile; that is, they are capable of movement, possessing one or more extracellular appendages called **flagella** (singular: flagellum) which enable them to swim.

A spherical or round bacterium is called a **coccus** (plural: cocci). This is typically a small cell and may occur singly, in pairs (**diplococci**), in clusters (**staphylococci**) or in chains (**streptococci**). Frequently, the grouping of the cocci is reflected in the naming of the organism. For example, *Streptococcus pyogenes* is an organism with a cellular arrangement consisting of chains of cocci.

A rod-shaped or cylindrical bacterium is called a **bacillus** (plural: bacilli). Most bacilli appear as single cells, but a few are joined end to end to form **diplobacilli** or **streptobacilli**. Some form palisades where the bacteria are arranged in a row like a fence (e.g. species of *Corynebacterium*).

Spiral bacteria may have one of three shapes. The **spirochaetes** have a corkscrew-like appearance and a strong axial filament running the length of the cell. Rotation of this filament propels the cell along. **Spirilla** (singular: spirillum) are not as tightly coiled and move by means of a flagellum, a propeller-like tail. **Vibrios** are slightly curved rod-shaped cells, resembling a comma or incomplete spiral.

Most bacteria grow in a characteristic shape and this can be a useful means of identification. However, the actual size of the cell can be influenced by the availability of nutrients in the medium. A few bacteria occur in more than one shape (e.g. some species of *Rhizobium* and *Corynebacterium*), which makes identification more difficult. These bacteria are termed **pleomorphic** (*pleo* = many).

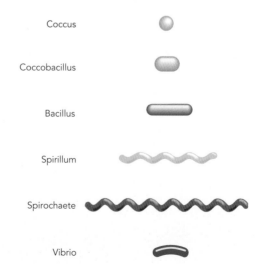

Coccus

Coccobacillus

Bacillus

Spirillum

Spirochaete

Vibrio

Figure 4.1

Representative bacterial shapes (morphology)

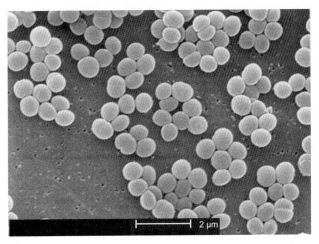

(a)

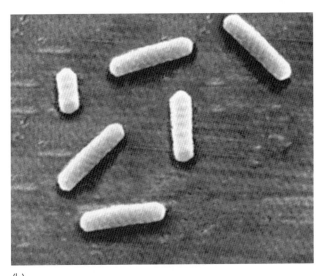

(b)

Figure 4.2

(a) Spherical and (b) rod-shaped bacteria

Structure of bacteria

A typical procaryotic cell is shown diagramatically in Figure 4.4 together with an electron micrograph of a typical *E. coli* cell. The following sections describe the structure of bacterial cells in detail.

EXTERNAL STRUCTURES OF BACTERIAL CELLS

Glycocalyx

Some bacteria are surrounded by a **glycocalyx**, a sticky, polysaccharide-containing layer that is secreted onto the cell surface. Depending on its structure and function it is referred to as a **capsule** or **slime layer**. These layers protect the cell from drying out.

Bacterial capsules are composed of polysaccharide and/or polypeptide molecules. They are usually synthesised inside the cell and excreted to the cell surface where they form an organised gelatinous layer firmly attached to the cell wall. An important function of the capsule is to help the bacterium adhere to host cell surfaces. The capsule possesses specific molecules which bind to complementary receptor molecules on the surface of the susceptible animal cell.

The capsule also has a protective function, allowing a bacterial pathogen to avoid ingestion by the white blood cells of the immune system (**phagocytosis**). The presence of a capsule is therefore considered to contribute to the **virulence** (ability to cause disease) of the organism. For example, encapsulated strains of *Streptococcus pneumoniae* are highly virulent whereas strains that lack a capsule are unable to produce disease symptoms.

The composition of the capsule is unique to the particular strain of bacteria in which it is found. The oral bacterium, *Streptococcus mutans*, forms a capsule containing **glucan**, a polymer of glucose, which is a major component of dental plaque. It helps bacteria to adhere to the tooth surface and cause dental decay.

Slime layers are composed of glycoproteins and polysaccharides and usually exist as a loosely attached, less defined structure than capsules. The presence of a slime layer assists in the attachment of the bacteria to host cells and appears to contribute to the formation of biofilms on medical devices.

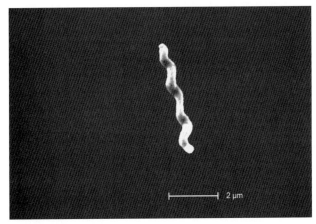

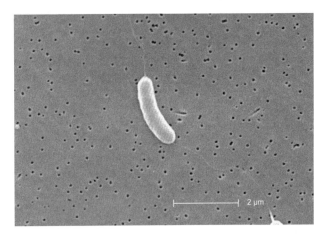

Figure 4.3

(a) Spiral bacteria, *Campylobacter*; (b) Comma-shaped bacterium, *Vibrio cholera*

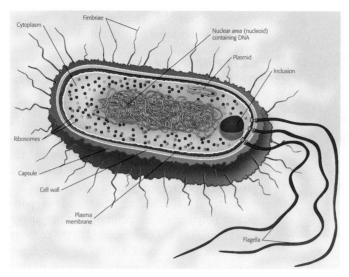
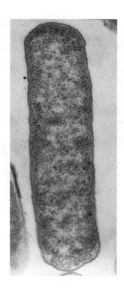

Figure 4.4

(a) Diagram of a typical procaryotic cell

(b) Electron micrograph of *E. coli* × 60 000 showing distinctive cell wall and membrane

Flagella

Many bacteria are motile, that is, capable of movement in a water environment. The most common way in which procaryotic cells move is by means of **flagella** (singular: flagellum), which are thin, rigid filaments that are usually many times longer than the cell itself. Some bacteria have only one flagellum located at one end of the cell; others have two, one at each end of the cell (see Figure 4.5). A few bacteria have numerous flagella, located all over the cell. Flagella consist of protein subunits arranged in a complex structure. They are attached to the cell membrane and wall of the bacterium by a structure called a **basal body**, a series of concentric protein rings which allow the flagellum to rotate. Movement of the bacterium is achieved by rotation of the flagella with a propellor-like motion, a process requiring energy in the form of ATP. Motile bacteria appear to respond to a stimulus in their environment and swim towards it. This phenomenon is called **chemotaxis**.

Pili and fimbriae

Pili (singular: pilus) and **fimbriae** (singular: fimbria) appear as hair-like appendages on the outside of Gram-negative bacterial cells (see Figure 4.6). Each has a distinct function. The thicker sex pili (1 to 10 per cell) are located on the surface of the cell; they are involved in the joining together of bacterial cells to allow transfer of the genetic material, DNA, from one cell to another during conjugation (see page 76). There are several thousand fimbriae per cell (sometimes called attachment pili). They are thinner than pili and concerned mainly with the attachment of the bacteria to surfaces. The presence of fimbriae contributes to the ability of the organism to cause disease by enabling it to adhere to the host cell and colonise it. For example, strains of *Neisseria gonorrhoeae* that lack fimbriae are not as pathogenic as strains that have fimbriae to help attach the organism to the mucosal cells lining the host genital tract.

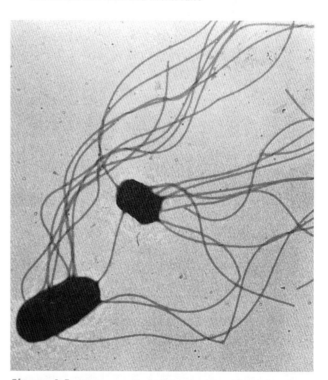

Figure 4.5

Bacterium with numerous flagella
Proteus vulgaris

CELL WALL

The most characteristic structure of bacteria is the cell wall (see Figure 4.7). It is a semi-rigid structure present in almost all bacteria and is responsible for determining the shape of the cell as well as some of its staining properties. It also provides mechanical support so that the cell does not burst when exposed to conditions of osmotic pressure that allow movement of water into the cell. Bacterial cell walls contain varying amounts of different macromolecules, which bestow certain characteristics on the cell. One

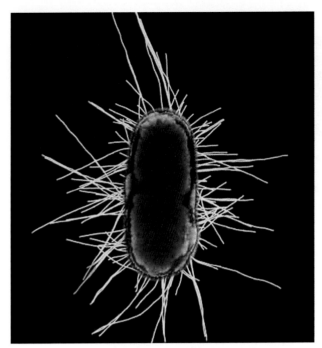

Scanning electron micrograph of *E. coli* showing fimbriae

of the major components is a complex substance called **peptidoglycan**, which consists of repeating units of a disaccharide molecule containing two glucose derivatives, N-acetylglucosamine and N-acetylmuramic acid. The disaccharide molecules are cross-linked by an interbridge of four or five amino acids to form a complex rigid network (see Figure 4.7(a)). Based on the composition of the cell wall, nearly all bacteria can be classified into one of two groups, Gram-negative or Gram-positive.

Structure of Gram-positive cell walls

Cells classified as Gram-positive have a defined cell wall structure which determines their reaction in the staining procedure developed by the Danish microbiologist HANS CHRISTIAN GRAM (see Chapter 2, Figure 2.15). The main component of Gram-positive cell walls is a thick layer of peptidoglycan. Attached to the peptidoglycan are other complex polysaccharides called **teichoic acids**. These teichoic acids have a strong negative charge which appears to influence the passage of materials in and out of the cell and contribute to the antigenic specificity of the cell wall (see Figure 4.7(b)).

Structure of Gram-negative cell walls

The group of bacteria classified as Gram-negative have a more complex outer structure than the Gram-positives (see Figure 4.7(c)). The cell wall consists of a thin layer of peptidoglycan covered by an outer membrane containing **lipopolysaccharides**, **lipoproteins** and **phospholipids**. The outer membrane has several functions. It provides a barrier to the entry of various substances (e.g. some antibiotics) into the cell and also prevents the action of certain enzymes that break down the cell wall (e.g. **lysozyme**). The lipopolysaccharide component, called the O-polysaccharide or O-antigen, has a distinctive structure in each strain of

bacteria. This is useful in serological tests to distinguish between different strains of bacteria (see Chapter 15). The lipid portion, known as **lipid A**, is an **endotoxin**. It is responsible for some of the toxic effects (such as fever and shock) that occur when certain Gram-negative bacteria containing lipid A infect the human body (see Chapter 10).

Acid-fast bacteria

Not all bacteria can be grouped as either Gram-negative or Gram-positive. Some bacteria (e.g. the mycobacteria) have an outer layer composed of peptidoglycan, similar to the Gram-positive wall, but covered by a thick waxy layer that interferes with the Gram-stain procedure. The presence of mycobacteria (e.g. the causative agent of tuberculosis, *Mycobacterium tuberculosis*) is usually detected in sputum or lung biopsies by using the **Ziehl-Neelsen acid-fast stain** (see Chapter 2). Mycobacteria are often referred to as 'acid-fast bacilli' (AFB).

Damage to the cell wall

An intact cell wall is important to the structural integrity of the bacterial cell and its ability to survive in the environment. Thus the bacterial cell is particularly vulnerable to substances that destroy or damage the wall. Among these substances is the enzyme **lysozyme**, which occurs in egg white as well as in human tears and saliva. Lysozyme exerts an antibacterial effect by damaging the cell walls of Gram-positive bacteria by breaking the bonds in the peptidoglycan layer. When the wall is destroyed, the cell is left surrounded by only the plasma membrane. This structure is called a **protoplast** and it is very vulnerable to rupture by osmotic pressure. Lysozyme does not have such a dramatic effect on the cell walls of Gram-negative bacteria because it is unable to penetrate the outer layers of the cell wall and so cannot destroy the peptidoglycan layer.

Certain antibiotics specifically target the cell wall. **Penicillin** exerts its effect by inhibiting the formation of the cross-linking amino acid interbridges during the synthesis of peptidoglycan in rapidly growing cells (see Figure 4.7(a)). For this reason, rapidly multiplying Gram-positive bacteria are particularly susceptible to the action of the penicillin group of antibiotics. Gram-negative organisms are not as readily affected because their outer membrane interferes with the entry of penicillin to the cell and they contain only a thin layer of peptidoglycan. Some of the semi-synthetic penicillins, which are able to penetrate the outer membrane, are more effective against Gram-negative organisms (see Chapter 12).

CELL MEMBRANE

All bacterial cells have a **cell membrane**, or **plasma membrane**, which lies just underneath the cell wall. Bacterial membranes have a structure that is essentially similar to the membranes of all other living cells. It consists of a double layer of phospholipid molecules (a **phospholipid bilayer**) with an irregular arrangement of proteins embedded in the lipid layers. Bacterial cell membranes consist only of proteins and phospholipids whereas eucaryotic cell membranes also contain sterols

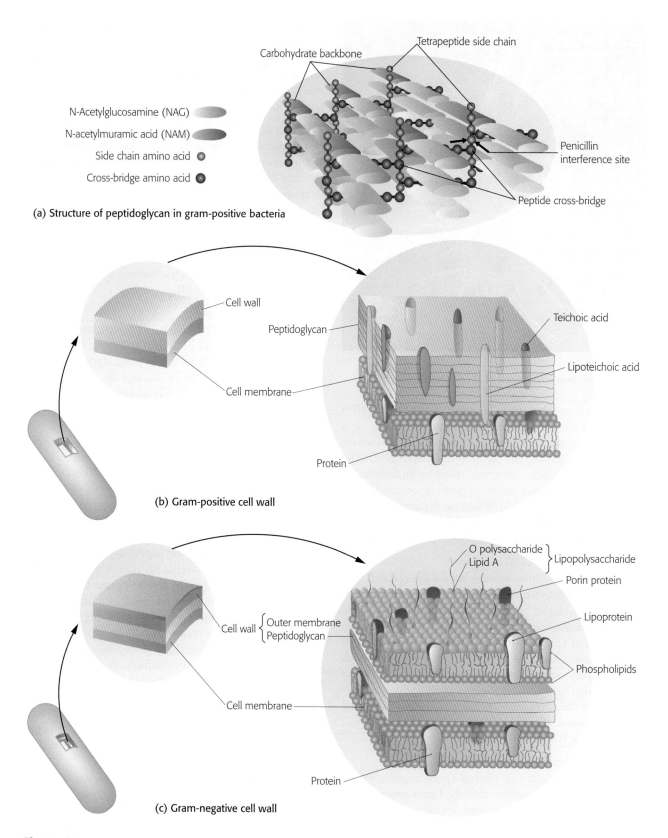

(a) Structure of peptidoglycan in gram-positive bacteria

N-Acetylglucosamine (NAG)
N-acetylmuramic acid (NAM)
Side chain amino acid
Cross-bridge amino acid

Carbohydrate backbone
Tetrapeptide side chain
Penicillin interference site
Peptide cross-bridge

(b) Gram-positive cell wall

Cell wall
Peptidoglycan
Cell membrane
Teichoic acid
Lipoteichoic acid
Protein

(c) Gram-negative cell wall

Cell wall { Outer membrane, Peptidoglycan }
Cell membrane
O polysaccharide
Lipid A
Lipopolysaccharide
Porin protein
Lipoprotein
Phospholipids
Protein

Figure 4.7

Bacterial cell walls

(a) The structure of peptidoglycan in Gram-positive bacteria. Together the carbohydrate backbone (glycan portion) and tetrapeptide side chains (peptide portion) make up peptidoglycan. The frequency of peptide cross-bridges and the number of amino acids in these bridges vary with the species of bacterium. The small arrows indicate where pencillin interferes with the linkage of peptidoglycan rows by peptide cross-bridges.
(b) Structure of the Gram-positive cell wall.
(c) Structure of the Gram-negative cell wall.

and carbohydrates that bestow additional properties on the eucaryotic membrane. The structure of the membrane is uniquely suited to its function in the cell. When examined under the electron microscope, it appears as a double layer consisting of phospholipid molecules arranged in a particular orientation (Figure 4.8(a)).

Phospholipids are compounds consisting of a molecule of glycerol esterified with two long-chain fatty acids (see Chapter 3). Fatty acids are long hydrocarbon chains that are **non-polar** (i.e. do not have any charged groups) and so are insoluble in water. They are therefore described as **hydrophobic**, or 'water-hating'. The phosphate group, which is attached to the third hydroxyl group of the glycerol molecule, is **polar** (i.e. charged) and is usually joined to another charged molecule such as ethanolamine or choline, or another molecule of **glycerol**. This part of the phospholipid molecule is termed **hydrophilic** ('water-loving'). Phospholipids therefore have two distinct regions – a polar, water-soluble, hydrophilic 'head' and a non-polar hydrophobic 'tail' (see Figure 4.8(c)).

In the cell membrane, two layers of phospholipids are arranged so that the polar, hydrophilic 'heads' are oriented towards the 'outside' water environment, while the non-polar fatty acid 'tails' are oriented towards the hydrophobic interior of the membrane. Embedded in the phospholipid bilayer are protein molecules which carry out various functions. This widely accepted model of membrane structure is usually called the *Singer-Nicholson model* or **fluid-mosaic model**. The term 'fluid-mosaic' describes a major characteristic of this membrane structure. The nature of the fatty acids allows the lipid and protein molecules to move sideways within the lipid matrix (see Figure 4.8(b)).

FUNCTIONS OF BACTERIAL CELL MEMBRANES

Movement of substances in and out of the cell: osmosis

Osmosis is the passage of a solvent (usually water) from one side of a membrane to another. Usually, the cell

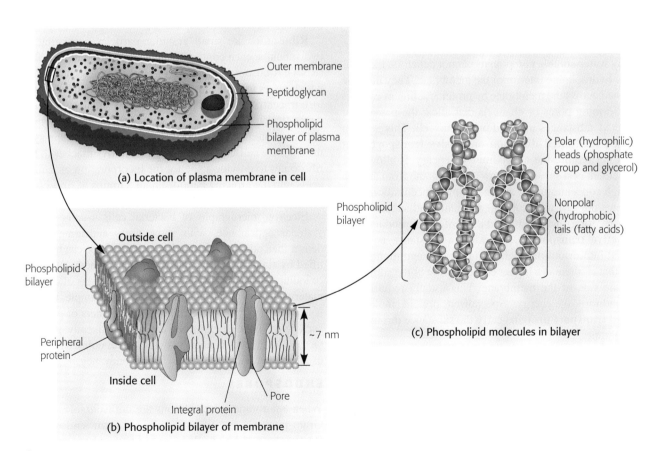

Outer membrane

Peptidoglycan

Phospholipid bilayer of plasma membrane

(a) Location of plasma membrane in cell

Outside cell

Phospholipid bilayer

Peripheral protein

Inside cell

Pore

Integral protein

~7 nm

(b) Phospholipid bilayer of membrane

Phospholipid bilayer

Polar (hydrophilic) heads (phosphate group and glycerol)

Nonpolar (hydrophobic) tails (fatty acids)

(c) Phospholipid molecules in bilayer

Figure 4.8

Plasma membrane

(a) A diagram showing the position of the phospholipid bilayer which forms the inner plasma membrane of Gram-negative bacteria.

(b) A portion of the inner membrane showing the phospholipid bilayer and proteins. The outer membrane of Gram-negative bacteria is also a phospholipid bilayer.

(c) Space-filling models of several molecules as they are arranged in the phospholipid bilayer.

membrane allows unrestricted movement of small molecules such as water, oxygen and carbon dioxide. The water molecules move from an area of 'high' water concentration (i.e. a dilute solution) to an area of 'low' water concentration (e.g. a more concentrated solution inside the cell). **Osmotic pressure** is the pressure required to prevent the flow of water molecules across a selectively permeable membrane.

Unlike human cells, which use homeostatic mechanisms to maintain a constant environment, bacterial cells can be subjected to different kinds of solutions in their environment. This may create differences in the osmotic pressure exerted on the cell. If the overall concentration of salts and ions (solutes) in the solution outside the cell is the same as inside, the solution is said to be **isotonic** (and water enters and leaves the cell at the same rate). If the solute concentration is higher outside the cell than inside, the solution is said to be **hypertonic**. Water leaves the cell and the cell dehydrates. If the solute concentration is lower outside than inside (e.g. as in distilled water), the solution is said to be **hypotonic**. Water passes through the membrane into the cell and the cell may burst. The rigid cell wall plays an important part in protecting bacteria from the effect of variations in osmotic pressure.

Passive and active transport

The main function of the plasma membrane in procaryotic cells is to act as a selectively permeable barrier for the cell. Many water-soluble compounds cannot penetrate the non-polar hydrophobic interior of the membrane. They must be assisted across the membrane by proteins acting as carriers and forming pores or channels that allow the passage of selected substances into and out of the cell. This is often termed **facilitated diffusion** or **passive transport** as it does not require the expenditure of energy. It allows the movement of a substance across a membrane from an area of high concentration to an area of low concentration. This enables the cell to absorb the nutrients and substances it requires for growth and to rid itself of waste products.

Active transport occurs when a substance is transported into or out of a cell *against* a concentration gradient; that is, there is a higher concentration of the substance on one side of the membrane. This usually requires the expenditure of energy. Specialised protein molecules called **transport proteins** carry the substance through the membrane.

Specialised functions of bacterial cell membranes

Procaryotic cells lack other cellular membranes, so the plasma membrane in bacteria is the site of proteins that carry out additional functions normally performed by the organelles in eucaryotic cells. These include:

- synthesis of cell wall components
- cellular respiration and synthesis of ATP
- secretion of proteins and enzymes, which are released from the cell as extracellular enzymes or toxins.

The membrane is a vital part of the cell and as such is very susceptible to damage. Some antimicrobial compounds exert their effect by disrupting the structure of the membrane. These include disinfectants, such as alcohol and the quaternary ammonium compounds, and the polymyxin group of antibiotics.

INTERNAL STRUCTURES OF BACTERIAL CELLS

The **cytoplasm** of bacterial cells is about 80% water and contains the proteins, carbohydrates, lipids and salts that are essential for the activities of the cell. The nuclear area of the cell contains a single circular chromosome, consisting of a double strand of DNA (deoxyribonucleic acid) which carries the genetic information necessary for the structure and function of the cell. Bacteria often carry one or more extra pieces of DNA, small circular structures called **plasmids**. Plasmids vary in size and replicate independently of the main chromosomal DNA. They appear to carry information that is not essential for the growth of the cell, such as genes for resistance to antibiotics or the production of toxins.

The gene for the production of the sex pili, which are involved in the transfer of genetic information from one bacterium to another during conjugation, is also carried on a plasmid. The transfer of genetic information by plasmids is used by scientists in the process of genetic engineering, described later in this chapter.

Ribosomes are small granular particles consisting of two subunits, each containing protein and ribonucleic acid (RNA). Ribosomes of procaryotic cells are designated **70S** which refers to their rate of sedimentation when subjected to ultracentrifugation. They are slightly smaller and less dense than the ribosomes of eucaryotic organisms which are designated **80S**. Ribosomes are the site of protein synthesis in the cell. Messenger RNA (mRNA) attaches to the ribosomes to provide a site for the incorporation of amino acids into the growing peptide chain. Groups of ribosomes attached to messenger RNA are called **polyribosomes**.

Electron micrographs of bacterial cells usually have a granular appearance, with some areas appearing to be denser than others. The granules, or **inclusions**, can be identified by staining with simple dyes such as methylene blue or iodine. These inclusions are usually polymers of cellular material and act as storage for the cell. For example, **volutin** is a polymer of phosphate molecules. Polymers of glucose, such as **glycogen** or **starch**, are also frequently present. Occasionally, cells contain **vesicles**, or **vacuoles**. These are usually filled with gas to give the cell buoyancy.

ENDOSPORES

When environmental conditions are unfavourable, certain Gram-positive bacilli are able to form endospores. Bacterial sporulation does not occur when cells are growing rapidly, but only when growth ceases due to the exhaustion of essential nutrients. An **endospore** is a specialised type of resting cell which is formed inside the bacterial cell membrane. It is surrounded by a **spore coat**, consisting of thick layers of peptidoglycan and protein, to provide protection. Bacterial endospores can survive conditions that destroy normal **vegetative** (growing) **cells**, such as boiling for up to five hours, freezing, desiccation (dehydration) and exposure to chemicals and radiation. The endospore develops inside the bacterial cell membrane and can be located by special staining procedures (see Figure 4.9).

The spore has a lower water content than vegetative cells and does not carry out metabolic reactions. It contains nucleic acid and the various cellular enzymes and substances that are essential for spore germination to occur when conditions become favourable. When this happens, water enters the spore, germination occurs and the vegetative cell that is produced resumes normal growth and metabolism. Endospore formation is *not* a method of reproduction – one bacterial cell gives rise to only one endospore, which then germinates into a single cell again. It is, however, a very important method of survival for

certain species of bacteria and has important clinical significance.

Bacterial endospores have been shown to survive in the soil for many years and there are even reports of their being found in fossils. Spores of *Bacillus anthracis* – the organism responsible for anthrax, a disease that affects humans as well as cattle – were found more than 20 years later at a site where diseased animals had been buried.

Many of the Gram-positive bacteria that form endospores are important pathogens. These include members of the genus *Clostridium* – *Clostridium perfringens* (food poisoning and gas gangrene), *Clostridium tetani* (tetanus) and *Clostridium botulinum* (botulism).

In the food industry, spores may survive the normal cooking process and cause food poisoning. An example is *Clostridium perfringens*, which is common in the environment. Spores of *Clostridium* may be ingested in food,

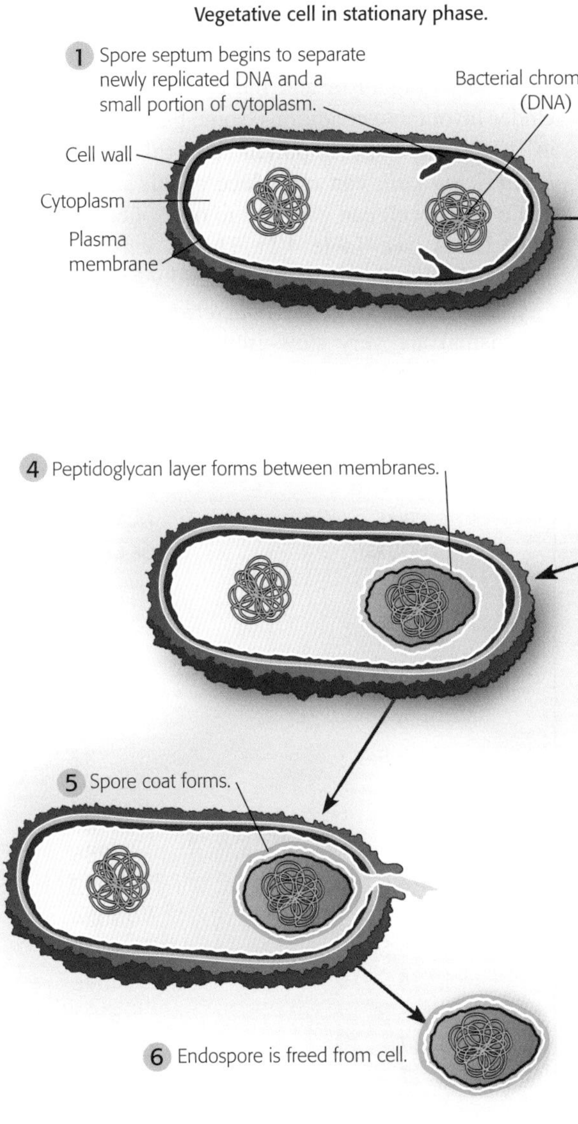

Vegetative cell in stationary phase.

1 Spore septum begins to separate newly replicated DNA and a small portion of cytoplasm.

Bacterial chromosome (DNA)

Cell wall

Cytoplasm

Plasma membrane

2 Plasma membrane surrounds DNA and cytoplasm, forming protoplast.

3 Spore septum surrounds separated protoplast forming prospore.

4 Peptidoglycan layer forms between membranes.

Two membranes

5 Spore coat forms.

6 Endospore is freed from cell.

(a)

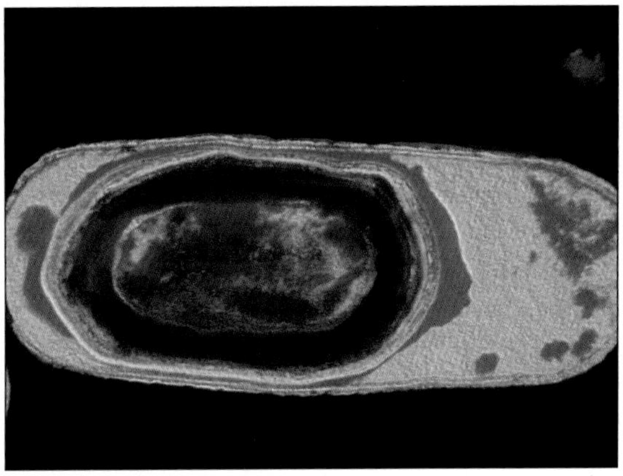

(b)

Figure 4.9

Formation of endospores by sporulation
(a) Diagrammatic representation of endospore formation
(b) Coloured scanning electron micrograph of spore formation in *Bacillus subtilis*

germinate in the intestine and produce symptoms of gastroenteritis (stomach cramps and diarrhoea) 12–24 hours later. This organism is also the cause of gas gangrene. If wounds containing dead tissue are contaminated with *C. perfringens*, either from the environment or from unsterilised medical equipment, gangrene may develop.

Clostridium botulinum spores are widespread in nature and may sometimes be found in preserved or canned foods that have not been adequately sterilised. The organism grows in the food under anaerobic conditions, producing a powerful neurotoxin (poison).

Clostridium tetani is a common inhabitant of the large intestine of humans and animals. Tetanus spores are frequently found in faeces or in soil where manure is spread. When introduced into deep puncture wounds, the spores germinate, grow anaerobically and produce the tetanus toxin responsible for spasms, paralysis and death. A vaccine is available against tetanus.

Knowledge of the existence of highly resistant forms of bacteria is important for the development of adequate methods of sterilisation and disinfection in hospitals, and methods of preservation in the food industry. Because they survive in soil or in dust, these resistant bacteria can contaminate hospital areas such as operating theatres unless strict attention is paid to hygiene. Contamination of deep surgical wounds can give rise to serious infections as the organisms can grow anaerobically. As discussed above, bacterial endospores are resistant to heat because of their comparatively low water content, and require treatment at 121°C for 15 minutes in an autoclave to be killed. The complex nature of the spore coat also makes them highly resistant to most germicides.

Reproduction in bacterial cells

Growth is usually defined as an increase in size. However, when microbiologists speak about bacterial growth, they are usually referring to an increase in numbers of bacterial cells. This may appear confusing until it is realised that bacteria do not increase in size very much during their lifespan. As soon as a bacterial cell has approximately doubled in size, it divides to form two identical daughter cells. Bacterial growth is therefore defined as *an increase in cell numbers*.

Cells use the energy derived from the metabolic breakdown of nutrients to produce new cellular components. In most bacteria, as the cell elongates, the genetic information contained in the chromosome is duplicated and one new chromosome moves to each end of the cell. The membrane and cell wall begin to grow inwards at a point about halfway along the cell, until a septum forms. The cell then splits, forming two new cells that contain identical components to the parent cell. This whole process is called **binary fission** (Figure 4.10).

The two daughter cells are identical; they are both completely new cells – not one old cell and one new cell. The time taken for the cell to reproduce itself is called the

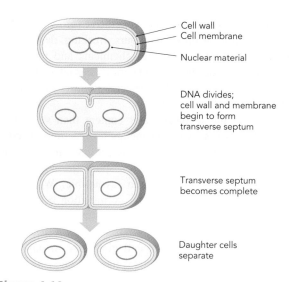

Figure 4.10
Binary fission in a bacterium

generation time; this can vary enormously, depending on the type of organism and the environmental conditions. Under favourable conditions, some bacteria can reproduce in 20–30 minutes. Important clinical species, such as *Escherichia coli*, can reproduce at this rate. This means that a single cell can give rise to over one million cells in 8–10 hours (see Table 4.1). This is why an apparently slight infection in a patient can rapidly become serious.

Other species (e.g. *Mycobacteria* and some anaerobic organisms) are very slow-growing and may take up to 12 hours to reproduce even when conditions are optimal.

Table 4.1
Bacterial growth

TIME (HOURS)	NUMBER OF CELLS
0	1
0.5	2
1	4
1.5	8
2	16
2.5	32
3	64
3.5	128
4	256
4.5	512
5	1024
5.5	2048
6	4096
6.5	8192
7	16 384
7.5	32 768
8	65 536
8.5	131 072
9	262 144
9.5	524 288
10	1 048 376

The time required to culture and identify an organism from a clinical specimen depends very much on the growth rate. Many bacteria produce visible growth in an overnight culture (18 hours), but some bacteria take days or even weeks. It is important to be aware of differences in growth rate when trying to identify a specimen in the laboratory. Cultures must be incubated for long enough to enable cells to multiply and be identified, otherwise the presence of a pathogen may be missed.

Requirements for bacterial growth

The rate at which bacteria reproduce is determined by both physical and chemical factors in their environment. Physical factors include temperature, pH, osmotic pressure and the presence or absence of oxygen. Chemical or nutritional factors include availability of water, a suitable carbon source, nitrogen, phosphorus, sulphur, trace elements and minerals. Some bacteria have an absolute requirement for a particular compound or growth factor. Overall, bacteria can grow in a wide range of environments, but each species has its own set of optimal conditions that allow it to achieve maximum growth rate. For most human pathogenic bacteria, these conditions are very similar to those found in the human body.

Most bacteria are free-living and can reproduce without using another cell. The exceptions, which replicate inside a host cell, are species of *Chlamydia* and *Rickettsia*, which are bacterial obligate intracellular parasites, and the mycoplasmas, which do not have a cell wall and so are vulnerable to changes in osmotic pressure.

PHYSICAL FACTORS

Temperature
Most bacteria will grow at the environmental temperatures usually encountered in temperate zones, 10°C to 39°C, but each will have a minimum, maximum and optimum temperature. Organisms that grow at moderate temperatures (25–35°C) are called **mesophiles**. Those that thrive in low temperatures (optimum 10°C) are called **psychrophiles** (cold-loving) and those that like high temperatures (optimum 60°C) are termed **thermophiles** (heat-loving). See Figure 4.11.

The rate of growth of most bacteria is greatly reduced at temperatures below 10° C, such as occur in a domestic refrigerator (4°C), a common method of preserving food. However, some bacteria will survive long periods of storage in the cold and even withstand freezing. Although food spoilage is greatly reduced at low temperatures, the bacteria are not killed and it is important to remember that food may still be contaminated by pathogens that were present before refrigeration.

Pathogenic bacteria usually have an optimum growth temperature similar to the human body (i.e. 37°C).

pH
The level of acidity or alkalinity of the culture medium (pH) is very important for bacterial growth. For most bacteria, the pH optimum, at which maximum growth occurs, is close to neutral – that is, pH 7. Most bacteria do not grow at all above pH 8 or below pH 6. Some bacteria produce organic acids during metabolism, causing a drop in pH that inhibits further growth. An important group of bacteria that can tolerate acid conditions belongs to the genus *Lactobacillus*. They produce lactic acid by fermentation of lactose and are responsible for the souring of milk to make products such as yoghurt. These bacteria can only tolerate moderate levels of acid (i.e. pH 4) so when the pH drops below 4 the culture stops growing. This is an excellent method of preserving milk products – spoilage is inhibited because most other bacteria cannot tolerate even mildly acid conditions.

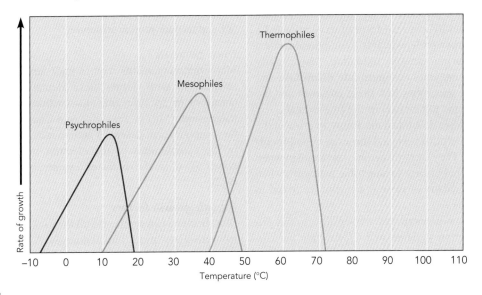

Figure 4.11

Typical growth rates of different types of microorganisms in response to temperature
Optimum growth (fastest reproduction) is represented by the peak of the curve. Notice that the reproductive rate drops off very quickly at temperatures only a little above the optimum. At either extreme of the temperature range, the reproductive rate is much lower than the rate at the optimum temperature.

Water and osmotic pressure

Bacteria grow best in an environment that is saturated with water. Although many bacteria can survive dry conditions, they require water to reproduce. They obtain all their nutrients from their surroundings so the composition of substances in the water environment will affect their growth. The dissolved substances exert osmotic pressure on the bacterial cell, which will be able to reproduce optimally if the growth medium is isotonic. This means that, if a bacterial cell is placed in a hypotonic solution such as distilled water, water moves into the cell which swells up and becomes turgid. If the pressure becomes too great to be contained by the rigid structure of the bacterial cell wall, the cell bursts and is destroyed (cell **lysis**).

If the cell is placed in a hypertonic solution – that is, a solution with a higher salt concentration (osmotic pressure) than the bacterial cytoplasm – water tends to move out of the bacterial cell into the surrounding medium, causing the cell membrane to shrink away from the wall. This greatly slows down or inhibits growth. This phenomenon is useful in food preservation. High concentrations of salt or sugar (hypertonicity) in foodstuffs prevent the growth of bacteria and subsequent food spoilage. Some examples are salted or cured meat and fish, jams and fruit syrups.

Oxygen

Bacteria can be divided into groups according to their requirement for molecular oxygen for growth. Organisms that use oxygen are called **aerobes**. Those that *require* oxygen for growth are called **obligate aerobes**. Obligate aerobes such as *Mycobacterium tuberculosis* are often found as pathogens in areas of high oxygen tension, such as the lungs. Bacteria that reproduce in the absence of oxygen are called **anaerobes**. Some of them are termed **obligate anaerobes** because they are not only inhibited, but destroyed, in the presence of oxygen. These obligate anaerobes are killed by a special form of oxygen called a **free radical**, or **superoxide**, which is a compound formed in most cells during aerobic oxidation, but usually destroyed by two enzymes – **superoxide dismutase** and **catalase**. Obligate anaerobes lack these enzymes and the cells are killed by the toxic effect of the free radicals.

Some bacteria have developed the ability to grow in the presence or absence of oxygen and these are called **facultative anaerobes**. They carry on aerobic metabolism when oxygen is present but change to anaerobic pathways when oxygen is limited. Many of these organisms are found in the human intestine.

Two pathogenic organisms that are sensitive to oxygen are *Clostridium tetani* (tetanus) and *Clostridium perfringens* (gas gangrene). Tetanus and gangrene are infections that occur in deep puncture wounds or necrotic tissue where the supply of oxygen is depleted. Both infections are sometimes treated by placing the patient in a hyperbaric oxygen chamber. Tissues are saturated with oxygen in an attempt to kill the causative organisms.

The oxygen requirement of pathogenic organisms is an important factor to consider when collecting specimens for laboratory diagnosis. Even a short exposure to oxygen (10 minutes) is sufficient to kill some anaerobes. Special techniques have been developed to collect and transport sensitive organisms (see Chapter 15).

NUTRITIONAL REQUIREMENTS

Carbon

The essential element in all living cells is carbon. Most bacteria need to be supplied with a suitable simple organic carbon compound in the medium. The bacteria break down these carbon compounds into smaller molecules which they use to synthesise their own cellular requirements. A few bacteria are **autotrophic** and are able to use carbon dioxide from the air as their sole carbon source.

Nitrogen

Nitrogen is an essential element for the synthesis of enzymes and other cellular proteins as well as the nucleic acids, RNA and DNA. Nitrogen is usually obtained from nitrogenous compounds such as nitrates and ammonium compounds in the environment, but some bacteria are capable of 'fixing' nitrogen from the air – that is, converting gaseous nitrogen into compounds such as nitrates which can be utilised by plants for growth. These bacteria usually live in nodules on the roots of plants.

Phosphorus

Phosphorus is needed for nucleotides, the nucleic acids RNA and DNA, the energy storage molecule, ATP, and for the structural phospholipids of the cell membrane.

Sulphur

Sulphur is an essential component of some amino acids, and of the sulphur-containing vitamin, **biotin**. The sulphur-containing amino acids form disulphide linkages between different parts of polypeptide chains and contribute to the folding of the chains into the correct secondary and tertiary protein structure.

Trace elements

Many microorganisms require trace amounts of minerals in order to grow. Often these elements are needed as cofactors in specific enzyme reactions – for example, magnesium (Mg) or zinc (Zn) (see Chapter 2). They may be components of essential compounds, such as iron (Fe) in the cytochromes of the electron transport chain, or cobalt (Co) in the cofactor cyanocobalamine (vitamin B12).

Organic growth factors

Most bacteria can synthesise all their cellular requirements from a variety of nutritional sources. A few have requirements for specific organic compounds which must be added to the medium for growth to occur. These may be vitamins, which act as coenzymes. Often the requirement will be for a specific amino acid that the bacterium is unable to synthesise for itself, but is essential for the formation of protein. This inability may be inherent in the species, or it may be the result of a mutation which has given rise to a particular strain of bacteria that has lost the ability to produce the enzymes required to make this compound for itself. This condition is described in more detail under Bacterial Genetics (see page 68).

Identification of bacteria in the laboratory

It can be seen from the preceding sections that much is known about the growth requirements of bacteria. Specialised techniques have been developed to isolate and identify bacteria in the laboratory by growing them on different media. A wide variety of media is used, differing in composition according to the nature of the specimen being examined. Most media consist of a solution of salts and nutrients in water, adjusted to the correct pH. The solution is prepared and sterilised in order to kill any unwanted bacteria. If a solid medium is required, a solidifying agent is added; this is usually **agar**, a complex polysaccharide extracted from seaweed. The medium is poured into a petri dish, or 'plate', and allowed to set before being inoculated with a clinical specimen.

CLINICAL SAMPLES

In order to identify a particular bacterial species from a clinical sample of blood, sputum or pus, it is first necessary to isolate it as a pure culture – that is, a culture containing only one type of bacterium. Microorganisms that occur in clinical samples are almost invariably a mixture of normal flora and the invading pathogen. To isolate individual bacterial types, clinical specimens are usually grown on an agar plate and 'streaked out' to obtain single colonies for identification. Various methods are used to quantitate and identify the bacterial cells present (see Chapter 15) .

PATTERN OF BACTERIAL GROWTH

Phases of growth

When bacteria are grown in the laboratory in liquid medium, the medium becomes cloudy or turbid. It is possible to measure the increase in numbers of bacteria at various time intervals and plot the values on a graph representing a growth curve. When cells are first inoculated into fresh medium containing all the nutrients they require, they take a short time to adapt before they start to divide. This is termed the **lag phase**. The cells then begin to duplicate their contents and undergo binary fission, doubling the cell numbers with each generation.

Thus, for each cell present initially, there are two cells after one generation, four (or 2^2) cells after two generations, eight cells (2^3) after three generations, and so on. In other words, the number of cells increases by a power of 2 each generation time. Mathematically, this is described as a **logarithmic**, or **exponential**, **increase**. It can be seen from the calculation in Table 4.1 and the graph in Figure 4.12 that a huge number of bacterial cells can be produced in a short time. This phase of growth is termed the **logarithmic**, or **log**, **phase** when the cells are gener-

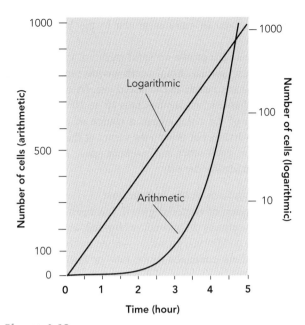

Figure 4.12

Rate of growth of bacterial culture

ally reproducing at a maximum rate. This type of growth rate is very sensitive to environmental conditions.

The logarithmic rate of bacterial growth continues only while conditions are optimal. As the number of bacteria increases, nutrients are used up and there is an accumulation of waste products. These may inhibit essential enzyme reactions in the cell, or cause a change in the pH of the medium, both of which will slow growth. As the density of cells in the culture increases, the availability of oxygen may decrease. The rate of cell division therefore slows down and eventually cell division ceases, or some cells may die instead of dividing. When the rate of cell division equals the rate at which cells are dying, the culture is said to be in the **stationary phase** of growth. Many important secondary metabolites are produced under the limited nutritional conditions encountered in the stationary phase (see Chapter 3, page 47).

Gradually, the rate of cell division stops completely and some of the cells die, so the number of viable cells is reduced and the culture enters the **decline** or **death phase**. Figure 4.13 illustrates the four phases of growth that are

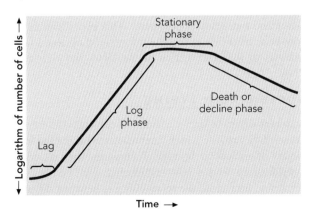

Figure 4.13

Typical growth curve for a bacterial culture

usually observed in cultures grown in the laboratory in liquid medium.

When cells are grown on solid medium, the dynamics of growth are similar. Single cells divide rapidly until a colony becomes visible to the naked eye. (A colony about 0.1 mm in diameter usually contains 10^4 to 10^5 cells.) Cells at the edge of the colony have a source of nutrients, so continue to divide, but cells in the centre of the colony pile up on top of each other and, without space or access to nutrients, gradually die off.

Pattern of growth in the human host

Our description of bacterial growth has been confined to laboratory cultures in closed or limited environments; under these conditions, growth is limited by the volume of culture medium contained in the tube or flask. The composition of this medium is continually being altered by the depletion of nutrients and accumulation of wastes. The rate of growth therefore slows down.

In the human body the bacteria causing an infection may be in an environment where there is a continuous supply of nutrients and oxygen via the bloodstream. Under these conditions there is no limit to growth and the infection develops unchecked. In the laboratory it is possible to devise a vessel called a **chemostat** which allows continuous additions of fresh medium and removal of spent medium and cells. Cells can also be harvested so that bacterial growth can be maintained in the logarithmic phase. Large quantities of bacteria can be produced by this method. A chemostat is used for experiments to determine the effect of limiting the amount of various nutrients on the growth of a culture, or to prepare large quantities of bacterial cells for research or commercial use, or to encourage the formation of secondary metabolites.

Classification of bacteria

A number of different criteria can be used to classify bacteria into groups. The formidable task of classifying bacteria was undertaken by a team of microbiologists and published under the title of *Bergey's Manual of Systematic Bacteriology*. The original basis for the classification included properties such as spore formation, cell wall structure, Gram stain, shape, motility, oxygen requirements and biochemical properties. This classification has now been modified to include information obtained from analysis of the composition of the DNA and ribosomal RNA.

NUCLEIC ACID TYPING

Different strains of bacteria usually have slight differences in their DNA profile which can be detected using the techniques of molecular biology. Techniques such as cross-hybridisation and DNA sequencing can be used to determine how close the relationship is between different strains of bacteria. This information will no doubt lead to some revision of bacterial classifications in the future. Ribosomal RNA is also used to identify bacterial strains.

PHAGE TYPING

A useful method of differentiating between strains of bacteria should be mentioned here. Some bacteria are attacked by viruses that are specific for a particular strain of bacteria within a species. A bacterial virus is called a **bacteriophage**, or **phage**. Bacteria isolated from different sources can be tested for their susceptibility to a particular phage. This helps to identify the strain of bacteria and can assist in epidemiological studies when clinicians are trying to identify the source of an outbreak of infection. For example, *Staphylococcus aureus* is frequently isolated from the noses of health personnel. Phage typing of the strain of *Staphylococcus* and comparison with the phage type of the outbreak can help to identify the source or carrier of the infection (see Figure 4.14).

It is beyond the scope of this text to discuss the details of bacterial classification, but it is important for students to be aware of the enormous diversity of microorganisms. Some of this diversity is shown in the photographs in Figure 4.15, and some bacteria of medical importance are described in the following sections.

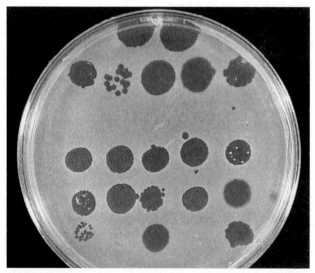

Figure 4.14

Phage typing of *Staphylococcus aureus*
A culture of the strain to be tested is spread over the whole plate and different phages inoculated in rows on the plate. The development of areas of lysis, or 'plaques', indicates that the strain of *Staphylococcus* is sensitive to infection by some of the phages and allows identification of the strain.

Bacteria of medical importance

There are literally thousands of different bacteria, but relatively few are pathogenic. Some of the more common bacteria are described here, grouped for convenience by their spore-forming ability, Gram-staining characteristics, shape and oxygen requirements. In the future these groupings may be changed to reflect new information about similarities in ribosomal RNA or base composition of DNA.

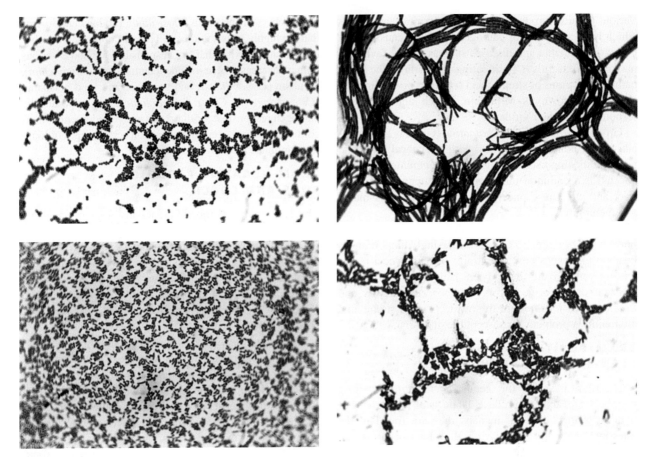

Figure 4.15
Diversity of bacterial morphology
The differences in size, shape and arrangement of cells can be seen in Gram-stained preparations
(a) *Staphylococcus aureus*; (b) *Bacillus subtilis*; (c) *Klebsiella pneumoniae*; (d) *Clostridium tetani*.

GRAM-POSITIVE COCCI (NON-SPORE-FORMING)

Many of the medically important bacteria are Gram-positive cocci. The **staphylococci** and **streptococci** which are responsible for many skin and wound infections belong to this group.

Staphylococci appear as grape-like clusters when viewed under the microscope. They are very tolerant in their growth requirements, surviving in conditions of relatively low moisture and high osmotic pressure (e.g. high salt concentration). *Staphylococcus aureus* and *Staphylococcus epidermidis* are two common inhabitants of the human body, and are found in areas of low moisture such as the nose or skin. *Staphylococcus aureus* is a common cause of wound infections in hospitals where it poses a serious threat because of its ability to quickly develop a resistance to antibiotics. It has also been identified as the agent responsible for toxic shock syndrome and for scalded skin syndrome.

Because of their tolerance of salt and dry conditions, staphylococci are often present in salted or preserved meats, such as bacon. Some strains of *Staphylococcus aureus* produce toxins which contribute to their pathogenicity. They are a common cause of food poisoning, producing an enterotoxin that causes diarrhoea and vomiting.

Staphylococcus aureus can be distinguished from *Staphylococcus epidermidis* (also a major cause of wound infections) by its ability to produce the enzyme, coagulase, and also by growth on the differential medium, mannitol salt, in which it produces a yellow colour due to a pH change in the medium (see Figure 3.17).

Streptococci are Gram-positive cocci that usually occur in chains of varying length (although *Streptococcus pneumoniae* typically occurs in pairs). They are responsible for a wide variety of diseases: wound and throat infections, scarlet fever, glomerulonephritis, pneumonia etc. (described in Unit IV). They are often classified by their growth on blood agar. Beta (β)-haemolytic streptococci produce an enzyme that lyses red blood cells, creating clear areas of haemolysis on blood agar plates. Alpha (α)-haemolytic species reduce haemoglobin to methaemoglobin, causing a greenish colour change on blood plates. Gamma (γ) or non-haemolytic streptococci have no effect on red blood cells.

In 1930 REBECCA LANCEFIELD discovered that the carbohydrates (antigens) in the cell walls of streptococci stimulated the formation of different antibodies. This method of identification is the basis of a system of classification whereby streptococci are placed in one of 14 groups using an alphabetical system (A,B,C, etc). Human disease is often associated with the Group A streptococci, of which *Streptococcus pyogenes* is the most common.

Various strains produce different enzymes and toxins which have a number of pathogenic effects, causing sore throat, septicaemia and diseases such as scarlet fever and necrotising fasciitis ('flesh-eating' bacteria). The most pathogenic strains of streptococci contain a protein in their cell walls known as M-protein, which appears to be responsible for their virulence.

Group B *Streptococcus agalactiae* (GBS) is the organism most commonly associated with **puerperal fever** and neonatal meningitis. *Streptococcus pneumoniae* (pneumococcus) is a common inhabitant of the upper respiratory tract and can cause pneumonia, bronchitis, otitis media and meningitis.

Enterococci are common inhabitants of the large intestine. They are becoming increasingly important as hospital pathogens now that strains of enterococci resistant to vancomycin have been isolated (vancomycin-resistant enterococci, VRE). *Enterococcus faecalis* and *Enterococcus faecium* are the most common strains and are mainly a problem for susceptible, high-risk patients.

GRAM-POSITIVE RODS (NON-SPORE-FORMING)

This group includes the genus *Lactobacillus*, whose members are able to produce lactic acid during carbohydrate fermentation. In humans they are found in the intestinal tract and oral cavity; they also occur in the vagina where they maintain a protective, slightly acid environment. They are used extensively in the food industry in the production of cheese, soured milk products and pickles, the lactic acid acting as a food preservative.

Listeria monocytogenes is a Gram-positive rod that sometimes contaminates dairy products. It poses a serious threat to pregnant women, causing damage to the foetus and sometimes resulting in stillbirth.

Some organisms are **pleomorphic** (i.e. their shape varies, often with the age of the cells). Best known are the **corynebacteria**, which tend to be mainly club-shaped. *Corynebacterium diphtheriae* is the causative agent of diphtheria. *Propionibacterium acnes* is found on the skin and is thought to be implicated in the skin infection, acne. Members of the genus *Actinomyces* are commonly found in the mouth and throat of humans and animals. They often form branched filaments. *A. viscosus* is involved in the colonisation of tooth surfaces, as a prelude to plaque formation by *Streptococcus mutans* and subsequent tooth decay. *Nocardia asteroides* causes skin abscesses and lung infections.

ENDOSPORE-FORMING GRAM-POSITIVE RODS

Some organisms form endospores as a means of survival under adverse environmental conditions. Some of these organisms are important pathogens. The two most important genera are *Bacillus* and *Clostridium*. *Bacillus anthracis* is the agent responsible for anthrax, a serious disease of cattle which can also affect humans. *Bacillus thuringiensis* is an insect pathogen.

Members of the genus *Clostridium* produce endospores that are highly resistant to heat. They are obligate anaerobes and produce toxins that are responsible for some serious human diseases. These include tetanus (*Clostridium tetani*), botulism (*C. botulinum*) and gangrene and food poisoning (*C. perfringens*). *Clostridium difficile* is an opportunistic pathogen responsible for diarrhoea and pseudomembranous colitis, which can occur in patients on certain types of long-term antibiotic therapy (see page 425).

GRAM-NEGATIVE AEROBIC RODS AND COCCI

This is a very large group of organisms, some of which are important human pathogens.

The genus *Neisseria* comprises non-endospore-forming diplococci which only grow well at body temperatures. It includes two important pathogens: *Neisseria gonorrhoeae* (see Chapter 21), the causative agent of gonorrhoea, and *Neisseria meningitidis* (meningococcal disease) (see Chapter 20).

The genus *Pseudomonas* consists of highly motile flagellated aerobic rods that exist mainly in water and soil. Many of them synthesise distinctive pigments ranging in colour from blue through greenish-yellow to brown. *Pseudomonas aeruginosa* is an important opportunistic pathogen. It is often responsible for serious infections in immunocompromised patients, especially in burns units. Its ability to grow in water with only minimal nutrients and its resistance to many disinfectants, antiseptics and antibiotics mean that it poses a particular threat in the hospital environment. *Burkholderia pseudomallei*, a small bacillus found in watery environments in Northern Australia, causes melioidosis which may start as a suppurative skin infection and develop into bacteraemia and pneumonia.

Legionella is a genus only recently discovered after an outbreak of atypical pneumonia in the United States. It is the cause of Legionnaires' disease and is spread mainly in water as aerosol droplets dispersed by wind from reservoirs such as the water-cooling towers of air-conditioning plants, where the bacteria are growing.

Moraxella, which causes conjunctivitis, and *Acinetobacter* are both aerobic coccobacilli. *Acinetobacter baumannii* can occur as a hospital pathogen and exhibits resistance to many antibiotics.

Bordetella pertussis, the causative organism of whooping cough, is a Gram-negative rod. Despite the availability of a vaccine, there are still hundreds of cases of whooping cough in Australia each year.

Other important pathogenic organisms in this group include *Brucella* (brucellosis) and *Francisella tularensis*, a fastidious organism that requires media enriched with blood or tissue extracts for growth, and causes tularaemia.

Pasteurellaceae are very small Gram-negative bacilli and coccobacilli. They are non-motile and are very fastidious in their nutritional requirements. *Pasteurella* species infect mainly animals but can be transmitted to humans (often by animal bites).

Haemophilus influenzae is a small coccoid bacillus and an important human pathogen. Although it is often present as part of the normal flora in the upper respiratory tract, it is a common cause of middle ear infections and is responsible for potentially fatal meningitis and epiglottitis in young children (see page 397). A vaccine for *Haemophilus influenzae* type b (Hib) is recommended in the childhood immunisation schedule in Australia.

The Vibrionaceae are a family of curved Gram-negative rods. The most important members are *Vibrio cholerae*, which causes cholera, and *Vibrio parahaemolyticus*, which is often found in shellfish and causes a form of gastroenteritis.

GRAM-NEGATIVE AEROBIC HELICAL BACTERIA

These are slender helical Gram-negative rods that do not have an axial filament but use flagella for motility. *Campylobacter jejuni* is an important pathogen responsible for food-borne gastrointestinal infections. *Helicobacter pylori* has been shown to be associated with gastric ulcers in humans (see Chapter 18, page 431).

FACULTATIVELY ANAEROBIC GRAM-NEGATIVE RODS

The **Enterobacteriaceae** (**enterics**) form a large group of very important organisms, many of which inhabit the human intestine as part of the normal flora. The most important genera are *Escherichia*, *Salmonella*, *Shigella*, *Klebsiella*, *Serratia*, *Proteus*, *Yersinia* and *Enterobacter*.

Escherichia coli (*E. coli*) is one of the predominant inhabitants of the human intestine. Its presence in water is often used as an indication of faecal contamination ('coliform' count). It is generally considered to be part of the normal flora and relatively non-pathogenic, unless it is transferred to body sites other than the colon. It is one of the most common causes of urinary tract infections. Some strains produce enterotoxins that can cause diarrhoea or haemolytic uraemic syndrome (see Chapter 18, pages 421ff).

Almost all the members of the genus *Salmonella* are pathogenic. *Salmonella typhi* is responsible for typhoid fever. Other *Salmonella* are responsible for various gastrointestinal diseases associated with food poisoning. The different strains are identified on the basis of their surface antigens which are referred to as 'serovars' or 'serotypes'. Species of *Shigella* are responsible for a severe type of diarrhoea called bacillary dysentery, or shigellosis, caused by the ingestion of contaminated food.

Among other enterics, *Klebsiella pneumoniae* is a major cause of pneumonia, especially in children and susceptible patients. *Proteus* is an inhabitant of the large intestine and a common cause of urinary tract and wound infections; it has a distinctive 'swarming' appearance when grown on plates in the laboratory and an unpleasant odour. *Enterobacter cloacae* and *E. aerogenes* are opportunistic pathogens which may cause urinary tract infections. *Serratia marcescens* grows at room temperature with the production of a distinctive red pigment. In recent years it has been recognised as a significant cause of opportunistic hospital-acquired infections.

The most pathogenic of all the enterics is *Yersinia pestis*, the cause of bubonic and pneumonic plague (see Chapter 19).

ANAEROBIC GRAM-NEGATIVE RODS

Bacteroides, which live in the human gastrointestinal tract, are anaerobic Gram-negative rods that are non-motile, do not form endospores and are often responsible for infections due to puncture wounds or surgery, and for peritonitis.

SPIROCHAETES

The **spirochaetes** are long (10μm) Gram-negative helical bacteria with two or more axial filaments for motility, giving them a distinctive corkscrew-like appearance. Some are free-living, occurring in sewage, mud and decaying organic matter. Others inhabit humans and animals as part of the normal flora. Among the spirochaetes is the causative organism of the sexually transmitted disease, syphilis – *Treponema pallidum* (see Chapter 21). Members of the genus *Borrelia*, which are usually transmitted by ticks, are responsible for relapsing fever and Lyme disease (see Chapter 19). *Leptospira* species are often acquired from water contaminated with animal faeces or urine and cause a disease characterised by kidney and liver damage.

INTRACELLULAR BACTERIA

Rickettsias are very small, obligate intracellular parasites and were not at first classified as bacteria because they can only reproduce inside a living cell. They are rod-shaped bacteria or coccobacilli that are **pleomorphic** (have many forms). They are Gram-negative and non-motile and most of them are transmitted to humans by insects or ticks. Some of the diseases caused by rickettsias include epidemic and endemic typhus, Rocky Mountain spotted fever in the United States, and scrub typhus in Australia. **Q fever**, caused by the rickettsia *Coxiella burnetii*, is harboured by ticks but appears to be mainly transmitted person to person in aerosols and from contaminated cattle.

Chlamydias are also Gram-negative, non-motile intracellular parasites and are transmitted by close person-to-person contact. They have a complex developmental cycle. In the host cell they develop inside membrane-bound cytoplasmic vacuoles, forming large metabolically active reticulate bodies. These divide many times by binary fission, rupture and release the smaller infectious particle, or elementary body, which can attack other cells. *Chlamydia trachomatis* is the agent responsible for trachoma. The organism can also be sexually transmitted and is a primary cause of non-gonococcal urethritis and pelvic inflammatory disease.

Chlamydia pneumoniae is now considered to be the most prevalent of the chlamydiae and is a significant cause of pneumonia, especially in elderly patients. It is transmitted person to person and is thought to be responsible for some infections that were previously identified as *Chlamydia psittaci*, the agent responsible for psittacosis in birds.

MYCOPLASMAS

Mycoplasmas are very small bacteria that do not form cell walls. They are mainly aerobic or facultatively anaerobic. Since they are not bound by a rigid cell wall, they are capable of assuming many shapes (**pleomorphic**), often producing fungus-like filaments. *Mycoplasma pneumoniae* is the cause of atypical pneumonia. The mycoplasmas and the **ureaplasmas** are often inhabitants of the vagina and are thought to be involved in intrauterine infections in pregnancy which may result in abortion.

MYCOBACTERIA

Mycobacteria are aerobic rod-shaped organisms that occasionally form filaments. They do not stain well with the Gram stain as they are surrounded by a waxy outer layer. An acid-fast stain is used instead (see Chapter 2) so they are also known as **acid-fast bacilli** (AFBs). *Mycobacterium tuberculosis* causes tuberculosis and *Mycobacterium leprae* is the causative agent of leprosy. *Mycobacterium avium* and *Mycobacterium intracellulare* are important opportunistic pathogens found in immunosuppressed patients. *Mycobacterium ulcerans* is responsible for Bairnsdale ulcers, which occur in certain regions of Queensland and Victoria.

Bacterial genetics

The year 2000 marked the completion of the human genome project which involved the mapping of all the genes that make up the human chromosomes. Research in bacterial genetics contributed to this project by providing much of our early understanding of DNA structure, gene expression and protein synthesis, and by the development of methods of nucleotide analysis. A full description is beyond the scope of this book, but some aspects of this topic have special significance for the health professional.

This section examines the structure of the genetic material (genes), its method of replication, the way in which cells synthesise nucleic acids, their involvement in protein synthesis, and the way genes direct and control cellular function. The effect on the cell when the composition of the DNA is altered by mutation or manipulation by scientists is discussed. The material presented here is an overview of the topic to help demystify some of the jargon that is used, and show how an understanding of genetic processes can assist in the control and treatment of disease.

GENES

The genetic material, or genes, determines all the characteristics of bacterial cells. What are genes and how do they control cellular activity?

A gene is a linear sequence of nucleotides of DNA (deoxyribonucleic acid). Each gene consists of a specific sequence of nucleotides and is responsible for determining a particular characteristic of the cell. **Nucleotides** consist of nitrogen-containing compounds called 'bases', joined to a sugar molecule, deoxyribose, and to phosphate. The nucleotide bases are the purines, **adenine** and **guanine**, and the pyrimidines, **thymine** and **cytosine** (see Figure 4.16(a)).

A number of genes are joined together to form a structure called a **chromosome**. In bacteria, all the genetic material is contained in a single circular chromosome containing many thousands of genes. Some bacteria contain one or more additional pieces of DNA called **plasmids**. Eucaryotic cells usually have more than one chromosome and the DNA exists in association with proteins called **histones**.

STRUCTURE OF DNA

The name 'nucleic acid' is derived from early studies which showed that the substance carrying hereditary traits was located in the nucleus of the cell. When DNA was first isolated in the 1940s and the bases were chemically analysed, it was found that the amount of thymine present was approximately the same as the amount of adenine and the amount of cytosine was approximately equal to guanine. However, the significance of this finding was not readily apparent and it was necessary to further elucidate the unique structure of DNA in order to understand that the pairing of these bases was crucial to the structure, providing a mechanism for genetic information to be preserved and transferred accurately during cell division.

Careful research by English scientists Max Wilkins and Rosalind Franklin, using X-ray crystallography of DNA, led James Watson and Francis Crick in 1952 to propose a structure for DNA that has laid the basis for our understanding of genetic inheritance.

The double helix

DNA consists of two strands of nucleotides twisted around each other into a double helical structure. The nucleotide bases are arranged in a specific sequence in each strand. The strand has a backbone of sugar and phosphate from which the bases protrude (see Figure 4.16(a)).

To enable the two strands to fit together into a double helix, the bases have to be held together by hydrogen bonds between the opposing strands, with adenine opposite thymine and guanine opposite cytosine. This explains the equal ratios of adenine to thymine and guanine to cytosine.

Figure 4.16(b) shows the simple, elegant structure proposed for DNA. It explains the unique properties of the genetic material and, in particular, allows for the exact replication of the nucleotide sequence. The sequence of nucleotides in one strand exactly complements the sequence in the other strand, but runs in the opposite direction.

NUCLEIC ACID SYNTHESIS

The elucidation of the structure of DNA showed how genetic properties could be preserved during cell division.

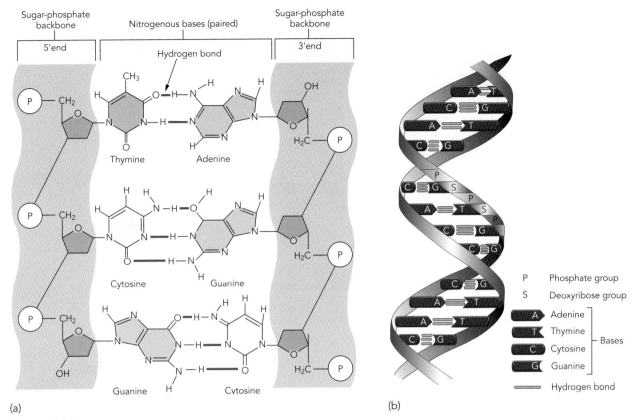

Figure 4.16

Structure of DNA

(a) pairing of nitrogenous bases in sugar-phosphate backbone; (b) helical structure of DNA.

DNA replication involves the separation of the two strands of DNA and the building up of a new strand of DNA on each of the original strands. The sequence of nucleotides in each strand acts as a pattern, or **template**, for the synthesis of the new strand. Base pairing ensures that two new identical double helices are formed (see Figure 4.17). In this way the genetic properties of the cell are preserved from one generation to the next. The same process occurs in all living cells.

PROTEIN SYNTHESIS

Most activities of the cell are carried out by proteins. Enzymes are proteins, as are many of the structural components of the cell. Proteins consist of long chains of amino acids arranged in a specific sequence and folded in various ways in order to carry out their function in the cell (see Chapter 3, Figure 3.13). The information needed for the synthesis of these proteins is contained in the DNA, so the cell needs a way of using this information to direct the synthesis of the correct protein structure. This is done by involving another type of nucleic acid called **RNA (ribonucleic acid)**. Ribonucleic acid differs from DNA in that the sugar molecule in the nucleotides is ribose and one of the bases, thymine, is replaced by the closely related purine molecule, uracil. In addition, RNA does not occur as a double helix, but usually in single strands.

There are three distinct types of RNA, varying in molecular size and function.

1. **Ribosomal RNA (rRNA)** is a large molecule that combines with protein to form particles called ribosomes, which are the site of protein synthesis in all cells.
2. **Messenger RNA (mRNA)** is a single strand of RNA that is synthesised on the DNA template and carries the information or 'message' from the chromosome to the site of protein synthesis. Messenger RNA is bound to the ribosomes and provides a template for the correct sequence of amino acids to form the protein.
3. **Transfer RNA (tRNA)** is a relatively small molecule, the function of which is to transfer amino acids to the mRNA strand on the ribosomes, and ensure that the correct amino acid is added to the growing peptide chain.

Mechanism of protein synthesis

The synthesis of a functional protein with the correct amino acid sequence is dependent on the information in the DNA being correctly transferred to the finished protein. Special terms are used to describe this process – transcription and translation.

Transcription is the term applied to the synthesis of mRNA on the DNA template – that is, the formation of a single strand of ribonucleic acid with a base sequence complementary to the base sequence of the DNA. The DNA is *transcribed* into a different form. The process could be likened to changing handwritten information into a typewritten form, but keeping the same language.

During transcription, the double strands of DNA are pulled apart and an enzyme called RNA polymerase binds

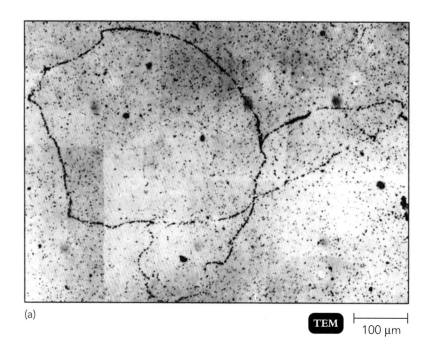

(a)

TEM 100 µm

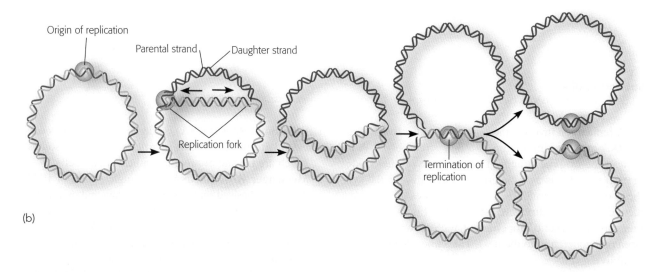

Origin of replication

Parental strand   Daughter strand

Replication fork

Termination of replication

(b)

Figure 4.17

Replication of bacterial DNA

(a) An *E. coli* chromosome in the process of replicating; (b) a diagram of the bidirectional replication of a circular bacterial DNA molecule. The new strands are shown in red.

to one of the strands of DNA at a site called the promoter. RNA nucleotides are then paired with the complementary DNA bases – adenine with thymine, uracil with adenine, and guanine with cytosine. As the messenger RNA is synthesised, the section of DNA that has been transcribed rejoins. When a terminator **codon** is reached, the RNA polymerase and the new mRNA are released. The mRNA that is produced may be a sequence containing the information from only one gene or from several closely related genes. The newly formed mRNA moves from the DNA to the ribosomes, where it is attached and acts as a template or pattern for the formation of protein molecules.

Translation refers to the formation of a protein, or polypeptide, composed of a chain of amino acids, using the mRNA as a template or pattern to ensure that the correct amino acid is inserted into the correct place. The product here is a long chain composed of amino acids instead of the nucleotides of the RNA and DNA. This process, therefore, can be likened to translating a message from one language to another (English to French, for example). In this case the information in the nucleic acid is *translated* into protein.

The process can be summarised as follows:

$$\text{DNA} \xrightarrow{\text{transcription}} \text{mRNA} \xrightarrow{\text{translation}} \text{protein}$$

During translation, the mRNA has to be able to direct the incorporation of amino acids into polypeptide chains in a specific sequence. How is this achieved?

In the 1960s several scientists working in the United States realised that the sequence of the four nucleotide bases in the nucleic acid molecules could determine which amino acid was incorporated into the protein. They were able to show that a specific sequence of three nucleotide bases, called a **codon**, was responsible for the binding of each particular amino acid.

There are four different nucleotides. It can be calculated that, if there are three nucleotides in each codon, they can be arranged in $4 \times 4 \times 4 = 64$ different ways (codons) – more than enough for the 20 amino acids found in proteins. We now know that some amino acids have more than one codon and some codons contain other messages, such as 'stop' and 'start'. Table 4.2 shows the nucleotide codon for each amino acid.

One further discovery was necessary to complete the picture. It was already known that small molecules of RNA, called **transfer RNA** (tRNA), could bind to amino acids. It was found that there was a specific tRNA for each amino acid and that this tRNA had a corresponding sequence of three nucleotides that could recognise the correct codon on the messenger RNA (see Figure 4.18). It was now possible to visualise a scheme whereby the genetic information in the DNA could be translated into functional proteins (see Figure 4.19).

Gene expression and repression

The accurate transfer of the genetic information contained in the DNA of the cell into functional proteins is of primary importance in all living cells. It is sometimes said that a gene is **expressed** or **not expressed**. This refers to whether or not the cell is actually producing a particular protein for which it has the gene. Most cells carry information for characteristics (proteins) which they do not need to use all the time. Bacteria, especially, are very small and there is no space in the cell for proteins that are not actually carrying out a function. Thus, although the bacteria may carry the gene, it may not necessarily be expressed. It is rather like having a book full of recipes (the DNA) which are only used when required. This char-

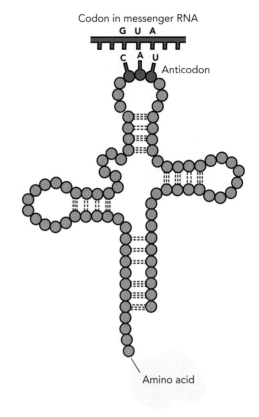

Figure 4.18

Structure of transfer RNA
The two-dimensional structure of a molecule of transfer RNA. The anticodon end will pair up with a codon on a strand of messenger RNA and deliver the desired amino acid, which is bonded to its other end. The molecule is maintained in its cloverleaf pattern by hydrogen bonding between strands that form the arms (dotted lines).

acteristic enables bacteria to make best use of their nutritional environment. This property of bacteria was discovered when it was found that *E. coli* only synthesised the enzymes necessary for the metabolism of lactose when it was grown in a medium containing lactose.

The mechanism that hinders the expression of a gene is called **repression** and is usually mediated by special proteins called **repressors**, which interfere with the transcription of the gene to mRNA. On the other hand,

Table 4.2

The genetic code
Codons are written with the 5′-terminal nucleotide on the left. Note that most amino acids are represented by more than one codon and that variation at the third nucleotide in a codon is common.

Amino acids are written as follows:

Ala	Arg	Asp	Asn	Cys	Glu	Gln	Gly	His	Ileu	Leu	Lys	Met	Phe	Pro	Ser	Thr	Trp	Tyr	Val	Stop
GCU	CGU	GAU	AAU	UGU	GAG	CAG	GGU	CAU	AUU	CUU	AAG	AUG	UUU	CCU	UCU	ACU	UGG	UAU	GUU	UGA
GCG	CGG	GAC	AAC	UGC	GAA	CAA	GGG	CAC	AUC	CUG	AAA		UCC	CCG	UCG	ACG		UAC	GUG	UAG
GCC	CGC						GGC		AUA	CUC				CCC	UCC	ACC			GUC	UAA
GCA	CGA						GGA			CUA				CCA	UCA	ACA			GUA	
	AGG									UUG					AGU					
	AGA									UUA					AGC					

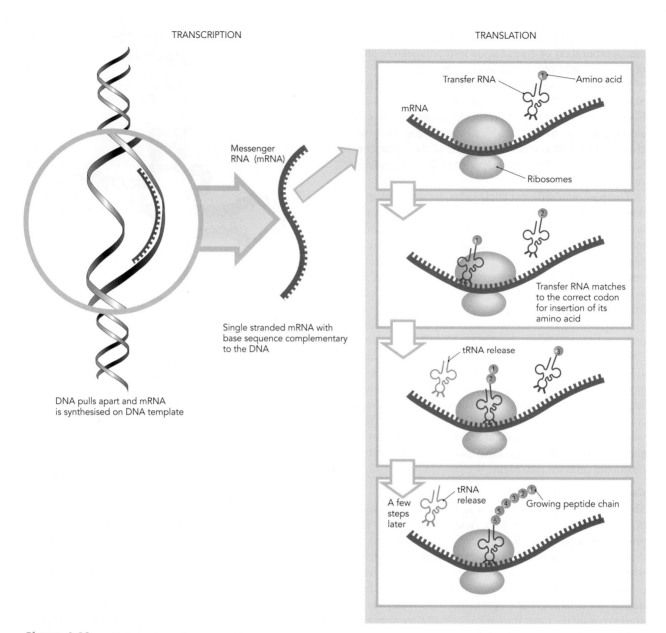

Figure 4.19

Main steps in protein synthesis

Diagrammatic representation of the events in protein synthesis. Genetic information encoded in DNA is transcribed into messenger RNA. The mRNA attaches to ribosomes in the cytoplasm and acts as a template for the insertion of the correct sequence of amino acids into the growing peptide chain by matching the codons on the transfer RNA.

substances such as lactose act as **inducers** to induce the transcription of the genes responsible for coding of enzymes necessary for lactose metabolism. Such enzymes are termed **inducible enzymes** because they are not part of the normal cellular makeup and are synthesised only when required.

Mutation

A **mutation** is defined as a permanent change in the sequence of the nucleotide bases in the DNA. From the foregoing discussion it can be seen that a change of even one base is likely to result in the formation of a protein with an altered amino acid sequence. Some mutations involve the change of only one base, a **point mutation**. Others involve a more dramatic change; for example, a **frame-shift mutation** occurs when the reading of the code misses a base or bases and gets out of phase. The protein formed as a result of a mutation may be non-functional or, on the other hand, it may have useful properties. Another outcome of mutation could be the formation of a **'nonsense' codon** which would give a 'stop' signal, resulting in the synthesis of an incomplete peptide chain. In fact, many mutations do not have any observable effect, as there is no significant alteration to the cellular proteins, but some are lethal (see Spotlight box, page 73). The possible effect of base substitution are illustrated in Figure 4.20.

Sickle cell anaemia

The inherited genetic disorder known as sickle cell anaemia is due to a single-base substitution in the DNA which gives rise to a haemoglobin molecule with one altered amino acid. The non-polar amino acid, valine, is substituted for glutamic acid. This change in the amino acid composition gives the molecule a different electric charge and so the haemoglobin molecules stick together under conditions of low oxygen tension, causing the red blood cell to change shape, or sickle, and become stuck in the capillaries.

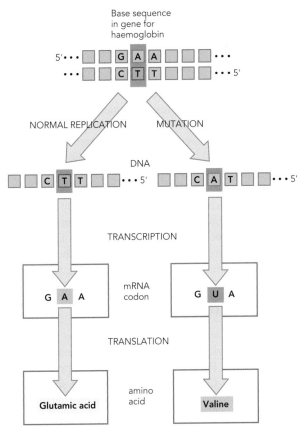

Figure 4.20

Possible effect of base substitution in a gene coding for a protein

The substitution of one base in the DNA sequence of the gene for haemoglobin gives rise to a different mRNA codon and leads to the insertion of the non-polar amino acid, valine, instead of the charged amino acid, glutamic acid.

HOW DO MUTATIONS OCCUR?

Many mutations occur spontaneously when the cell makes a mistake in the replication of the DNA during cell division. In bacteria the rate of spontaneous mutation is considered to be 1 in every 10^9 cell divisions. This may not seem very great but, considering the enormous rate at which bacterial cells divide, mutation is a very common event. Many of these mutations are not noticed because the change produces a cell that is not viable. Sometimes, the mutation results in the appearance of a cell with a characteristic that allows it to survive better, and so these cells flourish and multiply. A particularly important example is the development of resistance to antimicrobial drugs or antibiotics. Mutants that have resistance to a particular drug will survive and multiply in the presence of the antibiotic. Therapeutic or prophylactic use of the antibiotic, therefore, has the potential to select for antibiotic-resistant mutants. Continued exposure to antibiotics, especially in the hospital environment, has led to the emergence of a population of resistant microorganisms (see Chapter 12).

Chemical mutagens

Some chemicals damage DNA and cause an alteration to the nucleotide sequence. These chemicals are called **mutagens**. The chemical may act by altering the structure of the base so that it is incapable of pairing with its correct partner. This results in an abnormal DNA being formed with different properties to the DNA of the parent cell. Chemicals that cause damage to human cells so that they mutate and become cancerous are called **carcinogens**.

Much of our current knowledge about mutation has come from research with bacteria. A useful test for determining the potential carcinogenic properties of a chemical substance is the **Ames test**. A specific test strain of bacteria is exposed to the chemical. If it causes an observable change to the properties of the bacterial strain, then it is considered to have properties that are potentially mutagenic or carcinogenic for humans and requires further testing.

Radiation

Ionising radiation, such as X-rays and gamma rays, causes damage to the DNA by producing errors in replication. These rays penetrate tissue easily and can break the DNA chain, destroying chromosomes and leading to the death of the cell. Non-ionising radiation, such as UV light, also causes significant damage to cellular DNA by the production of **thymine dimers**. These distorted molecules are incapable of correct replication, and this may lead to the death of the cell or an alteration in its properties. UV light is used to destroy bacteria in clinical areas. The UV rays do not have great penetrating power but are useful for disinfecting air spaces and surface areas (see Chapter 11). Bacteria and some other organisms have enzymes that can repair radiation damage. Sometimes, an error occurs during the process of repair and gives rise to a mutant cell. The enzymes that are involved in DNA synthesis and repair have been isolated and are used by scientists in the process of genetic engineering (see below).

Damage or alteration to DNA has a profound effect in all types of cells. UV radiation damage to the DNA in skin cells may produce mutations that cause the cell to become cancerous, leading to the development of skin cancer, or melanoma.

Transfer of genetic material

The simplest kind of transfer of genetic information occurs during asexual cell division. In this process, the DNA molecule replicates itself exactly and each new DNA molecule moves into one of the two new daughter cells. However, in nature there are many variations on this simple process, and these are described below. DNA replication may involve any of the following processes: genetic recombination, 'crossing over', transformation, transduction, conjugation.

RECOMBINANT DNA

Genetic recombination is the term used to describe the transfer of genes from one DNA molecule to another, thus forming a new pattern of genes on a chromosome. In eucaryotic cells, recombination usually takes place during **meiosis** when chromosomes containing DNA molecules from each parent are lined up beside each other. If these chromosomes break and then rejoin, DNA from one chromosome can be transferred to the other in a process called '**crossing over**'. This is an ordered process that occurs regularly during sexual reproduction in eucaryotes and gives rise to the necessary genetic diversity observed in higher organisms (see Figure 4.21).

In bacteria, reproduction is usually asexual, so genetic recombination occurs relatively infrequently and requires special conditions. However, research into the mechanisms of DNA replication and transfer in bacteria has contributed greatly to our knowledge of the whole genetic process. DNA transfer between bacteria can occur under certain circumstances and always requires a donor cell and a recipient cell. The new DNA formed in the recipient cell is referred to as **recombinant DNA** (see below).

TRANSFORMATION IN BACTERIA

In the 1940s Griffith's experiments with pathogenic bacteria were responsible for identifying DNA as the carrier of genetic information. Heat-killed bacteria from a pathogenic encapsulated strain of *Streptococcus pneumoniae* were mixed with live bacteria from a non-pathogenic strain that did not form a capsule. Growth was allowed to take place and it was found that a live, encapsulated pathogenic strain was produced. This showed that a heat-resistant 'factor' from the killed bacteria, which carried the information for capsule formation and pathogenicity, had somehow entered the non-pathogenic cells and 'transformed' them into a pathogenic strain. This 'factor' was identified as DNA, which is not destroyed by heat, and the phenomenon that had occurred was termed **transformation** (see Figure 4.22).

Considerable research has been carried out since these early experiments and it is now known that, under certain conditions, live bacteria are able to take up fragments of DNA from their environment and incorporate them into their cellular DNA, thus 'transforming' their genetic properties. These fragments usually come from the lysis of dead cells. Not all bacteria are capable of undergoing transformation and it usually occurs only between cells of the same genera. *Bacillus*, *Haemophilus*, *Streptococcus* and *Staphylococcus* are some of the genera that have been shown to readily undergo transformation. Other cells have walls that do not easily allow the entry of large DNA molecules. The transformed cell, containing the recombinant DNA, continues to replicate and so the transferred genes are passed on to subsequent generations.

TRANSDUCTION

Bacteriophage, or **phage**, is the name given to viruses that attack bacteria. Viruses are very simple, consisting of genetic material, RNA or DNA, enclosed in a protein coat. As discussed in Chapter 5, viruses are quite specific for the cell they infect and this specificity can be used to target a particular strain of bacteria.

Lytic cycle and generalised transduction

When a bacterium is infected by a phage, the phage first attaches to a specific receptor site on the outside of the cell. It then injects its DNA into the cell, leaving its protein coat outside. The nature of viral replication is such that the virus uses the host cell's metabolic machinery in order to replicate. Once inside the cell, the phage DNA directs the synthesis of phage nucleic acid and proteins and assembles them into new phage particles. Eventually, the infected cell ruptures (lyses), releasing the new phage particles, and the cell is destroyed. This is termed a **lytic cycle**. During this process, phage enzymes break the bacterial chromosomal DNA into small fragments.

When the newly synthesised phage particles are being assembled, some of the bacterial DNA fragments may be

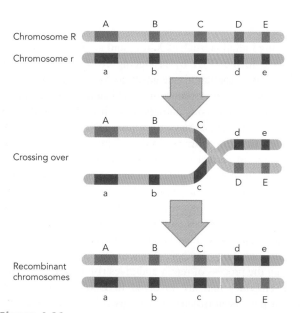

Figure 4.21

Genetic recombination between two adjacent chromosomes
The two homologous chromosomes *R* and *r* carry a copy of the genes *A* to *E* and *a* to *e* respectively. When the DNA strands break, cross over and rejoin, two recombinant chromosomes are formed carrying information from each parent.

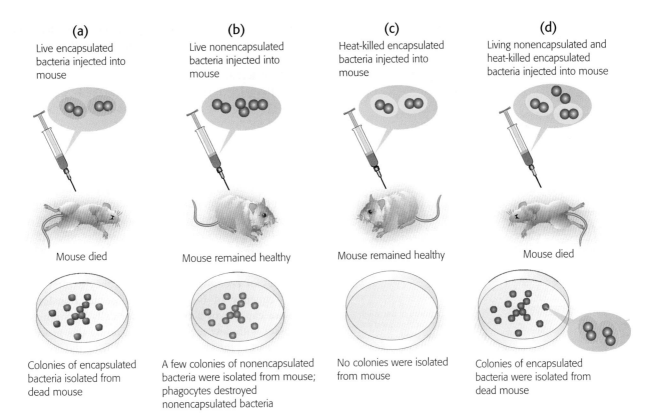

(a)
Live encapsulated bacteria injected into mouse

Mouse died

Colonies of encapsulated bacteria isolated from dead mouse

(b)
Live nonencapsulated bacteria injected into mouse

Mouse remained healthy

A few colonies of nonencapsulated bacteria were isolated from mouse; phagocytes destroyed nonencapsulated bacteria

(c)
Heat-killed encapsulated bacteria injected into mouse

Mouse remained healthy

No colonies were isolated from mouse

(d)
Living nonencapsulated and heat-killed encapsulated bacteria injected into mouse

Mouse died

Colonies of encapsulated bacteria were isolated from dead mouse

Figure 4.22
Transformation
The classic experiment by Griffith using pathogenic and non-pathogenic strains of *Streptococcus pneumoniae* which showed that genetic information in the DNA could be transferred from one cell to another. Pathogenic encapsulated bacteria were isolated from a dead mouse, heat killed and mixed with live unencapsulated, non-pathogenic cells. When injected into an experimental mouse, the animal died, showing that the heat-treated DNA had entered and transformed the non-pathogenic cells.

included at the expense of some of the phage DNA. Thus, when the phage particle is released and infects another cell, it may take with it some bacterial DNA that has been accidentally included. This phenomenon is referred to as **generalised transduction**. It involves the transfer of genetic material from one bacterial cell to another by a lytic phage and allows the transfer of bacterial characteristics from a donor to a recipient cell. Because the phage is carrying slightly altered DNA, some phage genes are lacking and it may not kill the cell it attacks. The phage DNA becomes incorporated into the recipient bacterial cell which acquires new characteristics from the donor cell (see Figure 4.23).

Specialised transduction

A different type of transduction, **specialised transduction**, occurs under some circumstances. **Temperate phages** are phages which, instead of lysing the host cell, insert their DNA into the bacterial chromosome. The inserted phage DNA is called a **prophage** and replicates along with the bacterial DNA, a state called **lysogeny**. The phage DNA may confer additional characteristics on the infected cell. For example, pathogenic strains of

Corynebacterium diphtheriae contain a temperate phage that carries the gene for toxin production. The toxin is largely responsible for the symptoms of diphtheria. Strains that do not carry the phage are not pathogenic.

A bacterial cell infected with a temperate phage may revert spontaneously to a lytic cycle, in response to an external stimulus. The phage DNA is then replicated, producing phage DNA and proteins and assembling them into new phage particles. These particles may contain fragments of bacterial DNA that will be transferred to the next bacterial cell the phage infects. The difference between these two types of transduction is that, in specialised transduction, the bacterial DNA carried to the new cell will usually be the DNA that was adjacent to the prophage DNA when it was in the lysogenic state. This phenomenon can be used to provide information about the location of specific genes on the bacterial chromosome, and can also be used to select particular genes to be transferred.

Transduction has been used by scientists to manipulate the DNA composition of bacterial cells. Bacteria that have a desired characteristic are infected with phage and the phage allowed to reproduce. Then the newly synthesised phages are transferred to another bacterial cell which can

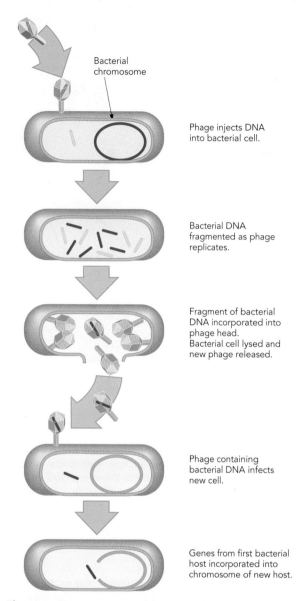

Bacterial chromosome

Phage injects DNA into bacterial cell.

Bacterial DNA fragmented as phage replicates.

Fragment of bacterial DNA incorporated into phage head.
Bacterial cell lysed and new phage released.

Phage containing bacterial DNA infects new cell.

Genes from first bacterial host incorporated into chromosome of new host.

Figure 4.23

Generalised transduction

Bacteriophage infection of a host bacterium breaks the bacterial chromosome into fragments which are carried (transduced) to the next bacterium the phage infects.

be tested to see whether the desired characteristic has been transferred – that is, whether transduction has occurred.

CONJUGATION

Conjugation is another important method whereby genetic information is transferred from one bacterial cell to another. It differs from transformation and transduction in that it requires the two bacterial cells, the donor and the recipient, to come into actual contact with each other. This is achieved by the formation of a **sex pilus**, a tubular structure that forms a bridge or channel between two cells to allow the passage of pieces of DNA from one cell to the other.

Very often, the DNA that is transferred is in the form of a plasmid. As mentioned earlier, **plasmids** are small, circular, extra-chromosomal pieces of DNA that occur in

some bacteria and replicate independently of the bacterial chromosome. They are not essential for growth of the cell, but have been shown to code for a number of other important characteristics.

The first plasmid to be described was the **F⁺ plasmid** of *E. coli*. F stands for fertility factor and refers to its ability to direct the formation of a sex pilus. Cells containing a plasmid that codes for a sex pilus are called F⁺ and those that cannot form a pilus are F⁻.

Figure 4.24 illustrates the mechanism whereby the F⁺ plasmid transfers its genes to another cell during conjugation. In the recipient cell, the plasmid either continues to replicate independently of the chromosomal DNA or it may fuse (recombine) with the chromosome. If this occurs, the recombinant DNA will then carry the genes for conjugation. These cells are called **Hfr strains** (**H**igh **f**requency of **r**ecombination) because they exhibit a very high frequency of bacterial chromosomal transfer. Hfr cells are capable of acting as donor cells in conjugation processes with new recipient cells. During this process, a copy of part of the chromosomal DNA from the donor cell is usually transferred and incorporated into the recipient cell DNA.

Transfer of plasmids during conjugation is an important method of transfer of genes from one bacterial cell to another. Plasmids containing the genes for a number of important properties have been described. Some carry genes for the production of toxins or virulence factors (see Chapter 10). A plasmid-containing strain of *E. coli* is responsible for the toxin production associated with 'traveller's diarrhoea'.

For clinical microbiologists, the most important plasmids are those carrying **resistance factors (R)**. These are genes that enable the cell to display resistance to various antibiotics, either by interfering with the entry or action of the antibiotic or by destruction of the antibiotic molecule. For example, most strains of *Staphylococcus aureus* currently isolated in hospitals carry an R plasmid with a gene that codes for the formation of the enzyme beta-lactamase, which destroys penicillin.

Resistance plasmids may carry genes for resistance to more than one antibiotic and, as described above, can be rapidly passed from cell to cell. Transfer can also occur between closely related genera, which gives rise to populations of organisms that are highly resistant to a range of antibiotics. Whereas mutation usually gives rise to resistance to one antibiotic at a time, plasmid transfer allows for the development of resistance to several antibiotics in one step. This is of increasing importance in the hospital environment (see Chapter 12).

Genetic engineering

The above description of the ways in which genetic information can be transferred between bacterial cells is given as an introduction to the subject of genetic engineering. Scientists have developed laboratory techniques that enable them to transfer genes from one cell to another and

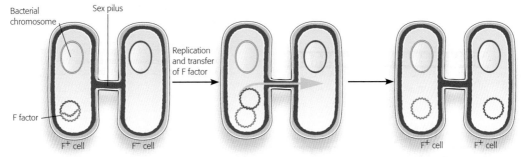

(a) When an F factor (a plasmid) is transferred from a donor (F⁺) to a recipient (F⁻), the F⁻ cell is converted into an F⁺ cell.

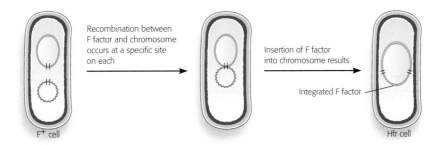

(b) When an F factor becomes integrated into the chromosome of an F⁺ cell, it makes the cell a high frequency of recombination (Hfr) cell.

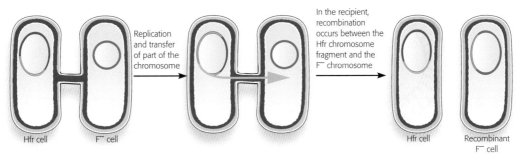

(c) When an Hfr donor passes a portion of its chromosome into an F⁻ recipient, a recombinant F⁻ cell results.

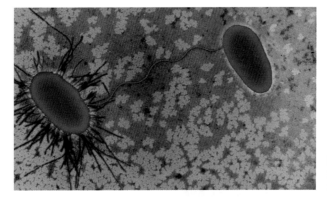

Coloured scanning electron micrograph of sex pilus formation in *E. coli*

Figure 4.24
Conjugation in *E. coli*

to manipulate the activities of microbial cells in order to obtain desired products. These techniques are based on the types of transfers described above and use many of the enzymes from bacterial cells.

Of particular use is a group of enzymes found only in bacteria, called **restriction endonucleases**. These enzymes recognise a particular sequence of nucleotides in the DNA molecule and hydrolyse (break) each strand at a specific point in the sequence. Because the DNA is a double strand, the break is always jagged, exposing a 'sticky' end. The enzymes are usually named after the

bacteria from which they were isolated. For example, Eco I comes from *Escherichia coli* (*E. coli*) and hydrolyses the sequence GAATTC between guanine and adenine, giving rise to two fragments each with the sequence AATT on the end of a single strand (the 'sticky' end). New pieces of DNA (genes) can be inserted into these breaks (see Figure 4.25).

Genetic engineering often involves the use of plasmids as vectors, or carriers, to introduce a foreign piece of DNA carrying the desired gene into a cell. A restriction enzyme is used to cut both the plasmid and the foreign DNA. This

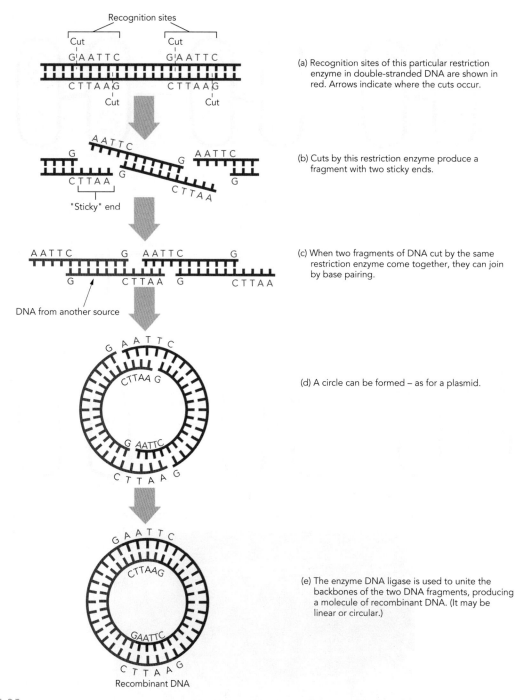

(a) Recognition sites of this particular restriction enzyme in double-stranded DNA are shown in red. Arrows indicate where the cuts occur.

(b) Cuts by this restriction enzyme produce a fragment with two sticky ends.

(c) When two fragments of DNA cut by the same restriction enzyme come together, they can join by base pairing.

(d) A circle can be formed – as for a plasmid.

(e) The enzyme DNA ligase is used to unite the backbones of the two DNA fragments, producing a molecule of recombinant DNA. (It may be linear or circular.)

Figure 4.25

The role of restriction enzymes in making recombinant DNA

gives rise to fragments of DNA from both sources which have corresponding sticky ends, with the sequence coding for the particular gene somewhere in between. When these are mixed, some of the foreign DNA can be inserted into the plasmid. An enzyme called DNA ligase is added to join the nucleotides together and the result is a plasmid vector carrying the desired gene. In the laboratory the plasmid is usually introduced into the recipient cell by transformation (see Figure 4.26). If the host cell does not normally take up DNA, the cell wall can be modified by chemical treatments.

Viruses are sometimes used as vectors for animal cells.

RECOMBINANT DNA TECHNOLOGY

The procedures used in genetic engineeering result in the formation of DNA molecules that have been modified in some way; that is, they have become 'recombinant DNA'. **Recombinant DNA** is a term widely used to refer to DNA that has been produced using DNA from two different sources. It can mean:

- the DNA produced by spontaneous crossing over during cell division; or
- the DNA produced in the laboratory by genetic engineering.

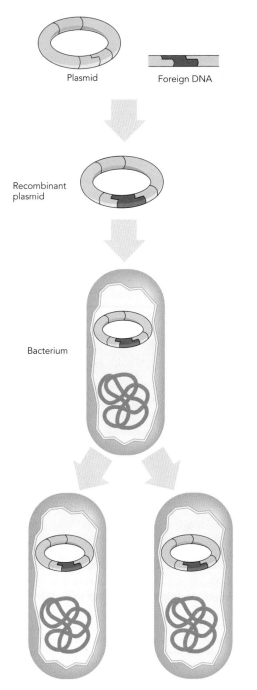

Figure 4.26

Insertion of foreign genes into a bacterium using a plasmid as the vector

Foreign DNA and plasmid DNA are cut with a restriction enzyme. The foreign DNA is inserted into the plasmid. The recombinant plasmid is introduced into a new bacterial cell which acquires the characteristics coded for by the foreign DNA and can be cloned.

Scientists have developed ways of using genetic engineering to benefit humans. For example, a gene from a eucaryotic cell can be inserted into a bacterial cell. The recipient bacterial cell containing the recombinant DNA can then be induced to express this gene. Because of the rapid rate of growth of bacterial cells, large amounts of the substance coded for in the eucaryotic gene can be produced quickly in a relatively pure form. One of the first examples of the use of this technique was the production of human insulin by cells of *E. coli*. The gene for insulin production was isolated from human pancreatic cells and inserted into *E.coli*.

Vaccines such as the one for hepatitis B, hep B surface antigen (HBsAg), have also been genetically engineered. The gene responsible for the synthesis of one particular sequence of the hepatitis B viral protein coat (the 'surface antigen') is introduced into a yeast cell. The yeast produces multiple copies of this fragment of the protein coat, which are then isolated, purified and used as a vaccine in humans to stimulate production of protective anti-hepatitis-B antibodies.

There are several advantages to the use of recombinant DNA in the production of compounds such as hormones or vaccines for human use. Previously, many of these compounds had to be derived from human or animal tissue. The presence of animal proteins often gave rise to an adverse immune reaction (see Chapter 9). The need to use blood or tissue from human sources limited the amount of the substance that could be produced and increased the cost. There was also a slight risk of transferring another human pathogen that might be present in the extracts. There is some evidence that this occurred with the use of preparations of human growth hormone from pituitary extracts from cadavers. Some patients treated with these hormone preparations have developed Creutzfeldt-Jakob syndrome, a disease of the nervous system (see Spotlight box, page 240).

The use of purified genetically engineered products, synthesised by microbial cells, minimises the risk of adverse effects from preparations contaminated with human pathogens or other substances that may cause hypersensitivity reactions.

Biotechnology is the term used for the many and varied techniques involving manipulation of genes or genetic information. Table 4.3 lists some of the microbial products of biotechnology.

DNA analysis

The techniques developed for genetic engineering are also of use in identifying DNA from various sources. This is described in more detail in Chapter 15. Analysis of DNA is used to identify microorganisms that may be difficult or slow to grow in the laboratory. Often a new species of bacteria can be identified because it has a different DNA composition from known bacteria. For example, DNA typing has been used to distinguish between different species of *Chlamydia*, an organism that cannot be grown in the laboratory. These studies have identified *Chlamydia pneumoniae* as a significant cause of pneumonia.

DNA analysis can be used in epidemiological studies to trace the occurrence of a particular strain of bacteria. It is also used for the identification of human tissue. No two humans (except identical twins) look exactly alike. This is

Table 4.3

Microbial products of genetic engineering

PRODUCT	ORGANISM	COMMENT
Medical		
Insulin	*E. coli*	Treatment for diabetes
Interleukin 2 (IL-2)	*E. coli*	Stimulates immune system
Interferon α and γ	*E. coli*	Possible therapy for viral diseases
	S. cerevisiae	
Tumour necrosis factor	*E. coli*	Attacks cancer cells
Human growth hormone	*E. coli*	Corrects growth deficiencies
Colony stimulating factor (CSF)	*E. coli*	Stimulation of immune system and treatment
	S. cerevisiae	of infections
Vaccine		
Hepatitis B	*S. cerevisiae*	HBsAg for vaccine
Modified organisms		
Genetically modified plants	*Pseudomonas syringae*	Prevents frost damage to plants
	Bacillus thuringiensis	Resistance to insect pests and herbicides

because every person has a different complement of DNA in his or her genes. DNA fingerprinting is used in forensic science to compare, for example, the DNA in a sample of semen with the DNA in a blood sample to help establish the identity of a criminal, or determine paternity.

DNA FINGERPRINTING

Methods have been developed to compare DNA samples obtained from different sources. The DNA analysis involves the use of special enzymes to cut the DNA sample into small fragments (**RFLPs – restriction fragment length polymorphisms**) which are then separated by gel electrophoresis. In electrophoresis the sample is placed in a special compartment or 'well' in an agarose gel in a buffer solution, and an electric current passed through the gel. **Pulse field gel electrophoresis** (**PFGE**) is one method that provides good separation. The fragments of DNA move through the gel and separate into bands depending on their size, the larger ones remaining behind and the smaller ones migrating quickly to the opposite pole. A pattern, or fingerprint, of the DNA is obtained which is visualised by staining or using radioactive probes (see Figure 4.27).

This technique is very useful in epidemiological investigations. Isolates of bacteria obtained from different sources can be compared to see whether they are the same strain. For example, the anthrax samples that were sent through the mail in the United States in 2002 were analysed in this way to try to identify the source of the organism.

SEQUENCE ANALYSIS

Very often, a genetic characteristic can be ascribed to a particular nucleotide sequence or gene. Techniques are now available which allow the determination of the sequence of nucleotides in a piece of DNA. In other words, it is now possible to detect the presence or absence of a particular gene. This method was developed in exper-

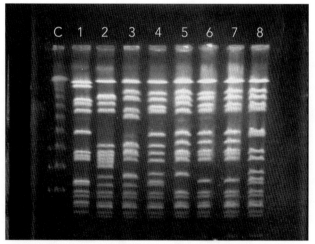

Figure 4.27

Pulse field gel electrophoresis of DNA from different isolates of MRSA

The bacterial isolates were collected from the same hospital ward over a period of six months. It can be seen that only two of the isolates (6,7) exhibit the same pattern (i.e. are the same strain), which indicates that a number of different strains are present in the hospital and it is not possible to identify the source of the infections.

Samples 1–4   July 1996
Sample 5   October 1996
Sample 6   December 1996
Samples 7,8   November 1996

iments with microorganisms – the complete sequence of nucleotides in the chromosome of *E. coli* (its 'genetic map') being one of the first to be completed. The development of automated sequencing machines has enabled these studies to be extended to an analysis of the genetic composition of higher organisms.

The human genome project is a worldwide cooperative study by scientists which has mapped the complete sequence of the 100 000 genes that make up the human chromosomes. This has required the determination of the sequence of about three billion nucleotide pairs. It is now theoretically possible to screen individuals and determine their exact genetic makeup. DNA analysis also allows scientists to test for defective genes that may be responsible for a particular disease. There are many ethical issues about how this information should be used. Attempts have been made to introduce DNA into embryonic cells in order to correct genetic defects, but these experiments are in the early stages and are also the subject of much discussion about the ethics of such procedures.

Analysis of ribosomal RNA has been used for the classification of organisms into domains and kingdoms, as described above.

AMPLIFICATION OF DNA

The determination of the nucleotide sequence in DNA samples requires relatively large amounts of DNA which may not always be available. In this case, a method of DNA amplification such as the **polymerase chain reaction**, or **PCR**, is used. In this technique, fragments of the DNA of interest are copied until enough molecules are obtained to carry out an analysis such as fingerprinting or sequencing (described above). PCR can make billions of copies of a particular nucleotide sequence in just a few hours.

The piece of DNA to be copied is heated so that the double helix separates into single strands. The solution is then cooled and the four DNA nucleotides and enzymes are added. The nucleotides are incorporated, pairing with their corresponding bases on the exposed single strand. The new DNA strand is then 'zipped up' by the action of a polymerase enzyme, effectively doubling the amount of DNA each time (see Figure 4.28).

PCR must be carried out under very strictly controlled laboratory conditions, as it is an extremely sensitive technique. It is important to ensure that the equipment and solutions are not contaminated with any external DNA from another source. Other amplification methods have been developed (see Chapter 15).

DNA PROBES

Another important technique is the use of DNA probes to see whether a particular nucleic acid sequence is present in a sample. This is very useful in diagnostic microbiology. Some microorganisms are either very difficult to grow or grow very slowly in the laboratory. A number of DNA 'probes' have been developed commercially and can be used to identify an organism or detect its presence in a clinical specimen or tissue. The **probe** consists of a small fragment of DNA containing a nucleotide sequence which is specific to the particular organism being looked for. In the '**dot blot**' method, the DNA to be tested is first amplified by PCR if necessary, applied to a filter paper and heated to pull the strands apart. The probe, which has been labelled with a radioactive or fluorescent marker, is then introduced and the DNA strands allowed to rejoin. If the complementary sequence of nucleotides is present in the test DNA, then the probe will combine with it, giving a radioactive or fluorescent product that can be detected by X-ray film or visualised with UV light.

SOUTHERN BLOTS

Southern blot is another technique used to determine whether a particular nucleotide sequence is present in a DNA sample. The DNA is hydrolysed and then subjected to gel electrophoresis. The fragments obtained are transferred to a nitrocellulose membrane by 'blotting' and the membrane is then treated with a radioactive probe. If the desired sequence of nucleotides is present the probe will bind to it and can be detected by exposure to an X-ray film. This method is useful when trying to identify a particular nucleotide sequence (gene) in a complex mixture.

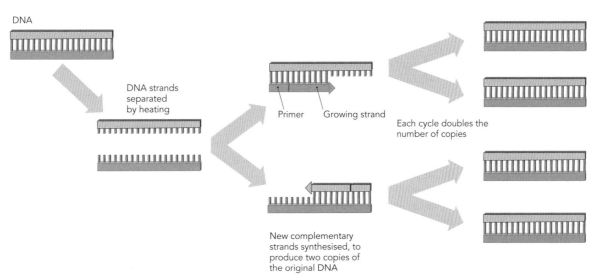

Figure 4.28
Polymerase chain reaction

The future of biotechnology

In the future there will be increasing use of nucleic acid amplification and detection techniques to test for the presence of bacteria in a sample when the concentration of cells is too low to be detected by any other means. This is already having a major impact on diagnostic microbiology. As more probes become available commercially, these methods are being used increasingly in clinical laboratories to reduce the time required for identification (see Chapter 15). In agriculture, recombinant DNA technology is being used to produce genetically modified (GM) crops that are resistant to frost or drought, have an increased yield or resistance to insects.

The last 20 years have seen an explosion in our knowledge of genes and our ability to manipulate genetic characteristics. However, this has been accompanied by many legal and ethical questions. Should scientists be allowed to release genetically modified organisms into the environment? Are genetically modified crops safe to eat? Should doctors manipulate the genes in unborn babies?

The use of techniques of DNA analysis means that it is now possible to test people for genetic defects, to help in the identification of human remains by comparison with the DNA of living relatives, to solve cases of missing persons and to assist in criminal forensic investigations. However, confidentiality issues are a major cause of concern.

The use of bacteria to produce vaccines and other substances of benefit to humans is expanding at an incredible rate. One of the strategies currently being investigated to produce an AIDS vaccine involves the use of recombinant DNA technology to modify the *Vaccinia* virus to carry HIV antigen. This creates a virus with the antigenic properties of HIV but not HIV-DNA, so it should theoretically stimulate the immune response without causing disease.

SUMMARY

STRUCTURE OF BACTERIA

- Bacteria occur in three main shapes – spherical (cocci), rod-shaped (bacilli) and spiral (spirilla, spirochaete or vibrio).
- Some bacteria are surrounded by a polysaccharide-containing capsule, the glycocalyx, which allows the bacteria to bind to surfaces and evade phagocytosis.
- Flagella are thin, rigid filaments which enable the bacteria to swim.
- Pili are short, hair-like appendages which aid in the attachment of bacteria to mucosal cells. Some are involved in bacterial conjugation.
- Bacterial cell walls are complex, semi-rigid structures.
- Depending on the structure of the wall, bacteria are classified as Gram-positive or Gram-negative.
- Mycobacteria have a waxy outer layer that necessitates their identification by the acid-fast stain.
- The cell wall can be damaged by certain chemicals or enzymes such as lysozyme. The synthesis of peptidoglycan is inhibited by penicillin.
- Bacterial cells have a plasma membrane, consisting of a phospholipid bilayer with proteins embedded in it.
- The membrane is a semi-permeable barrier, controlling the passage of substances into and out of the cell.
- Bacterial cell membranes are the site of metabolic reactions which occur in the organelles of eucaryotic cells.
- The cytoplasm contains water, enzymes, ribosomes, inclusion granules and a single, circular chromosome of DNA.
- In some bacteria, additional genetic information is carried on a plasmid.
- Ribosomes are the site of protein synthesis.
- Some Gram-positive bacilli form resistant endospores when environmental conditions are unfavourable.

REPRODUCTION IN BACTERIAL CELLS

- Bacterial growth is defined as an increase in cell numbers.
- Bacteria reproduce by binary fission.
- The time taken for a cell to reproduce itself is called the generation time.

REQUIREMENTS FOR GROWTH

- Bacteria require various physical factors for growth, including correct temperature, correct pH, correct osmotic pressure and the correct amount of oxygen.
- Nutritional requirements include water, the elements carbon, nitrogen, sulphur and phosphorous, and various trace elements. Autotrophic bacteria use carbon dioxide from the atmosphere. Some bacteria require specific organic compounds.

IDENTIFICATION OF BACTERIA IN THE LABORATORY

- Bacteria can be grown, isolated and identified in the laboratory by growing them on defined media.
- When grown in the laboratory under controlled conditions, bacteria have four phases of growth: lag, logarithmic, stationary and death.

CLASSIFICATION OF BACTERIA

- Bacteria can be classified on the basis of their cell wall structure, Gram stain, shape, motility, oxygen requirements, biochemical properties and analysis of ribosomal RNA.
- Phage typing and DNA typing are used to differentiate bacterial strains.
- Many bacteria are of medical importance.

BACTERIAL GENETICS

- The characteristics of bacterial cells are determined by their genetic material or genes, which are linear sequences of nucleotides of DNA.
- DNA consists of two strands of nucleotides twisted around each other to form a double helix.
- In protein synthesis, the genetic information contained in the DNA is first transcribed to messenger RNA, which then acts as a template for the synthesis of proteins.

MUTATION

- Mutation (which can occur as a result of exposure to chemicals or radiation) is a change in the nucleotide bases in the DNA that gives rise to different properties in the cell.
- Favourable mutations, such as the development of drug resistance, allow some bacteria to survive instead of others.

TRANSFER OF GENETIC MATERIAL

- Genetic recombination refers to the exchange of DNA between two molecules.
- Transformation, transduction and conjugation are different ways in which one bacterial strain acquires the characteristics of another strain.

GENETIC ENGINEERING

- Recombinant DNA technology is being used in a number of ways to develop products that are of benefit to humans.
- Biotechnology is used to determine genetic characteristics and identify samples based on their DNA composition.

STUDY QUESTIONS

1. Describe the major shapes of bacterial cells.
2. What is meant by morphology?
3. How does the structure of Gram-positive cell walls differ from the structure of Gram-negative cell walls?
4. What is meant by an acid-fast bacillus?
5. Where is the genetic information in bacterial cells located?
6. What is the function of these extracellular bacterial structures – glycocalyx, flagella and pili?
7. What are the main requirements for bacterial growth?
8. Describe the four phases of bacterial growth.
9. What are the properties used to classify bacteria by Bergey's method of classification?
10. How are proteins synthesised in bacterial cells?
11. What is meant by the term 'gene expression'?
12. What happens when a mutation takes place in a bacterial cell?
13. What is meant by 'recombinant DNA'?
14. Describe the ways in which recombinant DNA technology is being used to benefit humans.

TEST YOUR UNDERSTANDING

1. How does the structure of the plasma membrane control the passage of substances into and out of the cell?
2. Why is correct osmotic pressure important for bacterial cell growth?
3. Why is it important to use methods of sterilisation that destroy endospores?
4. Why is tetanus and/or gangrene sometimes treated by placing the patient in a hyperbaric oxygen chamber?
5. How can phage typing help to identify the source of an infection?
6. How is the information for antibiotic resistance transferred from one bacterial cell to another? What are the implications for the control of infectious diseases?
7. How does the use of nucleic acid analysis (NAA) contribute to the classification of bacteria?

Further reading

Holt JG (ed.) 1994, *Bergey's Manual of Systematic Bacteriology*, 9th edn, Baltimore: Williams & Wilkins. (A standard reference for identification and classification of bacteria.)

For an interactive introduction to genetics visit <www.dnai.org>.

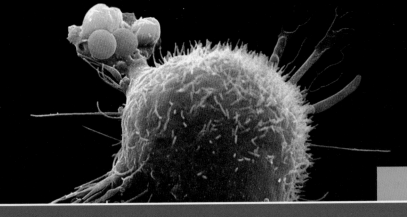

Viruses and
Viral Diseases

[CHAPTER FOCUS]

- *What are the special characteristics of viruses?*

- *How do viruses replicate inside cells?*

- *What are the different clinical outcomes of viral infection in humans?*

- *What are the major routes of transmission of viral diseases?*

- *How are viral diseases diagnosed, treated and prevented?*

Why are viruses important?

Many of the significant diseases that affect our society are caused by viruses and new ones, such as AIDS and SARS, are constantly emerging. Most of the viruses responsible for these diseases have been identified in the last 60 years. Before then, many unexplained illnesses were attributed to the effects of toxins or poisons, or to exposure to 'bad air'.

The word **virus** means venom, or poison, and the original name given to the infective agents that caused these diseases was 'filterable viruses'. This was because samples obtained from diseased animals or plants were still infectious after being passed through a filter that was known to retain bacteria. There are many different kinds of viruses and they cause disease not only in humans but also in other animals, plants and even bacteria. In this chapter we describe the unique properties of viruses and examine the way in which they cause disease in a susceptible host.

Characteristics of viruses

Viruses are among the smallest infectious agents known. They range in size from the tiny polio virus (20 nm diameter) to the large pox virus which is 400 nm in diameter. This is still smaller than even the smallest bacteria which are 1000–2000 nm (1–2 μm) in diameter. For comparison, human erythrocytes are 7–8 μm in diameter. Viruses cannot be seen under the light microscope, requiring the higher resolution of electron microscopy for their structure to be visible.

We now know that viruses lack most of the enzymes necessary for the metabolism and synthesis of complex molecules and so can replicate (grow) only inside a living (host) cell. Viruses have to use the metabolic machinery of the host cell and, as a result, have been called *obligate intracellular parasites*. In most instances, viruses damage the cells in which they replicate, causing the cells either to burst (lyse) or to die gradually

Structure of viruses

Viruses have a simple structure consisting of only one type of nucleic acid enclosed in a protein coat called a **capsid**. Some of the more complex viruses have, in addition, a protein core enclosing the nucleic acid. Others have an additional outer layer called an envelope (see Figure 5.1). Viruses are not cells and they are unable to carry out any metabolic functions without the involvement of a host cell. Each virus has a distinctive shape and structure that can be used in classification (see Figure 5.2).

NUCLEIC ACID

Each virus possesses only one type of nucleic acid, which carries its genetic information. This is either single-stranded RNA (ss-RNA), double-stranded RNA (ds-RNA), single-stranded DNA (ss-DNA) or double-stranded DNA (ds-DNA). The size of the viral genome is limited and does not carry all the information necessary for the synthesis of a complete virus. Instead, the viral genes code mainly for structural viral proteins and a limited number

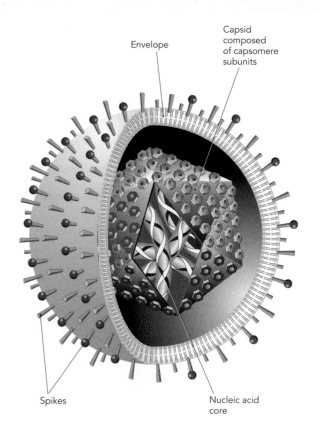

Figure 5.1

Schematic diagram of a virus

(a) Naked virus

(b) Enveloped virus

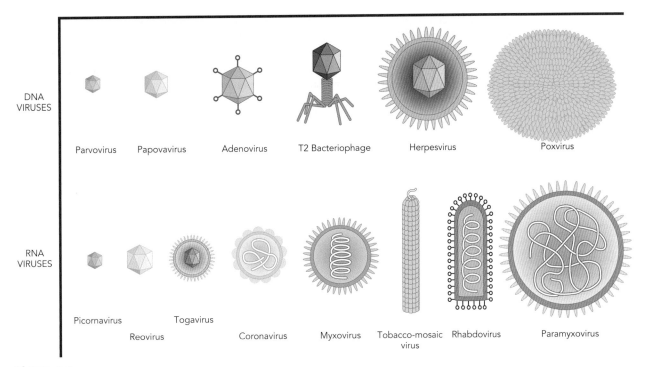

Figure 5.2
Relative sizes and shapes of different viruses

DNA VIRUSES: Parvovirus, Papovavirus, Adenovirus, T2 Bacteriophage, Herpesvirus, Poxvirus

RNA VIRUSES: Picornavirus, Reovirus, Togavirus, Coronavirus, Myxovirus, Tobacco-mosaic virus, Rhabdovirus, Paramyxovirus

of viral enzymes, as well as regulatory genes which direct the host cell pathways to produce new viral particles.

THE VIRAL CAPSID

The protein coat covering the nucleic acid is called a **capsid** and is made up of repeating protein units called **capsomeres**. These are often arranged in symmetrical patterns which enable the purified virus particles to be crystallised. Capsids occur in distinctive shapes (see Figure 5.2). Many consist of a regular polyhedron such as the icosahedral (20-sided) structure found in, for example, the adenovirus. Others are helical, forming hollow cylinders which may be either rigid or flexible. Some (e.g. the pox viruses) have a complex structure.

Although viral capsids contain only a minimum number of protein molecules, the capsid proteins have a number of important functions. They may have antigenic properties (i.e. they possess a distinctive molecular structure which stimulates the production of a corresponding antibody, see page 193) and they participate in the attachment and entry of the virus particle to the host cell during infection (see below). They also protect the nucleic acid against inactivation by nuclease enzymes.

ENVELOPE

Some viruses are surrounded by an envelope. This usually consists of a lipid bilayer derived from the membrane of the host cell, into which some specific viral proteins and glycoproteins have been inserted. The viral glycoproteins may appear as 'spikes' protruding from the envelope. The structure of the envelope assists the virus to attach to the host cell. For example, the spikes on the influenza virus enable it to attach to the surface receptors on the cells of the respiratory epithelium and also to similar receptors on red blood cells, causing agglutination (see Figure 5.1b).

Viruses that lack envelopes are called **naked viruses**. They are generally more resistant to environmental conditions than enveloped viruses because the envelope is easily damaged by chemicals or extremes of pH or temperature.

The surface protein components of enveloped viral particles participate in the attachment of the viral particle to the specific receptor site on the susceptible cell. They also determine the antigenic characteristics of the virus. The immune system of the host produces antibodies directed against the proteins and glycoproteins present on the viral surface (see Chapter 9).

VIRAL ENZYMES

Viruses do not have all the enzymes required to carry out metabolic processes outside the host cell. However, some viruses contain genes for the production of enzymes that are important for the infective process. Most of these are involved with nucleic acid transcription – for example, reverse transcriptase carries out the initial step in the replication of the retroviruses, the synthesis of DNA from viral RNA. Neuraminidase, an enzyme located in the spike of the influenza virus, is important for the release of new viral particles. These enzymes are not generally found in the host cell so they are good targets for antiviral therapy (see Chapter 12).

TERMINOLOGY

A number of different terms are used to describe viruses.

- **Virion** is used to describe an entire mature virus particle consisting either of nucleic acid and capsid (naked virus) or nucleic acid, capsid and envelope (enveloped virus). Virions are found outside the host cell and are capable of transmission from one host to another.

- **Virus**, or **viral particle**, refers to the intracellular infectious particle consisting of nucleic acid and a protein coat.
- **Nucleocapsid** refers to the protein–nucleic acid complex of the virus – it may also be a subunit of a more complex virus.
- The **viral genome** is the genetic information of the virus, either RNA or DNA.
- **Viroids** are infectious agents that lack a capsid and consist only of a closed circular RNA molecule. They are usually plant pathogens and are not discussed further in this text.
- **Prions** are unusual infective particles that consist only of protein.

PRIONS

Prions are infective particles that have been implicated in some unusual transmissible neurodegenerative disorders, known as **transmissible spongiform encephalopathies (TSEs)**. These include kuru and Creutzfeldt-Jakob disease (CJD) in humans, scrapie in sheep, and bovine spongiform encephalopathy (BSE), or 'mad cow disease' (see Chapter 20, page 500). They were first thought to be a kind of virus; however, they appear to consist only of protein, without any nucleic acid. It is thought that the diseases they cause are due to a conformational change in the proteins in brain cells, initiated by the prion protein. Prions are particularly resistant to procedures that normally destroy cells such as treatment with disinfectants and autoclaving.

Classification of viruses

The clinical classification of viruses, based on the disease they produce or the part of the body they affect, is useful but not completely satisfactory for the scientist who is interested in other properties. Viruses with very different structures may cause diseases that are superficially similar. For example, hepatitis A, B, C, D and E all affect the liver but belong to quite different viral families. Some of the viruses responsible for known diseases have not yet been isolated or seen under a microscope (e.g. hepatitis C virus) and others have not been cultured in the laboratory (e.g. HPV, human papilloma virus).

New techniques in immunology and molecular biology are providing information about the structure of viruses. This knowledge may give rise to different grounds for classification. At present, viruses are separated into major groups or families, based on the type of nucleic acid they contain, their shape and structure and their method of replication.

Table 5.1 lists the major families of viruses responsible for human infections.

Host range and specificity

Viruses are often highly selective for the range of hosts and the type of cells they infect. In general, plant viruses infect only plants, bacterial viruses infect only bacteria and animal viruses infect only animals. Within these broad categories, most viruses will attack only one type of animal or plant (its host range) and may even be specific for only one kind of cell or tissue within that organism (**tissue tropism**). However, some viruses are able to cross the species barrier and infect birds as well as animals (e.g. avian influenza virus, H5N1, and influenza A).

The ability of a virus to infect a particular kind of cell is dependent on the presence of an attachment site for the virus on the surface of the host cell. **Ligands** (chemical groups) in specific proteins (**viral attachment proteins**) on the surface of the virion bind to receptor molecules on the surface of the plasma membrane of the target cell. For some viruses the chemical structure of the ligands and corresponding receptor molecules has been determined. For example, orthomyxoviruses bind to a terminal sialic acid molecule located on a side chain of a membrane glycolipid or glycoprotein. The gp120 attachment protein of the human immunodeficiency virus, HIV, binds to the CD4 receptor molecule on the membrane of T4 lymphocytes.

The recognition of specific receptors by particular viruses is not absolute. Sometimes, unrelated viruses use the same receptor, which means that a cell with that receptor may be vulnerable to attack by a number of different viruses. On the other hand, similar viruses may use quite different receptors. In addition, certain viruses are able to recognise more than one kind of receptor. If the receptors are on different types of cells this will extend the **tissue tropism** (i.e. the range of cells the virus can attack) or even the host range of the virus. For example, the rabies virus can attach to the acetyl choline (ACh) receptor as well as sialyted gangliosides, and this greatly extends its range of susceptible cell types. The more common the receptor molecule, the wider the range of cells the virus can attack.

In general, it appears that viruses have evolved in such a way as to make maximum use of the available glycoprotein molecules on the host cell membrane as their receptors. It should be noted, however, that these molecules are an integral part of the host cell membrane and have functions other than merely serving as attachment sites for viruses. The presence or absence of these receptor molecules is a fundamental determinant of the susceptibility of the host cell to viral attack. The polio virus, for example, binds to specific receptors that are present in primate cells but not in other animals. Hence the polio virus can attack humans and monkeys, but not mice. However, replication of the polio virus occurs only in neuronal and muscle cells so it appears that the existence of appropriate receptors on primate cells is not the only determinant of successful infection. Other kinds of primate cells may be non-permissive for other reasons.

Table 5.1

Viruses that affect humans classified into families by chemical and physical properties

VIRAL FAMILY	CAPSID SYMMETRY	VIRION NAKED OR ENVELOPED	SIZE (NM)	NUCLEIC ACID
DNA viruses				
Parvoviridae	Icosahedral	Naked	18–26	ssDNA
Polyomaviridae	Icosahedral	Naked	40	dsDNA (circular)
Papillomaviridae	Icosahedral	Naked	55	dsDNA (circular)
Adenoviridae	Icosahedral	Naked	70–90	dsDNA
Herpes viridae	Icosahedral	Enveloped	150–200	dsDNA
Hepadna viridae	Icosahedral	Enveloped	40–48	dsDNA (circular)
Poxviridae	Complex		230 × 400	dsDNA
RNA viruses				
Reoviridae	Icosahedral	Naked	60–80	dsRNA (segmented)
Picornaviridae	Icosahedral	Naked	20–30	ssRNA
Calciviridae	Icosahedral	Naked	27–40	ssRNA
Astroviridae	Icosahedral	Naked	28–30	
Togaviridae	Icosahedral	Enveloped	50–70	ssRNA
Flaviviridae	Unknown	Enveloped	45–60	ssRNA
Arenaviridae	or	Enveloped	50–300	ssRNA (segmented)
Coronaviridae	complex	Enveloped	120–160	ssRNA
Retroviridae		Enveloped	80–100	ssRNA (diploid)
Bunyaviridae	Helical	Enveloped	80–100	ssRNA (segmented)
Bornaviridae	Helical	Enveloped	80–125	ssRNA
Orthomyxoviridae	Helical	Enveloped	80–120	ssRNA (segmented)
Paramyxoviridae	Helical	Enveloped	150–300	ssRNA
Rhabdoviridae	Helical	Enveloped	75 × 80	ssRNA
Filoviridae	Helical/filamentous	Enveloped	80 × 1000	ssRNA

Source: Data derived from Brooks GF, Butel JS & Ornston LN. *Jawetz, Melnick & Adelberg's Medical Microbiology*, 2004, McGraw-Hill.

It is thought that, after penetration of the host cell by the virus, viral replication depends on the activity of a number of regulatory factors, determined by the host cell genome and viral genome, and variously called promoters, enhancers or transcriptional activators. These regulatory factors may be restricted to certain types of cells and tissues where they exert an important role as an additional determinant of successful viral infection.

Few viruses cause disease in both humans and other animals because viruses are host-specific. Those few viruses that do, usually occur under conditions that allow transmission from the animal reservoir to humans, and use receptor molecules that are found in a wide variety of cells. One of these is the rabies virus, which is widespread throughout the animal kingdom and can be transmitted to humans by the bite of an infected animal.

Other viruses that persist in nature in an animal reservoir can be transmitted to humans by close contact with the animal or infected droppings. Among these, the han-

tavirus, which was responsible for a serious outbreak of an influenza-like disease in New Mexico in 1993, was linked to a plague of deer mice. Hendra virus (previously named equine morbillivirus), which was identified as responsible for the death of a horse trainer and 14 racehorses in Australia in 1994 (see Spotlight box, page 157), is another example of a virus that can apparently cross the species barrier. The virus has been found in fruit bats, which are thought to be the main animal reservoir. The recently identified bat lyssavirus is a rabies-like virus that is also found in fruit bats. The rabies vaccine is used to treat people infected with lyssavirus.

Menangle virus which has been found in New South Wales, and Nipah virus which occurs in Malaysia, are also carried by fruit bats and infect both pigs and humans. West Nile virus and the avian influenza virus, H5N1, are recently identified viruses that infect birds and humans.

Some viruses that persist in animal or bird reservoirs are transmitted to other animals or humans by the bite of insects such as mosquitoes. These viruses cause a subclinical infection in the animal host and multiply in both the vertebrate host and invertebrate vector. They are called **arboviruses** and are described later in this chapter.

Viral replication

As was mentioned earlier, viruses do not contain the genetic information required to produce all the enzymes necessary for the synthesis of new viral particles. Instead, they use the host cell DNA and some host cell enzymes to produce viral components. The assembly of the new components into viral particles is under the direction of the viral genes.

REPLICATION OF BACTERIAL VIRUSES

Although we are not primarily concerned in this text with the infection of bacteria by viruses, a brief description is included here as they provide a simple model for investigating the mechanisms of viral infection. Viruses that infect bacteria are called **bacteriophage**, or **phage**. They have been extensively studied, and have provided much information about the important processes that occur during the infection of animal cells. A bacterial culture contains many millions of identical cells. It is easy to infect a culture of bacteria with phage and observe the results in a uniform population.

Phage exert the same specificity for their host cell as the

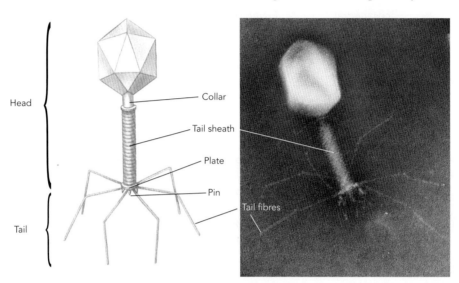

(a)

(b)

Figure 5.3

Bacteriophage

(a) Diagram and electron micrograph of T-even bacteriophage; (b) diagrammatic representation of lytic and lysogenic cycles of bacteriophage infection.

viruses that infect higher organisms. This property is often used to differentiate strains of bacteria, using a technique known as phage typing (see Chapter 4, page 64). The first step in the infection of a bacterium by a phage involves the attachment of the phage to a specific receptor site on the bacterial cell wall. Since the bacterial cell is relatively small, only the viral nucleic acid is injected into the bacterium during infection. This is illustrated in Figure 5.3.

Once the phage DNA has entered the cell, a number of different events may occur. The most usual outcome is that the phage takes over the cell machinery, produces many new phage particles and then causes lysis of the cell as the new phage are released into the surrounding medium. This is called the **lytic cycle**.

Sometimes, the phage enters the cell but, instead of reproducing itself, the phage DNA is incorporated into the host cell DNA. In this state, called **lysogeny**, the phage is **latent** and does not produce new phage or cause lysis. The phage DNA that has been inserted into the bacterial chromosome is called a **prophage**. When the bacterium divides, the phage DNA is also copied, with the result that all the bacterial daughter cells contain the phage genes. One possible outcome of lysogeny is that the host cell may exhibit new properties.

For example, *Corynebacterium diphtheriae*, the bacterium that causes diphtheria, is only pathogenic when it is carrying the prophage that has the gene for the production of the diphtheria toxin. Scarlet fever, a possible complication of a streptococcal infection, occurs only when the particular strain of streptococcus is carrying the gene for the erythrogenic scarlet fever toxin on its prophage DNA.

Lysogeny can also give rise to **specialised transduction**, in which bacterial genes are transferred with the phage DNA to another bacterial cell (see Chapter 4). A similar process to lysogeny can occur in animal cells, and may involve the transformation of the animal cell by the incorporation of viral DNA into the host cell genome. This usually results in the production of abnormal or cancerous cells. However, it also has the potential to be used clinically or therapeutically. Research is continuing into virus-mediated gene therapy which would allow the insertion of a desired gene into a cell that has a defective gene. This is discussed further on page 99.

REPLICATION OF ANIMAL VIRUSES

Of more interest to health professionals is the sequence of events that takes place when an animal (human) cell is infected by a virus. This process can be broken down into six steps.

1. **Adsorption**. The first step in viral infection is the attachment of the virion to a specific receptor site on the outside of the host cell. The part of the viral capsid or envelope that binds to the host has a specific chemical structure and is often a glycoprotein spike or other part of the viral antigen.
2. **Penetration**. After the virion has attached to the host cell, the whole virion enters the cell by one of three processes – direct penetration, membrane fusion or phagocytosis (a process in which the host cell membrane engulfs the viral particle). Animal cells are so much larger than viruses that there is plenty of room for the whole virion to enter.
3. **Uncoating**. The virus is then dismantled, the envelope and capsid removed and broken down into their component amino acids, and the nucleic acid is released into the cytoplasm.

Adsorption, penetration and uncoating occur very rapidly, usually taking only a few minutes.

4. **Synthesis**. The nucleic acid is then copied many times, the viral genes directing the synthesis of viral messenger RNA and new viral capsid proteins and enzymes. The process of nucleic acid replication and protein synthesis differs for different viruses, depending on the type of nucleic acid involved – single- or double-stranded RNA or DNA (see below).
5. **Assembly**. The viral nucleic acid and the newly synthesised capsomeres are assembled in either the nucleus (for DNA viruses) or the cytoplasm (RNA viruses) of the cell.
6. **Release**. Naked viruses are released from the host cell, usually resulting in cell lysis and death. Enveloped viruses 'bud' out through the cell membrane, acquiring their envelope from the host cell membrane which has been modified by the insertion of viral glycoproteins (see Figure 5.4).

The complete cycle may occupy several hours.

When many viral particles are synthesised and released at once, lysis and death of the host cell inevitably occurs. Sometimes, virus formation is slower and the new virions are released continuously. This does not necessarily cause the immediate death of the cell.

SYNTHESIS OF VIRAL PARTICLES

Synthesis of new viral components takes place in the nucleus and cytoplasm of the host cell. The actual method

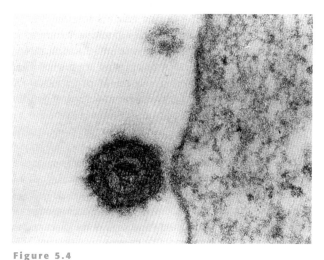

Figure 5.4

Herpes budding out of cell

of viral replication varies, depending on whether the viral nucleic acid is RNA or DNA, and whether it is single- or double-stranded. The replication of double-stranded DNA (dsDNA) viruses essentially follows the usual pathways for nucleic acid and protein synthesis, the host cell providing most of the necessary enzymes. The viral DNA is first integrated into the host cell genome and then directs the synthesis of viral messenger RNA and proteins and the assembly of the viral components into new viral particles. This process is illustrated in Figure 5.5 for a DNA-containing virus.

The details of replication of the different RNA viruses are quite complex. Most RNA viruses contain single strands of RNA (ssRNA) which are described as either positive or negative sense strands. The single RNA strands synthesise new viral RNA and viral protein via a series of steps involving positive and negative sense RNA strands. Positive (+) sense strands can function directly as messenger RNA (i.e. as a template for protein synthesis). The viruses containing double-stranded RNA (dsRNA) first synthesise viral messenger RNA which then directs the synthesis of the viral enzymes needed to make new dsRNA for assembly into new viral particles.

A completely different pathway of synthesis occurs in an important family of single-stranded RNA viruses known as **retroviruses**. Replication in these viruses initially involves a reverse process whereby viral DNA is first synthesised from the single-stranded viral RNA, using a viral enzyme called **reverse transcriptase**. The viral DNA is then transcribed into viral messenger RNA, protein and new viral RNA. A number of very important pathogens belong to this group, including the human immunodeficiency virus, HIV. Figure 5.6 illustrates the steps involved in the synthesis of a retrovirus.

Figure 5.7 shows a human T cell under attack by the AIDS virus.

An understanding of the different pathways of viral synthesis allows scientists to identify critical steps that could be the target for antiviral drugs (see below and Chapter 12).

Pathogenesis of viral infections in humans

It is important that health professionals understand the characteristics of viral infection in humans and the outcome for the host in order to appreciate the implications for transmission, treatment and prevention of viral disease. A knowledge of the methods of viral replication and the course of viral diseases can aid in the development

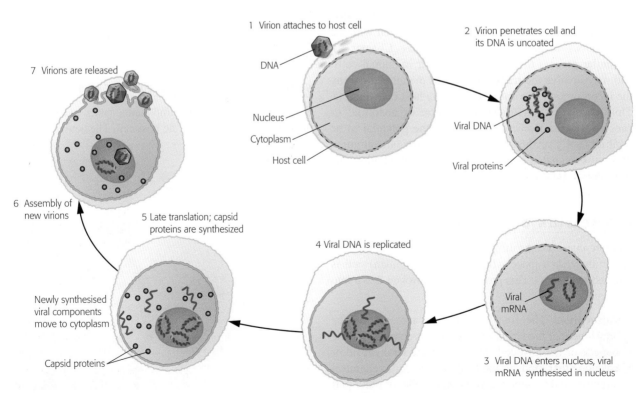

Figure 5.5

Multiplication of a DNA-containing virus

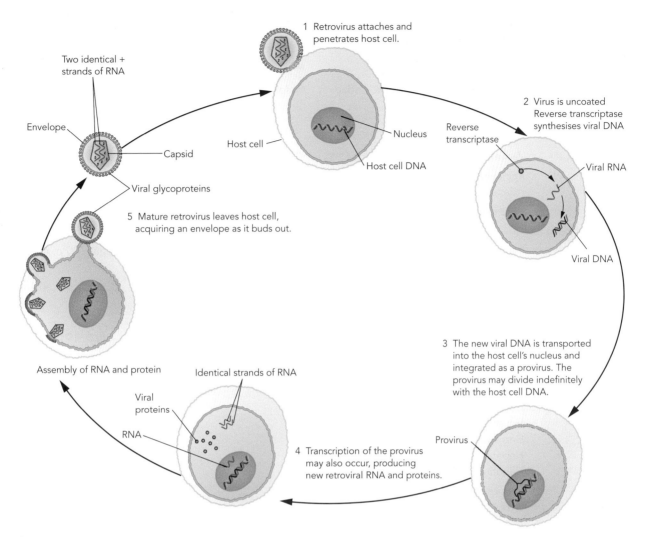

1 Retrovirus attaches and penetrates host cell.

Two identical + strands of RNA

Envelope

Capsid

Host cell

Nucleus

Reverse transcriptase

2 Virus is uncoated
Reverse transcriptase synthesises viral DNA

Viral glycoproteins

Host cell DNA

Viral RNA

Viral DNA

5 Mature retrovirus leaves host cell, acquiring an envelope as it buds out.

Assembly of RNA and protein

Identical strands of RNA

Viral proteins

RNA

4 Transcription of the provirus may also occur, producing new retroviral RNA and proteins.

Provirus

3 The new viral DNA is transported into the host cell's nucleus and integrated as a provirus. The provirus may divide indefinitely with the host cell DNA.

Figure 5.6
Retroviral infection and multiplication

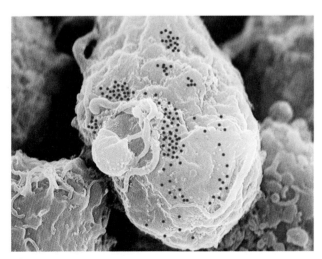

Figure 5.7

Coloured scanning electron micrograph of T-lymphocyte under attack by AIDS virus (blue dots)

of suitable treatments or preventative measures. When a virus infects a cell the response to the infection may vary widely, from no apparent effect to significant cellular damage leading to cell death, hyperplasia or cancer.

Table 5.2 is a list of common viral infections of humans. New viruses are constantly being described so a table such as this requires continual updating. The diseases listed are described in detail in other chapters of this book under the affected body system (see references in table).

For arboviral infections, see Table 5.4.

Viral disease is a result of the viral infection – the signs and symptoms make up a syndrome that is typical of a particular viral infection. The severity of the symptoms and the outcome of the infection may vary and are determined by the type of virus and the susceptibility of the host. Some viruses produce a range of disease symptoms (e.g. measles) and the same apparent disease can be produced by a number of different viruses (e.g. the

Table 5.2

Some common viral infections of humans

DISEASE	VIRUS	FAMILY	MAJOR ORGANS AFFECTED	REFERENCE
Bronchiolitis	Respiratory syncytial virus Human metapneumovirus	Paramyxoviridae	Respiratory tract	Chap. 17 p. 400
Chickenpox	Varicella zoster	Herpes viridae	Generalised symptoms/skin rash	Chap. 16 p. 375
Common cold	Rhinovirus Adenovirus	Picornaviridae Adenoviridae	Respiratory tract	Chap. 17 p. 394
CMV	Cytomegalovirus	Herpes viridae	Generalised/salivary glands	Chap. 19 p. 469
Ebola, Marburg*		Filoviridae	Haemorrhagic	
Encephalitis	Various/some arthropod-borne		Nervous system/brain	Chap. 20 p. 491
Gastroenteritis	Rotavirus Norovirus Enterovirus	Reoviridae Calciviridae Picornaviridae	Gastrointestinal system	Chap. 18 p. 421ff
Glandular fever (infectious mononucleosis)	Epstein-Barr	Herpes viridae	Immune system	Chap. 19 p. 467
Hantavirus	Hantavirus	Bunyaviridae	Respiratory system	
Hepatitis	Hepatitis A Hepatitis B Hepatitis C Hepatitis D Hepatitis E	Picornaviridae Hepadnaviridae Flaviviridae ? Calciviridae	Liver	Chap. 18 p. 436ff
Herpes	Herpes simplex type 1, type 2	Herpes viridae	Skin	Chap. 16 p. 376 Chap. 21 p. 519
HIV/AIDS	Human immunodeficiency virus	Retroviridae	T4 cells of immune system	Chap. 19 p. 459ff
Influenza	Influenza type A, type B Parainfluenza	Orthomyxoviridae Paramyxoviridae	Generalised/respiratory system	Chap. 17 p. 401
Lassa fever *	Lassa	Arenaviridae	Haemorrhagic	
Measles	Rubeola	Paramyxoviridae	Generalised/skin rash	Chap. 16 p. 374
Meningitis	Various		Nervous system/meninges	Chap. 20 p. 490
Mumps	Mumps	Paramyxoviridae	Salivary glands	
Polio	Polio	Picornaviridae	Nervous system	Chap. 20 p. 498
Rabies	Rabies, Lyssa	Rhabdovirus	Nervous system	
Rubella (German measles)	Rubella	Togaviridae	Generalised/skin rash affects foetus	Chap. 16 p. 373
SARS	Coronavirus	Coronaviridae	Severe acute respiratory syndrome	Chap. 17 p. 407
Shingles	Herpes zoster (latent form of varicella zoster)	Herpes viridae	Skin/nervous system	Chap. 16 p. 375
Warts	Papilloma	Papillomaviridae	Skin/mucous membranes	Chap. 16 p. 376
Yellow fever†	Yellow fever	Flaviviridae	Generalised/ liver	Chap. 19 p. 470

* Blood-borne haemorrhagic diseases, not seen in Australia
† Mosquito-borne disease endemic to South America and tropical areas

common cold is caused by adenoviruses, rhinoviruses, parainfluenza viruses, enteroviruses, etc.).

Viral infections can be described as acute, subclinical, latent, chronic (carrier), persistent, slow or oncogenic. The familiar acute, highly contagious viral illness that follows a defined course, is characterised by recognisable signs and symptoms and leads to complete recovery is only one of the outcomes of viral infection. Many viral infections do not produce recognisable symptoms of disease at all and are said to be **subclinical**.

We now look at each of these phenomena in some detail.

ACUTE LYTIC INFECTION

An acute lytic infection is typified by a disease with well-defined, recognisable symptoms – for example, the common cold, mumps or influenza. The virion gains entry to the host, attaches to its specific target cell, enters and takes over the host cell machinery, making many copies of the virus. The release of the new virions causes cell lysis and death. The new viral particles then infect neighbouring cells, producing typical disease symptoms. Eventually, the host immune response is successful in eliminating the invading virus, and immunological memory is established to protect against further infections by the same virus.

For many diseases (e.g. mumps) this acute infection will give rise to long-lasting immunity. However, some viruses, such as those responsible for influenza, have the ability to mutate and alter the structure of their outer envelope or capsid. This means that the antibodies produced against one particular strain of influenza virus will not recognise and be effective against another strain (see Chapter 9 for discussion of antigen-antibody reactions). Exposure to this new or altered strain of influenza virus will *apparently* give rise to the same disease again.

SUBCLINICAL INFECTIONS

Very often a person is infected by a virus but does not exhibit any recognisable clinical signs or symptoms. A general feeling of malaise, slight fever or **lymphadenopathy** ('swollen glands') may be the only signs that the patient is unwell. In this type of infection, the patient recovers, often unaware of having had any disease. Frequently, the only evidence of infection is that an immune response has been provoked, resulting in the production of antibodies and a cellular immune response to the virus. The antibodies can be detected by serological examination of the patient's blood. Depending on the level of antibodies present (the **antibody titre**), the patient may be considered to be immune – that is, protected from future attacks by the same virus.

Rubella (German measles) can be a very mild disease and is often subclinical. However, when this disease occurs during the first trimester of pregnancy it can cause serious congenital abnormalities in the foetus, even though the mother may experience few, if any, symptoms. Similarly, cytomegalovirus infection produces only very mild cold-like symptoms, but can cause serious congenital

defects in a developing foetus. Possible exposure of the mother to these viruses during pregnancy can be determined by measuring the level of recently formed antibodies (IgM) in the mother's serum, although additional tests are needed to clearly define the risks to the unborn baby (see Chapter 9).

Polio is another disease that can occur subclinically as well as in the more acute paralytic form. When the polio virus was first isolated and tests were developed for the detection of antibodies, it was found that a large percentage of the population was carrying antibodies to the virus without any previous history of the disease. It has been suggested that this was most probably the result of a subclinical infection in an earlier childhood exposure.

Other viral diseases that are known to occur subclinically include glandular fever (Epstein-Barr virus) and hepatitis B and C. These diseases can also have serious outcomes.

Persistence of viral infections

Many viral infections are self-limiting – that is, the host immune system overcomes the virus and it is completely eliminated from the body. However, sometimes the virus persists in the human host for long periods. This persistence may have a number of different outcomes, variously described as latent, chronic or slow infections. Oncogenic viruses also persist and transform the host cells into cancer cells.

LATENT VIRAL INFECTIONS

In some cases the virus remains latent (dormant) in some of the host cells and can be reactivated at a later stage, causing a recurrence of the disease. Latent infections are caused by all viruses in the herpes family as well as the human immunodeficiency virus, HIV.

The virus generally produces an initial recognisable disease, followed by apparent recovery. However, instead of the virus being completely cleared from the host by the immune system, some viral particles remain. They often 'hide' in cells that are not the usual target of attack. Reactivation of the virus may occur when the physiological state of the host is altered. This may be due to conditions of physical or psychological stress, immunosuppression or other illnesses.

The most familiar example of a latent infection are the blisters produced by herpes simplex virus (HSV), types 1 and 2. Many patients only ever report one initial attack of herpes. However, others suffer repeated attacks associated with colds ('cold sores', 'fever blisters'), exposure to UV light (sunburn) or other stress factors. The virus has been shown to be dormant in the nerve cells of the sensory ganglia. Other herpes viruses also produce latent infections. These include the varicella zoster virus which is responsible for **varicella** (chickenpox) and **zoster** (shingles). After an attack of chickenpox, the virus remains dormant in the sensory nerve ganglia and may give rise to shingles many years later.

Epstein-Barr virus (EBV), which is responsible for glandular fever, and cytomegalovirus (CMV) can also establish latent infections.

An important characteristic of latent infections is that they tend to be reactivated when the immune system is compromised. This may be a serious complication for elderly patients, for immunodeficient patients or for those receiving immunosuppressive therapy or after transplant surgery. Infections such as shingles (reactivated varicella zoster virus, VZV) and cold sores (reactivated herpes simplex virus, HSV) are common in these patients.

Slow infections

In some types of latent infection, the virus responsible for the disease persists in the host and, many years after the initial infection, symptoms of a new disease occur, usually slowly and over a long period. These symptoms are not the same as the original disease. **Subacute sclerosing panencephalitis** (SSPE) is a rare late complication of measles infection, and usually occurs in teenagers and young adults. It has been attributed to the persistence of the measles virus, which lodges in the brain cells. The disease is characterised by slow (1–2 years), progressive

---

SPOTLIGHT ON
Hepatitis C

On a busy Friday night, the nurse attending a patient who had been admitted to the accident emergency department of a city hospital with a drug overdose suffered a needlestick injury. The patient subsequently tested positive for antibodies to hepatitis C.

Comment

This scenario is one that all health professionals could face. About 80% of people infected with hepatitis C in Australia are injecting drug users. A major route of transmission is the sharing of needles. People who received blood transfusions prior to 1990, when a screening test became available, make up 7–8% of those infected and in most other cases the source of the infection cannot be identified. The term 'epidemic' has been used to describe the occurrence of hepatitis C in Australia, but the epidemic is only real among injecting drug users and other groups who engage in high-risk behaviour. There is a high incidence among prison inmates, linked to needle sharing in injecting drug use and tattoos. Currently, the rate of new notifications is highest in the 20–39 age group with a male:female ratio of 1.7:1.

Hepatitis C is caused by the hepatitis C virus (HCV), which infects the liver, causing progressive damage over 20–30 years. In 10–20% of cases, significant cirrhosis occurs and about 2% of patients develop hepatocellular carcinoma. It is a blood-borne virus and the main route of transmission appears to be through parenteral exposure. Recent studies have shown the risk of sexual transmission is extremely low. An Australian study has shown that the risk of vertical transmission from a viraemic mother to baby is about 6% (compared with 70–85% for hepatitis B).

The disease was originally called 'post-transfusion' hepatitis and later, after tests for hepatitis A and hepatitis B became available, it was referred to as 'nonA, nonB', or NANB, hepatitis. The virus has not been isolated and has not been grown in the laboratory. Molecular biology has been used to develop a diagnostic test to detect antibodies to HCV, and measurements of viral RNA are made to detect the presence of live virus in blood samples and

determine the infectivity of the patient. In Australia, screening of blood for HCV since 1990 has eliminated transmission of the virus by blood transfusion.

Because the screening test has only been available since 1990, the true number of people who are infected is not known. In 75% of cases the infection is asymptomatic and may not be detected until the patient has a routine blood test, or presents with symptoms of liver damage. There are people living in the community who may have been infected many years ago when infection control measures were not as rigorous. Public health programs in many countries involved mass vaccination campaigns in which needles were reused. Others may have acquired the virus by blood transfusion before screening was available, or by medical procedures before the risks of transmission of blood-borne viruses were known.

Some of these people are now presenting with advanced liver disease and they make up a significant percentage of patients requiring liver transplants. Immigrants from countries such as Egypt and Vietnam, which have a high prevalence of hepatitis C, form a large part of this group. There are six main genotypes and numerous subtypes of the virus which occur in different parts of the world, so the origin of the infection can sometimes be determined.

It is estimated that over 75% of high-risk people exposed to large amounts of the hepatitis C virus will develop a chronic infection – that is, they become carriers of the disease. (This compares with 5–10% for hepatitis B). There is a large pool of infected people among injecting drug users and also in the prison population. The risk of transmission in these groups is therefore very high. The main treatment is interferon but it is only effective in about 20% of cases. A combination of ribavirin and interferon gives better results but the treatment is very expensive and there is still only a 35% success rate. Many people with chronic (undiagnosed) infections are not receiving treatment and it is expected there will be a significant increase in the burden of HCV-related liver disease on the health system in the future.

Further data are needed to determine the real risk of sexual and vertical transmission. The search for a vaccine and better methods of treatment is continuing.

mental deterioration and degeneration of the nervous system, and is invariably fatal.

CHRONIC VIRAL INFECTIONS (CARRIER STATE)

An important outcome of viral disease is when the virus remains in the host and gives rise to a continuous low level of viral production and shedding – the carrier state. This can occur after either an acute illness or a subclinical infection. Patients do not have any disease symptoms and are often unaware that they are chronic carriers of the virus and, therefore, infectious to others.

Infection with hepatitis B virus can have a number of outcomes. Exposure to the virus may cause an acute infection, leading either to complete recovery and development of immunity or, occasionally (1–2%), to a fulminant infection resulting in death. In most cases it results in a mild or subclinical disease that gives rise to a chronic carrier state in 5–10% of patients. Hepatitis B can also be acquired by vertical transmission from a carrier mother to her baby. The baby may not exhibit any symptoms of hepatitis, but has an 80–95% risk of becoming a carrier. Serological testing for the presence of the various hepatitis B antigens and antibodies is used to establish the infectious status of mother and baby. (See Chapter 18 for a discussion of hepatitis and the significance of the presence of the various viral antigens.)

Chronic active hepatitis B infection can cause long-term liver damage, **cirrhosis**, and in some cases **hepatocellular carcinoma**.

Hepatitis C is another virus that can persist as a chronic infection. A test for hepatitis C has only been available since 1990 and there is still much to be learnt about this virus. However, it is estimated that more than 75% of people who contract this virus become carriers. Hepatitis C also has long-term sequelae and can lead to liver cancer (see Spotlight box, page 96).

Human immunodeficiency virus (HIV) is the primary cause of AIDS (**A**cquired **I**mmune **D**eficiency **S**ydnrome). It is described as a chronic infection because the virus is considered to be transmissible throughout the illness.

ONCOGENIC VIRUSES

A number of viruses have been shown to cause tumours in animals and to be able to transform human cells into cancer cells in tissue culture. These viruses are termed **oncogenic**. Cancer cells are cells that have lost control of normal regulation of growth processes. One of the most important of these regulatory mechanisms is **contact inhibition**. Transformed cells replicate in an uncontrolled way, piling up on top of each other into a mass of cells (tumour). A number of agents, including mutagenic chemicals, ionising radiation and certain viruses, have been shown to be able to alter cellular DNA in such a way that the cell loses contact inhibition and multiplies uncontrollably. This phenomenon is called **neoplasia** and the tumour formed is a **neoplasm**. There are two ways in which it is thought that a virus can alter normal cells:

1. the oncogenic virus introduces a new 'transforming' gene into the cell; or
2. the virus induces or alters the expression of a pre-existing cellular gene (a 'proto' oncogene).

In both cases the DNA from the oncogenic virus is integrated into the host cell genome and replicates with the host cell DNA in a similar manner to lysogeny in bacteria.

Various types of cancers have been shown to be associated with a previous or current viral infection. They are listed in Table 5.3 on page 98.

There is a large amount of evidence linking certain types of papilloma virus to the occurrence of cervical cancer. Early changes in cervical cells can be detected by a Pap smear (see Spotlight box, page 98).

Other important oncogenic viruses are hepatitis B, hepatitis C, human herpes virus 8 (HHV8), human T cell lymphotrophic virus (HTLV1) and Epstein-Barr virus (EBV).

HOST RESPONSE TO VIRAL INFECTION

The human body has a complex system of non-specific and specific responses to invasion by foreign organisms. This is described in detail in Chapter 9.

The response to infection by a virus depends on the type of virus and the susceptibility of the host. After gaining entry to the body the virus is usually spread via the bloodstream or lymphatic system. In the early stages, large numbers of viral particles are present in the bloodstream – a state known as **viraemia**. Virions may be present in plasma or associated with a particular cell type.

Viral infection provokes several kinds of response by the host's immune system. The first is the production and release of interferon from infected cells. There are three different classes of interferons (α, β and γ), specific for the cells that produce them but not for virus type. They are called **cytokines** (proteins which modulate the immune response). The interferon binds to receptors on uninfected cells to prevent further viral replication.

The immune response also includes:

- activation of T cells, which identify and destroy infected cells
- production of lymphokines and other cytokines
- activation of B lymphocytes and the production of antibodies, which inactivate free viral particles
- production of memory cells to protect against new infection (see Chapter 9).

The activation of the immune system and the production of interferon and cytokines are responsible for many of the symptoms associated with viral infections – for example, swollen glands (lymphadenopathy), malaise, headache and myalgia. Treatment of most viral infections is aimed at relieving the symptoms. Bed rest and administration of analgesics and antipyretics are the main methods available. Recovery from the disease depends largely on the ability of the host's immune system to recognise the

Table 5.3

Human cancers related to viral infections

CANCER	VIRUS	FAMILY	GENOME
Adult T cell leukaemia	HTLV-I	Retroviridae	ssRNA
Skin carcinomas;	Papilloma, HPV 5,	Papillomaviridae	DNA
genital carcinomas	HPV 16,18	Papillomaviridae	DNA
Kaposi's sarcoma	HHV 8	Herpes viridae	DNA
Hepatocellular carcinoma	Hepatitis B	Hepadnaviridae	DNA
	Hepatitis C	Flaviviridae	RNA
Nasopharyngeal carcinoma	Epstein-Barr	Herpes viridae	DNA
Burkitt's lymphoma	Epstein-Barr	Herpes viridae	DNA

SPOTLIGHT ON

Cervical cancer

Mrs Y, a 32-year-old mother of two children, was admitted to hospital with advanced cervical carcinoma. Although she had been sexually active since she was 20, she had never had a Pap smear. A hysterectomy was performed to remove the diseased uterus, followed by radiation treatment and chemotherapy. However, the cancer had already spread through her body and she died 18 months later.

Comment

In Australia there is an average of 1000 new cases of cervical cancer and 350 deaths each year. More than 80% of cases are associated with a previous infection by the human papilloma virus (HPV), the cause of genital warts. All women who have ever been sexually active are at risk of developing cervical cancer, even if they have never suffered from genital warts. The risk is highest in women with multiple partners who do not use protection such as condoms or if they have other sexually transmitted infections.

There are more than 100 different types of human papilloma viruses that attack skin and mucosal cells. About 30 types have been associated with genital infections. Of these, types 16 and 18 are most frequently associated with abnormal Pap smears. Type 16 is most commonly associated with cancer in Australia and type 18 has been shown to have the highest risk of recurrence. Other types that have been implicated in various parts of the world are types 31, 33, 35, 39, 45, 51, 52 and 56.

HPV induces characteristic changes in the epithelial cells of the cervix. These can be detected by microscopic examination of a smear of cells obtained from the cervix (the Papanicolaou test – Pap test), and appear even before the first evidence of malignancy.

The changes to the epithelial cells progress through stages described as cervical intraepithelial neoplasias (CIN) to carcinoma in situ (CIS), which is a precancerous condition and can lead to invasive squamous cell carcinoma. The stages are described as:

CIN I   minor dysplasia
CIN II   moderate dysplasia
CIN III severe dysplasia – carcinoma in situ (CIS).

If abnormal cells are detected by a Pap smear, the patient is referred for colposcopy. This involves examination of the cervix after a painless application of 3% acetic acid (vinegar). The lesion appears as a flat white plaque and can be removed by laser treatment. If detected early, the treatment is successful, but the woman is advised to have regular follow-up Pap smears. If the disease has progressed further, a cone biopsy can be performed. Early treatment of cervical cancer is very successful and in all countries where routine Pap smears are available the mortality from the disease has been reduced.

The Pap test is not always accurate and incorrect results may sometimes occur because of poor sampling or from laboratory error. Approximately 20% of tests may return false negative results. However, the benefit of regular screening far outweighs problems with diagnosis. Recently, some laboratories have introduced computerised scanning of microscope slides to improve the accuracy of diagnosis. Women are advised to have a Pap test at least every two years, or more frequently if there are abnormal symptoms, as the disease can be cured if detected early. Women who live in rural and remote areas or who are immigrants to Australia are less likely to be aware of, or to comply with, screening programs.

Some states have established a central register to encourage women to return for regular checkups. Research is continuing into the development of a vaccine against HPV.

foreign invader and produce antibodies and T cells to combat it.

The age of the patient and the status of the immune system are important determinants of the patient's susceptibility to viral infections. It is well known that the immune system matures in the first year of life and that it is less effective in the aged. On the other hand, there seems to be an age-related difference in susceptibility to some viral infections. The so-called childhood diseases, such as mumps and chickenpox, are usually much more severe in adults.

During pregnancy, the mother's immune system is also somewhat compromised to accommodate the foetus. This may explain the ability of viruses such as rubella and cytomegalovirus to cross the placenta and cause congenital defects. A very high level of maternal mortality is associated with hepatitis E infection in pregnancy.

Viral evasion mechanisms

Viruses are true parasites and need to establish a balance with their host and its immune system or they would not survive. They use various strategies to escape detection and to avoid killing their host, thus ensuring their own survival. These include 'hiding' in infected cells, so that the viral antigen is not expressed on the outside of the infected cell and is thus protected from attack by cytotoxic T cells.

Some viruses continually change their appearance (outer structure) so that previously formed antibodies are no longer effective. Other viruses become latent (e.g. the herpes zoster virus persists in nerve cells) and manipulate the host immune system. HIV attacks and destroys the T cells of the cell-mediated immune system.

Transmission of viral diseases

Effective prevention and control of viral diseases depends on an understanding of the mechanisms of transmission of these infectious agents. Infections are transmitted from one host to another when complete viral particles (virions), shed by the infected host, reach a susceptible host. Most viruses do not survive for long periods outside living cells, so transmission usually requires direct transfer of body fluids or tissues, close contact between hosts, or transmission via an insect vector.

The rate and number of virus particles being shed varies during the course of the infection. Very often virus production and shedding is highest just before recognisable clinical symptoms develop (the **prodromal phase**). This fact helps to explain the occurrence of epidemics, since transmission can take place before patients are aware they have the disease (e.g. chickenpox outbreaks in schools).

AIRBORNE TRANSMISSION

Viruses are shed mainly from the area of the body where the infection is localised. Thus, infection of the mucosal cells of the upper respiratory tract by cold viruses (rhinoviruses, coronaviruses) results in virions being shed in aerosol droplets when the patient coughs or sneezes. These viruses do not survive for long outside the body. Other viruses that enter via the respiratory route are mainly shed in the same way.

Viral infections, such as chickenpox and herpes, that produce pustules or vesicles on the skin also shed virions into the air from these lesions. Transmission of herpes is thought to mainly occur when visible vesicles are present, although there is some evidence that, in genital herpes, virus shedding can occur when there are no apparent symptoms.

FAECAL-ORAL TRANSMISSION

Microorganisms that cause gastrointestinal infections are usually shed in the faeces. Many viruses are transmitted by faecal contamination of food or water – for example, hepatitis A, rotavirus and enteroviruses. Among these, rotavirus is of special concern as it can cause rapid, severe dehydration and death in infants. Special care must be taken to prevent transmission of rotavirus among babies and small children in hospitals and child-care centres. A vaccine for rotavirus that was developed has been withdrawn due to suspected side effects.

Outbreaks of food poisoning are often caused by noroviruses (previously called Norwalk-like viruses) (see Chapter 18, page 427). They are transmitted by faecal-oral contact and epidemics occur because they can easily be spread in aerosols. Personal hygiene (handwashing) is most important to prevent the spread of the virus. Symptoms may persist for up to three days and oral rehydration is the main treatment. Exposure to noroviruses does not always give protection against reinfection as different strains circulate at different times.

The polio virus (another enterovirus) is also shed in faeces. A worldwide vaccination campaign has eradicated polio from many parts of the world. Viruses transmitted by the faecal-oral route are still a cause for concern in areas where sanitation is poor and they remain a major cause of death in developing countries.

TRANSMISSION IN BODY FLUIDS

In recent years considerable attention has focused on viruses that can be transmitted in blood or other body substances. These include hepatitis B virus (HBV) and hepatitis C virus (HCV), and human immunodeficiency virus (HIV). The discovery in the 1980s of a previously unknown and potentially fatal virus (HIV) drew attention to the possible presence of other unidentified viruses in body substances. A system of infection control procedures designed to minimise the risks of transmission of viral infections has been developed to prevent the spread of these viruses in hospitals and health-care facilities (see Chapter 13).

Occasionally, viruses can be transmitted by organ transplantation if screening procedures are not used on the donor organs.

TRANSMISSION BY VECTORS

An important method of transmission for some viruses is by **arthropod vectors** – that is, by insects and other arthropods which carry the virus from an infected host to a susceptible human. These viruses are called **arboviruses** (**ar**thropod-**bo**rne). Transmission by arthropods requires the ingestion of the virus from an infected human or animal reservoir while the insect is feeding. The virus replicates in the gut of the insect vector, spreads to the salivary glands and is injected into a susceptible host during the next blood meal. The replicative phase may take several days and the rate is affected by the ambient temperature.

Approximately 80 arboviruses are known that are capable of infecting humans, although only a limited number occurs in Australia. Most arboviruses are maintained in nature in animal hosts that usually sustain a subclinical infection and develop immunity. One of the most common arthropod vectors is the mosquito, and specific breeds of mosquito act as vectors for different viruses. An outbreak of a viral disease can occur if there is a pool of infected hosts present in the community, together with favourable breeding conditions for the particular type of mosquito. Control is best achieved by mosquito eradication programs.

Some important viral diseases that are endemic to Australia and transmitted by mosquitoes include Ross River fever, Murray Valley encephalitis and dengue fever. Of these, Ross River fever is the most widespread and the mosquito vector (*Aedes* species) is found throughout the eastern states. Other serious arboviral diseases found outside Australia are yellow fever, Lassa fever and Japanese encephalitis.

Table 5.4 lists the major arboviral infections occurring in Australia see also Spotlight box, page 336.

FOETAL AND NEONATAL TRANSMISSION

Viral infections in the mother can have serious repercussions for the foetus or neonate. These include vertical transmission of infection to the neonate, congenital effects that are present at birth, teratogenic (mutational) effects and the acquisition of viral diseases during birth.

Teratogenic effects

Several viruses have been proven to have serious effects on the unborn foetus. One of the earliest to be recognised was the effect of rubella (German measles) virus on the foetus during the first trimester of pregnancy. The connection was first observed in Sydney in 1941, when a severe epidemic of German measles was followed by a very high incidence of congenital abnormalities. These included congenital heart defects, total or partial blindness, and growth or mental retardation. Work carried out by Sir Norman Gregg at the Royal Alexandra Hospital for Children in Camperdown, Sydney, correctly identified the rubella virus as the causative agent. A vaccine to prevent rubella is now available and is given routinely in combination with measles and mumps vaccine (MMR) to all children (male and female) at 12 months of age, and again at 4 years of age. Some recent cases of congenital rubella in Australia have occurred mainly in unvaccinated immigrant women.

Another virus that has been shown to cross the placenta and cause congenital abnormalities is cytomegalovirus, CMV. The extent of damage caused by CMV depends on the state of gestation at which infection occurs and is worse if the mother acquires the infection for the first time during pregnancy. *In utero* infections may result in death or premature birth. Growth retardation and developmental malformations such as congenital heart defects, cataracts, deafness and central nervous system defects may also result. No vaccine is available for CMV. Despite a high level of immunity in the community from previous, mainly subclinical, exposure, CMV remains the most common cause of congenital malformations in Australia and other developed countries.

Recent studies have shown that there is also a slightly increased risk of congenital defects if the mother acquires chickenpox during pregnancy. Another viral infection, parvovirus B19, is generally a mild disease but there is a slight risk of damage to the foetus if contracted during the first half of pregnancy. Viral infection during pregnancy is suspected of being associated with the occurrence of other birth defects, and of causing severe foetal damage leading to abortion. However, not enough data are avail-

---

Table 5.4
Major arboviral infections in Australia

FAMILY	VIRUS	MOSQUITO VECTOR	REFERENCE	
Flaviviridae	Murray Valley encephalitis (MVE)	*Culex annulirostris*	Chapter 20	p. 491
	Kunjin (KUN)	*Culex annulirostris*	Chapter 20	p. 491
	Dengue	*Aedes aegypti*	Chapter 19	p. 467
Togaviridae (Alphavirus)	Ross River (RR)	25 species including *Aedes vigilax* and *Aedes camptorynchus*	Chapter 19	p. 466
	Barmah Forest (BAR)	*Culex annulirostris*	Chapter 19	p. 466
	Sindbis (SIN)	*Culex annulirostis* *Aedes normanensis*		

able at present to link specific viruses with specific outcomes.

Vertical transmission of infection to the neonate

The blood-borne viruses, hepatitis B, HIV and, to a lesser extent, hepatitis C, can be transmitted vertically to the neonate.

If the mother is infected with hepatitis B (HBV), there is a significant risk of the infection being passed on to the baby. It is not certain whether the virus crosses the placenta during the last few weeks of pregnancy, or whether the virus is acquired by the neonate when blood from mother and baby mix at the time of delivery. Probably both situations occur. If there is no intervention, the baby has a 70–85% risk of being infected and this often leads to a chronic infection. In Australia, babies born to mothers who are known hepatitis B carriers are given anti-hepatitis B immunoglobulin antibodies at birth. The hepatitis B antibodies neutralise any live virus particles transmitted at, or just prior to, birth. The baby is then started on a course of hepatitis B vaccination to prevent development of the disease by future exposure to the maternal carrier. Usually breast feeding is not recommended in this situation. Babies treated this way have a very good chance of not acquiring hepatitis B, and of not suffering any ill effects. Since 2001, all babies born in Australia have been given free hepatitis B vaccination, beginning at birth.

Babies born to HIV-positive mothers are usually antibody-positive at birth because they are carrying IgG antibodies which have been transferred across the placenta from the mother. It will be 6–12 months before the maternal antibodies disappear from the neonate and it is therefore not possible, during this period, to test specifically for neonatal antibodies to find out whether the baby is infected with the virus. Tests for the virus itself are useful in detecting HIV in the baby, but may not be conclusive as the virus may be 'hiding' inside a white blood cell or lymph node, rather than being free in the bloodstream. Breast feeding by HIV-infected mothers is usually not recommended.

Present data indicate that the risk of vertical mother-to-baby transmission in Western countries is less than 2% if mothers are treated with combination (three-drug) antiviral therapy during pregnancy, particularly just before birth (parturition). The risk is influenced by the stage of illness and level of viraemia in the mother. Unfortunately, drug treatment is expensive and not readily available in developing countries where there has been an explosion of HIV infection in the heterosexual community and as many as 50% of babies born to HIV-positive mothers are infected.

The risk of transmission for hepatitis C is very low although additional data are still being collected.

Viral diseases acquired at birth

Viruses acquired during the birth process may also pose a serious risk to the neonate. The most serious of these is herpes simplex. If the mother has an active genital herpes infection at the time of birth, the baby may acquire the virus during passage through the birth canal. Usually the eyes are infected first, but in severe cases **herpes encephalopathy**, viral infection of the brain, may result. This can be fatal. If the mother has had a long-established genital herpes infection, the baby will already have maternal IgG antibodies that will provide some protection. The greatest risk to the neonate is from a recently acquired active maternal infection. In such cases, lower segment caesarean section (LSCS) is often performed to avoid exposure of the baby to the virus during passage through the birth canal. Infected babies are treated with intravenous aciclovir, but relapse can occur even after successful treatment.

Inactivation of viruses

There is great variability in the length of time that a virus particle (virion) can survive outside the host cell, as well as in the range of physical and chemical conditions it can withstand. In order to prevent transmission of viral infections it is necessary to be familiar with methods that can be used to inactivate them.

- Most viruses are destroyed by heating at 60°C for 30 minutes although some, such as the hepatitis B and papova viruses, can withstand much higher temperatures. Many viruses can survive for several days in the cold (4°C).
- Some viruses are stable in the presence of salt solutions and buffers, which means that the virus can persist in food or body substances for significant periods of time. Viruses are usually stable at neutral pH (pH 5–9) but most are destroyed by alkaline conditions. Some viruses, like the enteroviruses, are resistant to acid pH, which allows them to survive the acidity of the stomach.
- Disinfectants such as quaternary ammonium salts, organic iodine compounds and alcohols are not very effective against viruses. Higher concentrations of chlorine are needed to kill viruses than are required to kill bacteria. Treatment of viruses with the chemical, formaldehyde, has been used in the preparation of some viral vaccines, such as the Salk polio vaccine, as the antigenic properties of the capsid proteins are retained but the virus is no longer infective.

Methods of sterilisation and disinfection are described in Chapter 11.

Diagnosis of viral infections

Most viral infections are diagnosed by signs and symptoms. Very often, a general feeling of malaise and slight fever is suddenly explained when a distinctive rash appears (e.g. chickenpox). Usually, by the time these symptoms appear in an acute infection, the body's immune system has already responded. Treatment of the patient is therefore largely symptomatic.

Sometimes, however, it is important to have an accurate diagnosis as early as possible. It may be necessary to determine the level of infectivity of the patient and the consequent risk of transmission to other patients. Blood samples or specimens from the affected tissues of the patient are taken, and various methods are used to detect and identify the virus. Significant developments in the diagnosis of viral infections have occurred in recent years, due to the development of techniques for nucleic acid amplification and identification. These are discussed in detail in Chapter 15.

A brief overview of the use of each technique is given here.

IMMUNOFLUORESCENCE

If large numbers of viral particles are present in the specimen, they can often be detected by reaction with a fluorescent labelled antibody, followed by observation with a fluorescence microscope (see Figure 5.8). This method can give a quick definitive answer in 2–3 hours, but is limited to viruses for which appropriate labelled antibodies are commercially available.

NUCLEIC ACID ANALYSIS

Tests for the presence of live viruses in serum or tissue may require the use of nucleic acid amplification and detection techniques (e.g. PCR) and DNA or RNA typing. The use of DNA or RNA probes (i.e. specific nucleotide sequences) can detect viral nucleic acid sequences which correspond to the presence of viral particles in clinical specimens. For example, probes for the detection of the various types of human papilloma virus in cervical cells are available commercially. The use of these probes can confirm the presence or absence of the viral types (16,18) linked to cervical cancer in abnormal Pap smears. Patients who test positive for hepatitis C antibodies can be tested for HCV-RNA to find out whether virus is present and to determine their level of infectivity.

SEROLOGY

Serology is the detection of viral antigens, and antibodies to those antigens, in body tissues. It requires the presence of a measurable level of antigen or antibody in serum. A blood sample is taken from the patient and tested for the presence of antibodies to the suspected virus. The presence of specific IgM antibodies generally indicates a recent infection, although in some cases (e.g. CMV) they can persist for months to years in serum. IgG antibodies indicate that the infection occurred at an earlier time. The method is limited by the time (several days) required after infection for the body to mount an immune response and produce detectable antibodies. It is useful mainly for the determination of a patient's immune status, in screening blood and tissue products and in epidemiological studies. The most common method involves the use of EIA (enzyme immunoassay), an automated colour reaction.

CELL CULTURE

Culture of viruses in the laboratory is more difficult, expensive and time-consuming than the culture of bacteria, because viruses must be grown inside a living cell. When insufficient virus particles are present in the specimen to detect by immunofluorescence, a sample is usually inoculated into a cell culture and grown for 2–5 days. The cells are then observed for **cytopathic effects (CPE)** (see Figure 5.9). This method is slow and mainly used now for confirmation of other test results, for research or if other identification methods have not been successful.

The cell culture can also be tested for the presence of a specific virus by immunological methods and molecular methods (see Chapter 15). These include the direct enzyme-linked immunosorbent assay (**ELISA**), which

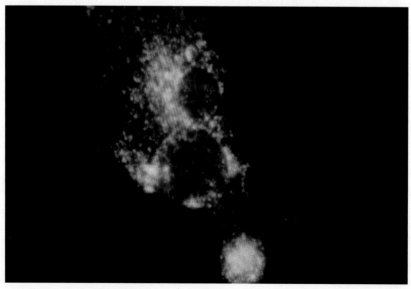

Figure 5.8

Detection of virus particles by immunofluorescence

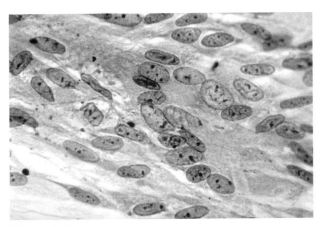

Figure 5.9
Cytopathic effects of viral infections in cell culture
This photomicrograph reveals the presence of multinucleated giant cells along with intranuclear inclusions in cell cultures inoculated with varicella virus. Magnified 500×.

produces colour reactions linked to antibody-antigen reactions, and the immunofluorescent antibody method described above.

Growth of viruses in the laboratory

Viruses can only replicate (grow) inside a living cell. This characteristic places severe limitations on the methods that can be used to cultivate viruses. In general, viruses are grown in the laboratory for one of the following reasons:

- diagnosis of infection
- research
- preparation of a vaccine.

The actual method employed depends on the number of viral particles required and the availability of suitable cell cultures. Early attempts to grow viruses relied on the use of animals or embryonated eggs. The inoculation of viral specimens into live animals is costly and in many cases inconclusive. It is used mainly for the primary isolation of 'new' viruses or for studies of *in vivo* pathogenesis or oncogenesis.

Growth of viruses in embryonated eggs is a convenient and cheap alternative to whole-animal experiments for viruses such as influenza. Several different membranes in the egg are able to support the growth of viruses. The effects of viral infection are measured by death of the embryo or production of typical lesions or other damage. Early vaccine preparations were made from viruses harvested from egg cultures. However, there were problems associated with this method as the vaccine sometimes contained residual egg proteins which provoked an allergic response in some individuals. Most viral cultures are now carried out using the techniques of cell culture (tissue culture). Some vaccines (e.g. hepatitis B) are produced by genetic engineering (see page 76).

Cell cultures are preparations of animal (usually human) cells grown in a special cell-culture medium under strictly controlled aseptic conditions. The cells adhere to the walls of the flask and spread out to form a confluent monolayer. Viral specimens are inoculated into the culture and the effect of the virus on the host cell can be observed microscopically. The changes that occur in infected cells are called **cytopathic effects** and are usually typical of the infecting virus. These effects include:

- production of 'inclusion bodies' – granules in the cytoplasm of the infected cell
- fusion of several cells, forming giant, multi-nucleated or 'syncytial' cells
- transformation of the cell into a spindle-shaped cell that does not exhibit contact inhibition
- cell death.

Cell culture is the main method used in specialist viral laboratories. The cells are grown in special culture flasks, and may also be grown in small volumes in the wells of microtitre plates. Different dilutions of the virus preparation are inoculated into the wells to observe the cytopathic effects produced by the virus infection and to quantify the amount of virus present (see Figure 5.9 and Chapter 15). After the virus has been allowed to multiply in the cells, it may also be further identified by the ELISA test or by reaction with specific fluorescent antibodies, as described above.

Treatment and prevention of viral infections

Viral infections provoke a number of responses in the host which are usually treated symptomatically – bed rest, fluids, analgesics. There are very few effective antiviral drugs available, and they are of most use in chronic infections.

ANTIVIRAL DRUGS

An understanding of the methods of viral replication is important in order to appreciate the difficulties associated with finding suitable antiviral drugs. One of the basic requirements for a safe, effective drug is **selective toxicity** – that is, the ability to kill the pathogen without harming the host cell. Since viruses use the host cell machinery to replicate, any drug that inhibits or interferes with viral multiplication is also likely to have an adverse effect on the host cell. Most drugs that interfere with viral replication are too toxic to be used therapeutically. It is therefore necessary to identify steps in the replicative process that are unique to the virus, or to identify and target one of the few virus-specific enzyme reactions. This is why antibacterial antibiotics are not effective against viruses.

A limited number of antiviral drugs has been developed for herpes viruses, influenza viruses, HIV and hepatitis C.

At present, the most successful antiviral drugs are those that are analogues of the various nucleotide bases found in viral DNA – that is, they have a structure that is similar, but not identical, to the naturally occurring base. They can be incorporated by the viral enzymes into viral DNA, but the DNA is inactive and cannot be replicated. Other possible antiviral targets include the attachment site of the virus to the host cell the translation of viral mRNA to viral proteins, and assembly and release of new virions.

Zidovudine (AZT), an analogue of thymine, was one of the first nucleotide analogues to be used; it is incorporated into the DNA of the AIDS virus by an enzyme unique to retroviruses, called **reverse transcriptase**. This enzyme is used by the virus to synthesise DNA from RNA. Incorporation of the analogue into the viral DNA gives rise to an inactive DNA which cannot be replicated and so prevents further viral replication. However, although zidovudine is readily incorporated into viral DNA by reverse transcriptase, it is also incorporated to some extent by DNA polymerase into normal cell DNA, causing severe side effects in the host, such as bone marrow depression. Other nucleotide analogues have also been used successfully.

Currently, the best results are being obtained with combination therapy using protease inhibitors as well as nucleotide analogues. This helps to minimise the problems of development of drug resistance.

Another useful drug is **aciclovir**, an analogue of guanosine. This compound is phosphorylated by thymidine kinase, an enzyme present only in herpes viruses, to produce an inactive nucleotide triphosphate that, when incorporated into viral DNA, interferes with DNA replication. Aciclovir has been used successfully for the treatment of a number of infections caused by the herpes family of viruses, including shingles and genital herpes.

Interferons are naturally occurring antiviral proteins that are produced by animal (host) cells in response to viral infection. There are several different interferons, commonly grouped into three classes: alpha interferon (α-IFN), beta interferon (β-IFN) and gamma interferon (γ-IFN). They appear to act by stimulating the synthesis of antiviral proteins which block the translation of viral messenger RNA into viral protein, thus preventing the further production and spread of virus after the initial infection has occurred. Interferons are host-cell specific, not virus-specific. There are, however, serious limitations in their therapeutic use since they have a very short half-life in the human body, and a number of toxic side effects. They have been used with some success in the treatment of chronic viral infections such as hairy cell leukaemia, hepatitis B and hepatitis C. Combination therapy of interferon with ribavirin is being used with more success.

A major breakthrough in the development of antiviral drugs was the synthesis of compounds that specifically inhibit the neuraminidase enzyme of the influenza virus. This enzyme is involved in the release of new viral particles from infected cells. Two drugs are approved in Australia – **zanamivir**, which is administered by inhalation, and **oseltamavir**, which is taken orally. When given within the first 48 hours, use of these drugs can reduce the duration of the illness by 1–2 days.

Antiviral drugs are discussed in more detail in Chapter 12.

VACCINATION

The observation by Edward Jenner in the 18th century that milkmaids who had recovered from cowpox did not usually contract smallpox laid the basis for our modern vaccination programs. Vaccination (or immunisation) is the major weapon available against viral disease, and is the means whereby smallpox has been eradicated worldwide.

Vaccination involves the exposure of a person to a modified pathogen in order to elicit an immune response without causing the disease. The aim is to produce antibodies and B lymphocyte and T lymphocyte memory cells specific to the pathogen, without producing any clinical symptoms of disease. These antibodies and memory cells protect the patient against subsequent exposure to the virulent form of the disease-causing agent. The mechanism of the immune response is discussed in Chapter 9.

It has been possible to derive attenuated (weakened) forms of many viruses for use in vaccines. Other vaccines consist of killed or inactivated viral preparations which retain their antigenic properties; that is, they are still able to stimulate an immune response. Recent developments in genetic engineering have seen the production of vaccines consisting of fragments of the virus produced by cloning a part of the viral DNA in a yeast or bacterial cell. Hepatitis B vaccine is one example of this type of vaccine. One of the major advantages (apart from the ease of production) is that there is no risk of causing the actual disease since the vaccine consists of only part of the viral coat.

Prevention of viral disease by mass immunisation campaigns is an important aspect of primary health care. Table 5.5 lists the viral diseases for which vaccines are currently available. Because the ability of the influenza virus to mutate the composition of the influenza vaccine has to be modified each season to provide adequate protection against the strains of the virus circulating in the community. Figure 5.10 illustrates the dramatic fall in the incidence of some important diseases since the introduction of vaccines.

It is theoretically possible to eradicate viral diseases such as measles and polio, for which humans are the only reservoir, and which are caused by viruses that do not survive for long periods outside the human body, by effective vaccination campaigns. Smallpox has officially been eradicated worldwide. Polio has been eradicated from America and the Western Pacific region, which includes Australia (see Spotlight box, page 499). The campaign against measles has not been as successful, due partly to poor compliance with vaccination programs (see Chapter 14).

Future directions in virus research

It has become apparent in recent years that many viruses are yet to be discovered. Some of these may be responsible for presently unexplained illnesses. People in Africa were dying from 'wasting disease' long before HIV was identified as its cause, and 'post-transfusion hepatitis' was

Table 5.5

Viral diseases for which vaccines are available

DISEASE	RECOMMENDED SCHEDULE IN AUSTRALIA
Chickenpox	Recommended for health-care workers and at risk individuals.
Hepatitis A	Three doses: two 1 month apart, and a booster at any age.
Hepatitis B	Three doses: 1, 2, 6 months apart, can be given at any age. Now included in childhood immunisation schedule at birth, 2, 4, 6, and 12 months with a booster at 10–13 years.
Influenza	Different vaccine produced each year for prevalent strain. Recommended for elderly and 'at risk' patients.
Measles	MMR: two doses, 12 months, 4 years.
Mumps	MMR: two doses, 12 months, 4 years.
Rubella	MMR: two doses, 12 months, 4 years. Booster may be required before becoming pregnant. Antibody titre should be checked.
Polio	Sabin oral vaccine (OPV) or Salk IPV: 2, 4, 6 months; boosters at 18 months, 5 years, 15 years.
Rabies	Usually only after exposure to rabies virus, or bat lyssavirus.
Yellow fever	Recommended when travelling to endemic countries.

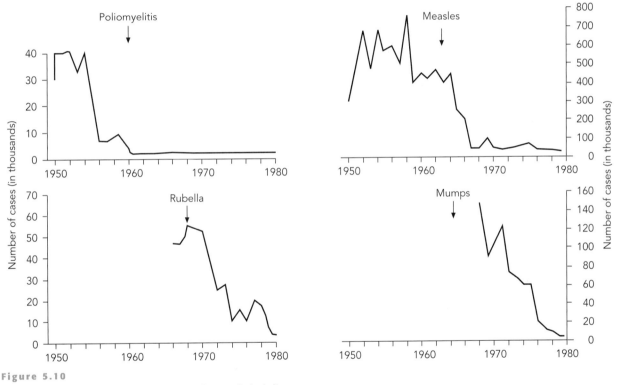

Figure 5.10

Effect of introduction of vaccines on incidence of viral diseases

The fall in incidence of poliomyelitis, measles, rubella and mumps in the United States following the introduction of vaccination against diseases (arrows). Inactivated poliovirus vaccine was introduced in 1954, live vaccines in 1963. The other three, for measles (introduced in 1963), mumps (1967) and rubella (1969), are live vaccines. (From DO White and F Fenner 1994, *Medical Virology*, 4th edn, Academic Press.)

described long before it was shown to be caused by the hepatitis C virus. New techniques in molecular biology make it possible to identify a viral genome without isolating or culturing the virus itself, as has been the case for hepatitis C. This virus has still not been observed microscopically or cultured in the laboratory, despite the fact that sophisticated tests are available to detect the presence of both viral antibodies and viral RNA in blood.

The ability to amplify fragments of viral RNA or DNA by the polymerase chain reaction (PCR) has far-reaching consequences for diagnostic virology. The sensitivity of PCR means that it is easier to probe for the viral nucleic acid than to try to isolate the virus itself. The discovery of new viruses such as SARS, Hendra virus and bat lyssavirus indicates that there are probably many other still unidentified viruses.

Human metapneumovirus (HMPV) was only identified in respiratory secretions in 2001 but has now been isolated from clinical samples from as early as 1953. TTV (transfusion-transmitted virus) is another virus that was cloned from blood in 1997 but its effect (if any) on the human body is not yet clear.

Genetic analysis of a virus can yield information about its antigenic structure that may be useful in determining public health programs. For example, viruses that have stable antigens on their surface (e.g. measles and polio) are more easily controlled by vaccination (as the antibodies required for neutralisation also stay the same). Other viruses that exist as many genetic types (cold viruses, rhinoviruses) or change their outer coat frequently (influenza A) are difficult to control by vaccination. It is also difficult to develop a vaccine for viruses that persist and mutate in the host (e.g. HIV) because the immune response that is induced is effective only against the original virus structure.

Despite our detailed understanding of viral replication, we still have a lot to learn about how viruses cause disease. Cytopathic effects, leading to the destruction of infected cells, are obvious consequences, but there are more subtle physiological changes that appear to be due to non-cytocidal viruses. The ability of some viruses to evade host defences, to undergo specific mutations, or to lie dormant and be reactivated under certain conditions has far-reaching implications for human health in general. Persistent viral infections, such as measles and polio, which produce symptoms many years after the patient has apparently fully recovered from the disease, pose a particular challenge. The World Health Organization is mounting a worldwide campaign aimed at eradicating both these diseases. This requires education and the cooperation of both individuals and governments.

The significance of the role that viruses play in multifactorial diseases such as hepatocellular carcinoma has yet to be fully elucidated. One of the most interesting aspects of viral infection that needs further study is the involvement of viruses in autoimmune reactions and the possible viral suppression of the immune system with consequent reactivation of, or superinfection by, other microbial species.

SUMMARY

STRUCTURE OF VIRUSES

- Viruses are the smallest type of infectious particle.
- Each virus possesses only one type of nucleic acid – RNA or DNA – enclosed in a capsid made up of capsomeres.
- Capsids occur in distinctive shapes (e.g. icosahedral, helical).
- Some viruses are enclosed by an envelope that helps the virus attach to the host cell.
- Viruses use the host cell enzymes for synthesis.

CLASSIFICATION OF VIRUSES

- Viruses are classified into groups or families based on the type of nucleic acid they contain, their shape, structure and method of replication.

HOST RANGE AND SPECIFICITY

- Viruses are specific for the type of organism and the type of cell they infect.
- This specificity depends on the presence of a suitable receptor for viral attachment to the susceptible cell.

VIRAL REPLICATION

- Viruses always replicate inside another living cell.
- Bacteriophage infect bacteria, resulting in lysis, lysogeny or specialised transduction.

Replication of animal viruses

- Viral infection of animal (human) cells involves six steps: adsorption, penetration, uncoating, synthesis, assembly and release.
- The method of replication inside the host cell depends on the type of nucleic acid the virus contains.

PATHOGENESIS OF VIRAL INFECTIONS IN HUMANS

- Many common human diseases are caused by viruses.
- Viral infections may be acute, subclinical, chronic, latent, slow or oncogenic.

HOST RESPONSE TO VIRAL INFECTION

- Viral infections usually activate the immune system with the production of cytokines, T cells and B cells that produce antibodies to protect the host against subsequent infection.
- The susceptibility of a person to viral infection is influenced by age and immune status.

TRANSMISSION OF VIRAL DISEASES

- Viruses are shed mainly from the area where the infection is localised.
- Control of the spread of virus disease is helped by an understanding of the method of transmission of the virus.
- Transmission may be via the airborne route as aerosol droplets, from vesicles or pustules, via the faecal-oral route, or in blood and other body fluids.
- A system of infection control procedures for the handling of blood and body substances has been introduced to prevent the transmission of blood-borne pathogens.
- Arboviruses are transmitted by insects, the most common of which is the mosquito.
- Some viruses are transferred vertically from mother to baby, transmission occurring *in utero*, during birth or through breast milk.
- Some viruses are teratogenic, causing congenital defects in the foetus when the mother contracts the infection during pregnancy.

INACTIVATION OF VIRUSES

- Most viruses are destroyed by heat, detergents and chlorine.
- Many viruses are stable in the presence of salt solutions and buffers, and between pH 5 and pH 9.
- Treatment of viruses with formaldehyde destroys their infectivity but leaves their antigenicity intact.

DIAGNOSIS OF VIRAL INFECTIONS

- Viral diseases are diagnosed mainly by signs and symptoms.
- The presence of virus particles in tissues can often be detected in the early stages of infection by reaction with fluorescent antibodies.
- Viruses can be grown in cell culture which is observed for cytopathic changes.
- The presence of antibodies to the virus in the patient's blood indicates infection.
- Some viruses are identified by DNA or RNA typing, using nucleic acid probes.

GROWTH OF VIRUSES IN THE LABORATORY

- Viruses may be grown in the laboratory in animals, embryonated eggs or cell culture.

TREATMENT AND PREVENTION OF VIRAL INFECTIONS

Antiviral drugs

- It is difficult to find antiviral drugs that do not also harm the host cell.
- The most successful antiviral drugs are analogues of DNA bases which react with specific viral enzymes.
- Interferons are naturally occurring antiviral compounds.

Vaccination

- Vaccines are available for many serious viral diseases.
- Effective mass vaccination campaigns can lead to the eradication of some viral diseases.

STUDY QUESTIONS

1. Describe the structure of a virus.
2. What type of nucleic acid occurs in viruses?
3. Where do viruses replicate?
4. What is meant by 'virus specificity'?
5. What is (a) a capsomere, (b) a capsid?
6. Describe the major shapes of viral particles.
7. How does the newly synthesised virus acquire its envelope?
8. What is (a) a virion, (b) a prion?
9. How are viruses classified?
10. What are bacterial viruses called?
11. Differentiate between 'lysis' and 'lysogeny' when applied to viral infection of bacterial cells.
12. List the six steps involved in the replication of a virus in an animal cell.
13. What is meant by a 'subclinical infection'?
14. List the viruses that can cause latent infections.
15. List the major routes of virus transmission.
16. What is meant by 'viral shedding'? When and where does it occur?
17. How can you control the transmission of blood-borne viruses?
18. What is meant by an arbovirus? Give examples.
19. Which viruses have teratogenic effects?
20. What are the most effective ways of inactivating viruses?
21. How are viral diseases diagnosed?
22. What are interferons?
23. What is meant by an 'attenuated' virus?
24. What is the most effective way of preventing viral diseases?

TEST YOUR UNDERSTANDING

1. How does the replication of the retroviruses differ from other RNA-containing viruses?
2. Differentiate between the processes that occur in the host during an *acute* and a *chronic* viral infection.
3. What types of viral infections elicit an immune response?
4. What are the major advantages of being vaccinated against measles rather than acquiring the disease naturally?
5. How are viruses able to transform normal cells?
6. Why is it difficult to design antiviral drugs?

Further reading

Dore GJ, M Law, M MacDonald & JC Kaldor 2003, Epidemiology of hepatitis C infection in Australia. *Journal of Clinical Virology*, 26(2): 171–184.

Lee LM & DK Henderson 2001, Emerging viral infections. *Current Opinion in Infectious Diseases* 14(4): 467–480.

Radford AD, RM Gaskell & AC Hart 2004, Human norovirus infections and the lessons from animal calciviruses. *Current Opinion in Infectious Diseases* 17(5): 471–478.

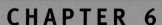

CHAPTER 6

Eucaryotic Microorganisms: Fungi, Protozoa and Multicellular Parasites

[CHAPTER FOCUS]

- ■ *What are the main properties of fungi?*

- ■ *Which are the most important infections caused by fungi?*

- ■ *What are the main characteristics of protozoa?*

- ■ *How do parasitic diseases caused by protozoa and helminths differ from other infectious diseases?*

- ■ *What factors affect a patient's susceptibility to fungal and protozoal diseases?*

- ■ *What is the role of insects in the transmission and cause of infections?*

Eucaryotic microorganisms

A significant number of diseases are caused by eucaryotic organisms that are either microscopic (e.g. fungal spores, yeasts and protozoa) or have a microscopic stage in their life cycle (e.g. some fungi, worms and other parasites).

Some of these eucaryotes cause only minor diseases in healthy individuals, but can have serious effects on a person whose immune system is compromised in some way. They are then referred to as opportunistic pathogens. **Opportunistic infections** are defined as infections caused by microorganisms that would not normally cause disease in individuals whose immune system is intact, but may do so in people with altered defence mechanisms. Opportunistic infections caused by protozoa or fungi are a major cause of mortality in AIDS patients.

Eucaryotic microorganisms have very similar properties to their host (human) cells, which means that it is often difficult to find drugs that can destroy them without having significant side effects on the host. This is of special importance in the treatment of systemic infections, when the infection is spread throughout the body and various body organs. In these cases, administration of an antimicrobial drug may mean that susceptible host cells are also exposed to the drug.

In this chapter we look at the properties of these organisms and discuss briefly the diseases they cause and the implications for health care.

Characteristics of fungi

Fungi are a large, diverse group of eucaryotic organisms that are widely distributed in nature. They exhibit a range of morphology (appearance). Fungi comprise two major groups – yeasts and moulds.

There are thousands of different types of fungi, ranging from microscopic single-celled yeasts to multicellular, filamentous moulds and large fleshy moulds, or mushrooms. All fungal cells are surrounded by a cell wall, consisting of carbohydrate, polysaccharides and lipids, and this determines their shape. They are distinguished from plants and algae in that they do not contain chlorophyll and cannot carry out photosynthesis. They differ from animal cells because they have cell walls.

Most fungi can grow under conditions where bacteria are not able to thrive. For example, many moulds grow on substances with a very low moisture content (e.g. bread and cereals) and are resistant to extremes of osmotic pressure (e.g. they are able to grow in high sugar or salt concentrations). Many prefer an acid pH and can tolerate cold conditions (e.g. the household refrigerator). They are described as heterotrophic; that is, they require an organic source of carbon for growth. Many of them are saprophytes, feeding off dead, woody plant materials that are not readily decomposed by bacteria. Thus, they play an important role in the decomposition of organic matter.

Many fungi are beneficial to humans. Some species are a source of antibiotics (e.g. penicillin and cephalosporin) and other drugs (e.g. the immunosuppressive drug, cyclosporine). Yeasts are important in the food industry for making bread, wine, beer and soy sauce. Moulds are used to give special flavour to some cheeses. The large fleshy mushrooms are a source of food.

However, fungi also account for a significant amount of food spoilage and, in agriculture, fungal diseases of crops cause important economic losses.

TYPES OF FUNGI

Yeasts

Yeasts occur widely in the environment and are found on the surfaces of plants and fruit. They are able to ferment sugars with the production of alcohol. Strains of the yeast *Saccharomyces cerevisiae* are used in bread making and in wine and beer production. *S. cerevisiae* has also been used by molecular biologists for the production of genetically engineered products, such as the vaccine for hepatitis B (see Chapter 4). The yeast *Candida albicans* occurs as part of the normal flora in humans.

Yeasts are unicellular organisms, usually spherical to oval in shape and bounded by a cell wall. They are slightly larger than bacteria, varying from about 3 to 15 μm, and contain various subcellular organelles. A number of pathogenic strains exhibit **dimorphism** – that is, the ability to grow in two different forms. Dimorphic fungi are usually filamentous at room temperature but grow as yeast cells in the body or when incubated in the laboratory at 35°C on an enriched medium such as blood agar.

Candida albicans, the organism responsible for thrush, exhibits several forms of growth, at 28°C and also in the host tissues. At 28°C it may exhibit a single-celled budding yeast form, or produce rudimentary filaments called pseudohyphae, or even true **hyphae**. The production of pseudohyphae appears to aid in the invasion of the muco-cutaneous host tissues and indicates a pathogenic rather than commensal role for the organism (see Figure 6.1).

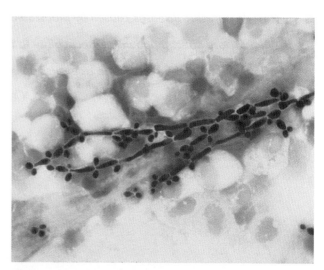

Figure 6.1

***Candida albicans* in tissue phase showing blastoconidia budding from pseudohyphae**

Reproduction in yeasts is mainly asexual, by a process called *budding*. A small outgrowth, or bud, appears on the parent cell; it gradually enlarges and then separates, forming a new daughter cell, which then rapidly increases in size (Figure 6.2). Some non-pathogenic yeasts exhibit sexual reproduction, in which two haploid cells fuse to form a zygote, followed by the production of spores.

Moulds

The moulds are filamentous fungi that are capable of growth in many different habitats. They are commonly found growing on stale bread, cheese, cereals and vegetables. They consist of long filaments or **hyphae** (singular: hypha) which grow by extending the terminal cell at the tip of the filament. As they grow, the hyphae branch and form a dense mat of filaments called a **mycelium**, which is usually visible to the naked eye. The cells of this vegetative structure often contain more than one nucleus. After the dense mycelial mat has formed, **aerial hyphae** are produced and extend up into the air above the mycelial mat.

The most common method of reproduction in moulds is by the production of asexual spores in specialised structures on the ends or off the sides of these aerial hyphae. Asexual spores are produced by mitotic division of the parent cell. There are two main types (see Figure 6.3).

1. **Sporangiospores** are produced inside a sac, or **sporangium**, on the tip of a stalk, or **sporangiophore**. These spores are released when the sporangium ruptures.
2. **Conidia** (**conidiospores**) are not enclosed in a sac. They develop by being pinched off from the tip of an aerial hypha. Conidiospores are the most common type of asexual spore. They are usually pigmented, ranging in colour from blue or green to black or red, so the

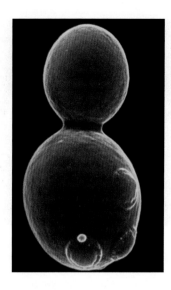

Figure 6.2
Yeast reproducing by budding
Circular scars can be seen on the surface of the larger cell, representing sites of previous budding.

growing fungus changes in appearance from a white mat to its own particular colour with a dusty surface.

The structure of the spore-bearing hyphae is distinctive for each mould and is useful for identification. Their production is essential for survival. They are dispersed on air currents and carried to a new site where they germinate and grow into new hyphae. Some typical moulds are illustrated in Figure 6.4.

Some filamentous fungi produce chemicals with antibacterial properties. The most important of these is penicillin, which is produced by several species of *Penicillium* (see page 48).

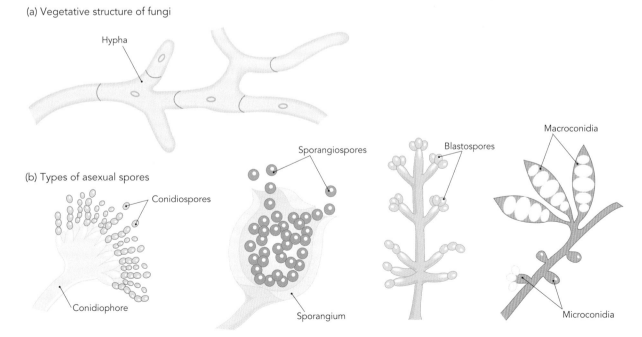

(a) Vegetative structure of fungi

Hypha

(b) Types of asexual spores

Conidiospores

Conidiophore

Sporangiospores

Sporangium

Blastospores

Macroconidia

Microconidia

Figure 6.3
Structure of filamentous fungi

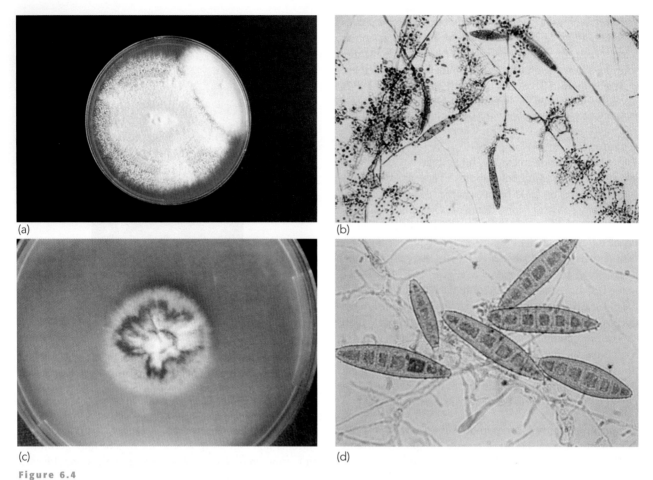

(a)

(b)

(c)

(d)

Figure 6.4

Structure of moulds

(a) Distinctive appearance on agar plate of dermatophyte; (b) microscopic appearance of spores of *Trichophyton* mentagrophytes; (c) growth of *Microsporum cookei* on agar; (d) microscopic appearance of spores of *M. cookei*.

Mushrooms are filamentous fungi in which the aerial hyphae form a fleshy structure called a fruiting body. During most of its life, the mushroom exists as a mycelium of hyphae in the soil; when conditions are favourable a fruiting body or 'mushroom' is formed. Spores are produced on the coloured gills underneath the cap, and are dispersed when the mushroom matures and dries. The various members of the mushroom family are an important food source.

FUNGAL INFECTIONS

Although many fungi are responsible for plant infections, there are only about 100 species of fungi that actually cause disease in humans. Very few are truly pathogenic. The fungi that cause human disease belong to two main groups: (1) the **yeasts** and (2) the **filamentous fungi**. Most fungal infections are cutaneous, affecting only the upper layers of the skin, or mucosa, and do not cause severe illness. However, some fungal infections can become systemic, spreading throughout the body and causing life-threatening conditions.

For many years, infections caused by fungi were regarded as a nuisance rather than life threatening. More recently, however, fungal infections have become increasingly important, especially when they occur in patients with serious underlying diseases or compromised host defences. Such people are not necessarily confined to hospital. Many of them live in the community. They include transplant patients who are being treated with immuno-suppressive drugs, patients with leukaemia, other cancer patients and diabetics, as well as people suffering from immune disorders such as AIDS. All these individuals are likely to suffer severe morbidity (illness) if they contract a fungal infection, even though it may not be serious in a healthy person.

An infection caused by a fungus is called a **mycosis**. Depending on its location in the body, it may be classified as **superficial**, **cutaneous**, **subcutaneous** or **systemic**. Most superficial and cutaneous infections are not life-threatening, although they are often resistant to treatment and tend to persist for long periods with associated inflammation and discomfort.

Superficial mycoses

The most common of the superficial mycoses is pityriasis versicolor (**tinea versicolor**), caused by the fungus *Malassezia furfur* (see Figure 6.5). It is a mild infection of the skin and produces lesions that range from white, or non-pigmented (usually seen in darker-skinned people – e.g. in New Guinea it is colloquially called 'white spot')

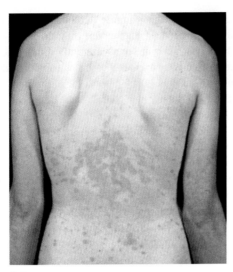

Pityriasis versicolor
Distinctive rash caused by the dermatophyte *Malassezia furfur*.

through to brown, which is more common in fair-skinned people. The lesions are purely cosmetic. No inflammatory response is involved and the infection responds to topical antifungal treatment, such as selenium.

Cutaneous mycoses

Cutaneous mycoses comprise the familiar skin infections commonly referred to as **tinea** or **ringworm** (see also Chapter 16, page 377). They are caused by fungi called **dermatophytes** which invade keratinised tissue (skin, hair and nails). The most important of these are organisms belonging to the genera *Microsporum*, *Trichophyton* and *Epidermophyton*. Dermatophyte infections may be identified by microscopic examination of skin scrapings. The arrangement of their hyphae and the structure of their conidiospores are distinctive for each species. In the laboratory they can be identified by culture on Sabouraud's agar. See Figure 6.4.

Cutaneous fungal infections are transmitted by person-to-person contact or by the shedding of infected skin scales or hair clippings. Tinea infections can occur on any part of the body and are named accordingly.

- **Tinea pedis (athlete's foot)** is the most common dermatophyte infection. Usually, the skin between the toes becomes infected, followed by the development of small vesicles that burst and cause peeling and cracking of the skin (Figure 6.6). *Tinea pedis* is frequently contracted from fungal cells present in communal showers and change rooms.
- **Tinea corporis** may occur anywhere on the body. The lesion usually consists of a central scaly patch surrounded by a circular border of vesicles that are red and inflamed, giving the appearance of a ring – hence the name 'ringworm'. See Figure 6.7.
- **Tinea cruris** (jock itch) occurs in the groin.
- **Tinea capitis** is the name given to infections on the scalp. These may also involve the roots of the hair.

Subcutaneous mycoses

Subcutaneous infections occur when a fungus penetrates beneath the skin and establishes an infection. They are usually caused by soil or plant microorganisms that are introduced when the skin is broken or damaged, such as when a thorn or splinter penetrates the skin while gardening. Many of the fungi associated with plants cause this type of infection – for example, *Sporothrix schenckii*, which lives on wood and plants and produces a chronic granulomatous infection that can spread along the lymphatic system.

Paronychia or **onychomycosis** is an infection that occurs under the finger- or toenail. It is caused by any of the soil or plant fungi but can also be caused by the yeast, *Candida albicans* (Figure 6.8a, b). Subcutaneous mycoses are difficult to treat and can persist for long periods.

Systemic mycoses

Systemic (deep) fungal infections are caused by pathogenic fungi or by opportunistic fungi that have invaded an immunosuppressed patient. Very few fungi are truly pathogenic; that is, very few will cause an infection in an

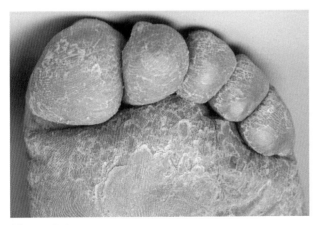

Figure 6.6
Tinea pedis **showing severe scaling**
Ringworm of the foot, or athlete's foot (*Tinea pedis*). Moisture between the toes favours fungal infections.

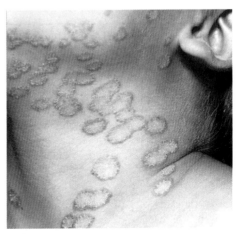

Figure 6.7
Tinea corporis **or ringworm**
The infection has circular scaly lesions with distinct raised erythmatous borders.

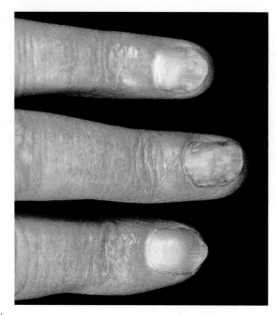

(a)

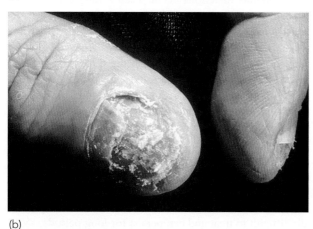

(b)

Figure 6.8

Effects of *Candida albicans*

(a) Mild paronychia due to *Candida albicans*—fungal infections of the nails are very difficult to eradicate.
(b) Chronic onychomycosis (paronychia) of the fingernail—destruction of tissue due to *C. albicans*.

individual with normal immune defences. Table 6.1 is a list of true pathogenic fungi which may give rise to systemic infections. They are predominantly dimorphic, free-living soil organisms and tend to be restricted to defined geographical habitats. These fungi are a common source of infection in the United States (see Table 6.1). They are rarely seen in Australia, with the exception of *Histoplasma*, a few cases of which have been reported.

In endemic areas these pathogenic fungi are usually introduced into the body by inhalation of spores. In the majority of cases the result is a mild lung infection. In a small percentage of cases, the fungus may be disseminated (spread) through the body, affecting other body organs and progressing to a full-blown, sometimes fatal, disease. Patients' ability to withstand invasion by these fungi depends on the integrity of their cell-mediated immune response (see Chapter 9). Although these fungi may infect any individual exposed to them, they have much more serious consequences in immunosuppressed patients and are commonly found as opportunistic infections in AIDS patients in the United States.

Apart from the pathogens described above, the major cause of systemic mycoses are opportunistic fungi, which occur mainly in immunodeficient patients.

Opportunistic fungal infections

A number of fungi are opportunistic pathogens; that is, they cause disease only when the host defences are weakened (see Table 6.1). Among these, the yeast *Candida albicans* and related *Candida* species are the most common. *Candida* is a **commensal** of human mucosal surfaces, especially the mouth, vagina and intestinal tract, but may become pathogenic when the body's defence mechanisms are impaired or when the balance of microbial flora is disrupted.

Candida infections may be either **mucocutaneous** or **systemic**. **Thrush** is the name commonly given to mucocutaneous infections of the mouth or vagina. Outbreaks of thrush are usually indicative of a local or systemic weakness in the immune system. A number of factors can con-

Table 6.1

Systemic fungal infections

ORGANISM	DISEASE	DISTRIBUTION/HABITAT
Pathogenic fungi		
Blastomyces dermatitidis	Blastomycosis	North America
Coccidioides immitis	Coccidioidomycosis	Soil; south-west United States, Mexico
Histoplasma capsulatum	Histoplasmosis	Central and eastern United States, South America, Africa
Paracoccidioides brasiliensis	Paracoccidioidomycosis	Soil; Latin America
Opportunistic fungi		
Candida spp.	Candidiasis	Normal human flora
Aspergillus spp.	Aspergillosis	Ubiquitous; soil, grains
Cryptococcus neoformans	Cryptococcal pneumonia Cryptococcal meningitis	Birds
Rhizopus, Mucor	Zygomycosis	Soil, plants
Scedosporium spp.		Environment, dust

tribute to the proliferation of *Candida* and production of disease (candidiasis). For example, oral thrush is frequently seen in neonates (especially low birth weight infants) where the immune system is immature and the population of protective normal flora has not yet been established. Oral thrush is commonly associated with the use of corticosteroid puffers for asthma. Thrush often occurs after long-term treatment with broad spectrum antibiotics, which alters the composition of the normal bacterial flora.

Chronic mucocutaneous candidiasis (CMC), which presents first in childhood but is also seen in adults, is usually an indication of an underlying deficiency in cellular immunity. See Figure 6.9.

Vaginal candidiasis in adult females is often associated with diabetes, pregnancy or the use of the contraceptive pill. Alterations in the body's physiological state, such as hormonal imbalance or stress, appear to favour the growth of the yeast cells. Prolonged antibiotic therapy can also destroy the normal flora in the vagina. Species of *Lactobacillus*, a normal inhabitant of the vagina, help to maintain an acid environment, limiting the growth of *Candida* which prefers a neutral pH (pH 7). Destruction of the lactobacilli by prolonged broad spectrum antibiotic therapy allows the pH to rise and an overgrowth or **super-infection** of *Candida* may result.

Candida can also cause skin infections in obese or diabetic patients. The yeast flourishes in the warm moist parts of the body (axillae, skin folds, under the breasts in females), causing inflammation and red weeping vesicles. It can also be a cause of skin infections in elderly patients, who may have problems with hygiene and adequate care. Nappy rash in babies due to the constant moisture on the skin can also be caused by *Candida* (see Figure 6.10).

Mucocutaneous candidiasis can be treated with topical antifungal preparations, although some species (e.g. *Candida glabrata*) are exhibiting increased drug resistance.

Systemic candidiasis (**candidaemia**) is an invasive fungal infection that is a significant cause of health-care-associated infections (HCAI). It generally occurs in asso-

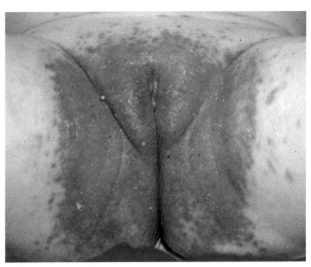

Figure 6.10

Nappy rash due to *Candida albicans*

ciation with another severe underlying disease such as leukaemia or other cancer and has a mortality rate as high as 40%. The incidence of systemic infection is also high in patients subjected to traumatic medical procedures, such as organ transplantation with consequent immuno-suppressive therapy. Invasive procedures, such as intravenous therapy with **total parenteral nutrition (TPN)**, or **endotracheal intubation**, increase the risk of systemic infections. *Candida* infections are frequently associated with central lines and Hickman catheters. Severely compromised babies in intensive care may develop systemic *Candida* infections, often with a significant mortality rate.

The ability of *Candida* to develop into a systemic infection is related to the immune status of the patient. *Candida* typically grows in the extracellular spaces and is subject to phagocytosis by neutrophils and macrophages. **Neutropenia** (a deficiency of neutrophils) appears to render a patient more susceptible to systemic *Candida* invasion. However, *Candida* infections also occur in association with a reduction in T cells and the cell-mediated immune response (see Chapter 9). Mucocutaneous candidiasis is commonly seen in patients with the human immunodeficiency virus (HIV-positive) but it does not appear to be readily disseminated in patients who have progressed to AIDS.

Pneumocystis pneumonia (**PCP**) is a major cause of illness and death in people with impaired immunity. It is caused by an unusual fungus, *Pneumocystis jiroveci*, which was originally classified as a protozoan and named *Pneumocystis carinii*. DNA testing in recent years has confirmed that the organism is a fungus. It is an obligate parasite, and has not been grown successfully in the laboratory. The usual diagnosis is by observation of clinical symptoms, X-ray of the lungs or examination of an induced sputum specimen (see Figure 6.11). *Pneumocystis* is thought to be present in the respiratory tract of many healthy individuals, but only becomes invasive in immunosuppressed patients. It is a primary cause of

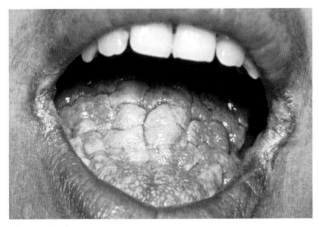

Figure 6.9

Chronic oral mucocutaneous candidiasis of tongue and mouth in adult with underlying immunodeficiency

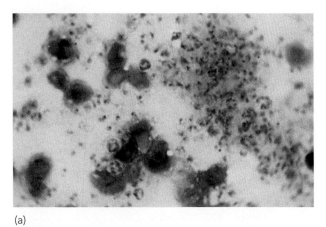

(a)

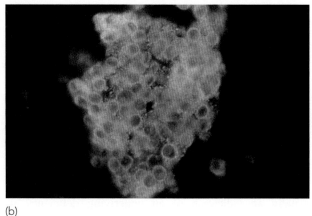

(b)

Figure 6.11

Pneumocystis jiroveci

(a) Conventional stain where structures are difficult to identify; (b) fluorescent antibody stain clearly showing the cysts that block the alveoli.

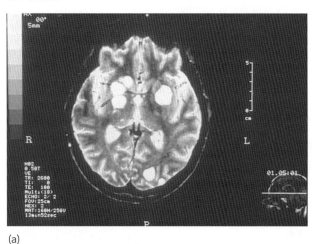

(a)

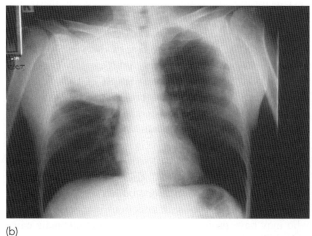

(b)

Figure 6.12

***Cryptococcus neoformans* infection**

(a) MRI scan showing multiple cryptococcomas (white masses) in the brain; (b) X-ray showing pulmonary cryptococcal infection in upper right lobe.

pneumonia in AIDS patients and responsible for a large number of AIDS deaths.

Cryptococcal infections are caused by *Cryptococcus neoformans* var. *neoformans*, an encapsulated yeast found in the excreta of pigeons and other birds in most parts of the world. The organism enters the body via the respiratory tract and is responsible for causing a mild, largely asymptomatic pneumonitis in humans. However, in immunosuppressed patients, the organism can become invasive and cause severe cryptococcal pneumonia. It may also spread to the brain, causing cryptococcal meningitis. See Figure 6.12. This occurs in about 80% of AIDS patients. Cryptococcal infections are frequently seen in patients receiving steroids or in transplant patients on immunosuppressive drugs.

The variety, *C. neoformans* var. *gattii*, is found mainly in areas where the Australian river red gum (*Eucalyptus camaldulensis*) is growing. It occurs in certain parts of Australia and in other countries to which the tree has been exported. Infections seem to occur mainly during the flowering season. Aborigines who live in dry river beds in Northern and Central Australia are often infected with this variety. It is rarely seen in immunocompromised patients in urban areas.

Aspergillus infections are opportunistic infections caused predominantly by *Aspergillus fumigatus*. Members of the *Aspergillus* genus are widely distributed in nature and release spores that are inhaled into the lungs. See Figures 6.13 and 6.14. If the fungus invades the lung tissue it is able to enter the bloodstream and be disseminated throughout the body, causing potentially fatal abscesses in various body organs. In health facilities, invasive aspergillosis is a major problem for immunosuppressed patients and transplant patients, especially bone marrow recipients. Infections are usually traced to contaminated air-conditioning ducts.

Fusarium species are common soil organisms and plant pathogens which can also cause superficial mycoses, especially of the skin and eyes. Disseminated *Fusarium* infections that occur in leukaemia or transplant patients are difficult to treat and have a high mortality rate. Scedosporium is another mould that sometimes causes infections in hospitalised patients.

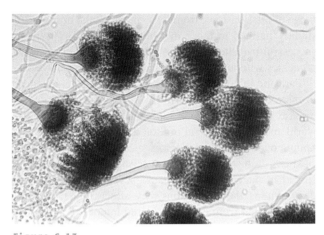

Figure 6.13

Microscopic morphology of _Aspergillus fumigatus_ showing typical conidial heads

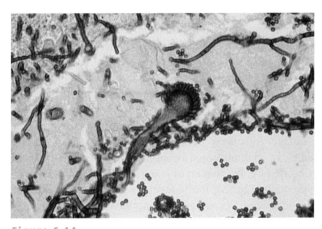

Figure 6.14

Silver stained section of lung tissue showing infection with _A. fumigatus_

TRANSMISSION OF FUNGAL INFECTIONS

Most fungi live in the soil or on plants and are transmitted to humans by contact with the fungus or its spores. In health facilities fungal spores may be carried on air currents from contaminated air-conditioning units. They are frequently inhaled (e.g. _Aspergillus_ spores and _Cryptococcus_), but they can also enter through broken skin. Some of the cutaneous mycoses are transmitted by contact with infected skin scales, or by direct contact with a lesion on the skin of an infected human or animal (e.g. ringworm on cats).

A notable exception is _Candida_. Since _Candida_ species are normal human commensals, they tend to cause infection when there is a lowering of the host resistance, as described above.

FACTORS CONTRIBUTING TO FUNGAL INFECTIONS

It should be noted that most fungal infections are of only minor importance in healthy individuals. The overall integrity of the host immune system is of utmost importance in avoiding fungal infections.

A number of factors contribute to patient susceptibility.

Neutropenia is a predisposing factor for many infections. Certain medical procedures also affect susceptibility, including:

- Transplant surgery with administration of immuno-suppressive drugs.
- Prolonged broad spectrum antibiotic therapy which destroys the normal flora.
- Other invasive therapies such as intravenous total parenteral nutrition (TPN). This involves the use of solutions containing high concentrations of glucose which inhibit bacterial growth but favour the growth of fungi such as _Candida albicans_. The use of fat emulsion in TPN also encourages the growth of _Malassezia furfur_, an otherwise harmless superficial fungus.
- **CAPD** (**C**ontinuous **A**mbulatory **P**eritoneal **D**ialysis). This therapy is used as an alternative to haemodialysis for patients with renal failure. The main problem with this therapy is the risk of fungal infections as well as bacterial infections through the indwelling cannulae.
- Fungal infections may also occur in prosthetic devices. The organisms originate from contaminated equipment or materials.

Approximately 10% of hospital-acquired infections are due to fungi.

DIAGNOSIS OF SYSTEMIC INFECTIONS

Diagnosis of systemic fungal infections is difficult because the symptoms are often not definitive and laboratory growth of fungi is very slow. Fungal infections are usually suspected if the patient is immunocompromised and does not respond to empirical antibacterial therapy. Careful collection and processing of specimens is very important.

TREATMENT OF FUNGAL INFECTIONS

Cutaneous fungal infections are treated with topical antifungal preparations. Systemic infections are more difficult to treat as there are few antifungal drugs that do not have serious side effects on the host. Amphotericin is the most effective drug for neutropenic patients. Candidiasis and cryptococcosis in AIDS patients (who are usually not neutropenic) are treated with fluconazole. Antifungal drugs are described in more detail in Chapter 12. No vaccines are available for any of the fungal infections.

HARMFUL EFFECTS OF FUNGI

Apart from causing infections, fungi can have other harmful effects. These include the induction of allergic responses to fungal spores and the harmful effects associated with the ingestion of fungal toxins.

Mould-related health problems

It is becoming increasingly apparent that the growth of moulds in damp or poorly ventilated buildings can give rise to a number of minor or serious health problems. The release of spores, mould fragments or volatile products (toxins) into confined areas can have harmful effects on the people working in these buildings ('sick building syndrome'). Some of the symptoms produced include respiratory problems, difficulty breathing, sore throats, cough, nasal and sinus congestion, eye irritation, allergic reactions, skin irritation, headaches and central nervous system problems. Many of these symptoms are transient but, as with all fungal infections, they may cause serious problems in immunocompromised patients.

The release of dust and mould spores during building works and renovations also creates a potential hazard, especially in the hospital environment where mould and spores can be drawn into the ventilation system and reach susceptible patients.

Allergic reactions

Allergic bronchopulmonary reactions may result from the repeated inhalation of mould spores. Workers in farm industries are particularly at risk of occupational exposure due to inhalation of spores of fungi such as *Aspergillus* species, which are commonly found in grain storage bins, haystacks, silos and sugar cane piles (bagasse). The introduction of spores into sensitised lungs causes a hypersensitivity reaction, usually associated with severe breathing difficulties (farmer's lung).

Fungal toxins

Some fungi produce chemicals that are toxic to humans. The poisonous effects of eating some species of mushroom (commonly called toadstools) are well known. Symptoms such as nausea, severe diarrhoea, damage to body systems, muscle spasms and death may occur. Other fungi infect food and produce toxins that are ingested with the food. Among these is **aflatoxin**, produced by the mould *Aspergillus flavus* when it grows on peanuts and some grains. It has been linked to the occurrence of liver cancer.

Ochratoxin A is produced by a number of fungi and, in Australia, has been isolated from *Aspergillus carbonarius*, a fungus found on grapes. It is suspected of being carcinogenic and teratogenic (affecting the foetus), and of having harmful effects on the immune system.

Another interesting toxin is ergotamine, produced by *Claviceps purpurea*, a mould that infects rye grain. It is a chemical similar to LSD (lysergic acid diethylamide) and produces hallucinogenic effects. It has been suggested that some of the witchcraft incidents of the Middle Ages were due to the ingestion of this mind-altering toxin in contaminated rye bread. It is important to have strict health controls to prevent the contamination of food with fungal toxins. The presence and possible harmful effects of fungal toxins in animal feed is also of concern to farmers.

Parasites

A **parasite** is defined as an organism that derives its nutrients from another living organism, its host. Parasitic diseases usually refer to those caused by protozoa, helminths and arthropods, which live at the expense of their host. As we explain in Chapter 7, parasitism encompasses a wide range of relationships, from those in which the host is only slightly harmed to those in which it is killed. The most successful parasites are those that maintain their own life processes without killing their host.

Parasitic infections are often given very little coverage in microbiology courses. However, each year they cause disease in more than one billion people throughout the world and lead to several million deaths, mostly in developing countries. Major diseases such as malaria, sleeping sickness, schistosomiasis and leishmaniasis are widespread in many areas, and cause severe debilitation and death among the populations they affect. Other parasitic infections that were once considered minor are becoming more important because of their occurrence in immunocompromised individuals. These include the infections caused by the protozoa *Toxoplasma* and *Cryptosporidium*.

In Australia, serious parasitic diseases are still relatively uncommon. However, an increasing number of individuals in our community are immunocompromised and therefore potentially susceptible. These include AIDS patients, cancer patients and transplant patients on immunosuppressive therapy. There is also a significant number of people who are susceptible because of their lifestyle and other contributing factors. Many indigenous Australians in remote communities have an increased susceptibility to parasitic infections because of pre-existing conditions such as malnutrition, alcoholism and diabetes. Their lifestyle (e.g. the custom of going barefoot) places them at risk of contracting the parasitic worms, hookworm and strongyloides, which gain entry to the body by burrowing through the skin.

Scabies is endemic in the indigenous community and the resulting irritation and scratching provides a portal of entry for more serious streptococcal infections.

Parasitic infections differ from those caused by bacteria or viruses in several ways.

- Parasites frequently have a complex life cycle involving the formation of resistant cyst forms of the organism. These cysts can survive for long periods outside the host.
- The life cycle may involve an insect vector (carrier) that is essential for the transmission of the disease. Elimination of the vector should effectively control the spread of the disease, but this has proved impossible in most cases.
- Some parasites are capable of infecting both humans and other animals. In this case, both animals and humans can act as reservoirs for the infection. This is especially true for many of the protozoal infections carried by insects.
- Many of the helminths (worms) have two or more hosts in their life cycle. The **definitive host** harbours the mature adult form of the parasite, and the **intermediate host** has the immature or larval form. Frequently, humans are an 'accidental' host, obtaining the parasite by eating infected meat (e.g. the beef tapeworm).
- Many parasites have life cycles that need sufficient time

for the various stages to mature, either in soil or in an insect or host.

In the following sections we describe the properties of the protozoa and helminths and discuss the problems associated with the prevention and control of the infections they cause.

Protozoa

CHARACTERISTICS

Protozoa are single-celled eucaryotic organisms ranging from 20 to 50 μm in size, containing various subcellular organelles and surrounded by an outer membrane rather than a cell wall. Some have flagella for movement (see Figure 6.15(a)). They are mostly found in water habitats, but a number exist as parasites in animals (including humans) and insects. Protozoa obtain their nutrients by absorption of small molecules, or ingestion of food particles or even microorganisms from their environment. Some protozoa have a clearly defined gullet and anal pore (e.g. the paramecia, see Figure 6.15(b)). Others obtain food by phagocytosis. The cell surrounds the food particle and engulfs it, drawing the food inside the cell where it is contained in a vacuole, or sac, and then digested (e.g. amoeba, see Figure 6.15(c)). Intracellular parasites obtain their food by absorption of nutrients from the host cytoplasm through their outer layer.

CLASSIFICATION OF PROTOZOA

Protozoa are usually classified into four main groups, depending on the way they move: the sarcodina, mastigophora, ciliata and sporozoa.

Mastigophora (flagellates)

These protozoa move by the action of flagella, whip-like tails that propel the organism through water environments. Mastigophora are usually oval in shape and reproduce asexually by longitudinal binary fission. Most of them are able to form cysts for survival. Several of the flagellates are important human pathogens.

Ciliates

The third group of protozoa are the ciliates. These organisms have cells with a large number of small hair-like appendages that move in a synchronised wave to propel the cell along. There are many ciliates in the environment (e.g. paramecia) but the only human pathogen is *Balantidium coli*, a large protozoan that causes diarrhoea. Although it is widely distributed throughout the world, infections are rare.

Sarcodina (amoebae)

This group consists of the **amoebae**, large cells surrounded by a membrane and lacking a definitive shape. They move by extending the cell membrane and allowing the cytoplasm to flow into this extension, called a **pseudopod** (false foot). Amoebae absorb nutrients from their

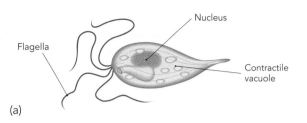

(a)

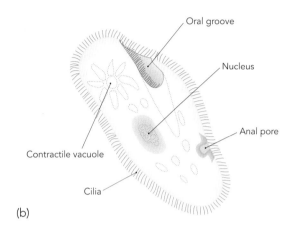

(b)

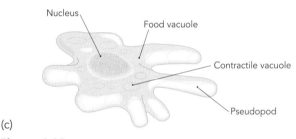

(c)

Figure 6.15

Protozoa
Diagrammatic representation of three different protozoa: (a) flagellate; (b) ciliate; (c) amoeba.

environment through their membrane, or engulf food particles by phagocytosis.

Sporozoa

Sporozoa are non-motile protozoa; that is, the adult forms do not have any mechanism or appendages to enable them to move. This group contains several important human pathogens.

REPRODUCTION

Many of the protozoa have a complex life cycle involving a number of different forms or stages – for example, the malaria parasite, *Plasmodium*. The simplest form of reproduction is asexual by a process of budding, binary fission or **schizogony** of the infective stage (**trophozoite**). In schizogony, or multiple fission, the nucleus undergoes multiple divisions before the cell divides. Cytoplasm forms around each new nucleus before division takes place, giving rise to multiple daughter cells. Sexual reproduction occurs mainly in protozoa that have an insect vector stage, although *Cryptosporidium*, which is a cause of diarrhoea in humans, can undergo sexual reproduction.

Most protozoa are capable of encystment – that is, the production of a resistant cyst form of the cell. **Cysts** are surrounded by a protective layer that is resistant to drying and enables them to survive for long periods (even years) in the soil. Some cysts are also resistant to the chlorine compounds used in water purification, and to stomach acid.

PROTOZOAL INFECTIONS

Protozoa are responsible for causing some important human diseases. They may be found as intracellular or extracellular parasites in blood, intestines and other organs. Like opportunistic fungi, protozoal infections have a more serious outcome in immunocompromised patients (e.g. *Cryptosporidium* in AIDS patients).

Most protozoal infections are acquired by one of two main routes.

- The first route of transmission is by the ingestion of the parasite in contaminated food or water; or, as is the case for *Toxoplasma*, by the inhalation of dried oocysts.
- The other route of transmission is via the bite of a blood-sucking insect. In some cases the insect acts purely as a vector, in others the parasite multiplies and undergoes a developmental stage in the insect (e.g. malaria).

The incidence of a disease and ease of transmission depend on a number of factors, including climatic conditions and the distribution of the appropriate insect vector.

A knowledge of the stages in the life cycles of the pathogenic protozoa is important for the prevention of transmission of the organisms and for the development of vaccines. For example, patients suffering from diseases that require an insect vector for transmission are not considered infectious to other patients or health workers, unless a suitable vector is present. The development of a vaccine for malaria has proved particularly difficult because of the existence of multiple stages in the life cycle of the parasite (see page 475).

The protozoa that cause infections in humans are listed in Table 6.2. Not all these protozoa are found in Australia. Several of the more serious infections are transmitted by insect vectors, and so their incidence is limited to the geographical regions where these insects are found. A successful life cycle also depends on climatic conditions of temperature and humidity that favour the survival and replication of the insect vectors and the different stages of the parasitic life cycle. The references in the table are to the pages of this text where the diseases are discussed in more detail.

Pathogenic amoebae

Several different species of amoeba may inhabit the human intestine. Many of these are non-pathogenic (e.g. *Entamoeba coli*). They form cysts in the host that are excreted in the faeces and can then be ingested by another host (human) in contaminated food or water.

The pathogenic amoeba, *Entamoeba histolytica*, is the major cause of amoebic dysentery worldwide, with most infections occurring in tropical and subtropical regions. The disease may range from mild diarrhoea to severe dysentery or ulcerative colitis, characterised by blood, pus and mucus in the faeces. It is only rarely seen in Australia, but travellers to endemic tropical areas may contract it

Table 6.2

Protozoal infections in humans

PHYLUM	ORGANISM	DISEASE	HABITAT SOURCE/VECTOR	REFERENCE	
Sarcodina (amoebae)	*Entamoeba histolytica*	Amoebic dysentery	Contaminated water	Chapter 18,	p. 428
Mastigophora (flagellates)	*Giardia intestinalis*	Giardiasis	Contaminated water	Chapter 18,	p. 427
	Trichomonas vaginalis	Vaginitis	Vagina	Chapter 21,	p. 522
	Trypanosoma brucei gambiense	Sleeping sickness	Tsetse fly	Chapter 6,	p. 121
	Trypanosoma cruzi	Chagas disease	Kissing bug	Chapter 6,	p. 121
	Leishmania spp.	Cutaneous leishmaniasis Visceral leishmaniasis (kala-azar)	Sandflies	Chapter 6,	p. 121
Ciliata	*Balantidium coli*	Balantidial dysentery	Contaminated water	Chapter 6,	p. 121
Sporozoa	*Plasmodium* spp.	Malaria	Anopheles mosquito	Chapter 19,	p. 471
	Toxoplasma gondii	Toxoplasmosis	Cat faeces	Chapter 19,	p. 475
	Cryptosporidium	Diarrhoea	Humans/animals	Chapter 18,	p. 427
	Microsporidium	Diarrhoea	Humans/animals	Chapter 18,	p. 420

there. Despite treatment, some individuals become asymptomatic carriers and continue to shed cysts of *E. histolytica* in the faeces, thus contributing to the spread of the disease.

Pathogenic flagellates

Giardia intestinalis (*Giardia lamblia*) is a common intestinal parasite found throughout the world, including Australia (see Spotlight box at right). It exists in two forms: the infective trophozoite stage, which has four pairs of flagella and a 'sucker' that allows it to attach to the wall of the intestine; and the resistant cyst stage which is shed in the faeces and is able to survive for weeks in a moist environment (see Figure 6.16).

Contaminated drinking water is the main source of infection. Symptoms may take several weeks to appear so it is often difficult to establish when and where the infection was contracted. *Giardia* is notoriously difficult to diagnose. Symptoms may range from abdominal pain and prolonged bouts of diarrhoea to weight loss and general lack of energy. Examination of faeces is often inconclusive as the cysts and trophozoites tend to be shed intermittently. Physicians who are aware of the high incidence of *Giardia* infections often treat patients who have prolonged gastrointestinal symptoms empirically with drugs like metronidazole or tinidazole.

Drinking water should be filtered and chlorinated to remove *Giardia* cysts, as outbreaks frequently occur when drinking water supplies become contaminated with sewage. In urban areas, broken water pipes or an overflow of sewage during storms can cause problems. In rural areas, water supplies are often derived from natural creeks which may have become contaminated with sewage. There is some evidence that other animals can harbour the same species that infects humans. Bushwalkers should avoid drinking unboiled water from creeks and water courses.

Trichomonas is a flagellated protozoan that occurs as a commensal in a large percentage of the population. *Trichomonas hominis* is found in the large intestine and *Trichomonas vaginalis* is a frequent inhabitant of the female genital tract. Vaginitis due to *Trichomonas* is

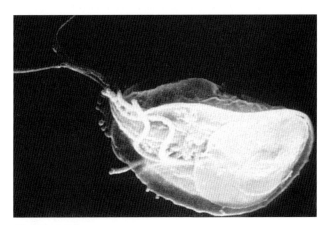

Figure 6.16

Scanning electron micrograph of the flagellate protozoan *Giardia lamblia*

SPOTLIGHT ON
Water quality and public health

A safe water supply is essential for public health so there was alarm in July 1998 when part of Sydney's water supply was found to be contaminated with high levels of *Giardia* and *Cryptosporidium*. Initially, the contamination was thought to be in only one section of pipes serving a small section of the Sydney CBD, but over a period of days it was found to extend to most areas of Sydney supplied by the Sydney Water Corporation. Heavy rainfalls that filled the storage dams added to the problem. Residents were advised not to drink water unless it had been boiled for at least one minute.

Cryptosporidium and *Giardia* are protozoal parasites that are carried by many animals as well as humans and are excreted as oocysts in the faeces. Presumably, they enter the water supply in run-off from catchment areas. *Giardia* is often contracted by bushwalkers drinking from contaminated streams or by travellers in developing countries, and causes diarrhoea, stomach cramps and general malaise. It can be difficult to treat and may persist for months.

Cryptosporidium causes gastrointestinal infections with watery diarrhoea which can be serious and even fatal for immunocompromised people. Outbreaks are sometimes associated with children's wading pools. In Milwaukee, USA, in 1993 there was a breakdown in water treatment standards; over 405 000 people were infected with *Cryptosporidium* and a number of immunocompromised patients died.

Water treatment plants are designed to filter and disinfect the water before it is supplied to the public. However, there are problems associated with measurements of water quality. Protozoal cysts are much more resistant to the usual methods of water treatment than bacteria, and there is no accepted standard for the levels of contamination that may pose a health hazard. There are difficulties in measurement as the methods currently available do not distinguish between living (viable) and dead parasites.

The high levels of contamination were detected in Sydney's water for nearly two months and during this time residents were advised to boil their water. Sales of bottled water soared. Curiously, there was only a slight and probably not significant increase in reports of infections, despite the fact that surveys indicated less than 100% compliance with the 'boil water' alert. The reasons for this are not clear – it may be that the cells detected were not viable or that the strain of *Cryptosporidium* was one that did not infect humans.

However, the events served as a timely reminder of the importance of a safe water supply and provided the incentive for a review of water treatment methods and standards in New South Wales.

characterised by a smelly greenish vaginal discharge. It may occur when the pH of the vagina becomes less acid, allowing *T. vaginalis* to multiply (see Chapter 21). The organism is sexually transmitted, so treatment should include both partners.

The **haemoflagellates** are a group of flagellated protozoa responsible for a number of serious diseases with a high morbidity and mortality rate. They are the cause of millions of deaths in some parts of the world. *Trypanosoma brucei gambiense*, found in West Africa, and *Trypanosoma brucei rhodesiense* in East Africa, are both carried by the tsetse fly and are the cause of African sleeping sickness. The protozoa affect the nervous system, leading to coma and death. *Trypanosoma cruzi*, the cause of Chagas disease, is also carried by an insect vector, the reduviid or kissing bug. This flightless insect is found in South America, usually in areas of poor quality housing. The disease has a slow progression with increasing debilitation and eventual death, often due to myocarditis. None of these diseases occurs in Australia as the appropriate insect vectors are not found in this country.

The *Leishmania* are a group of haemoflagellates that are spread by sandflies and are responsible for the serious illness **leishmaniasis**. They are distributed over South and Central America, India, the Middle East and Africa. The disease takes two forms. Some species attack the skin, causing cutaneous leishmaniasis which is not usually fatal; others that affect the liver and spleen, cause visceral leishmaniasis (also called kala-azar). Untreated kala-azar is invariably fatal. Several different drugs are used, but in many Third World countries access to treatment is difficult and the cost of drugs prohibitive. Prevention of these diseases depends on an effective campaign to control the sandfly vectors. Animals other than humans can serve as a reservoir for *Leishmania*, so it is very difficult to limit the incidence of the disease.

Leishmaniasis is only seen in Australia if the patient has contracted the disease outside Australia. However, cutaneous leishmaniasis was reported recently in Australian kangaroos, which raises the possibility of its transmission to humans via sandfly bites.

Pathogenic sporozoa

Sporozoa belonging to the genus *Plasmodium* are responsible for causing **malaria**. There are four species – *Plasmodium falciparum*, *P. vivax*, *P. ovale* and *P. malariae*. They are non-motile protozoa and require an insect vector, in this case the Anopheles mosquito, for transmission. It is estimated that worldwide there are 200 million cases of malaria annually and between one and two million deaths. The disease is widespread in tropical areas, but is not endemic in Australia at present. However, the north of Australia (above latitude 19°S) is a receptive area where Anopheles mosquitoes are found.

The malaria parasite has three distinct stages in its life cycle. The first involves the injection of the **sporozoite** into the human host via the bite of an infected female Anopheles mosquito. The sporozoite migrates to the liver

where, over a period of several days or weeks, it replicates asexually, producing hundreds of **merozoites**.

The second asexual stage occurs in the red blood cells of the human host. The merozoites that were released from the liver into the bloodstream invade the red cells and multiply, causing haemolysis and releasing hundreds more merozoites into the bloodstream. It is this stage that produces the typical symptoms of malaria – headache, nausea, fever and chills. These symptoms occur at regular intervals, coinciding with the synchronised release of the merozoites from the red cells. As the life cycle continues, some merozoites produce **trophozoites** which develop into male and female gametes.

The gametes are ingested by the feeding Anopheles mosquito and undergo the third, and sexual, stage in the mosquito, which takes 7–10 days. Gametes fuse to form a zygote which matures into a sporozoite that is released through the salivary glands of the mosquito when it bites a new host, thus completing the cycle. Malaria is described in more detail on page 471.

There is an interesting relationship between the occurrence of red blood cell disorders and susceptibility to malaria. Individuals who carry the genetic trait (i.e. are heterozygous) for sickle cell anaemia appear to have an increased level of immunity to malaria (see Spotlight box, page 73). The red blood cells of these carriers are not as susceptible to *Plasmodium* as are normal blood cells. This also seems to apply to other genetically inherited blood disorders – thalassaemia and glucose-6-phosphate dehydrogenase deficiency.

Programs for the prevention of malaria have been aimed at control or eradication of mosquitoes. These have not been very successful, partly because of bureaucratic inefficiency, but also because the mosquitoes have become resistant to pesticides such as DDT. Another serious problem is the widespread appearance of strains of *Plasmodium* that are resistant to the antimalarial drugs currently in use.

Research into a vaccine for malaria has so far been unsuccessful. It is difficult because the complex nature of the life cycle means that each stage of the parasite has a different antigenic structure. To be effective, a vaccine would have to be active against more than one stage in order to eliminate the parasite. The sexual stage of the life cycle also allows for genetic variation to occur, so that there is a continual change in the antigenic structure of the parasite.

Toxoplasma gondii is a sporozoan responsible for a mild flu-like illness in humans, **toxoplasmosis**. The life cycle of the parasite and characteristics of the disease are described in detail in Chapter 19. Humans can be infected by the accidental ingestion of oocysts that have been shed in cat faeces, or by the consumption of undercooked meat containing cysts.

Like many of the parasites discussed in this chapter, *Toxoplasma* has much more serious effects in patients whose immune system is deficient. These include the foetus during pregnancy, and immunocompromised patients such as those with AIDS.

Toxoplasma produces congenital defects when a non-immune mother is infected during pregnancy. The type of congenital abnormality depends on whether infection occurs during the first, second or third trimester of pregnancy. The outcomes of infections during the first trimester are the most serious and include stillbirth and neurological defects such as blindness. If infection occurs later in pregnancy, the effects are not so severe and may not be clinically apparent until later in life. Neurological problems and learning difficulties are sometimes an outcome of late prenatal toxoplasmosis. *Toxoplasma* is widely distributed and many Australians carry antibodies to the protozoan. Women considering pregnancy can be tested to determine their level of immunity and, if not immune, should avoid contact with cat faeces and undercooked meat (see Chapter 19).

In patients who are immunodeficient (AIDS) or immunosuppressed (transplant), latent *Toxoplasma* can be reactivated to a fulminating fatal infection. Other serious consequences of reactivation include retinitis, encephalitis and pneumonia.

Cryptosporidium and *Microsporidium* are non-motile protozoa that commonly inhabit the intestines of some native animals and birds. They can enter the water supply and are then transmitted via the faecal-oral route. They are a probable cause of transient mild diarrhoea in humans, which can be quite serious in children and immunodeficient people. There have been reports of outbreaks of diarrhoea due to *Cryptosporidium* in day-care centres, and reports that were traced to public wading pools. In the United States a serious outbreak was linked to a contaminated water supply (see Spotlight box, page 121).

In individuals who are HIV-positive, *Cryptosporidium* and, more recently, *Microsporidium* have been found to be responsible for chronic diarrhoea with loose watery stools. *Cryptosporidium* can be identified in faecal specimens using a special staining technique or by immunofluorescence. See Figure 6.17.

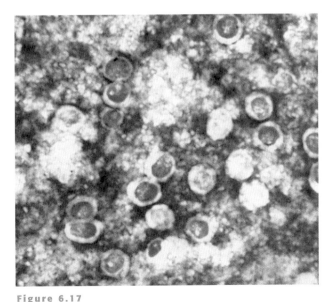

Figure 6.17

Cryptosporidium parvum
A Zeihl-Neelsen stain of oocysts.

Helminths

Helminths, or worms, are a common cause of parasitic infection throughout the world. In general, their occurrence in humans is linked to low socioeconomic conditions and poor sanitation. Although infections are widespread, especially in developing countries, they are rarely fatal on their own. Many individuals carry a significant worm 'load' without apparent ill effect, but in some cases the parasites contribute to significant morbidity.

Many helminths have a complex life cycle, often involving more than one host. Some require an insect vector for transmission. An understanding of the life cycle of each parasite is essential in order to develop appropriate strategies for prevention and treatment of infection. The **definitive host** harbours the sexually mature adult form of the parasite, while the cyst or larval stages are found in the **intermediate host**. The human host is not necessarily an essential part of the life cycle of the parasite. Very often humans are an 'accidental' host – that is, they acquire the parasite by ingestion of contaminated food or water.

With rare exceptions, helminths do not replicate within their human hosts. However, the production of eggs in the human intestine, with subsequent shedding in the faeces, contributes to the continuation of the life cycle.

CLASSIFICATION

The parasitic helminths that occur in humans belong to two phyla – the **Platyhelminthes**, or flatworms, which include the **trematodes** (flukes) and cestodes (tapeworms); and the **Aschelminthes**, which contain the **nematodes** (roundworms). Helminths are usually large organisms with a complex body structure. However, the larval stages may be quite small, only 100–200 μm in size, and the eggs are microscopic.

DISTRIBUTION

Table 6.3 lists the common species of worms that cause human infections in Australia. Other serious parasitic helminth infections – such as filariasis, onchocerciasis and schistosomiasis – occur in many parts of the world but are not usually seen in Australia. This can be due to lack of the appropriate insect vector, lack of a suitable intermediate host for the parasite, or to the absence of a reservoir of infection. Many of these infections are associated with tropical climates and poor sanitary practices. This section concentrates on helminth infections that are prevalent in Australia.

FLATWORMS

The **cestodes**, or **tapeworms**, live as intestinal parasites in their definitive host. They consist of a head, or **scolex**, and a long body made up of segments, or **proglottids** (Figure 6.18). The scolex has hooks or suckers, enabling the worm to attach to the mucosal cells lining the intestine. The worm obtains its food by absorption of predigested nutrients directly from the intestine of the host, through pores on the surface of the proglottids. Each segment

Table 6.3

Endemic helminth infections in Australia

ORGANISM	DEFINITIVE HOST	INTERMEDIATE HOST	TRANSMISSION TO HUMANS	MEDICATION
Taenia saginata (beef tapeworm)	Humans	Cattle	Ingestion of undercooked beef	Praziquantel Niclosamide
Echinococcus granulosis (dog tapeworm)	Dogs	Humans/Tissues (hydatid cysts)	Ingestion of eggs	Albendazole
Hymenolepis nana (dwarf tapeworm)	Humans intestine		Ingestion of eggs	Praziquantel
Ascaris lumbricoides (roundworm)	Humans intestine		Ingestion of eggs	Mebendazole
Enterobius vermicularis (pinworm)	Humans intestine		Ingestion of eggs	Albendazole
Ancylostoma duodenale *Necator americanus* (hookworm)	Humans intestine		Penetration of skin by larvae	Albendazole
Strongyloides stercoralis	Humans intestine/other tissues		Penetration of skin by larvae	Thiabendazole
Trichuris trichiura (whipworm)	Humans		Ingestion of eggs	Mebendazole

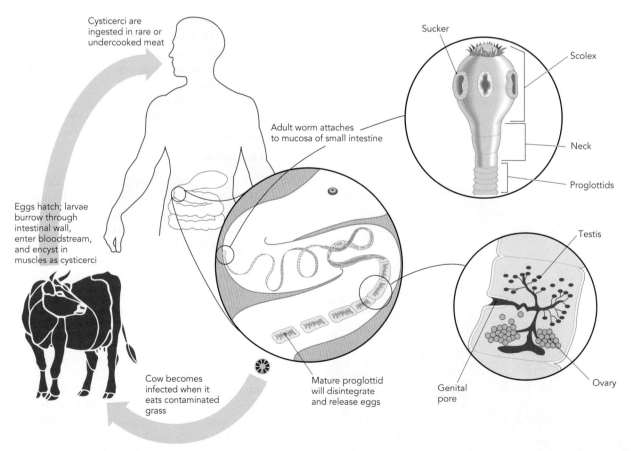

Figure 6.18

Beef tapeworm, *Taenia saginata*

The adult tapeworm has suckers to attach to the mucosa of the host intestine. Eggs are excreted in faeces and eaten by the cow which is the intermediate host. Humans are infected by eating contaminated meat.

contains both male and female sexual organs and is thus capable of egg production. Mature proglottids containing thousands of eggs are shed in the faeces. Other animals ingest vegetation or water contaminated with the eggs. In the new host, the eggs hatch into larvae which bore through the intestinal wall and establish cysts in the tissues of the infected animal (intermediate host). Ingestion of cysts in meat by the definitive host completes the cycle.

Humans act as the definitive host for the beef tapeworm, *Taenia saginata*, and the pork tapeworm, *Taenia solium*. Of these, only the beef tapeworm occurs in Australia, mainly in cattle-raising areas. Strict meat inspection procedures at abattoirs prevent contaminated meat from reaching the markets and, up to now, quarantine regulations have prevented the pork tapeworm from reaching Australia. Humans can often unknowingly harbour large tapeworms without any apparent symptoms.

The dwarf tapeworm *Hymenolepis nana* is sometimes found in Northern Australia. It is unusual in that it does not require an intermediate host. Ingested eggs can develop into mature worms in the human intestine.

Humans are the intermediate host for the dog tapeworm, *Echinococcus granulosis*, giving rise to a condition known as **hydatid cysts**. Dogs and cats are the definitive hosts for this tiny tapeworm, which is 2–8 mm in length. Eggs are shed in the faeces and may be transmitted to humans from faeces on the fur or tongue of the animal. The eggs hatch in the human intestine and migrate to various parts of the body, where they form large fluid-filled sacs of larvae, called hydatid cysts. Cysts may form in any tissue but those that form in the liver, lungs and brain are the most common and have the most serious consequences (see page 435). Hydatids can be avoided by worming domestic animals regularly and not feeding them raw meat.

The **trematodes**, or **flukes**, have a flat, leaf-shaped body and a rudimentary digestive system consisting of a mouth and intestine but no anus. Most of the body is taken up by a complex reproductive system. On the outside surface of the fluke are muscular suckers that enable it to attach to host tissue (see Figure 6.19). Two main groups of flukes cause disease in humans:

- The tissue flukes attach to the lungs (e.g. *Paragonimus westermani*) or liver (e.g. *Clonorchis sinensis*, *Opisthorchis felineus*, *Opisthorchis viverrini* and *Fasciola hepatica*).
- The blood flukes (e.g. *Schistosoma*) reside in the vascular system of their human hosts.

The life cycle of all the flukes is very complex, often involving more than one intermediate host. They all require a species of freshwater snail which is usually specific for each of the fluke species and occurs only in certain habitats. Tissue flukes usually have a second intermediate host, a crustacean or fish, which acts as a source of infection for the definitive human host. The schistosomes (blood flukes) are released from the snail as the free-swimming fork-tailed infective form, **cercariae**,

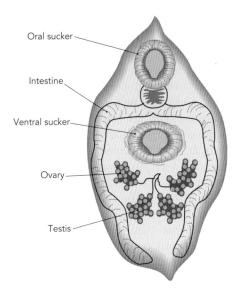

Figure 6.19
Flukes
This generalised diagram of the anatomy of an adult fluke shows the oral and ventral suckers. The suckers attach the fluke to the host. The mouth is located at the centre of the oral sucker. Flukes are hermaphroditic; each animal contains both testes and ovaries.

which invade humans by direct penetration through the skin. **Schistosomiasis** is a major world health problem and is discussed further in Chapter 19.

With the exception of *Fasciola hepatica*, infections by flukes do not occur in Australia. Good sanitation, combined with the absence of the specific snail hosts, keep the parasite out of this country. However, cases of schistosomiasis, acquired from contaminated water or fish, have been seen recently in Australia in travellers returning from endemic tropical areas.

ROUNDWORMS

Nematodes, or roundworms, are widely distributed throughout the world. They are long, cylindrical worms with a complete digestive system comprising a mouth, intestine and anus. Male and female sex organs are located on different organisms, the female worm often being significantly larger than the male. In general, nematodes have a less complex life cycle than flatworms. Several roundworms are able to parasitise humans and other animals, as well as insects and plants. For humans, the important parasites include the common roundworms, hookworms and threadworms. Many of these occur in Australia (Table 6.3).

The common **pinworm**, or **threadworm**, *Enterobius vermicularis*, is universally distributed. The tiny (0.5 cm) worm lives in the large intestine, the female emerging at night to lay eggs around the anus. The main symptom is anal pruritis (itching) due to irritation of the skin. Transmission of the worm occurs when the eggs are picked up on the fingers and ingested by the same host (reinfection) or another host. Eggs are frequently shed into clothing and bedding, which can also serve as a source of infection. Most children are infected at some time and the itching may cause disturbance to their sleep. Threadworm infections do not really have any major adverse effects on the host, and are usually easily treated.

Strongyloides stercoralis is another threadworm infection, commonly seen in tropical and subtropical regions, especially in Aboriginal people. It is acquired by larval penetration of the skin. The adult worms, which are only 2–3 mm long, are found lodged in grooves in the intestinal mucosa, but the larvae circulate constantly through the body. The worm is unusual in that it can replicate within the human host, so the infection may persist for long periods. If only a few worms are present, patients may be asymptomatic but, with heavy infestations, symptoms such as abdominal pain, rashes and pruritis occur. Immunocompromised or debilitated patients often have more severe symptoms and treatment may need to be repeated at regular intervals (Figure 6.20).

The roundworm *Ascaris lumbricoides* is a large worm that may reach 30 cm in length. It usually lives in the small intestine, producing mild symptoms of abdominal discomfort. Occasionally, a bolus of worms may cause intestinal obstruction in children. The female worm produces thousands of eggs that are passed in the faeces. They can survive for long periods in the soil. When ingested by another host, the eggs hatch in the intestine, mature in the lungs and then migrate back to the intestine. Occasionally, adult worms are excreted in the faeces.

Hookworm infections are caused by *Ancylostoma duodenale* and *Necator americanus*. Hookworms are about 1 cm in length and have a mouth with hooks or suckers which enable them to attach to the wall of the intestine and suck blood. Depending on the level of infection (worm load), symptoms may range from slight discomfort to anaemia and abdominal pain. Eggs are shed in the faeces and develop into larvae in the soil. Infection takes place when the larvae burrow through the skin, enter the blood vessels of the host and are carried to the lungs. The larvae are coughed up in sputum, swallowed and finally arrive in the intestine where they attach to the mucosal cells and establish an infection.

Hookworm occurs mainly in remote areas of Australia, when sanitation is poor. The Aboriginal population is particularly susceptible because of chronic malnutrition and the practice of walking barefoot. See Figure 6.21.

Trichinosis is a serious infection caused by the roundworm *Trichinella spiralis*. It is acquired by eating raw or undercooked pork that is contaminated with cysts of the worm. Although widespread in America, trichinosis is not a problem in Australia; the pork sold in Australia is currently free of this parasite.

Several other roundworms that do not occur in Australia are responsible for severe infections in other parts of the world. Among these are the **microfilariae**, tiny worms that are carried by insects. **Filariasis**, or **elephantiasis**, is caused by *Wuchereria bancrofti* and transmitted by mosquitoes (see Chapter 19). The worm blocks the vessels of the lymphatic system, preventing drainage of fluid from the tissues and causing gross distortion of parts of the body – for example, legs, arms, breasts, vulva and scrotum. Filariasis is common in the Pacific Islands.

Onchocerca volvulus is a tiny worm carried by the black fly and is responsible for river blindness, a debilitat-

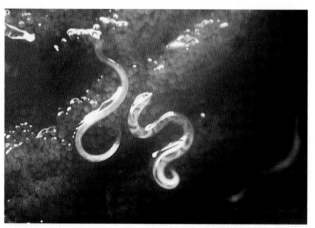

Figure 6.21

Hookworms attached to the intestinal mucosa
Barely visible larvae penetrate the skin (often through bare feet), are carried to the lungs, go through the respiratory tract to the mouth, are swallowed and eventually reach the intestine. The journey takes about a week.

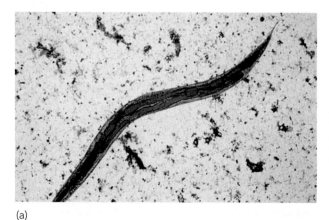

(a)

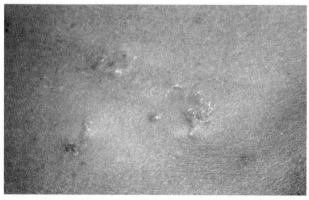

(b)

Figure 6.20

***Strongyloides* infection**
(a) Worm; (b) a patient with disseminated *Strongyloides* infection; trails under the skin indicate the migrations of the worms.

ing blindness that affects many thousands of people in developing countries. Guinea worm (*Dracunculus medinensis*) is another nematode acquired from contaminated drinking water; it produces large painful abscesses when the worm emerges from the body.

The cat and dog roundworms, *Toxocara cati* and *Toxocara canis*, are transmitted to humans, mainly children, by the ingestion of eggs in dog or cat faeces. After ingestion, the eggs hatch and the larvae migrate to various body organs, including the eye, when blindness may result. The worm occurs in Australia although it is more widespread in other parts of the world. Regular worming of pets is an effective control.

TREATMENT AND PREVENTION OF HELMINTH INFECTIONS

In recent years the attitude of the medical profession to the treatment of helminth infections has altered significantly. This is due to a number of factors.

- We now know that most helminths do not replicate inside their definitive human host.
- It is now recognised that worms only cause significant damage to their host when the infestation is very heavy and that, in general, most infected individuals do not carry a sufficient population of worms to cause disease.
- More importantly, in recent years a number of effective antihelminthic drugs have become available. These are listed in Table 6.3.

For Australia, this means that there are safe, effective drugs available to treat any worm infestations that may occur. These drugs, combined with education about proper sanitation and improved awareness of the importance of nutrition, should improve the health of people in remote areas.

In developing countries, there has been a shift in the strategies employed for the control of helminth diseases. It should be apparent from this discussion that the life cycles of the various helminths are very complex. Attempts to prevent worm infections by destruction of intermediate hosts, elimination of vectors, or alteration of environmental conditions to destroy larvae are all very costly and have not proved effective. The availability of inexpensive, effective drugs means that public health measures aimed at prevention and treatment now concentrate on the administration of these drugs at regular intervals.

Worldwide policy for the treatment of worm infestations in children in developing countries now involves regular administration of antihelminthic drugs at yearly intervals. Since 1993 this has been implemented for school children in developing countries, along with the administration of nutritional supplements. The program has seen a marked reduction in worm load, accompanied by significant improvements in general health and development.

Ectoparasites

A number of arthropods (insects) are capable of existing in a parasitic relationship on the outside surface of the human body. These are called **ectoparasites**. The most common are fleas, ticks, lice, and mites such as scabies (see Figure 6.22).

SCABIES

Scabies is an itchy skin infection caused by a tiny mite about 0.4 mm in diameter, called *Sarcoptes scabei* (Figure 6.22). The female mite burrows under the surface of the skin, forming a tunnel in which she lays two or three eggs each day. The infection is visible as a red, inflamed line, caused by an allergic reaction to the faeces left in the tunnel by the mite. Infection may occur anywhere on the body but is most common on the hands and forearms, or in warm, moist areas such as the armpits or groin. The mites are transmitted directly from person to person, but they are also found on bedding and clothing and can survive for 2–3 days away from a human host.

Treatment with benzyl benzoate or a cream containing 5% permethrin is effective, but eradication requires that all clothing and bed linen is washed and household contacts are also treated.

Scabies is endemic within Aboriginal communities in Northern Australia, and also occurs in urban areas where there is close human contact, such as in nursing homes (see Figure 6.23). Prevalence rates in Northern Territory Aboriginal school children are 30–65%. One of the major problems associated with scabies infection is that the itching and subsequent scratching allow secondary bacterial infections to occur.

Staphylococcal and group A streptococcal infections are commonly associated with scabies. They can be readily treated with antibiotics, but if the scabies infection is not eliminated the bacterial infection may recur and antibiotic-resistant strains of bacteria may arise. If untreated, group A streptococci can give rise to bacteraemia, rheumatic fever and kidney diseases such as acute post-streptococcal glomerulonephritis (see Chapter 14).

FLEAS

Fleas are blood-sucking insects that live parasitically on any warm-blooded animal. Occasionally, they will move

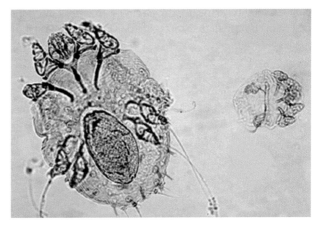

Figure 6.22
Scabies
Adult scabies mite with an egg and newly hatched mite.

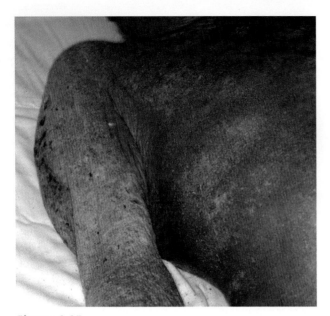

Scabies
Crusted scabies in an elderly nursing home resident.

from their usual animal host (cats, dogs, rats, wild animals) to humans. Usually, they do not create a problem, other than a brief irritation, and can easily be removed by improved hygiene or, if necessary, treating houses with insecticides. Fleas are the carrier (vector) of the bacterium that causes bubonic plague, *Yersinia pestis*. Usually, the infection occurs in rodents (rats, squirrels) but when the animal dies the infected fleas may move to a human host. Plague is not endemic in Australia although there have been outbreaks in the past (see Chapter 19).

LICE

The louse, *Pediculus humanus*, is a small insect that lives on the outside of the body, particularly on the scalp and in the hair. The bite causes redness, itching and some lymph exudate which can provide a medium for secondary bacterial infections. Lice infestation is easily diagnosed by the presence of small white eggs (nits) attached to the hair shaft. The lice are transmitted directly by person-to-person contact. Outbreaks of lice are common in school children and can be treated with preparations obtained from the pharmacist. Bedding and clothing should also be disinfected.

The crab louse, *Phthirus pubis*, is found mainly in the pubic region and is transmitted by sexual contact (see Figure 6.24).

ARTHROPOD VECTORS

A number of ectoparasites – ticks, mites and lice – can harbour rickettsia-like organisms in the cells of the alimentary canal. The insect acquires the organism by biting an infected animal or human and transmits the infection by biting or by faecal excretion onto the skin of another host. Scratching the bite allows the organism to penetrate the skin and enter the new host. Of these infections the most serious is epidemic typhus, which is carried by the human body louse. The disease is limited to developing countries or conditions of poor hygiene.

Ticks carry rickettsias such as *Rickettsia honei* (which causes Flinders Island spotted fever). Spotted fever was first reported in 1991 and is characterised by fever, headache, myalgias, arthralgias, a maculopapular rash and focal skin lesions.

Mites are responsible for carrying scrub typhus, which occurs in Northern Queensland and the Northern Territory. A number of diseases are carried by insects and other arthropods. See Tables 5.4 and 8.4.

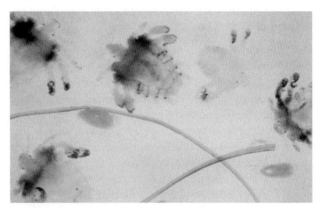

Pubic louse
False-colour SEM of the pubic louse, *Phthirus pubis*, also known as a crab louse, clinging to a pubic hair. The lice suck blood, feeding about five times a day.

SUMMARY

- A number of infectious diseases are caused by eucaryotic microorganisms.
- Patients who are immunocompromised are very susceptible to opportunistic infections caused by protozoa and fungi.

FUNGI

- Fungi comprise two groups: yeasts and moulds. Fungal cells are surrounded by a cell wall; they lack chlorophyll and cannot carry out photosynthesis.
- Fungi can grow at extremes of pH, temperature and osmotic pressure and are important for the decomposition of organic material.
- Yeasts are unicellular organisms that reproduce by budding. Some pathogenic yeasts (e.g. *Candida*) exhibit dimorphism.
- Moulds are filamentous fungi; they grow by producing a mat of hyphae called a mycelium as well as aerial hyphae that extend up above the mycelium.
- Asexual reproduction takes place by the formation of spores on the tips of the aerial hyphae.

FUNGAL INFECTIONS

- A fungal infection (mycosis) may be superficial, cutaneous, subcutaneous or systemic.
- Cutaneous infections (tinea) are caused by fungi called dermatophytes.
- Subcutaneous infections occur when the fungus is inoculated beneath the skin.
- Systemic mycoses are caused by pathogenic fungi, or fungi that have invaded an immunocompromised patient.
- Most serious fungal infections are opportunistic.
- *Pneumocystis jiroveci* is an opportunistic fungus that causes atypical lung infections in immunocompromised patients.

Transmission of fungal infections

- Fungi can be transmitted by direct contact with an infected lesion or skin scales.
- Fungal spores are spread throughout the atmosphere on wind currents.
- Patient susceptibility to fungal infection is affected by use of immunosuppressive drugs, invasive procedures, IV therapy and prolonged antibiotic therapy.

Treatment of fungal infections

- Topical antifungal preparations are useful for cutaneous infections.
- Systemic infections are difficult to treat as most drugs have side effects.

Harmful effects of fungi

- Allergic bronchopulmonary reactions occur from repeated inhalation of fungal spores.
- Some fungi produce toxins that are poisonous to humans.

PARASITES

- Parasites are organisms that derive their nutrients from another living organism.
- Parasites often have a complex life cycle, involving two or more hosts. The definitive host harbours the mature adult form of the parasite. The intermediate host has the immature or larval form.
- Serious parasitic diseases are relatively uncommon in Australia.
- Lifestyle factors and deficiencies in the immune defences increase susceptibility to parasitic infections.

PROTOZOA

- Protozoa are single-celled animals surrounded by a cell membrane. They are found mainly in water habitats.
- Reproduction is mainly asexual by binary or multiple fission.
- Protozoa form cysts that are able to survive for long periods under adverse conditions.
- Protozoa can exist as intracellular or extracellular parasites in humans and animals.
- Protozoal infections can be acquired by ingestion of the parasite or via the bite of a blood-sucking insect.
- Protozoa are classified by the way they move.
- Sarcodina (amoebae) move by extending the cell membrane to form a pseudopod and allowing the cytoplasm to flow into it.
- Protozoa that move by means of flagella include *Giardia*, which is responsible for gastrointestinal infections, and *Trichomonas vaginalis*, a sexually transmitted pathogen.
- Ciliates move by hair-like appendages called cilia.
- Sporozoa are non-motile protozoa.
- The genus *Plasmodium* is the cause of malaria and requires the Anopheles mosquito for transmission.
- *Toxoplasma gondii* is a non-motile sporozoan carried by cats. It has serious effects on immunosuppressed patients and can cause congenital defects.
- *Cryptosporidium* and *Microsporidium* cause chronic diarrhoea in immunodeficient patients.

HELMINTHS

- Helminths (worms) include the phylum *Platyhelminthes* (flatworms, i.e. flukes and tapeworms) and the phylum *Aschelminthes* (roundworms).
- Many helminths have a complex life cycle involving an intermediate and a definitive host.
- Cestodes (tapeworms) consist of a head (scolex) and a body made of proglottids (segments) with both male and female organs on each segment. Eggs are produced and excreted in the faeces.
- Trematodes (flukes) have a flat body with muscular suckers for attachment.
- Nematodes (roundworms) are cylindrical worms with male and female organs located on different worms.

Treatment and prevention of helminth infections

- Several antihelminthic drugs are available.
- Adequate nutrition and good sanitation are effective control measures.

- Arthropods such as scabies mites, fleas and lice can exist on the surface of the human body, causing skin irritation and carrying infection.

STUDY QUESTIONS

1. How do opportunistic infections differ from other infections?
2. Name the two main groups of fungi.
3. Describe the structure and method of replication of yeasts.
4. Describe the structure of moulds and their method of asexual reproduction.
5. What is a mycosis?
6. Differentiate between superficial, cutaneous and subcutaneous mycoses.
7. What is tinea?
8. Under what conditions is *Candida albicans* likely to cause infections?
9. How are fungal infections transmitted?
10. List two harmful effects of fungi other than mycoses.
11. What is a parasite?
12. What are some of the predisposing factors that allow parasitic infections to occur?
13. How do diseases caused by protozoa and helminths differ from those caused by bacteria or viruses?
14. What is the difference between an intermediate host and a definitive host?
15. What are protozoa?
16. How do protozoa reproduce?
17. What is the importance of the cyst form of protozoa?
18. How are protozoa classified?
19. Describe the causative organism, transmission and symptoms of amoebic dysentery.
20. Describe two important flagellate diseases present in Australia.
21. What is the most important sporozoal infection worldwide?
22. What role does the domestic cat play in the transmission of *Toxoplasma*?
23. What is a common cause of diarrhoea in AIDS patients?
24. How are worms classified?
25. How do tapeworms reproduce?
26. What are the main differences between human infections due to the beef tapeworm and those caused by the dog tapeworm?
27. Why are infections due to flukes not commonly seen in Australia?
28. What is the most common roundworm infection of children?
29. Why are worm infestations more common in people of lower socioeconomic status?
30. Which helminth infections are carried by insects?
31. How are helminth infections (a) prevented, (b) treated and (c) controlled?
32. What is scabies? Describe the major problems associated with scabies infections.
33. What is an ectoparasite? Give three examples.
34. Which diseases can be carried by ectoparasites?

TEST YOUR UNDERSTANDING

1. What is the difference between a cutaneous and a systemic mycosis?
2. Why are many hospitalised patients at risk of acquiring systemic fungal infections?
3. Why is it difficult to find an effective vaccine for malaria?
4. What other health problems would you suspect in a patient who is diagnosed with atypical pneumonia due to *Pneumocystis jiroveci*? Why?
5. Why should pregnant women avoid soiled kitty litter, sandpits and undercooked meat?
6. How do climate and environmental conditions influence the occurrence of parasitic infections? Explain your answer.
7. Discuss why effective drug therapy for diseases caused by eucaryotic organisms is difficult to achieve.

Host–microbe Interactions

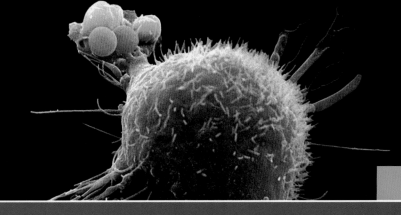

CHAPTER 7

Host–Microbe Interactions and Principles of Disease

[CHAPTER FOCUS]

- ■ *What kinds of relationships exist between living organisms?*

- ■ *What are the properties of the microorganisms that inhabit the human body?*

- ■ *What is an infectious disease?*

- ■ *What factors determine whether a microorganism will cause an infection?*

- ■ *What are the signs and symptoms of infectious diseases?*

- ■ *What are the stages in the progress of a disease?*

Introduction

In previous chapters we have described in some detail the properties of the major types of microorganisms and introduced some of the diseases they cause. But:

- What is the definition of disease?
- What determines whether an organism will cause disease?
- Why do some organisms cause disease and others do not?

There are microorganisms all around us in the environment and on the human body, so why do some people get sick and others do not?

Other questions also need to be answered.

- How do we know that microorganisms cause disease?
- How does disease spread from one person to another?

The chapters in this unit describe the interactions between humans and microorganisms that determine whether a state of health, disease, epidemic and/or death will occur. This interaction is complex and depends on a number of factors including the susceptibility of the human host, the risk of exposure to disease and the method of transmission of the organism. The virulence of the pathogen and the ability of the body's defences to withstand invasion by the microorganism also help to determine the outcome.

In this chapter we focus on what is meant by infection and infectious disease, pathogenicity and virulence, and discuss the ways in which the delicate balance between microorganisms and humans can be altered, thus giving rise to a state of disease. Other chapters in this unit discuss how diseases are spread, the properties of microorganisms that enable them to overcome human host defences and produce damage and disease, and the way in which the immune system protects the host against disease.

Symbiosis

The biological term used to describe two organisms living together is **symbiosis**. All living organisms exist in some kind of relationship with each other. Sometimes the organisms do not interact unless they are physically brought together, for example, humans and animals. Sometimes the relationship is very close, as with members of a family. The study of how organisms interact in an environment is called **ecology** and each defined environment is termed an **ecosystem**.

The human body can be regarded as a special type of ecosystem. At any moment in time, the human host may be interacting with numerous microorganisms and is subjected to physical, nutritional and traumatic alterations in environmental conditions that may have a marked influence on this interaction. Within this ecosystem, microorganisms live either permanently or transiently and, depending on various other factors, they may or may not cause an infection.

Not all symbiotic relationships are equally beneficial to both organisms. There are three broad categories of symbiotic association, based on the degree of benefit each organism receives – mutualism, commensalism and parasitism. In practice, the categories overlap to some extent, especially when applied to the human body, as the type of interaction may vary depending on physiological circumstances.

MUTUALISM

Mutualism usually refers to a situation where two independent organisms live together to their mutual benefit. The most commonly cited example is that of bacteria living in the stomach of ruminant cattle, where they aid in the digestion of cellulose in the animal's diet and in return receive a constant supply of nutrients. In humans, the bacteria living in the large intestine (colon) are of benefit to the host by producing vitamin K and some B vitamins; these are absorbed from the large intestine into the bloodstream and contribute to the host's requirements for those vitamins. The bacteria also help in the breakdown of waste material and the formation of faeces. In return, the bacteria benefit because they have a sheltered environment and an assured food supply.

COMMENSALISM

Commensalism is an association between two organisms where one benefits while not causing any harm to the other. This is the term normally used to describe the relationship between the human host and many of the microorganisms that reside in or on the human body (see 'Normal Flora' below). For the most part, these organisms are harmless, living on the body surfaces and making use of the waste products (oils and fatty acids) that are excreted through pores on the skin surfaces (see Figure 7.1). Indeed, by preventing colonisation by harmful bacteria, they may also be regarded as being of indirect benefit to the host. However, when environmental conditions alter, these commensals sometimes gain entry to other parts of the host and set up an infection. This situation is called **opportunism** and is discussed later in this chapter. The definition of commensalism is therefore not clear-cut as the relationship between host and resident microbes may vary with conditions.

PARASITISM

Parasitism is defined as a situation where one organism benefits at the expense of the other, usually larger, organism – the host. This usually means that the host is damaged or disadvantaged in some way. Most infections caused by microorganisms result in some degree of damage to the host cells. Parasitism, therefore, encompasses a wide range of relationships, from those in which the host is only slightly harmed to those in which it is killed. The most 'successful' parasites are those that maintain their own life processes without killing their host, which is their source of nourishment. Many bacteria are commensals and are usually only considered to be in a parasitic relationship when they cause an infection. However, other microorganisms, such as the viruses and some protozoa and

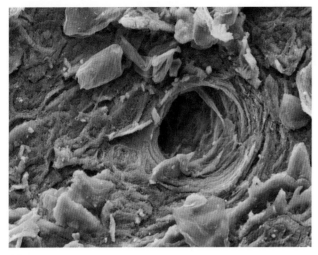

(a)

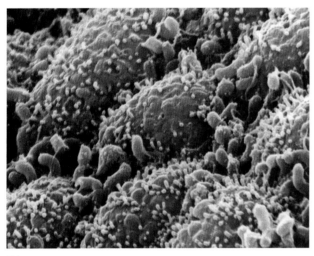

(b)

Figure 7.1

Normal flora

(a) Scanning electron micrograph of human skin showing uneven surface, skin scales and bacteria; (b) scanning electron micrograph of human intestine showing bacteria on mucosal surfaces. Most of the bacteria are commensals which indirectly benefit the host by competing with harmful organisms for nutrients and preventing them from finding a site to attach and invade the tissue.

helminths, are true parasites in that they are unable to live outside their host and so always cause an infection and produce some degree of damage (see Chapter 6).

As will become apparent in the following sections, the relationship between the microorganisms and their human host is complex and continually changing, due to alterations in the physiological and nutritional states of both. This relationship determines whether a clinically identifiable infection or disease will occur.

Microorganisms of the human body: normal flora (microbiota)

Before discussing the process of infection and disease, we should examine the human body as a habitat for micro-

organisms. Microorganisms are found everywhere in the environment and a rich population of microbes, especially bacteria, resides on the human body. These are called the **normal flora**, or **microbiota**, of the body.

The human foetus develops in a sterile environment in the uterus and at birth the neonate is free of microorganisms. However, within days, even hours of birth, a population of microorganisms, mainly bacteria, takes up residence on the various body surfaces. They are derived from the baby's immediate environment, usually the birth canal of the mother, the hands of the people who care for the infant, the surfaces in the hospital nursery and other parts of the hospital environment. Because of the different organisms to which they are exposed, babies who are bottle-fed tend to have different bacteria in the large intestine from those who are breast-fed.

For the rest of their lives, humans are constantly exposed to a changing population of microorganisms. Some of these take up permanent residence on the skin and on the mucosal surfaces of the upper respiratory tract, mouth, gastrointestinal system and genital tract. They are called normal or **resident flora**. Others (some of which may be pathogens) establish themselves briefly in suitable areas (e.g. nose and throat) and are said to **colonise** these surfaces. They are not permanent residents and, after some time, are excluded from the site by competition with the normal flora or by the host's immune defence mechanisms. Other microorganisms are **transient** and may be carried for a brief time on hands or other skin surfaces; they are usually considered to be **contaminants** and can be removed by physical means such as handwashing.

The human body provides an excellent shelter and source of nourishment for microbes. The various areas of the body have different conditions of temperature, moisture, pH, nutrients and oxygen so that different species can select the most suitable environment in which to reside. Most body surfaces (internal and external) that are exposed to the environment can, and do, harbour microorganisms. The bloodstream and the internal organs, however, are usually maintained in a sterile state by the various body defence mechanisms. When microorganisms enter these sites and persist, a state of disease exists.

The normal flora have a number of useful and protective effects. They occupy sites in the body and create an environment which inhibits colonisation by other organisms (e.g. lowered pH on the skin) so that harmful organisms cannot become established and cause an infection. Once established in a suitable area, they can modify their environment – they may alter the pH (e.g. lactobacilli in the vagina lower the pH to 5 which inhibits the growth of other bacteria and fungi), excrete chemicals with antibacterial activity (e.g. bacteriocins and organic acids in the large intestine) or produce vitamins that are of benefit to the host.

The value of the normal flora to the human host is apparent when their numbers are reduced by long-term, broad spectrum antibiotic therapy. A frequent side effect of such therapy is an overgrowth of undesirable organisms;

for example, *Clostridium difficile* may flourish in the large intestine, causing diarrhoea and pseudomembranous colitis. Vaginitis, or thrush, is caused by growth of *Candida albicans* in the vagina if the lactobacilli are destroyed. Cessation of antibiotic therapy usually allows the normal flora to become re-established.

The microbes that make up the normal flora are relatively stable but can be influenced by factors such as age, nutritional status, exposure to antibiotic therapy or a change in environment, such as a prolonged stay in hospital. Studies have shown that the composition of the microbial population alters very rapidly after a patient enters hospital, the normal flora being replaced with hospital strains that are generally resistant to antibiotics. Infection with these hospital strains has serious implications for the patient as they are usually more difficult to treat. Normal body flora can also be the cause of infections if the delicate balance between host and microbe is upset (see 'Opportunism', page 139).

NORMAL FLORA: TYPES OF ORGANISMS

By far the most predominant kinds of organism found on the human body are bacteria (see Figure 7.2). They can be easily identified by standard laboratory techniques and their role in maintaining the human ecosystem has been accepted for some time. The yeast, *Candida*, is the major fungal inhabitant and there are a few protozoa that appear to live in harmony with the human host (e.g. *Trichomonas intestinalis, Entamoeba coli*).

Because viruses are always thought of as disease-producing, they are not generally considered part of the normal flora. However, it may be that some viruses are able to reside in the human body without producing disease symptoms unless there is a change in the immune status of the host. An example of these would be latent viruses, such as members of the herpes family – herpes simplex, Epstein-Barr and cytomegalovirus (CMV) – but there may be others not yet identified (see Chapter 5).

NORMAL FLORA OF THE SKIN

The skin harbours a diverse population of microorganisms. Bacteria reside in or on the dead layers of skin, obtaining nutrients from the secretions of the sebaceous glands and hair follicles. There are two distinct cutaneous populations: contaminants and resident flora. The **contaminants**, or **transient** organisms, cling to the skin surfaces but do not usually replicate there. They include any organisms that the body (especially the hands) may have come into contact with during normal daily activities. Contaminants are greatly influenced by the personal hygiene of the individual. For health workers, the organisms carried on the hands are important in the transmission of disease.

The **resident flora** of the skin usually live in warm, moist areas of the body such as the axillae (armpits) and groin, in deep crevices in the skin layers, in hair follicles and in sweat glands. There are relatively few organisms present on the exposed, dry areas of the skin surface. The organisms usually present include species of *Staphylo-*

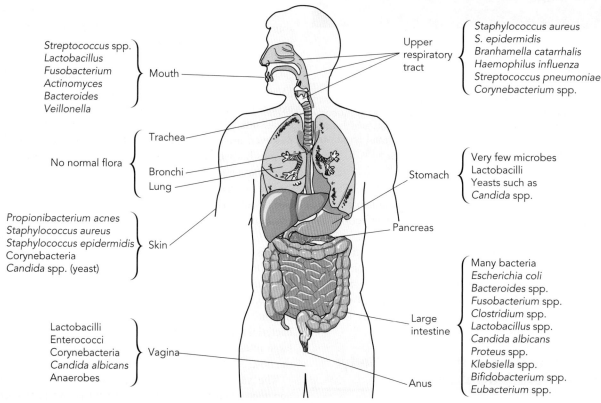

Figure 7.2

Location of normal flora on the human body

coccus, *Corynebacterium*, *Propionibacterium* and some fungi. *Staphylococcus epidermidis* is found mainly on dry areas of the skin, whereas *Staphylococcus aureus* prefers a moister environment such as the nasal passages. The organisms that populate the axillae metabolise the chemicals in sweat, producing breakdown products with a distinctive odour (body odour). Most commercial deodorants act by inhibiting the metabolic action of the bacteria or by drying the skin surface so that the bacteria cannot multiply.

NORMAL FLORA OF THE RESPIRATORY TRACT

The upper respiratory tract has a rich population of resident flora, including streptococci, staphylococci, diphtheroids and Gram-negative cocci. *Staphylococcus aureus* is found mainly in the nasal passages. Alpha- and beta-haemolytic streptococci and *Haemophilus influenzae* are frequently found in the throat. *Streptococcus pneumoniae* may be present and is often responsible for middle ear infections (otitis media). Other organisms that may be present include *Neisseria meningitidis*, *Moraxella (Branhamella) catarrhalis* and *Candida albicans*.

The bronchial tubes and lungs are relatively free of organisms in healthy individuals.

NORMAL FLORA OF THE GASTROINTESTINAL SYSTEM

The gastrointestinal system consists essentially of a long tube extending from the mouth to the anus. Varying conditions of oxygen tension, availability of nutrients and pH occur along this system and this is reflected in the different microbial populations that exist in each region.

The mouth contains a distinctive population of oral bacteria, the mucous membranes of the mouth supporting as many as 10^{11} bacteria per gram wet weight of tissue. These bacteria are usually present as commensals but can also be responsible for diseases in the mouth. The viridans group of streptococci are common members of the flora of the upper respiratory tract. They include the aerobes *Streptococcus mutans* and *Streptococcus sanguis* which can contribute to dental decay (**caries**) by secreting glucan, a sticky polysaccharide that attaches to the enamel of the tooth surface. **Plaque** consists of a film of bacterial cells anchored in a matrix of glycoproteins and polysaccharides that the organisms have secreted. This matrix provides a stable environment in which other oral bacteria thrive and metabolise sugars, producing acid that contributes to dental decay.

Other bacteria, including *Lactobacillus*, *Fusobacterium* and *Actinomyces*, which prefer an anaerobic environment, thrive on the gums or in crevices between the teeth. Sometimes these organisms are responsible for an infection of the gums known as **gingivitis**.

The pH of the stomach is acid due to the secretion of hydrochloric acid, and inhibits the growth of most microorganisms. A few acid-tolerant lactobacilli may be present in the gastric mucosa. *Helicobacter pylori*, a bacterium that has been shown to be involved in the occurrence of gastric ulcers, can also tolerate this environment, but is not considered part of the normal flora. The upper part of the ileum (duodenum) is slightly alkaline and is also relatively free of bacteria. The lower intestine, the caecum and colon, harbours a large population of bacteria (approximately 10^{12} bacteria per gram of intestinal contents) which can comprise up to 30% of the faecal volume.

The predominant flora are anaerobes or facultative anaerobes such as *Escherichia coli*, *Klebsiella* and *Enterobacter*, but strict anaerobes such as *Bacteroides* are also present in large numbers (see Table 7.1). The presence of *E. coli* in water samples is often used as a test for faecal contamination. Bacteria in the colon are of benefit to the host by digesting waste material and converting it to faeces, as well as the production of vitamins K and B and short-chain fatty acids (SCFA) which are important in maintaining the health of the colon. Anaerobic conditions in the colon result in the formation of gas (flatus) and various breakdown products with a strong, distinctive odour.

NORMAL FLORA OF THE GENITOURINARY TRACT

The major components of the urinary system – the kidneys, bladder and upper part of the urethra – are usually sterile. The lower portion of the urethra, especially in females, may harbour microorganisms that are representative of those present on the skin, vagina or colon. They are usually flushed out regularly by the flow of urine but if they persist can cause urinary tract infections.

The composition of the normal flora of the vagina illustrates how the flora change depending on age and physiological conditions. Before puberty, the pH of the vagina is about 7 and the main inhabitants are staphylococci, streptococci, diphtheroids and some coliforms. After puberty the hormone, oestrogen, stimulates the secretion of glycogen by the vagina. Fermentation of glycogen is carried out by lactobacilli with the production of acid, which lowers the pH to about 5. This acidic pH is protective, inhibiting the growth of many other organisms and establishing conditions suitable for fertilisation. If the lactobacilli of the vagina are destroyed by prolonged antibiotic therapy, or the pH is altered by hormonal or physiological disturbances, an overgrowth of other organisms frequently ensues (e.g. *Candida albicans*, causing thrush).

Infection and disease

Up to now we have been considering the microorganisms that live on the human body as a normal part of our environment. However, a delicate balance exists between a state of health and disease. Under certain conditions many of the normal flora, as well as organisms from the external environment, have the potential to cause disease.

The first step is for potential pathogens to become established or colonise the human body. They then have an opportunity to penetrate the host defences, invade the tissues, multiply and set up an **infection**. When the results

Table 7.1

Representative examples of normal human body flora[a]

Skin	*Propionibacterium acnes, Staphylococcus aureus, Staphylococcus epidermidis, Corynebacterium xerosis, Candida* spp. (yeast)
Eyes	*Staphylococcus aureus, Staphylococcus epidermidis,* diphtheroids
Upper respiratory tract	*Staphylococcus aureus, Staphylococcus epidermidis,* diphtheroids (mainly in nose)
Nose/throat	*Streptococcus pneumoniae, Haemophilus influenzae, Neisseria* in throat, *Moraxella* spp., *Micrococcus* spp.
Gastrointestinal system	
Mouth	*Streptococcus* spp., *Lactobacillus, Fusobacterium, Actinomyces, Bacteroides, Veillonella, Candida* (yeast)
Stomach	*Lactobacillus*
Large intestine	More than 300 species including *Bacteroides, Enterococcus, Enterobacter, Escherichia coli, Proteus, Klebsiella, Bifidobacterium, Candida* (yeast), *Clostridium perfringens*
Genital tract	*Lactobacillus, Streptococcus,* Corynebacterium, diphtheroids, *Staphylococcus, Candida* (yeast), *Trichomonas vaginalis* (protozoan)
Urinary tract[b]	*Staphylococcus, Streptococcus, Proteus, Enterococcus, Lactobacillus, Klebsiella*

[a] Unless otherwise indicated, these organisms are bacteria.

[b] In females, flora exist in the lower portion of the urethra. The population is similar to that found in the large intestine. In males, the urethra has a much smaller population of organisms.

of the infection produce clinical symptoms, a disease results. **Disease** is defined as any harmful alteration to the physiological or metabolic state of the host. An **infectious disease** occurs when this alteration is caused by a microorganism or its products, such as **toxins** (see Chapter 10). Any organism capable of causing disease is called a **pathogen**. The microorganisms responsible for the infection may come from anywhere in the environment or from the human body itself.

ENDOGENOUS AND EXOGENOUS INFECTIONS

Depending on the source of the causative organism, an infectious disease can be classified as endogenous or exogenous.

Endogenous infections occur when the source of the pathogen is the human host itself. Thus, diseases caused by normal flora are endogenous. The flora usually cause the infection when they are displaced from their normal habitat to a susceptible body site. For example, skin bacteria such as *Staphylococcus epidermidis* are a major cause of infection in surgical wounds and intravenous lines. Nasal carriers of *Staphylococcus aureus* can transfer bacteria from the nose to an open wound or sore. Cells of *E. coli* may be carried from the colon to the bladder and cause a urinary tract infection. Latent viral infections may be reactivated when the host immune defences are reduced.

Congenital infections are a type of endogenous disease that occur in the foetus or neonate when the source of the pathogen is the mother. Sometimes, the pathogen crosses the placenta during pregnancy and produces congenital defects such as occur with rubella, syphilis, cytomegalovirus and toxoplasmosis. If the mother is a carrier of a blood-borne virus, the baby may become infected late in pregnancy or at the time of birth, as occurs with hepatitis B and HIV. Sometimes, the foetus is infected *in utero* by flora from the vagina (e.g. group B streptococci or *Mycoplasma*). These latter infections have been implicated as a cause of premature labour.

Exogenous infections are caused by organisms from the external environment. They may be acquired by cross-infection from patients in the hospital environment, or from people in the wider community. Most infectious diseases are acquired in the community and are transferred from person to person by various routes (see Chapter 8). If the infectious disease is treated at home, the pathogen remains in the community. Sometimes the disease requires hospitalisation and so the pathogen is introduced into the hospital environment, where it may spread.

Exogeneous infections acquired during a patient's stay in hospital are called **health-care-associated infections (HCAI)**. They were previously called **hospital-acquired infections (HAI)** or **nosocomial infections** (see Chapter 13). It is not always possible to distinguish between a health-care-associated infection and one that is acquired in the community. Infections due to pathogens acquired in hospital are often very serious as the hospital environment harbours a large population of antibiotic-resistant organisms, and hospitalised patients are frequently very susceptible. The major risks to patients are from medical or surgical procedures or from contact with contaminated surfaces or the hands or clothing of health workers. When such infections can be largely attributed to invasive medical procedures they are called **iatrogenic**.

THE DISEASE PROCESS

Pathogenicity is defined as the capacity to produce disease. This capacity depends on certain characteristics of the organism, including the ability to:

- gain entry to the host
- attach to the host tissues and multiply
- evade the host defences
- damage tissue and produce disease symptoms.

Some diseases are not as serious as others, and this depends on the type of pathogen involved. The degree of pathogenicity of different types of microorganisms ranges from mild to serious or even fatal. For example, the cold virus is a pathogen, but the disease it causes is usually only mild, whereas infection with the influenza A virus is much more serious. An infection with the rabies virus is nearly always fatal.

Differences in pathogenicity are also related to the **virulence** of the organism or strain of that organism. Virulence refers to the intensity of the disease symptoms produced by a particular organism. It depends on a number of factors, such as how easily the organism invades the host cell and produces damage. Some organisms are able to carry this out more effectively than others and so are described as being very virulent. For example, encapsulated strains of *Streptococcus pneumoniae* are more virulent than unencapsulated strains. The presence of the capsule allows the bacterium to attach to and invade the host tissues, and also contributes to its ability to evade phagocytosis by the host's white blood cells.

Other virulence factors include the enzymes and toxins that damage the host cell. Different strains of the same organism may show a variation in virulence. For example, some strains of *Streptococcus pyogenes* are very invasive and cause rapid, severe, sometimes fatal infections (see Case History 7.1). Other strains are not as virulent and produce milder symptoms (e.g. 'strep throat'). Some strains of *E. coli* produce toxins which cause serious diseases such as 'travellers' diarrhoea' and haemolytic uraemic syndrome (see Chapter 18). The difference in virulence between strains is related to the virulence factors (and toxins) they produce. Some strains of influenza are more virulent than others, causing serious epidemics throughout the world.

The mechanisms used by pathogens to produce disease are discussed in detail in Chapter 10.

The virulence of a particular organism may be altered by its passage through a susceptible animal host. The mutational changes that give rise to new strains of influenza each winter tend to occur when the influenza virus enters the pig or duck population in Asian countries, giving rise to a more virulent strain. Sometimes this change occurs spontaneously, when influenza spreads through the human population. The strain of the virus isolated at the end of an epidemic is frequently more virulent than the original pathogen. The mutational changes that cause this alteration in virulence are not well understood.

In the laboratory, the virulence of a particular organism can often be decreased or *attenuated* by repeated passage through cell culture, or prolonged growth in artificial media. This technique has been used successfully to produce weakened strains of organisms which can then be

---

CASE HISTORY 7.1
Systemic disease related to tinea

In October 1999 a 34-year-old businessman who had recently arrived from London via Bangkok was admitted to a Sydney teaching hospital suffering from leg pain. On examination the leg was found to be swollen with a red blistered area on the left ankle, and the lymph nodes in the groin were enlarged. The patient had chronic tinea infection on both feet. Swabs and blood samples for bacterial culture were taken and the patient was started on IV antibiotics.

Over the next few days the patient remained febrile (40°C) and suffered headache, delirium, rigor and peripheral shutdown. *Streptococcus pyogenes* was identified from the swabs. The condition of the patient deteriorated, deep cellulitis was present and the ulcerated area affected 30 cm on the lower left leg. Antibiotic medication was increased but there was a real possibility that amputation would be necessary. Because he was a businessman who travelled extensively the loss of the leg would have had serious implications. Fortunately, the treatment was successful; the man recovered completely but required extensive rehabilitation.

Comment

The chronic tinea infection (see Chapter 6) provided an easy portal of entry for the streptococcal infection. Group A streptococci are found in the environment and may sometimes be part of the normal flora. They can survive for days or weeks outside the body. They are often the cause of local infections which can progress to systemic infection and rapidly cause serious disease. Not all strains are toxinogenic but some produce exotoxins that have been implicated in life-threatening diseases with a high mortality rate, such as necrotising fasciitis and toxic shock syndrome. The patient was given treatment for the tinea and advised about the importance of maintaining an intact skin to prevent infection.

Source: S. Greig, personal communication.

---

used as vaccines (e.g. the MMR vaccine contains attenuated strains of measles, mumps and rubella viruses).

Another important factor in determining whether a disease will occur is the **infective dose**, or the number of cells of the organism that are able to enter the human body and become established. If only a few cells are present, then the host defences may be able to destroy them. However, if the numbers are large they may overwhelm the defences. For example, the stomach acid may be sufficient to neutralise the few bacteria normally contained in food, but is not able to inactivate all the microbes in a heavily contaminated food sample. In general, the more virulent the organism, the fewer the number of cells that will be needed to establish an infection and produce disease symptoms. For example, a gastrointestinal infection due to

Shigella may require as few as 100 organisms to be present in contaminated food or on the hands, whereas one million *Salmonella* cells might be needed under similar circumstances.

OPPORTUNISTIC INFECTIONS

So far we have been describing the characteristics of true pathogens – that is, microorganisms that always overcome the natural host defences and cause disease in an otherwise healthy host. However, a significant number of diseases are caused by microorganisms that set up an infection because they have been moved from their normal habitat, or because the host defences are lowered or compromised in some way. For this reason, we define another type of relationship that may occur.

Opportunism refers to a situation where microorganisms that *would not normally cause an infection* do so because of an alteration in physiological conditions in the host, or a change in the environment where the organism is located. These organisms are called **opportunistic pathogens**. They are able to gain entry and set up an infection in a host when the host defences are lowered or compromised in some way. The seriousness of the infection and the ease of treatment depends on various factors including the immune status of the host, the site of infection and the properties of the particular organism causing the infection.

These infections may be caused by normal flora of the host that have been displaced from their usual habitat. For example, many of the infections in surgical wounds or those associated with intravenous catheters or central lines are due to *Staphylococcus epidermidis*, derived from the patient's own skin. Urinary tract infections are frequently caused by bacteria that are normally resident in the large intestine but which have been transported from the anus to the opening of the urethra, from where they can gain entry to the bladder.

An alteration in the physiological or hormonal state of a patient may encourage the overgrowth of one of the normal flora. For example, as mentioned before, the yeast *Candida albicans*, a normal inhabitant of the vagina, is often the cause of vaginitis, or thrush. Prolonged use of antibiotics destroys the normal flora of the bowel and allows overgrowth of organisms such as *Clostridium difficile* which causes severe diarrhoea and pseudomembranous colitis.

The most serious opportunistic infections occur when the normal defences of the host are lowered. This is probably of greatest importance in hospitals where many of the patients have a real or induced deficiency of their immune system, placing them at great risk of acquiring infection. Transplant patients on immunosuppressive drugs, cancer patients undergoing chemotherapy and AIDS patients are particularly vulnerable to opportunistic infections as their own immune system cannot function to fight the invading pathogens. Some of the common opportunistic infections seen in these patients are fungal infections such as systemic candidiasis and cryptococcal meningitis, reactivation of latent viral infections such as cytomegalovirus and herpes, and the atypical pneumonia due to *Pneumocystis jiroveci* (previously called *Pneumocystis carinii*).

HOST RESISTANCE OR SUSCEPTIBILITY

One of the most important factors to consider when discussing an infectious disease is the ability of the host to resist invasion by the pathogen. The human body has a complex system of specific and non-specific mechanisms to deal with foreign particles and microorganisms. These are discussed fully in Chapter 9. One of the most important of these is the mechanical barrier provided by an intact skin. Once this barrier is broken (e.g. in wounds, surgery or burns), microorganisms are able to gain easy access to the tissues. Table 7.2 summarises the risk factors that increase susceptibility to infection.

Table 7.2

Factors that increase susceptibility to infection

FACTOR	SUSCEPTIBILITY
Age	Neonates have immature immune system. Elderly have decreased immune system. Some pathogens have increased virulence in different age groups.
Pregnancy	More susceptible to some diseases, e.g. hepatitis E, malaria.
Nutrition	Malnutrition and alcoholism lower immune response.
Illness	Underlying illnesses, e.g. diabetes, cancer, liver disease, contribute to susceptibility.
Immunosuppressive drugs	Transplant patients have lowered immune response.
Chemotherapy	Cancer patients susceptible, due to effects of drugs.
Atmospheric pollution	Lung damage increases susceptibility to respiratory infections.
Surgery/Trauma	Provides portal of entry for pathogens.
Physical defects	Provide site for infection.
Stress	Lowers immune response.
Immune diseases, acquired or genetic	Lower immune response.
Gender/Genetic predisposition	Variable effect on susceptibility to different diseases.

The general health of the host is important in determining the outcome of exposure to a pathogen. A healthy person is often able to ward off an infection, whereas someone with an additional, often unrelated, illness may succumb. One of the most difficult problems for health workers is when a patient presents with an infection or infectious disease which is really an expression of a number of underlying diseases. This is especially true of patients in some remote areas of Australia, and among indigenous Australians and people in lower socio-economic groups. Underlying illnesses such as diabetes or anaemia may contribute to patient susceptibility. Those with a lowered white blood cell count (**neutropenia**) or suffering from leukaemia are at greater risk of infection.

Some treatments for other diseases affect the functioning of the immune system – for example, cancer patients receiving chemotherapy and transplant patients receiving immunosuppressive drugs to prevent rejection. Most of these drugs also interfere with the body's ability to fight foreign microorganisms, rendering these patients at risk from infectious diseases. Patients with immune disorders are obviously more susceptible to all types of infection.

General lifestyle and nutritional status affect the susceptibility of the host. Malnutrition and alcoholism both contribute to lowered body defence mechanisms. Injecting drug users are at risk of acquiring blood-borne pathogens such as hepatitis B, hepatitis C and HIV. Cigarette smokers tend to be at greater risk of lung infections and bronchitis. Many people who die from Legionnaires' disease have a previous history of lung problems associated with smoking.

Age is an important factor, as it often reflects the status of the immune system. Neonates and infants up to about one year of age have a poorly developed immune system and so are particularly susceptible to infection, even though they have some protection from maternal antibodies. As their immune system matures they are able to deal with invading pathogens and develop their own immunity. The system appears to decline in old age, so the elderly are at greater risk of infection. Males and females show a different pattern of susceptibility. For example, females suffer more urinary tract infections because of the comparative shortness of the female urethra and the proximity of the anus to the urethra. During pregnancy, the immune system is slightly compromised and so pregnant women tend to be more susceptible to some infections. Hepatitis E and malaria are two diseases with an increased risk of a fatal outcome during pregnancy.

There is considerable evidence that the genetic makeup of an individual plays a part in susceptibility to infection. The reason for this is not well understood at present, but there are documented cases of differences in the ability of various individuals to resist disease that can only be explained on the basis of genetic differences in their immune system.

PREDISPOSING FACTORS

As well as individual susceptibility, a number of external factors contribute to the likelihood of someone acquiring an infectious disease. High on the list is the environment in which they live and the general hygiene of their surroundings. The climate often has an effect, as it may favour the persistence of a pathogen or its vector. The weather, winds, temperature or natural disasters such as floods will facilitate the spread of microorganisms. Air pollution affects the lungs and lowers resistance to respiratory pathogens. An existing viral infection may predispose a patient to a secondary bacterial infection. Many infectious diseases have a seasonal occurrence; for example, influenza occurs more often in the winter months, chickenpox usually in spring.

Patients who are hospitalised are often at greater risk of acquiring an infection than they would be outside the hospital environment. This is largely due to their lowered resistance because of illness, but is also related to the invasive procedures they may have undergone. In the hospital environment, they are likely to be exposed to large numbers of microorganisms, many of which are resistant to antibiotics. Hospital-acquired infections are discussed in Chapter 13.

Koch's Postulates

How do we know that microorganisms cause disease? Today, we take it for granted that microorganisms are responsible for the clinical signs and symptoms of an infection. This was not always the case – in 1876, when the German microbiologist ROBERT KOCH proposed his **germ theory of disease**, he had to overcome significant opposition to his ideas. Koch investigated the cause of a disease, anthrax, that was killing the cattle in Europe and discovered that a bacterium he named *Bacillus anthracis* was responsible (see Figure 1.2, page 7). He subsequently went on to isolate other bacteria that were responsible for tuberculosis and cholera. Based on his research he put forward a set of criteria that should be met when deciding whether an organism is responsible for causing a particular disease.

They are called **Koch's Postulates** and can be summarised as follows:

- The organism must always be present in every case of the disease.
- It must be possible to isolate the organism from the diseased host and grow it in pure culture.
- The pure culture of the organism, when inoculated into a new susceptible host, must produce the same symptoms of disease.
- It must be possible to recover the organism from the experimental host.

Koch's work was important in developing the concept of 'one germ, one disease' – that is, that a single type of organism is responsible for causing a disease with a characteristic group of symptoms. These postulates provided a sound scientific approach to the problem of identification of the causative agents of infection and, in the 30 years following the publication of his postulates, scientists around the world adopted his methods and were successful in isolating and identifying the bacteria responsible for many of the major diseases then known (see Table 1.2, page 7).

These methods were very useful for bacterial diseases but, during the 20th century, diseases caused by viruses were identified. Although the basic principles of Koch's Postulates still stand, they need some modification in the light of our current understanding of the nature of infectious diseases, the type of pathogens that have been described in recent years and the new technology that is available for identification of microorgansisms. For example:

- Some organisms are difficult to grow in pure culture away from the host. *Mycobacterium leprae*, the causative organism of leprosy, has never been grown on artificial media, nor have the hepatitis C or human papilloma viruses. Viruses, chlamydiae and rickettsiae can be grown only in cell culture.
- In 1976 a previously unknown organism, *Legionella pneumophila*, was identified as the bacterium responsible for Legionnaires' disease. Although it is now possible to grow it in the laboratory on special medium, the bacterium was originally identified by an indirect method. Samples of lung tissue from infected patients were injected into guinea pigs to produce antibodies to the infectious agent. Patients who had had Legionnaires' disease were tested and found to have antibodies to the same bacteria that had produced the disease symptoms in the guinea pigs.
- Some diseases can be caused by more than one type of pathogen. For example, pneumonia, which is really an infection of the lungs, can be caused by any one of a number of organisms, some of which are listed in Table 7.3.
- Some organisms apparently cause more than one disease. For example, streptococci, which are responsible for 'strep sore throat', may also release bacterial antigens into the bloodstream and affect the heart, causing a post-streptococcal hypersensitivity response known as rheumatic fever.
- Sometimes a pathogen may enter the body, giving rise to a **subclinical infection** without any clinically identifiable disease symptoms (see page 149). This is often the case with diseases such as rubella (German measles) and glandular fever. Other pathogens, especially the viruses belonging to the herpes family, can remain in the body in a *latent* form and be reactivated when the physiological state of the host changes. Neither of these situations fulfils the criteria used by Koch.

However, even with these modifications, Koch provided a set of scientific principles that formed the basis for a sound experimental approach to the investigation of the **aetiology** (cause) of infectious diseases.

Table 7.3
Some microbial causes of pneumonia

Bacteria	*Streptococcus pneumoniae*
	Staphylococcus aureus
	Haemophilus influenzae
	Escherichia coli
	Klebsiella pneumoniae
	Pseudomonas aeruginosa
	Legionella pneumophila
	Mycobacterium tuberculosis
	Mycoplasma pneumoniae
Chlamydia	*Chlamydia* spp.
Rickettsia	*Coxiella burnetii*
Viruses	Influenza virus
	Respiratory syncytial virus
	SARS (severe acute respiratory syndrome)
Fungi	*Pneumocystis jiroveci**
	*Histoplasma capsulatum**

*in immunosuppressed patients

Signs and symptoms of disease

In the previous sections we distinguished between situations where microorganisms reside normally in or on the human body and those cases in which an infection or disease is present. To decide whether a state of infection or disease exists, it is usual to observe the patient for the presence of tell-tale signs or symptoms. These represent pathological changes or damage to the host cells and tissues; they are often characteristic of the type of infection and so are useful for diagnosis.

Signs are measurable changes in the patient that can be observed by examination of the patient or their body fluids. They include occurrences such as fever, swelling (oedema), rashes, vomiting and diarrhoea, as well as data derived from laboratory tests.

Symptoms are changes that are felt and reported by the patient, such as pain, headache, nausea, or a general feeling of illness (**malaise**). Sometimes these categories overlap. The combination of signs and symptoms that characterises a particular disease state is called a **syndrome** (e.g. AIDS stands for acquired immune deficiency **syndrome**).

FEVER

Fever (**pyrexia**) almost invariably accompanies serious infections and is one of the most useful early warning signs. Constant monitoring of a patient's temperature will often indicate that an infection is present, long before other symptoms appear. Human body temperature is maintained within narrow limits by the temperature-regulating centre in the hypothalamus in the brain. An increase in body temperature (fever) is produced when chemicals called **pyrogens** act on the hypothalamus and reset the thermostat to a higher temperature.

Endogenous pyrogens are produced within the human body as part of the immune response by the phagocytic white blood cells, monocytes and macrophages (see Chapter 9). The main ones are **interleukin-1** (IL-1) and **tumour necrosis factor** (TNF).

Exogenous pyrogens are products of infectious organisms and act by stimulating the release of endogenous pyrogens such as IL-1, which in turn act on the hypothalamus as described above. One of the most important is an endotoxin called lipid A, which forms part of the lipopolysaccharide found in the cell wall of some Gram-negative bacteria (see Chapter 4).

Fluids to be administered to patients (such as IV solutions) are frequently labelled 'pyrogen-free'. This means they do not contain any fever-producing substances such as fragments of dead microorganisms. Endotoxins can also cause other serious effects in the human host (see Chapter 10).

The body's immediate response to an increase in the temperature set point in the hypothalamus is to try to raise the body temperature by involuntary muscle contraction (shivering) and the narrowing of surface blood vessels to prevent heat loss (**vasoconstriction**). The effect is that the patient becomes pale and feels cold or chilled. When further fluctuations occur in the set point control, returning it to the normal lower temperature, the body responds by trying to increase heat loss to lower the body temperature. This involves sweating, and dilation of the surface blood vessels, causing reddening of the skin or flushing. The patient feels hot and has a fever.

Nearly all fever is caused by an infection. **Pyrexia of unknown origin (PUO)** is a term used to describe a situation where the patient has an unexplained fever. In more than 50% of these cases, an infection is present. There are a few non-infective causes of sustained fever, including some malignancies and some vascular diseases.

INFLAMMATION

Inflammation is a common non-specific response that occurs at the site of injury or infection. The syndrome, which consists of heat, pain, redness, vasodilation and swelling, is described in Chapter 9. When the host tissue is damaged, one of the first reactions is the activation of the inflammatory response, which is mediated by a number of chemicals released by the damaged cells and other cells of the immune system.

Important among these chemicals is **histamine**, which causes vasodilation and an increase in permeability of the blood capillaries. Fluids and white blood cells (phagocytes) move into the tissues, resulting in redness, swelling and pain. A localised increase in temperature at the site of inflammation is due to this vasodilation. Other chemicals released by the damaged cells attract phagocytic white blood cells (monocytes and macrophages) to the site. They may release pyrogens such as interleukin-1 (IL-1) which act on the hypothalamus (as described above) and produce a rise in temperature throughout the body (fever). The pus that forms at the site of an infection is a mixture of dead microbial cells, dead or damaged host cells and white blood cells.

Many of the signs and symptoms observed are actually a result of the host's own defence system attempting to counter the infection.

IMMUNE REACTIONS

The reaction of the body to infection involves an immune response that is discussed in detail in Chapter 9. Some of the signs of this immune response can be detected and serve as an indication of the presence of infection. Stimulation of the immune system results in increased activity in the lymph nodes or glands, causing **lymphadenopathy** (swollen glands) see Figure 7.3. Changes in the white blood cell population are typical of the body's response to infection and are indicative of certain kinds of disease. **Leukocytosis** is an increase in the white cell count, while **leukopenia** is a decrease in the number of white cells circulating in the bloodstream.

The specific immune response also results in the formation of **antibodies** to the organism responsible for the infection. These can be detected in the blood and their number and type are indicative of the progress of the disease in the patient. IgM antibodies indicate a recent infection whereas IgG antibodies are indicative of an old infection.

SKIN SIGNS

Skin rashes are often non-specific, but some are quite distinctive and play a major role in diagnosis (see Figures 7.4–7.9). For example, the pustular lesions of chickenpox are easy to identify. The reaction of the skin during infection can be described in various ways.

- **Lesion** – any area of damaged tissue.
- **Erythema** – reddening of the skin, due to dilation of the surface capillaries.
- **Macule** – a small, flat, reddish patch.
- **Papule** – a slightly raised red spot, such as a pimple.
- **Vesicles** – small blisters, often filled with clear, yellowish fluid (serum).
- **Pustule** – a lesion containing creamish opaque material (pus).

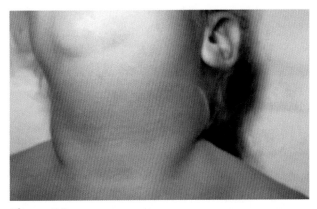

Figure 7.3

Child with typical swollen glands associated with mumps

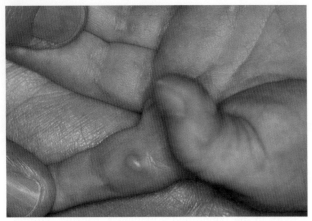

Figure 7.4

Distinctive blisters are a symptom of hand, foot and mouth disease, a viral infection caused by coxsackie virus and common in child-care centres

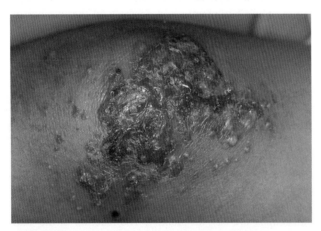

Figure 7.5

Impetigo, a skin condition usually associated with staphylococcal or streptococcal infection

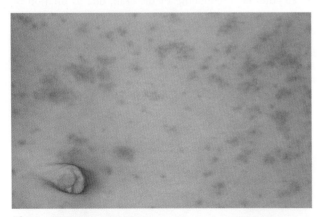

Figure 7.6

Maculopapular rash of measles

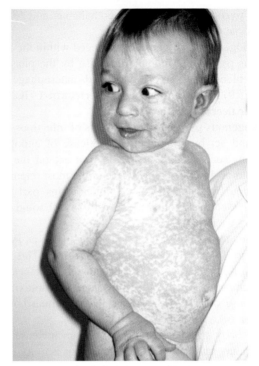

Figure 7.7

Non-specific viral rash on 12-month-old child
Children often present with this type of rash which is difficult to diagnose without other symptoms being present.

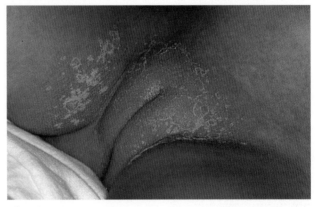

Figure 7.8

Rash associated with scarlet fever, caused by *Streptococcus pyogenes*

- **Ulcer** or **erosion** – a skin lesion that is deep and reaches subcutaneous tissue.
- **Abscess** – a localised collection of pus.

The signs and symptoms of disease are usually indicative of the body system that is affected. Infections of the gastrointestinal system typically cause nausea, stomach cramps, vomiting and diarrhoea. Headache, stiff neck and confusion indicate infection of the nervous system. Some symptoms are non-specific. For example, headache, nausea and fever may occur in a number of diseases. Frequently, the presence of a high fever will induce vomiting that may be unrelated to the true cause of the illness. To diagnose a disease correctly it is usually necessary to carry out laboratory tests.

LABORATORY TESTS

Laboratory examination of swabs or specimens plays an essential role in diagnosing the causative agents of an infection (see Chapter 15). Tests are carried out on specimens of blood, urine, cerebrospinal fluid (CSF) and other

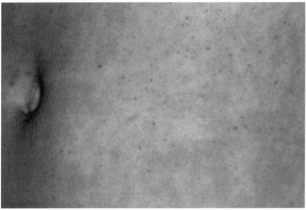

(a)

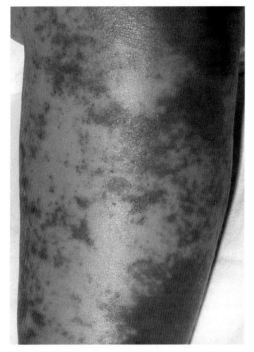

(b)

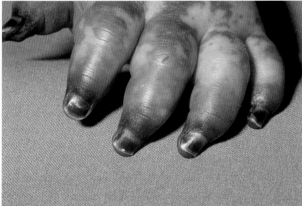

(c)

Figure 7.9

Meningococcal disease due to infection by *Neisseria meningitidis*

(a) Petechial rash on the trunk, typical of damage to blood vessels caused by endotoxins; (b) rash on leg showing more extensive damage; (c) damage to capillaries has caused necrosis and gangrene in the hand.

tissue samples in order to detect or confirm other signs of infection. The presence of microorganisms in a specimen or swab from a normally sterile body site usually indicates an infection is present. Cultures of blood specimens are used to detect systemic infections that are not visible on the body surface, since microorganisms responsible for infections in internal tissues can enter the bloodstream through breaks in the capillary walls.

The detection of bacteria (**bacteraemia**) or viruses (**viraemia**) in the blood is not necessarily significant unless other symptoms are also present.

Sepsis occurs when the organisms multiply in the bloodstream and may result in a **systemic inflammatory response (SIR)**, which can be fatal.

Development of disease

The course of infection and disease in the human body generally follows a defined pattern or sequence of events (see Figure 7.10). The initial incubation period is followed by the prodromal phase, the invasive or acute phase of disease (which sometimes involves a peak or crisis) and the convalescence. The outcome of the disease may be complete recovery, death, or the establishment of a latent or chronic infection (see below).

INCUBATION PERIOD

After successfully gaining entry to the body, the pathogen has to overcome the host defences in order to establish itself, multiply and cause disease. The **incubation period** is the time interval that occurs between the exposure of the host to the pathogen and the appearance of any signs or symptoms of disease. The incubation time is affected by a number of factors, including the properties of the pathogen, its virulence, the infective dose, the place of entry of the pathogen into the host relative to its target organ, and the resistance of the host. In gastrointestinal infections, the length of time before the onset of symptoms depends on the nature of the ingested pathogen (bacteria, bacterial endospores, viruses or preformed toxins).

Table 7.4 shows typical incubation times for some infectious diseases. During the incubation period, patients are often unaware that they have been exposed to the pathogen. However, during this period as well as the following prodromal period, they are usually infectious and thus able to spread the disease to others.

PRODROMAL PERIOD

As the pathogen continues to multiply, non-specific disease symptoms are produced such as headache, nausea and general malaise. This is termed the prodromal period and signals the beginning of disease. Sometimes the host defences overcome the pathogen at this stage and the symptoms disappear before a recognisable disease syndrome develops. The host may or may not be left with an acquired resistance (antibodies and memory cells) to the pathogen but, if antibodies are produced, the host is

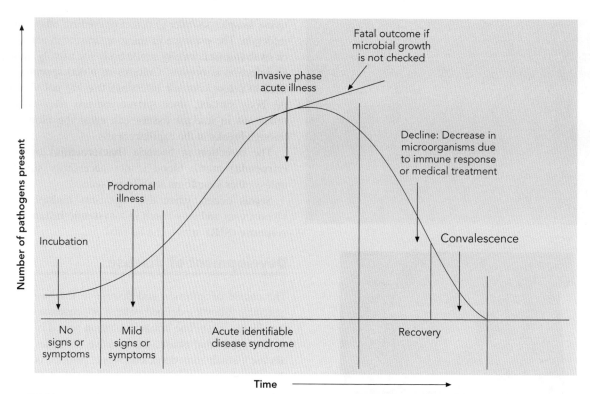

Number of pathogens present

Fatal outcome if
microbial growth
is not checked

Invasive phase
acute illness

Decline: Decrease in
microorganisms due
to immune response
or medical treatment

Prodromal
illness

Convalescence

Incubation

No
signs or
symptoms

Mild
signs or
symptoms

Acute identifiable
disease syndrome

Recovery

Time

Figure 7.10
Stages in the progression of disease

Table 7.4

Incubation times for some common infectious diseases

DISEASE	TIME
Chickenpox	2–3 weeks
Measles	8–14 days
Mumps	12–25 days
Diphtheria	2–6 days
Tuberculosis	4–12 weeks
Rubella (German measles)	14–21 days
Influenza	2–3 days
Food poisoning	12–36 hours
Gangrene	24–48 hours
Tetanus	24–48 hours after injury
Whooping cough	7–10 days
Glandular fever	4–6 weeks
Hepatitis A	3–5 weeks
Hepatitis B	2–6 months
Hepatitis C	6–8 weeks
HIV (appearance of antibodies)	Minimum 3 weeks; may be months or years
Gonorrhoea	2–5 days
Syphilis	2–3 weeks

ACUTE OR INVASIVE PHASE

If the early host defences do not overcome the pathogen, the prodromal stage is followed by a period of acute disease, the **invasive phase**, during which the pathogen invades and damages the host tissue. Fever and chills, caused by the presence of pyrogens, are typical symptoms of the invasive phase of the disease.

Some diseases, such as malaria, have repeated episodes of fever and chills, mediated by the synchronised release of merozoites from the red blood cells (Chapters 6, 19). Others have a longer period of sustained elevated temperature before a sudden drop or a slow decline. There is some evidence that a moderate increase in temperature (up to 40°C) is protective. The multiplication of some microorganisms is inhibited or slowed by higher temperatures. In addition, the higher body temperature may stimulate the rate of the inflammatory immune response.

Some invasive phases reach a crisis or peak over a short period of time, after which symptoms (especially fever) quickly subside. Other diseases are characterised by a longer invasive phase during which additional signs and symptoms occur, such as cough, diarrhoea, jaundice, loss of muscle control, swelling, pain and discharge. These additional symptoms may be due to the action of toxins produced by the pathogen (see Chapter 10). For example, the cough associated with whooping cough develops as the disease progresses and is due to inflammation and damage to the trachea caused by the toxins produced by the causative bacterium (*Bordetella pertussis*). The cough persists long after the invasive phase has ended and the patient is no longer infectious.

said to have experienced a subclinical infection (see page 149). Not all diseases have a prodromal phase. Many start suddenly with acute symptoms of pain and fever, reflecting the nature of the infection.

The ability of the host to overcome the invasive phase determines the outcome of the disease – that is, recovery or death (terminal outcome). A **fulminating disease** is an acute infection that progresses very rapidly, often with a fatal outcome. The symptoms appear suddenly and develop quickly into a serious infection (e.g. cerebral malaria, meningococcal meningitis or pneumonic plague). In this situation, the pathogen overcomes the host before protective immunity can develop.

DECLINE PHASE

If the immune system responds to the infection and overcomes the effects of the pathogen, the symptoms subside, the disease enters the decline phase and the patient begins to recover. In some cases, however, the host defences are unable to eliminate the pathogen completely from the body and the disease progresses to a latent or chronic state (see section below, 'Types of Infection').

EFFECTS OF DRUG THERAPY

The above description of the progress of a disease needs to be modified when drug therapy (antimicrobials, antipyretics, analgesics) is used. Often, the use of an appropriate antimicrobial drug will speed up the destruction of the pathogen and dramatically shorten the invasive phase, sometimes averting a fatal outcome. However, one of the undesirable outcomes of antibiotic use is that endotoxins may be released from the breakdown of certain types of dead Gram-negative bacteria. These endotoxins can produce serious, sometimes fatal, effects such as fever and septic shock, leading to haemorrhage, collapse of the circulatory system and sequential failure of essential body organs – as can occur in meningococcal meningitis (see Chapter 10).

There is considerable discussion about the merits of using antipyretics, especially aspirin, to reduce fever in the early stages of infection. As mentioned above, fever may sometimes be beneficial, provided body temperature does not exceed 40°C, when organ damage may occur. There is some evidence that the use of aspirin in children is associated with the development of **Reye's syndrome**, a sometimes fatal disease characterised by brain damage and degeneration of some internal organs. The use of paracetamol is considered preferable, although excess use can cause liver damage.

CONVALESCENCE

Convalescence is the time when the body repairs itself and regains strength. The energy that has been used to activate and support the immune response is directed back to the normal processes of cell regeneration and tissue repair. In today's busy society, many people fail to allow sufficient time for convalescence and so are frequently exposed to another pathogen before regaining their full strength. The result is a series of illnesses because the immune system is too weak to protect the body effectively.

Types of infection

When microorganisms invade host tissue an infection occurs. The type of infection depends on the nature of the invading organism, the site of entry and the susceptibility of the host. The definitions of many of the terms commonly used to describe infection and disease are listed in Table 7.5.

LOCALISED INFECTIONS

Infections that are confined to the site where the pathogen enters the body are said to be **localised**. Some examples are an infected wound (usually due to bacteria), cutaneous fungal infections, and warts (papilloma virus). In the case of cutaneous infections (warts and fungi), the infection remains localised because the pathogen preferentially attacks epidermal tissue. Other organisms remain on body surfaces because they prefer the lower temperature on the skin (33°C). *Mycobacterium leprae*, the causative organism of leprosy, is one such example, usually occurring only on the nasal mucosa, skin and superficial nerve cells of the limbs. See Figure 20.8.

Wound infections, ulcers and abscesses remain localised because they are contained by the inflammatory reactions described above. Inflammation involves fibrin deposition and causes swelling; this effectively walls off the site of the infection and prevents the escape of the infectious agent (usually bacteria) into the surrounding tissue and blood vessels. Large numbers of phagocytic cells are attracted to the infected site by chemotaxis and attack the pathogen.

Superficial localised infections can be treated with topical antiseptic or antimicrobial drugs. A combination of antiseptic treatment and the non-specific immune response often limits the pathogen to the original site of infection. More serious infections require **debridement** (removal of necrotic tissue and debris) and/or wound cleansing, which may be accompanied by the administration of oral or intravenous antibiotics.

DISSEMINATED INFECTIONS

A **disseminated infection** occurs when the pathogen escapes from its primary site of infection into the bloodstream or lymphatic system and spreads to other parts of the body where it establishes another infection. Disseminated infections include situations such as the spread of *Streptococcus pneumoniae* from the throat (pharyngitis) to the ears (otitis media) or lungs (pneumonia), or when opportunistic infections spread in immunocompromised patients (e.g. cytomegalovirus or tuberculosis in AIDS patients).

Minor skin infections due to streptococci can also be disseminated throughout the body (see Case History 7.1, page 139). Usually, the bacteria gain entry to the lymphatic system via a break in the skin and are carried to the lymph nodes. The inflammation that occurs in the lymph capillary may appear as a red line running from the site of the infection towards the lymph node. The stimulation of

Table 7.5

Definitions of infection and disease

TERM	DEFINITION
• Infection	Situation where microorganisms invade the host tissue and multiply.
• Disease	Harmful alteration to the physiological or metabolic state of the host.
• Infectious disease	A disease caused by a microorganism.
• Pathogen	A microorganism capable of causing disease.
• Infective dose	The number of cells of a pathogen that are required to produce disease symptoms.
• Virulence	The severity or intensity of the disease symptoms produced by a pathogen.
• Signs	Measurable changes in the patient as the result of an infection.
• Symptoms	Changes felt by the patient as a result of an infection.
• Syndrome	The combination of signs and symptoms.
• Bacteraemia	Presence of bacteria in the blood.
• Viraemia	Presence of viruses in the blood.
• Septicaemia	Multiplication of bacteria in the blood.
• Toxaemia	Presence of toxins in the blood.
Disease	
• Acute	Characteristic symptoms appear and the disease runs its course quickly.
• Fulminating	The symptoms appear suddenly and the disease proceeds rapidly, often to a fatal outcome.
• Chronic	The disease progresses slowly and persists for long periods with continuous shedding of the pathogen.
• Latent	The pathogen remains dormant in the host and may be reactivated under certain conditions.
• Subclinical	The infection produces an immune response without recognisable symptoms.
Infections	
• Localised	Confined to one area of the body.
• Systemic	The pathogen progressively affects more than one organ.
• Primary	The first sign of infection in a healthy host.
• Secondary	Develops when the defences are lowered by the primary infection.
• Superinfection	Results from overgrowth of opportunistic organisms, following destruction of normal flora.

the lymphocytes of the specific defence system in the lymph nodes causes swelling, producing 'swollen glands', which are an indication of the immune system being activated to fight the invading pathogen.

The presence of bacteria or viruses in the lymphatic system or bloodstream does not always lead to an infection or disease. Sometimes, microorganisms gain entry and circulate, producing transient viraemia or bacteraemia without any disturbance to body functions. However, serious infections may result when the bacteria lodge in susceptible locations such as the ends of growing bones, causing osteomyelitis, or on defective heart valves, causing endocarditis. Sometimes, infections from the ear or the lungs can spread to the brain and cause meningitis. *Streptococcus pyogenes* can spread from a localised infection on the skin to the kidneys and establish a serious condition known as acute post-streptococcal glomerulonephritis (APSGN), or to the heart and initiate a hypersensitivity reaction known as rheumatic fever. This type of spread is a major health problem among the indigenous population in the Northern Territory (see Chapter 14).

SYSTEMIC DISEASES

A **systemic disease** occurs when the pathogen affects several different organs or tissues in the body during the normal course of the infection (e.g. typhoid, measles, chickenpox). The pathogens gain entry to the body via the mucosal or skin surfaces of the respiratory or gastrointestinal tract and are then spread to other body organs via the blood or lymph. This may involve a stepwise invasion of various tissues before the final site of replication and disease production is reached.

For example, typhoid enters via the gastrointestinal system, then spreads via the blood and lymphatic system to the liver, spleen and bone marrow, causing fever, septicaemia, haemorrhage and diarrhoea. The measles virus enters via the upper respiratory system and spreads slowly via the lymphatic system to the lymph glands and then to the bloodstream. It finally invades various epithelial cells, causing cold-like symptoms in the upper respiratory tract, distinctive white patches (Koplik's spots) in the oral mucosa and a maculopapular skin rash. See Figure 7.6.

Some infections remain localised, but the pathogen produces toxins that have a systemic effect. For example, *Clostridium tetani*, the cause of tetanus, sets up an anaerobic infection at the wound site, and produces a powerful neurotoxin that circulates through the bloodstream and causes muscular spasms.

MIXED INFECTIONS

Some diseases are due to the effects of more than one pathogen; that is, they are mixed infections. In such cases the pathogens act *synergistically* (they help each other) by breaking down tissue or providing a favourable environment for another microorganism to multiply. For example, gas gangrene is often associated with the presence of more than one organism. The initial wound infection may involve a mixture of organisms but, once the tissue is infected and damaged, **necrosis** (death of tissue) occurs. This produces an anaerobic environment that favours the growth of *Clostridium perfringens*, the cause of gangrene.

PRIMARY AND SECONDARY INFECTIONS

Sometimes, the disease symptoms change or develop over a period of time. The first or **primary infection** may lower the host's resistance, allowing another or **secondary infection** to occur. Often, an upper respiratory tract infection (URTI), caused by one of the cold viruses, creates a favourable environment for a secondary bacterial infection such as bronchitis or a middle ear infection (otitis media) to develop. Diseases that involve itchy skin lesions (e.g. chickenpox, scabies) encourage scratching which allows easy access for secondary streptococcal or staphylococcal infections.

A **superinfection** is a type of secondary infection that occurs as a result of the destruction of the normal flora, usually by the prolonged use of broad spectrum antibiotics in the treatment of a primary infection. It involves the overgrowth of an opportunistic pathogen, which occurs when the normal flora are suppressed (e.g. *Candida albicans* in vaginal thrush, or *Clostridium difficile* in pseudomembranous colitis, see page 418ff).

SUBCLINICAL INFECTIONS

Although many infections are obvious and produce identifiable symptoms, it is sometimes possible for a pathogen to cause a **subclinical infection**. When this occurs, the patient/host does not exhibit any symptoms of the disease, but the pathogen multiplies in the host and elicits an immune response that can be detected by the presence of antibodies in the bloodstream. Many people in the community have antibodies in their blood to diseases such as hepatitis C, cytomegalovirus or glandular fever, without any previous history of disease symptoms. Before widespread vaccination programs were introduced, many people had subclinical infections of rubella (German measles) or polio.

PERSISTENT INFECTIONS

A number of infectious agents are able to persist in the human body for long periods after the original disease symptoms have disappeared. These are classified as **slow**, **latent** or **chronic**, depending on the activity of the pathogen over time. Many of these are viral and are described in more detail in Chapter 5.

Slow infections

An unusual persistent infection is the 'slow' infection called subacute sclerosing panencephalitis (SSPE). This is a fatal, degenerative nerve disease which occasionally occurs after infection with the measles virus. The virus stays in the brain and produces symptoms several years later. Creutzfeldt-Jakob disease (CJD), which was originally thought to be due to a slow viral infection, is now known to be caused by a prion (see Spotlight box, page 240).

Latent infections

Latent infections refer to the situation where the pathogen (usually a virus) remains in the body after disease symptoms have subsided (see Chapter 5). The viral DNA replicates inside the cell with the host cell DNA but mature viral particles are not formed or shed; in other words, the host is not infectious. Reactivation of the infection may occur when the host defences are lowered. During reactivation, the host again becomes capable of transmitting the disease. Many of the viruses belonging to the herpes family are capable of latency, the most common ones being herpes simplex types I and II, herpes zoster (the cause of chickenpox, which reactivates as shingles), Epstein-Barr (glandular fever) and cytomegalovirus.

Chronic infections

Chronic infections occur when multiplication and shedding of the pathogen continue at a low level without any symptoms of disease. The host is still capable of transmitting infection and in this situation is said to be a **carrier**. Typical examples are pathogens that lodge in the liver, such as typhoid, hepatitis B (HBV) and hepatitis C (HCV). In chronic hepatitis, the patient may have had a subclinical infection and be unaware of their carrier (infectious) status. In some patients HBV and HCV persist and after many years can cause permanent liver damage (**cirrhosis**), which may develop into liver cancer. HIV is also considered a chronic infection as the virus is always present and the patient is infectious even when no symptoms are apparent.

Oncogenic infections

Some viruses persist and cause transformation of the cells they infect into cancer cells. They include hepatitis B and C viruses (liver cancer), human papilloma virus (cervical cancer), Epstein-Barr virus (Burkitts lymphoma) and human herpes virus 8 (Kaposi's sarcoma). There is still much to be learnt about the way viral infections affect the host (see Chapter 5).

Spread of infectious diseases

In this chapter we have examined the characteristics of different types of infection and the factors that lead to the development of a state of disease. The spread of disease depends on the ability of the microorganism to move from one host to another, to gain entry and to cause damage to the host. This is discussed in the next chapter.

- The interaction between host and microorganisms determines whether an infectious disease will occur.
- The biological term used to describe two organisms living together is symbiosis.
- Mutualism occurs when two organisms live together to their mutual benefit.
- Commensalism is an association where one organism benefits without harm to the other.
- Parasitism is when one organism benefits at the expense of the other (host) organism.

MICROORGANISMS OF THE HUMAN BODY: NORMAL FLORA

- Normal flora are the microorganisms found on the human body. They may be present on the skin, or in the gastrointestinal, respiratory or genitourinary tract.
- Normal flora may protect the host from invasion by pathogens.
- Bacteria are the most common kind of organism found on the human body. Other organisms are the yeast *Candida*, some protozoa and latent viruses.
- Some microorganisms reside permanently. Others colonise surfaces. Some are transient or contaminants.
- Contaminant microorganisms cling to skin surfaces, but do not replicate there. Resident flora live in skin crevices, and comprise species of staphylococci, streptococci, corynebacteria and some fungi.
- Oral bacteria (e.g. *Streptococcus* spp.) are found in mucous membranes and in plaque attached to the teeth. The stomach, which has an acid pH, inhibits the growth of most bacteria; the lower intestine harbours a large population of bacteria.
- The upper respiratory tract has a large population of resident microorganisms, but the bronchial tubes and lungs are free of microorganisms in healthy individuals.
- The major components of the urinary system are sterile, but the lower region of the urethra may harbour organisms representative of those found in the genital tract and colon.
- The normal flora of the vagina may vary depending on factors such as hormonal influences, stress, puberty and antibiotic therapy.
- When normal flora are destroyed by long-term antibiotic therapy, opportunistic pathogens often flourish.

INFECTION AND DISEASE

- It is important to be able to define these terms: infection, disease, infectious disease, pathogen, pathogenicity, virulence, infective dose.
- Endogenous infections occur when the source of the pathogen is the human host (e.g. normal flora, congenital infections).
- Exogenous infections are those where the pathogen is derived from the external environment.
- Nosocomial infections (now known as health-care-associated infections) are acquired in hospital.

- Iatrogenic infections are due to medical procedures.
- Opportunistic pathogens are able to gain entry to the host and set up an infection when the normal host defences are lowered or compromised.
- The ability of the host to resist invasion by a pathogen determines whether a disease will occur.
- Factors that contribute to patient susceptibility include: underlying diseases such as diabetes or anaemia; immunosuppression; chemotherapy and diseases of the immune system; poor nutritional status; alcoholism and IV drug use; age; genetic makeup.
- Other factors that influence the occurrence of an infection include: general environment and hygiene; climatic conditions; air pollution; seasonal variations.

KOCH'S POSTULATES

- In the germ theory of disease, German microbiologist Robert Koch proposed a set of criteria to determine whether an organism was responsible for a particular disease. They are known as Koch's Postulates.

SIGNS AND SYMPTOMS OF DISEASE

- Signs are measurable changes in the patient.
- Symptoms are changes that are felt and reported by the patient.
- The combination of signs and symptoms is called a syndrome.
- Signs of infection include: fever; inflammation; lymphadenopathy; changes in white blood cell count; formation of antibodies; skin rashes.
- Signs and symptoms of a disease are usually related to the body system affected.

DEVELOPMENT OF DISEASE

- The pattern of disease consists of the incubation period, the prodromal phase, the invasive or acute phase, and convalescence.
- A fulminating disease develops very rapidly, often with a fatal outcome.
- Drug therapy modifies the progress of disease.

TYPES OF INFECTION

- Infections may be localised, disseminated or systemic.
- Some pathogens produce toxins that have systemic effects.
- Some diseases are due to the presence of more than one pathogen.
- Primary infections may lower the host's resistance, allowing a different or secondary infection to develop.
- Superinfections result from an overgrowth of opportunistic pathogens.
- Infections that do not have symptoms may be subclinical, latent or chronic.

STUDY QUESTIONS

1. What is meant by the terms: symbiosis, commensalism, mutualism, parasitism?
2. Define normal flora.
3. How does the presence of the normal flora benefit the human host?
4. List two bacterial species that may be found as normal flora of (a) the skin, (b) the gastrointestinal system, (c) the upper respiratory tract, and (d) the vagina.
5. What is a pathogen?
6. What characteristics are required for pathogenicity?
7. What is meant by virulence?
8. What is meant by the infective dose of a pathogen?
9. What is the difference between endogenous and exogenous infections? Give examples of each.
10. Define opportunism.
11. Give two examples of opportunistic infections.
12. Who was the microbiologist responsible for the germ theory of disease?
13. What criteria are used to determine whether an organism is the cause of a disease?
14. What is the difference between signs and symptoms of disease?
15. List four of the common signs of an infection or infectious disease.
16. Why is fever sometimes considered to be beneficial?
17. What is inflammation?
18. Describe each of these skin signs: erythema, vesicle, lesion, pustule, ulcer.
19. Describe the stages in the development of an infectious disease.
20. What is pyrexia of unknown origin (PUO)?
21. What is a fulminating disease?
22. What is meant by a systemic disease?
23. What is the difference between primary and secondary infections?
24. What is meant by the terms: superinfection, subclinical infection, latent infection, chronic infection?

TEST YOUR UNDERSTANDING

1. What external factors affect the composition of the normal flora?
2. A patient, Mrs B, is diagnosed with a urinary tract infection. The causative organism is *E. coli*. Explain the significance of this finding and how the infection may have occurred.
3. Why are some organisms more virulent than others?
4. How do opportunistic infections differ from those caused by other pathogens?
5. Describe the factors that contribute to a host's susceptibility to infection.
6. Discuss how the criteria in Koch's Postulates need to be modified in the light of current knowledge of infectious diseases.
7. How is fever produced in the course of an infectious disease?
8. What factors determine whether an infection remains localised?

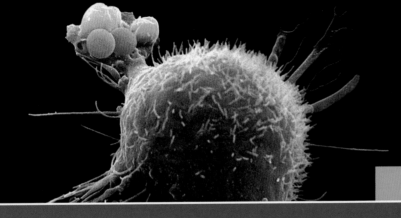

CHAPTER 8

Epidemiology – How Diseases are Spread

[CHAPTER FOCUS]

- **What is the difference between communicable and non-communicable diseases?**

- **What are the major reservoirs of infection?**

- **How do organisms gain entry to the human body?**

- **What are the major portals of exit from the human body?**

- **How are diseases transmitted from one person to another?**

- **How does the science of epidemiology help to control the spread of infectious diseases?**

Introduction

Epidemiology is the study of the origins and patterns of all types of disease. In this chapter we examine the occurrence, spread and control of infectious diseases. An infectious disease is one that can be transmitted (spread) from an infected patient to a susceptible host. Its spread depends on the ability of the pathogen to move from one host to another, to gain entry and to cause damage to the host. Some diseases are easily spread – others require a carrier or intermediate host. We describe the difference between communicable and non-communicable diseases and identify reservoirs and sources of pathogenic microorganisms. We also describe the ways in which different microorganisms gain access to the human body, how they are transmitted from one host to another and how outbreaks of disease occur. We examine how the science of epidemiology can improve public health outcomes through surveillance and the development of strategies for the prevention and control of infectious diseases.

Communicable and non-communicable diseases

Communicable diseases are infectious diseases that can spread from one host to another. Some spread more easily than others and are described as very infectious or **contagious**. The term 'contagious' is used to describe the *ease* of spread, not whether the disease can be spread or not. Communicable diseases include colds, influenza, measles, chickenpox, rubella, diphtheria and polio, as well as gastrointestinal diseases and sexually transmitted diseases. These diseases are transmitted in various ways:

- by contact with aerosols from an infected host
- via body fluids such as blood, urine, sputum and faeces
- by infected skin cells that have been shed into the environment
- from open lesions or wounds
- by contact with contaminated surfaces.

Non-communicable diseases are those that would not normally be spread from an infected host to a healthy person during the course of usual contact and normal daily activities. They include diseases that are acquired by the mechanical transfer of a pathogen from the environment into the host tissue, such as occurs with tetanus. Tetanus spores are usually carried on an implement into a puncture wound where they germinate, multiply and produce the toxin responsible for disease symptoms. Diseases such as cystitis (urinary tract infection), which are caused by the displacement of normal body flora from one site to another, are also not considered to be communicable.

Diseases transmitted by insects are unlikely to be communicable unless all the conditions for spread are ideal; that is, there is a large reservoir of infected hosts and an unlimited number of vectors. Parasitic diseases that require an intermediate host are not directly communicable from one definitive host to another.

Some diseases are caused by the ingestion of a pre-formed toxin produced by a microorganism. Strictly speaking, this should be defined as **intoxication** rather than infection. For example, the symptoms of botulism are caused by the ingestion of a preformed neurotoxin produced by the bacterium, *Clostridium botulinum*, which grows anaerobically in inadequately sterilised canned or bottled food. The bacterium does not multiply in the human body but is shed in the faeces. For transmission to occur, the spores have to find their way into unsterilised canned or bottled food.

In practice, there is some overlap between the strict definitions of 'communicable' and 'non-communicable' but it is a useful grouping that enables health workers to assess the risk of transmission of infection from a person with a disease to another individual – non-communicable diseases have essentially a low or negligible risk of transmission, communicable diseases have a high risk of transmission.

Reservoirs of infection

In order to acquire an infectious disease, an individual must be exposed to a reservoir or source of the pathogen and a situation must exist whereby the pathogen can be transmitted to the human body and gain entry in sufficient numbers to cause an infection.

By now it should be apparent that there are thousands of different types of microbes living in our environment and that humans are in constant contact with these organisms during the course of their normal daily activities. Some of these organisms are able to cause disease in healthy individuals (natural pathogens), while others cause disease only in immunocompromised people (opportunistic pathogens). Some are easily spread from one person to another, while others are only introduced into the human body by mechanical means. Many of the organisms that cause disease in humans survive for only a limited period outside the human body unless they are provided with a suitable alternative environment.

For a disease to be **endemic** (always present) in a community, there has to be a permanent reservoir of the infectious agent. This **reservoir** is a habitat where the microorganisms can persist for long periods. It may be a favourable environment where they are able to survive or even increase in numbers, or it may be an unfavourable environment where the organism survives in a resistant form – for example, protozoal cysts or bacterial endospores. It may be a human or other animal host or a non-living environment such as soil or water. For some infectious diseases, humans are the only reservoir (e.g. syphilis, gonorrhoea, the hepatitis viruses, smallpox and measles). Other pathogens (e.g. many kinds of bacteria) can survive in the external environment, in soil and water. Some microorganisms infect animals as well as humans, in which case the animal acts as the reservoir of the pathogen.

We can distinguish between a reservoir of infection and a source of infection. The **source** is the individual or object from which the infectious agent is actually acquired. The reservoir may also be a source if an opportunity exists for the microorganisms to pass directly from the reservoir to a susceptible host. For example, infected humans are both the reservoir and source for diseases such as measles and syphilis. However, sometimes the reservoir and source are different. For example, if the nose is colonised by staphylococci, it can be considered a reservoir of staphylococcal infection, but when the staphylococci from the nose are present as a contaminant in food, the food is the source of the infection.

A source may also be contaminated water, or a fomite. A **fomite** is an inanimate object that can carry microorganisms (usually bacteria) on its surface. In the hospital environment, fomites are important sources of infection. They include such items as medical equipment and instruments, soiled linen and dressings, keys and other utensils. Diseases such as polio or hepatitis A have human reservoirs, but the source of the infectious agent (virus) is usually food or water contaminated by infected human faeces. This applies to most diseases transmitted by the faecal-oral route (see page 166).

HUMAN RESERVOIRS

The most important reservoir of pathogenic microorganisms is the human body itself. Patients who are suffering from an infectious disease are constantly producing and shedding pathogens that can readily be spread to others during the incubation period and the early prodromal phase, as well as when the disease is fully established.

An individual with an obvious symptomatic infection is usually regarded as a reservoir for the pathogen and a potential source of infection. However, as we saw in Chapter 7, there are a number of situations where a person is infected without showing any apparent signs of illness. These include patients who have subclinical infections and people who are chronic asymptomatic carriers of a disease. Humans with latent viral infections are also important reservoirs for viral pathogens.

The normal flora of the human body also represent a significant reservoir of potential pathogens if they are displaced from their normal habitat or if their host is compromised in some way. For example, most urinary tract infections are caused by normal flora of the colon such as *E. coli*. A large number of the infections that occur in surgical or other wounds are caused by normal skin flora such as *Staphylococcus epidermidis*. *E. coli* may also be the cause of diarrhoea when toxin-producing strains of the bacteria are ingested in contaminated food or water (see Spotlight box on Haemolytic Uraemic Syndrome, page 423).

ANIMAL RESERVOIRS

Many animals, both wild and domestic, harbour microorganisms that can cause disease in humans. About 150 of these diseases – termed **zoonoses** (singular: zoonosis) – are known. In some cases (e.g. rabies), both animals and

humans suffer from a similar disease. In others (e.g. viral encephalitis), the animal does not appear to suffer from the disease but the organism is pathogenic for humans. The recently discovered SARS corona virus and the avian flu virus H5N1 appear to be of animal origin.

Transmission of many of these diseases from an animal reservoir to humans requires a vector in the form of a blood-sucking insect (e.g. plague is carried by fleas). For other diseases, transmission requires direct contact with the animal, its fur, feathers or body secretions. Some types of tinea (e.g. ringworm) are acquired from exposure to infected domestic animals or pets. Some of the protozoal and helminthic parasites have complex life cycles involving both animals and humans.

Humans may be either an accidental or a definitive host, while the animal may be an intermediate or definitive host for the parasite (see Chapter 6). For example, the beef tapeworm exists in the larval or cyst form in the muscle tissue (meat) of cattle, from where it is ingested by humans who are the definitive host. *Toxoplasma gondii* is harboured in the intestine of domestic cats and other animals and excreted as oocysts in their faeces. From there it may be ingested by animals, lodging in the muscle tissue which is then eaten by humans. An alternative route is the direct inhalation or ingestion of oocysts from soil or kitty litter. Most zoonoses are impossible to eradicate as to do so would require the destruction of all animal reservoirs. Table 8.1 lists some of the common zoonoses found in Australia.

Three new zoonotic viruses have recently been identified in Australia. They are the Hendra virus (HeV, previously called equine morbillivirus), Menangle virus and Australian bat lyssavirus (ABL). Flying foxes, commonly called fruit bats, are the natural reservoirs for these viruses (see Spotlight box, page 157).

NON-LIVING RESERVOIRS: SOIL AND WATER

Many microorganisms thrive in the external environment, especially in soil and water.

Soil

Bacteria may be present as vegetative cells or, in some cases, as resistant endospores. Some of the spore-forming bacteria are important pathogens, especially species of the genus *Clostridium*, which are commonly found in the soil. For example, spores of the tetanus bacillus (*Clostridium tetani*) are excreted in faeces and remain viable for long periods in the soil. They are transferred to humans when a person sustains an injury from an object contaminated with the tetanus spores. Gas gangrene (*Clostridium perfringens*) spores are also very resistant and widely distributed in the environment. If they gain entry to the body at the site of tissue injury or via surgical wounds they can cause gangrene but, if the spores are ingested in food, gastroenteritis may result.

Botulism is caused by the ingestion of poorly preserved food in which spores of *Clostridium botulinum*, commonly

Table 8.1

Selected zoonoses occurring in Australia

ORGANISM	DISEASE	ANIMAL RESERVOIR	TRANSMISSION
Bacteria			
Bacillus anthracis	Anthrax	Cattle	Contact with cattle or endospores
Brucella spp.	Brucellosis	Cattle	Direct contact
Borrelia spp.	Lyme disease	? Native animals	Tick bites
Chlamydia psittaci	Psittacosis (ornithosis)	Birds/parrots	Direct contact
Coxiella burnetii	Q fever	Cattle	Direct contact
Leptospira	Leptospirosis	Wild mammals, cats/dogs	Contact with urine/water
Listeria monocytogenes	Listeriosis	Domestic animals	Unpasteurised milk
Salmonella spp.	Salmonellosis	Poultry	Ingestion of contaminated food, water
Campylobacter	Gastroenteritis	Domestic livestock	
Bartonella henselae	Cat scratch fever	Cats	Scratching, contact
Rickettsia tsutsugamushi	Scrub typhus	Mites/ticks	Bites
Viruses			
Influenza virus	Influenza (some types)	Pigs, ducks	Direct contact
Flavivirus	Murray Valley encephalitis	Fowl/birds	Mosquitoes
Orf virus (parapoxvirus)	Orf	Sheep, goats	Direct contact
Alphavirus	Ross River fever	Native animals	Mosquitoes
Alphavirus	Barmah forest polyarthritis	Native animals	Mosquitoes
Hendra virus	Influenza-like illness	Flying fox	Contact with infected animals (horses)
Menangle virus	Fever/rash	Flying fox	Contact with animals (pigs)
Bat lyssavirus	Rabies-like illness	Flying fox	Bite, scratch by flying fox
Protozoa			
Toxoplasma gondii	Toxoplasmosis	Cats/other mammals	Ingestion of contaminated meat, contact with faeces
Fungi			
Trichophyton	Ringworm (tinea)	Domestic animals	Direct contact
Microsporum			
Helminths			
Echinococcus granulosis	Hydatid cysts	Dogs	Contact with faeces
Taenia saginata	Tapeworm	Cattle	Ingestion of contaminated meat
Toxocara spp.	Worm infestation of body organs	Dogs/cats	Ingestion of eggs

found in the soil, have germinated and grown under anaerobic conditions, producing the neurotoxin responsible for botulism. Anthrax spores are able to survive for many years in soil and infect animals or humans who come in contact with the contaminated soil. Species of Gram-negative pseudomonads are commonly found in soil and on plants and can be introduced into the hospital environment on flowers and plants. They are important opportunistic pathogens and a common cause of hospital infections, especially in burns patients.

Many protozoa form cysts as a stage in their life cycle and these survive for long periods in the soil before entering a human or animal host (e.g. *Toxoplasma*). Helminth eggs or larvae (e.g. hookworm) may be found in soil. Gardeners may be infected with *Legionella*, which is often present in potting mix (see Spotlight box, page 167). Soil containing bird droppings contaminated with *Chlamydi psittaci* can be the source of psitticosis or bird flu, an atypical pneumonia. Various soil fungi can be the source of hand and nail infections.

Water
Water is a reservoir for a number of pathogens that live and multiply best in an aqueous environment. These include protozoa such as *Giardia*, *Cryptosporidia* and *Entamoeba* which are frequently present in natural water

SPOTLIGHT ON

New zoonoses: viral infections linked to flying foxes

There are relatively few viruses that cross the species barrier and infect humans as well as animals. That is why, in September 1994, there was such interest when a racehorse in Brisbane, Queensland, died from a severe respiratory disease and, within days of the horse's death, a stablehand and the trainer who had cared for the horse became ill with an influenza-like illness. A number of other horses in the same stable became sick and, over a period of two weeks, a total of 14 horses died. The stablehand was ill for more than two weeks but gradually recovered fully. The trainer died about two weeks after becoming ill.

Extensive epidemiological investigations were carried out by the Queensland Health Department and the Queensland Department of Primary Industry (QDPI) to determine the cause of the illness.

A previously unidentified virus with characteristics of the Paramyxoviridae family was isolated from the lungs of six of the dead horses and from the kidneys of the trainer. It was identified at the CSIRO Australian Animal Health Laboratory (AAHL). It was at first named equine morbillivirus (EMV) and thought to belong to a group known as morbilliviruses, distantly related to measles, but has since been renamed Hendra virus. In October 1995, the death was reported of a man from Mackay in Queensland who had assisted at the autopsy of a horse in August 1994, before the Brisbane outbreak. He died from encephalitis, but blood tests showed the presence of antibodies to Hendra virus.

The virus appears to be transmitted by close contact with blood or secretions from the horse's nose or mouth. The severity of the symptoms and the final outcome probably depends on the level of exposure to the virus and the susceptibility of the patient. The virus is able to infect humans and horses and also some other animals, such as cats.

A number of animals were tested for the presence of antibodies to the virus and flying foxes (fruit bats) were identified as a natural reservoir of the virus. During the investigations another virus was isolated from a flying fox suffering from neurological symptoms. It was found to belong to the Rhabdoviridae (rabies-like) family of viruses and was named Australian bat lyssavirus (ABL). It was identified as the cause of death of two people who had been bitten or scratched by two different kinds of bat. Rabies vaccine is an effective treatment for exposure to the virus.

A third new virus was isolated in 1997 from stillborn piglets in New South Wales and named Menangle virus. It is morphologically a member of the Paramyxoviridae family. Two workers who had been exposed to animal secretions at the piggery suffered severe fever and rash and were found to have antibodies to Menangle virus.

Serological testing has established the presence of antibodies to Hendra virus, lyssavirus and Menangle virus in bat populations. It appears that flying foxes are the natural reservoir for all three viruses. At present the viruses have been found only in Australia but screening for them is being carried out in the Torres Strait Islands and Papua New Guinea.

Another new zoonotic virus, the Nipah virus, which also belongs to the Paramyxoviridae, was recently identified as the cause of encephalitis in pig farmers and pigs in Malaysia. Its natural reservoir is also the flying fox. Hendra, Menangle and Nipah viruses appear to be transmitted to humans via the secretions of infected domestic animals (pigs, horses). Lyssavirus is the only one that has been transmitted directly from bats to humans. The appearance of these viruses is an example of the effect of humans on the environment, leading to the emergence of new diseases by the transfer of the viruses from their natural hosts. Bats, including flying foxes, are widespread throughout Australia and play important roles in ecosystems by dispersing rainforest seeds, pollination or control of insects.

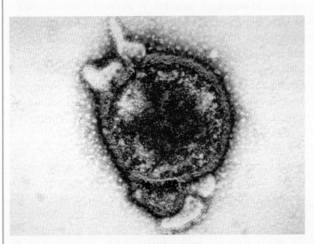 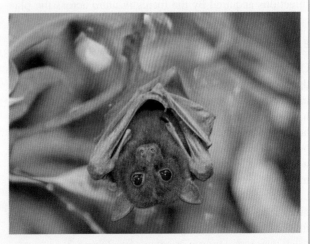

Figure 8.1

(a) Electron micrograph of Hendra virus. (b) A little red flying-fox *Pteropus scapulatus*.

environments, especially where sewage pollution occurs. Many different kinds of bacteria can be found in water. *Legionella* is found in natural streams and has been isolated from water in the cooling towers of air-conditioning plants. *Pseudomonas*, which has minimal nutritional requirements, is often present in the water in cooling towers, drinking water coolers and bubblers. Water contaminated with faeces can be the source of a large number of pathogens responsible for infectious diseases, including typhoid, cholera, polio and hepatitis A.

Leptospira may be found in water contaminated with animal urine. In tropical areas *Pseudomallei burkholderia*, which causes melioidosis, lives in water and enters through skin abrasions. The blood fluke *Schistosoma* has a free-living larval stage in water – the cercariae – and people swimming where these occur are at risk of acquiring the infection. Outbreaks of diarrhoea caused by *Cryptosporidium parvum* have been associated with children's wading pools.

Portals of entry

To cause disease, the infectious agent must first gain entry to the human body. The microorganisms may come from any of the reservoirs described above.

ENDOGENOUS INFECTIONS

Endogenous infections are caused by the microorganisms already present on the human body, which acts as the reservoir. They include infections such as:

* **cystitis**, an infection of the bladder, usually caused by normal flora from the colon
* **thrush**, an opportunistic infection caused by *Candida albicans*
* recurrent **herpes**, due to the reactivation of a latent infection
* disseminated infections such as those due to *Streptococcus* species, which spread from the throat and set up infections in the ears, lungs or kidneys.

Infections acquired by the foetus *in utero* across the placenta are also considered to be endogenous.

EXOGENOUS INFECTIONS

Other infections are caused by **exogenous** pathogens – that is, microorganisms derived from the external environment. An intact layer of skin provides a protective barrier for the body and anything that damages or penetrates this barrier allows the entry of microorganisms. Other major portals of entry are via the mucous membranes lining the walls of the respiratory, gastrointestinal and genitourinary tracts.

Most pathogens have a preferred **portal of entry**, one that gives ready access to an immediate environment suitable for the establishment of growth, or allows the pathogens to reach their target tissues or organs. See Table 8.2.

Sometimes the portal of entry is quite specific for the disease. For example, bacteria such as *Salmonella*, which cause gastrointestinal infections, enter via the mouth. In other cases, pathogenic organisms are able to gain entry to the body via more than one portal. *Mycobacterium tuberculosis* can enter via both the gastrointestinal and respiratory tracts.

Some diseases take different forms depending on the portal of entry. *Yersinia pestis*, the bacterium responsible for plague, produces buboes in the lymph glands (bubonic plague) when it is introduced via the bite of an infected flea. However, it can also be inhaled directly into the lungs, causing pneumonia and giving rise to a much more severe form of the disease (pneumonic plague).

SKIN AS A PORTAL OF ENTRY

Infections of the skin are described in Chapter 16. Intact skin is an important barrier to the entry of microorganisms (see Chapter 9). Cracks or splits in the skin, due to swelling, drying or cutaneous mycoses such as tinea, allow other microorganisms to enter and set up infections in the cutaneous or subcutaneous layers (see Case History 7.1). The herpes virus also enters through the skin and infects epithelial cells. Bacteria such as *Staphylococcus aureus* and *Streptococcus pyogenes* can infect hair follicles or sebaceous glands, causing pimples and boils. Damage to the skin caused by scratching itchy insect bites or scabies infections allows bacteria to enter, causing infections such as impetigo.

The conjunctiva of the eye provides protection against infection, so damage to the conjunctiva by dust or foreign bodies can allow entry of microorganisms. Pathogens such as *Neisseria gonorrhoeae* and *Chlamydia trachomatis* can infect the intact conjunctiva because they have attachment devices to avoid the flushing action of tears. Other important pathogens (e.g. hepatitis B) can gain entry via the conjunctiva as a result of splashes of blood or body fluids into the eyes.

The larvae of helminths such as hookworm enter the body by burrowing through the skin, as do the cercariae of *Schistosoma*. The bite of an insect vector that breaches the skin barrier and carries pathogens directly into the bloodstream is an important method of entry for many infectious agents. Mosquitoes can carry a variety of diseases – malaria, encephalitis, yellow fever, dengue fever and Ross River fever. Fleas carry plague, ticks carry Lyme disease and human body lice carry typhus.

The use of hypodermic syringes by injecting drug users breaks the skin and provides ready access for microorganisms. Sharing of needles and syringes allows the spread of blood-borne pathogens such as hepatitis B, hepatitis C and HIV, as well as bacterial infections.

Other microorganisms gain entry to the body through puncture wounds in the skin, and may lodge in wounds where there has been extensive tissue damage – for example, spores of the agents that cause tetanus and gangrene. They then reproduce under the favourable anaerobic conditions that exist in deep or necrotic tissue, causing disease by the production of harmful toxins.

The importance of intact skin is especially apparent in the hospital environment where breaks in the skin due to

Table 8.2

Preferred portal of entry for some common pathogens

PORTAL OF ENTRY	DISEASE	PATHOGEN
Skin		
Infections of skin and mucosal surfaces	Herpes	*Herpes simplex*
	Thrush	*Candida albicans*
	Skin infections	Staphylococci
		Streptococci
		Pseudomonads
Conjunctiva	Trachoma	*Chlamydia trachomatis*
	Gonorrhoea	*Neisseria gonorrhoeae*
Puncture wounds	Tetanus	*Clostridium tetani*
	Gangrene	*Clostridium perfringens*
IV drug users	Hepatitis B	Hepatitis B virus
Needlesticks	Hepatitis C	Hepatitis C virus
	AIDS	Human immunodeficiency virus
Burrowing parasites	Hookworm	Hookworms
	Schistosomiasis	*Schistosoma*
Insect-borne infections	Plague	*Yersinia pestis*
	Malaria	*Plasmodium*
	Arboviral infections	Various viruses (see Table 5.4)
Respiratory tract		
Localised infections of the respiratory tract and lungs	Diphtheria	*Corynebacterium diphtheriae*
	SARS	SARS- CoV
	Common colds	Various adeno, rhino viruses
	Tuberculosis	*Mycobacterium tuberculosis*
	Pneumonia	Various organisms (see Table 7.3), e.g. *Streptococcus pneumoniae*
Systemic infections	Whooping cough	*Bordetella pertussis*
	Chickenpox	*Varicella zoster* virus
	Measles	Morbillivirus
	German measles	Rubella virus
	Glandular fever	Epstein-Barr virus
	Influenza	Influenza virus
	Meningococcal meningitis	*Neisseria meningitidis*
Gastrointestinal tract		
Gastrointestinal infections	Gastroenteritis	Various organisms, e.g. *Shigella, Salmonella, Staphylococcus aureus, Campylobacter, E. coli, Cl. perfringens*, enteroviruses
	Cholera	*Vibrio cholerae*
	Hepatitis	Hepatitis A, hepatitis E viruses
Parasitic infections	Tapeworm	*Taenia saginata*
	Hydatids	*Echinococcus granulosis*
	Amoebic dysentery	*Entamoeba histolytica*
	Giardiasis	*Giardia intestinalis*
Systemic infections	Toxoplasmosis	*Toxoplasma gondii*
	Polio	Enterovirus
	Mumps	Paramyxovirus
	Typhoid	*Salmonella typhi*
Urogenital tract		
Sexually transmitted infections (STIs)	Gonorrhoea	*Neisseria gonorrhoeae*
	Syphilis	*Treponema pallidum*
	Trichomoniasis	*Trichomonas vaginalis*
	Chlamydia	*Chlamydia trachomatis*
	Genital warts	Human papilloma virus
	Herpes	*Herpes simplex*
	Thrush	*Candida albicans*
Systemic infections	Hepatitis B and C	Hepatitis B, hepatitis C viruses
	AIDS	Human immunodeficiency virus

surgical procedures provide an easy portal of entry, especially if the wound has a drainage device attached post-operatively. Even when correct aseptic techniques are followed, approximately 10% of all surgical wounds become infected while the patient is in hospital.

Invasive procedures such as the insertion of intravenous (IV) cannulas (in particular, central venous lines), and subsequent manipulation and care of these cannulas and catheters by nursing staff provide further opportunities for microorganisms to enter via breaks in the skin. Central venous lines pose an additional hazard when used for total parenteral nutrition, as the nutritious solutions used are an ideal growth medium for bacteria and fungi.

Burns patients may have large areas of damaged skin and are particularly vulnerable to infections by bacteria, of which *Staphylococcus aureus* and *Pseudomonas aeruginosa* are the most serious.

RESPIRATORY TRACT AS A PORTAL OF ENTRY

Infections of the respiratory tract are described in Chapter 17. The mucous membranes of the respiratory tract are a major portal of entry for many pathogens, which may be inhaled as aerosols or spores, or on dust particles. If they are not washed away by the mucous secretions, they adhere to the cells lining the upper respiratory tract and cause infections in the nasopharynx, tonsils, throat and larynx. They may then travel further – to the bronchial tubes, causing bronchitis, or to the lungs, causing pneumonia.

Common bacterial diseases that are acquired via the upper respiratory tract (URT) include whooping cough (*Bordetella pertussis*), diphtheria (*Corynebacterium diphtheriae*), meningitis (*Neisseria meningitidis*), streptococcal infections, tuberculosis (*Mycobacterium tuberculosis*), Legionnaires' disease (*Legionella pneumophila*). Tuberculosis enters via the URT and infects the lungs. The viruses of influenza, measles, chickenpox, rubella, mumps and the common cold also enter via the mucous membranes of the upper respiratory tract. From there, some of these organisms spread to other parts of the body and produce systemic symptoms, such as a skin rash or enlarged lymph nodes. Spores of fungi such as *Aspergillus* are able to infect the lungs (see Chapter 6). Certain infections that enter initially via the respiratory tract may be disseminated to other organs of the body, especially in immunocompromised patients.

Pneumonia is an inflammation of the lungs that can be caused by a number of different viruses and bacteria that enter via the respiratory tract and penetrate to the lung tissue (see Table 7.3, page 142). Among these, SARS (severe acute respiratory syndrome) is the most recent viral infection to be described. It enters via the mucosal surfaces of the URT and causes an atypical pneumonia (see Spotlight box, page 162). Hospitalised patients are particularly susceptible to colonisation by pathogens carried on air currents and aerosols around the hospital. Viral infections such as those caused by the respiratory

syncytial virus and influenza virus may be serious and even fatal to infants or elderly patients.

The use of respiratory equipment such as ventilators can create conditions that allow microorganisms to be introduced directly into the respiratory tract. Water from the humidification of the inspired air and the condensation of expired air collects in the ventilator tubing and may support the growth of bacteria, especially Gram-negative rods such as *Pseudomonas aeruginosa*. Tubes should be changed regularly to minimise this risk. Adequate cleaning and disinfection of all respiratory equipment is of the utmost importance.

Another hazard exists in the use of nebulisers for humidification as the equipment has the potential to spray the patient with contaminated water. Endotracheal intubation for mechanical ventilation bypasses the defence mechanisms normally present in the mouth and throat and allows entry of microorganisms directly to the lungs. The wound associated with the tracheostomy provides another portal of entry for infection as it may become colonised with organisms such as *Staphylococcus aureus* during handling of the tracheal tube. The maintenance of good oral hygiene is important in preventing the spread of bacteria from the mouth to the respiratory tract and lungs.

GASTROINTESTINAL TRACT AS A PORTAL OF ENTRY

Infections of the digestive tract are described in Chapter 18.

The ingestion of contaminated food or drink via the gastrointestinal tract (GIT) is a major way for pathogens to enter the body. To gain access by this route, the pathogen must be able to resist the acid conditions in the stomach (pH 1–2), as well as the other defences of the GIT. Resistant microbes may be ingested as eggs (e.g. helminths), cysts (e.g. *Giardia*) or endospores (e.g. *Clostridium perfringens*). In order for other kinds of organisms to enter by this route, they must be resistant to acid (e.g. cholera, some toxigenic *E. coli*, and enteroviruses), need only a low infective dose (e.g. *Shigella*) or be ingested in such large numbers that enough organisms survive to penetrate into the intestine. In some cases, the pathogens may be protected by the food in which they are carried. Most of the microorganisms responsible for gastrointestinal infections have specialised structures for attachment to the mucosal cells lining the intestine (see Chapter 10).

As well as being the entry route for the microorganisms that cause gastroenteritis, such as *Campylobacter*, *Salmonella* and *Shigella*, the GIT also acts as a portal of entry for various bacterial toxins that are produced in food before it is ingested. These include the neurotoxin of botulism and the enterotoxin of *Staphylococcus aureus*. These toxins are resistant to stomach acid and are absorbed in the small intestine, producing symptoms within hours of ingestion.

Other diseases that enter via the GIT, but are disseminated to other parts of the body, include hepatitis A which affects the liver, and polio which is absorbed in the intestine and affects other parts of the body including nerve cells.

UROGENITAL TRACT AS A PORTAL OF ENTRY

Infections of the urinary and genital systems are discussed in Chapter 21.

The lower section of the urinary tract, the urethra, is frequently contaminated with normal flora, similar to those found in the colon. In females these organisms are likely to ascend the relatively short urethra to the bladder, causing cystitis; if not treated they may reach the kidneys and cause pyelonephritis. A high percentage of all hospital-acquired infections are of the urinary tract and are associated with the use of urinary catheters. The use of indwelling catheters, especially in elderly or incontinent patients, gives bacteria ready access to the bladder, usually on the outside of the catheter. The infecting organisms are generally derived from the patient's own flora but, in hospitalised patients or patients undergoing long-term antibiotic treatment, there is the likelihood that these infections will be caused by antibiotic-resistant strains of bacteria. The most serious complication of urinary tract infections occurs when damage to the cells lining the mucosa of the urinary tract allows the organisms to gain access to the bloodstream, causing sepsis.

The genital tract is the main portal of entry for a number of infections, usually transmitted by intimate contact during sexual intercourse. Organisms responsible for diseases that enter this way include *Neisseria gonorrhoeae*, *Treponema pallidum* (syphilis), chlamydia, human papilloma virus (genital warts), herpes and *Trichomonas vaginalis*. Some of these microorganisms have special structures such as pili, which enable them to attach to the mucosal cells lining the genital tract and prevent their being washed away by urine or mucosal secretions (e.g. *Neisseria gonorrhoeae*).

Blood-borne viruses present in semen and vaginal secretions (e.g. hepatitis B and C, and HIV) can enter the bloodstream through breaks in the skin or the mucosal lining of the genital tract, although this is not considered their major portal of entry.

The prevalence of sexual practices other than vaginal intercourse means that sexually transmitted organisms can enter and infect other areas of the body such as the anus or mouth and throat, provided that specific attachment sites for the microorganisms exist in these areas. *Neisseria gonorrhoeae* is one such organism that can infect any of these sites as well as the genital tract.

CONGENITAL INFECTIONS

Microorganisms that infect the foetus, *in utero*, gain access by crossing the placenta. The placenta is usually an efficient barrier, allowing nutrients and waste to pass through, while excluding larger, possibly harmful, cells and molecules. However, some microorganisms are able to cross the placental barrier and infect the foetus. In the process, they can cause abortion or various degrees of foetal damage, depending on the type of organism involved and the stage

of pregnancy when the infection occurs. Organisms that can cause congenital defects include:

- rubella virus (congenital rubella syndrome)
- *Toxoplasma gondii* (toxoplasmosis)
- cytomegalovirus (congenital CMV)
- *Treponema pallidum* (syphilis)
- *Listeria monocytogenes* (congenital listeriosis).

Hepatitis B and HIV may also infect the foetus, but this usually occurs at the end of pregnancy or during birth and gives rise to a chronic infection in the neonate without congenital defects.

Perinatal infections (infections acquired at birth) are caused by microorganisms present in the mother's birth canal; they infect the baby by entering via any of the portals described above. Most serious for the neonate are herpes infections of the eyes (which can spread to the brain and cause herpes encephalitis), chlamydial and gonorrhoeal infections of the eyes, and pneumonia due to Group B streptococci or chlamydia. Thrush (*Candida albicans*), derived from the mother's genital tract, is a common infection of the mucosal lining of the mouth of the neonate.

Portals of exit

In earlier sections of this chapter we described the human body as an important reservoir for infectious microorganisms, and the body's secretions and excretions as a potential source of pathogens.

Microorganisms are continually being shed from the human body during such normal activities as coughing, sneezing, defecating and changing clothing. A healthy person sheds mainly normal flora which do not generally pose any special risk to other healthy members of the population. When a person is suffering from an infectious disease, the pathogens responsible for that disease are also shed in large numbers and may infect other susceptible people. Very often, the pathogen is shed from the same area (portal) by which it entered (see Table 8.3). In the hospital environment, it is important for the nurse to be aware of the way in which pathogens exit the human body in order to ensure the safe and effective disposal of contaminated material and to prevent cross-infection. Health workers also need to be aware of the potential risks to themselves of occupational exposure to pathogenic organisms (see Chapter 13).

UPPER RESPIRATORY TRACT: NOSE AND THROAT

Organisms that infect the nasopharynx, throat and lungs are usually present in large numbers in the watery mucosal secretions and in sputum. They are expelled as aerosols by talking, coughing and sneezing. The fine aerosol droplets allow rapid dispersal of pathogens such as the cold and flu viruses, which do not survive long outside the body. These aerosol droplets are able to infect other people, directly through inhalation, or indirectly by contamination of a fomite e.g. SARS (see Spotlight box on the next page).

In early March 2003, newspapers began to carry reports of an outbreak of atypical pneumonia in Hong Kong. The first death was of a doctor from Guandong province in China who had travelled to Hong Kong in February and stayed in a hotel, before being transferred to hospital. At least 17 other guests and visitors to the hotel became infected, some of whom travelled to Vietnam, Singapore and Toronto, where further transmission occurred. Hotel guests and their contacts were admitted to a number of hospitals in Hong Kong. In the first weeks of the outbreak in Hong Kong many of the cases occurred in health-care workers (HCW) who cared for the patients. In turn, they spread the infection to their household contacts.

An elderly woman who had stayed at the hotel in Hong Kong travelled back to Toronto. She died at home but her son was infected and hospitalised and became the index case for a major outbreak in Toronto which ultimately resulted in 361 cases and 41 deaths.

An outpatient at one of the Hong Kong hospitals became infected and transmitted the infection to a relative he visited in a block of apartments called Amoy Gardens, in Hong Kong. At Amoy Gardens 320 residents became ill – it is thought that the virus was shed in faeces and aerosols from contaminated sewage entered the bathrooms of other apartments through open U-traps. A resident of Amoy Gardens travelled to Taiwan and is thought to have infected a passenger on the train. Because there was no obvious connection with Hong Kong, SARS was not suspected when the passenger became ill, and this contributed to the extent of the outbreak in Taiwan. Travellers to Guandong province may also have carried the virus back to Taiwan.

In Toronto and Taiwan, it was at first thought that the patients were suffering from pneumonia so strict infection control precautions were not applied. This resulted in a large number of hospital-acquired infections, particularly among health-care workers and intensive care nurses.

By the middle of March it was apparent that health authorities were dealing with a serious new disease. It was named Severe Acute Respiratory Syndrome (SARS) and the World Health Organization (WHO) declared a global emergency. A team of epidemiologists, infectious disease specialists, public health physicians and microbiologists was assembled to study and contain the disease. Attention was also focused on Guandong province where, it was revealed, cases of a severe respiratory pneumonia-like disease had been occurring since November 2002.

The speed with which the world community reacted prevented the occurrence of a more serious pandemic. By the middle of April scientists had isolated the causative organism and identified it as a novel corona virus – it was named SARS-CoV. (Corona viruses are a family of enveloped, single-strand RNA viruses that usually cause mild infections such as the common cold in humans). The viral genome was sequenced and molecular techniques used to identify different strains of the virus and trace its spread.

By the time the epidemic was brought under control in June 2003, there had been over 8000 cases of SARS and 774 deaths worldwide, 21% of cases occurring in health workers. The overall case fatality rate was 9.6% (range 7–17%).

It is now known that the virus is spread through direct or indirect contact of the mucous membranes of the eyes, nose or mouth with infected respiratory droplets or fomites. Because many of the patients required ventilation, the use of procedures such as suctioning, endotracheal intubation, bronchoscopy and aerosolised medication all contributed to the generation of infected aerosols. Profuse watery diarrhoea is a symptom of the disease and the virus is shed in faeces. The virus can survive for days in faeces and when dried on surfaces.

The WHO and the Centers for Disease Control (CDC) developed a case definition and guidelines for infection control. The incubation period is 2–7 days, but may be up to 10 days. Early symptoms are non-specific and similar to respiratory illness – fever, coughing, shortness of breath and changes on X-ray similar to atypical pneumonia. Patients do not appear to be infectious during the incubation period. SARS is highly infectious to close contacts. Droplets and contact are the main routes of transmission and viral shedding is at a maximum at day 10 of the disease. Some patients may have only mild symptoms so an accurate case history, especially of international travel, is very important. Prevention in the health-care environment involves consistent handwashing, the use of protective clothing, particulate filter masks and disposable plastic gowns when caring for suspected SARS patients (see Chapter 13).

The global outbreak of SARS provided a fascinating study of the epidemiology of a new disease and an impressive example of the speed with which a disease can be identified and contained. This was due to the extensive collaboration between scientists and health authorities, the use of new technologies and an understanding of the viral transmission. SARS represents a continuing public health threat because of the particular characteristics of the disease. The reservoir of the viral pathogen is not known; early symptoms of the disease are non-specific yet the disease is highly infectious. Although there are infection control guidelines to prevent contact transmission of aerosols, it is not practical to use them for every patient who presents with a respiratory infection. Travel history is very important.

Figure 8.2 illustrates the spread of SARS.

continues

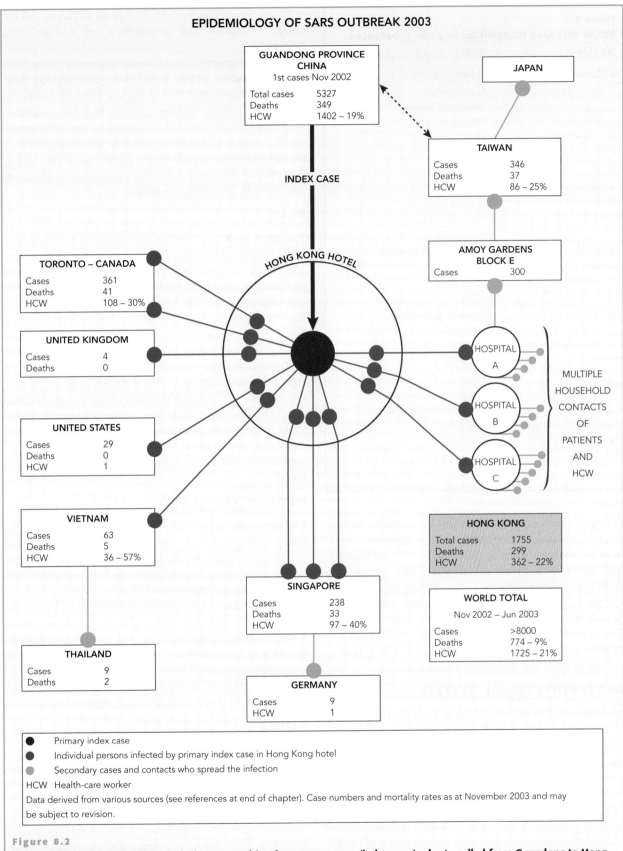

EPIDEMIOLOGY OF SARS OUTBREAK 2003

GUANDONG PROVINCE CHINA
1st cases Nov 2002

Total cases	5327
Deaths	349
HCW	1402 – 19%

JAPAN

TAIWAN

Cases	346
Deaths	37
HCW	86 – 25%

INDEX CASE

HONG KONG HOTEL

AMOY GARDENS BLOCK E

Cases	300

TORONTO – CANADA

Cases	361
Deaths	41
HCW	108 – 30%

UNITED KINGDOM

Cases	4
Deaths	0

UNITED STATES

Cases	29
Deaths	0
HCW	1

VIETNAM

Cases	63
Deaths	5
HCW	36 – 57%

THAILAND

Cases	9
Deaths	2

HOSPITAL A

HOSPITAL B

HOSPITAL C

MULTIPLE HOUSEHOLD CONTACTS OF PATIENTS AND HCW

HONG KONG

Total cases	1755
Deaths	299
HCW	362 – 22%

WORLD TOTAL
Nov 2002 – Jun 2003

Cases	>8000
Deaths	774 – 9%
HCW	1725 – 21%

SINGAPORE

Cases	238
Deaths	33
HCW	97 – 40%

GERMANY

Cases	9
HCW	1

● Primary index case
● Individual persons infected by primary index case in Hong Kong hotel
● Secondary cases and contacts who spread the infection
HCW   Health-care worker
Data derived from various sources (see references at end of chapter). Case numbers and mortality rates as at November 2003 and may be subject to revision.

Figure 8.2
Epidemiology of worldwide spread of SARS resulting from one person (index case) who travelled from Guandong to Hong Kong and infected other hotel guests.

Table 8.3
Major diseases transmitted in body substances

SECRETION	DISEASE
• Sputum, mucosal secretions	Tuberculosis
	Diphtheria
	Whooping cough
	Influenza
	Measles
	Rubella
	SARS
• Saliva	Mumps
	Glandular fever
	Hepatitis B (C?)
	Cytomegalovirus
• Semen/vaginal secretions	Sexually transmitted infections
	Hepatitis B
	AIDS
• Urine	Cytomegalovirus
	Leptospirosis
• Faeces	Polio
	Typhoid
	Cholera
	Hepatitis A, hepatitis E
	Gastroenteritis – bacterial and viral
• Blood	Hepatitis B
	Hepatitis C
	AIDS

Pathogens, such as those responsible for measles, chickenpox and tuberculosis, are also carried in respiratory secretions for short distances to their next host. Some bacteria, such as *Mycobacterium tuberculosis* (TB), persist in a dried form on dust particles and are carried by air currents for great distances. Viruses such as the mumps virus (which infects the salivary glands), herpes simplex virus, Epstein-Barr virus (glandular fever) and cytomegalovirus (CMV) are secreted and shed in saliva. CMV is also present in urine and other body fluids.

GASTROINTESTINAL SYSTEM

A major portal of exit of pathogens from the human body is via the bowel. Some of the pathogens responsible for gastrointestinal infections cause irritation of the lining of the large intestine and interfere with water absorption, giving rise to watery stools or diarrhoea. When this occurs, large numbers of the pathogens are shed in the faeces. Organisms responsible for other diseases such as cholera, typhoid, hepatitis A and polio, as well as protozoal cysts and helminth eggs and larvae are also excreted in faeces. When these pathogens contaminate the water supply, an epidemic can occur (e.g. cholera outbreaks often occur after natural disasters).

Faeces are a major source of potential pathogens so nurses need to be aware of the importance of hand-

washing, the correct method of disposal of faeces and the correct cleaning and disinfection of contaminated equipment.

In the community, faecal contamination of water is an important public health issue. Pathogens derived from faeces are frequently found in the sea water on Australian beaches and in stormwater run-off. In some countries, untreated sewage is used as a fertiliser for vegetable crops, which creates a serious health risk when unpeeled or unwashed fruit or vegetables are eaten. Faecal contamination of food and water is a major cause of gastrointestinal infections in developing countries.

SKIN

The dead outer layers of the skin (dermis) are constantly being shed as skin scales and may carry the bacteria that are resident or transient on the skin. Bacteria and viruses contained in dried particles from crusts or scabs of wounds and exudates from skin lesions, boils and pustular rashes (e.g. chickenpox) may also be shed in this way. In the hospital environment these dried particles and dust containing microorganisms can be disturbed by activities such as bedmaking, dry dusting or excessive movement of equipment and dispersed around the hospital on air currents. Other skin diseases in which microbes are shed into the environment include herpes, warts and syphilis. Some of these organisms survive for a long time in the environment (e.g. chickenpox) while others (e.g. syphilis) are quite fragile and do not survive for long outside the human body.

UROGENITAL TRACT

The organisms responsible for most sexually transmitted diseases are present in semen and vaginal secretions and so are discharged from the body in this way. Others such as herpes or warts, which infect the skin, are shed from lesions on the genital organs. Organisms that infect the bladder or kidneys are usually present in urine, but do not pose a significant health risk to others. Cytomegalovirus is a major pathogen shed in urine, but there is no evidence that HIV or hepatitis B or C viruses are present in urine in significant amounts. Urine from animals infected with *Leptospira* contains the bacterium and can be a source of infection when it contaminates water supplies.

BLOOD

Blood is not usually considered a portal of entry for pathogens unless contaminated blood is given in a transfusion. In Australia, the careful screening of blood donors and blood products has essentially eliminated the risk of transmission of these organisms by blood transfusion. However, blood is a significant portal of exit for several important blood-borne pathogens that are released when bleeding occurs, or when blood is removed from the body for some other purpose.

Viruses such as HIV, hepatitis B and hepatitis C are transmitted in blood, blood-tinged body fluids and blood products. They may be transmitted by the sharing of needles for injecting drug use, or through breaks in the skin or mucous membranes that allow blood containing the virus to enter the body. These pathogens can also be transmitted from an infected patient to another individual (patient or staff) during dental or medical procedures where bleeding occurs, if there is a breakdown in aseptic technique or if contaminated instruments are not adequately cleaned and sterilised.

Another risk for health workers is transmission occurring as a result of needlestick injuries (see Chapter 13).

Some diseases are transmitted in blood by the bite of a bloodsucking insect such as a mosquito. One of the most important of these is *Plasmodium*, the protozoan responsible for malaria, which is present in the blood of infected humans (see also page 169). In rare cases, malaria can be transmitted by a blood transfusion. The Ebola virus, responsible for outbreaks of haemorrhagic fever in Uganda, causes massive bleeding from body organs and is shed and transmitted in blood.

Transmission of microorganisms

So far, in this chapter, we have looked at the reservoirs of infection and the ways in which microorganisms enter and exit the human body. For a disease to spread, the causative organism or pathogen has to move or be transmitted from a reservoir or source to a susceptible host. A knowledge and understanding of the possible means of transmission is very important for health professionals, especially when working in a hospital, where there is a huge reservoir of pathogens and a population of susceptible patients. To prevent the spread of infection, it is important to be able to break the **chain of transmission**. This is discussed more fully in Chapter 13 (see Figure 13.6 on page 292). In this section we outline the major routes of transmission.

Transmission of microorganisms usually occurs horizontally – that is, from person to person. Organisms can be spread horizontally by **direct contact**, by **indirect contact** with the reservoir or source, by means of a **common vehicle**, or by a **mechanical vector** or **biological vector** (see Figure 8.3). Vertical transmission – that is, from mother to foetus – occurs across the placenta.

CONTACT TRANSMISSION

Many pathogens are too fragile to exist for any length of time outside their host. For these organisms to spread, there has to be direct or very close contact between the infected host and a suitable portal of entry in the next host. Organisms may be transmitted from one person to another by actually touching the skin or body secretions of the infected person, or by touching an object that has recently been contaminated with the pathogen.

Direct contact

Direct contact refers to close or intimate contact between the infected person and a susceptible individual. Exposure

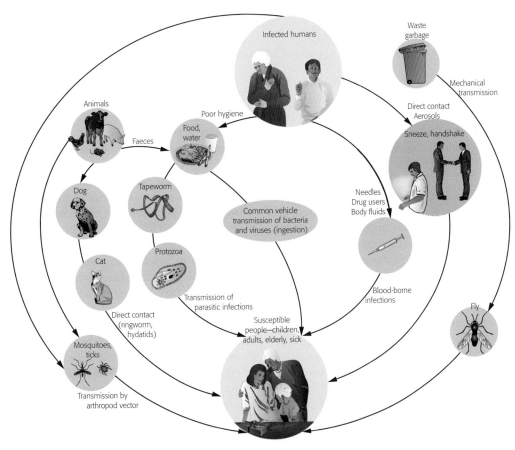

Figure 8.3

Methods of transmission

to skin and body secretions, such as occurs during kissing and sexual activity, is a major route of transmission of many infectious diseases. The transmission of pathogens present in the genital area, or in semen or vaginal secretions, can be prevented by adopting 'safe sex' practices, particularly the wearing of a condom. Skin infections such as herpes, cutaneous fungal infections and bacteria from infected wounds can also be transmitted by direct contact.

Infections may also be transmitted from one part of the body to another. For example, if the hands touch the genital region and then the eyes, infections such as gonorrhoea or herpes can be transferred from the genitals to the eyes. Similarly, normal flora from different parts of the body can be transmitted to an open wound. Once the hands are contaminated, organisms can be transmitted to other parts of the body or to another susceptible individual. Health workers should be aware of the need to wash their hands regularly, to wear gloves whenever caring for patients with a communicable infection, and to educate patients about personal hygiene.

Zoonoses are diseases of animals that can be transmitted to humans by direct contact with an infected animal. People working in the livestock industry may acquire the zoonoses, Q fever and brucellosis, which can be transmitted by direct contact with cattle as well as eating or handling contaminated meat. Although not found in Australia, rabies is a serious disease transmitted in the saliva of an infected animal, usually via a bite. Anthrax is transmitted by direct contact with the exudate from the lesions on an infected animal or by contact with or inhalation of anthrax spores. Other zoonoses transmitted by direct contact include tinea (ringworm), which is common in domestic cats and dogs.

A number of viruses (e.g. hantaviruses) that are endemic in the rodent population can find their way from wild rodents to domestic animals and then to humans. They are generally transmitted in saliva and urine by direct contact, or by indirect contact with dried urine or droppings.

Indirect contact

Indirect contact occurs when microorganisms from an infected host or other reservoir are deposited on an inanimate object, or **fomite**, and then transmitted to a susceptible host. This type of transmission can easily occur in the hospital environment unless health personnel take special precautions.

Fomites that can become sources of infection include medical equipment and instruments, eating utensils, bedpans, clothing, bedding, dressings, soap, taps, cupboard handles, refrigerators, sinks, telephones, computer keyboards, toilet bowls, keys, money and handkerchiefs. The pathogen leaves the human body by any of the portals described above and is deposited on a fomite. From there it can be spread directly to a new host. The pathogen may also be picked up on the hands of a health worker after handling the contaminated fomite and transferred to a susceptible patient.

Adequate cleansing and disinfecting procedures, careful handwashing and wearing of gloves are the main ways of preventing transmission by this route.

Faecal–oral transmission

Faeces contain a large number of microorganisms. Many pathogens are shed in the faeces and may be transmitted to another person by direct or indirect contact. Usually the pathogen is carried on the hands and may contaminate food which is then ingested. The bacteria and viruses responsible for gastrointestinal infections are easily transmitted person to person unless careful handwashing and good hygiene practices are followed.

Droplet transmission

Droplet transmission is also considered a form of contact transmission. Microorganisms contained in body secretions, usually from the upper respiratory tract, are expelled from the body by coughing, sneezing or talking and may immediately come into contact with a susceptible person. The major pathogens transmitted in this way are the viruses responsible for SARS, colds and influenza as well as whooping cough, measles and tuberculosis. The organisms are carried in droplets over a distance of less than one metre and inhaled directly into the respiratory tract of the new host. Simple actions like covering the nose and mouth when coughing or sneezing help to prevent the spread of these organisms.

COMMON VEHICLE TRANSMISSION

Microorganisms can be transmitted over a wide area by means of a vehicle such as air, water or food. When a number of people are infected with the same organism by one of these routes, it is called **common vehicle transmission**.

Airborne transmission

Airborne transmission occurs when disease-causing microorganisms are carried on air currents over distances greater than one metre. The pathogens must be able to survive outside the host and tolerate dry conditions. They include fungal spores, bacterial endospores and the cysts or eggs of various parasites. Certain bacteria, such as some staphylococci and the tubercle bacilli, are resistant to dry conditions and can remain viable (alive) for long periods. The oocysts of *Toxoplasma gondii* can be transmitted by inhalation of the dust from cat faeces in kitty litter.

Pathogens may also be present in fine water aerosol sprays that are too light to settle. The bacterium *Legionella pneumophila*, which is responsible for causing Legionnaires' disease (see Spotlight box on the next page), is transmitted in aerosol sprays derived from the exposed reservoirs of water-cooled air-conditioning plants and blown by wind currents over a wide area before entering a susceptible person via the respiratory tract.

Although pathogens are easily spread by the airborne route, they will only cause disease if they are able to gain access in sufficient numbers to a susceptible host through a suitable portal of entry. Organisms transmitted by the

Legionnaires' disease: an epidemiological investigation

Legionellosis or Legionnaires' disease is an atypical pneumonia, caused by bacteria of the *Legionella* species. Outbreaks occur from time to time, usually linked to public facilities such as shopping centres or other places where people congregate.

The discovery of *Legionella pneumophila* as the causative agent of an atypical pneumonia is a classic example of an epidemiological investigation. From time to time there is an outbreak of a disease that has not previously been described. This occurred in 1976 in the United States when 29 people from various parts of the country died from an unusual type of pneumonia. It might have gone unnoticed if it were not for the fact that all the victims were members of the American Legion and had recently attended their annual convention in Philadelphia. When reports of the sudden deaths of a number of their members simultaneously reached Legion headquarters, they decided to investigate the cause.

Epidemiologists from the Centers for Disease Control (CDC) in Atlanta, Georgia, were called in. A total of 182 people reported being ill and 29 died. The common link was that they had all been in or around the hotel where the convention was held. The investigation took on the character of a murder mystery. The hotel, its surroundings, the food that had been served, the water supply, and all the equipment and utensils that had been used were tested for microorganisms, food toxins and poisonous chemicals. There was a Senate inquiry and CDC scientists were accused of a cover-up! Finally, one of the scientists at CDC re-examined some tissue from one of the victims and found an unusual rod-shaped bacterium. DNA testing showed that it was a completely new genus. It was named *Legionella* (after the Legionnaires) *pneumophila* (lung-loving).

Outbreaks in other parts of the country helped to identify the reservoir of the infectious agent and the method of transmission. The bacterium was found growing in the open water tanks that were part of the air-conditioning system on the top of the Philadelphia hotel. Wind blowing across the tanks produced a fine aerosol spray carrying bacteria which were then blown around the street and into the foyer of the hotel. Anyone who happened to be present when the air currents were circulating in a certain way was at risk of inhaling the bacteria and contracting the infection.

Further investigations revealed that the bacterium occurs throughout the world, living in watery environments. Tests on stored blood and tissue samples of patients who had died from unidentified atypical pneumonia over a number of years revealed the presence of *Legionella*.

Over 40 different species of *Legionella* have now been identified. It is known that the disease has different forms depending on the species. The most severe form of pneumonia is caused by *Legionella pneumophila*, but there is a milder form known as Pontiac fever which is characterised by an influenza-like illness.

It has been shown that *Legionella pneumophila* is:

- transmitted by inhalation of the bacteria in fine aerosol sprays;
- not transmitted person to person within a household;
- sensitive to erythromycin.

One of the largest outbreaks of Legionnaires' disease in Australia occurred in April 2000 and was linked to the Melbourne Aquarium. The number of confirmed cases eventually reached 113, with two elderly patients dying from the disease.

The cases were confirmed by the identification of *Legionella pneumophila* serogroup1 antigen in urine samples from patients and the organism was isolated from cooling towers on the roof of the building. During 2000 there was a record number of 244 notifications in Victoria, with nine deaths.

Public health authorities have also reported that a number of cases of legionellosis occur each year, some of them fatal, after exposure to *Legionella longbeachae*. This particular strain of the bacterium is found in potting mix and soil in Australia and is associated with lower respiratory tract infections. Gardeners are warned to wear a mask and to keep the mix damp to avoid inhaling dust.

Note: Outbreaks of legionellosis occur from time to time in Australia. Usually, there are one or two deaths, mainly in older people who have associated illness or lung impairment. The disease can be successfully treated if diagnosed early. Health authorities require that all water tanks of water-cooled air conditioners be regularly cleaned and chlorinated. Deaths from *Legionnella* each year represent only a small percentage of the deaths from pneumonia caused by other organisms.

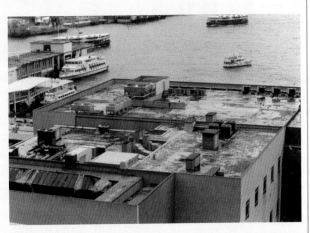

Figure 8.4

Water-cooled air-conditioning plants can be a reservoir for *Legionella*

airborne route do not multiply in air, but their spread is facilitated in modern air-conditioned buildings, such as hospitals, which have controlled temperatures and moist, recirculating air.

In the hospital environment there is a large reservoir of disease-causing microorganisms, constantly being shed in the form of aerosols, infected skin scales, and dried bacteria in crusts from infected wounds and herpes lesions. These organisms fall to the floor, some adhering to dust particles or to equipment and clothing. Activities such as cleaning, bedmaking or movement of equipment disturb them and they can then be carried on air currents throughout the hospital (see Figure 8.5).

The use of wet mops and dusters when cleaning can reduce the spread of pathogens by this route. Bed linen should be folded carefully and not shaken. The use of masks and special protective clothing helps to prevent airborne transmission in operating theatres, burns wards and intensive care units, where patients are particularly susceptible (see Chapter 13).

Water-borne transmission

Water is a major vehicle for the transmission of microorganisms. Faecal contamination of the water supply used for drinking or bathing is a major source of infectious agents. These include most of the bacterial and viral pathogens responsible for diarrhoeal infections, as well as the causative organisms of hepatitis A, hepatitis E, typhoid, cholera and polio. Protozoa such as *Giardia*, *Cryptosporidia* and *Entamoeba* live and multiply in fresh

water habitats and can be acquired by drinking or swimming in the water. As mentioned above, the bacterium *Legionella pneumophila* multiplies in water reservoirs and is dispersed in water aerosols. Water also acts as a vehicle for transmission of some parasites such as the cercariae of *Schistosoma* (blood flukes). The bacterium *Leptospira* is generally transmitted in water contaminated with animal urine.

A clean, uncontaminated water supply is essential for public health (see Spotlight box, page 121). In developed urban areas, government authorities are responsible for ensuring the quality of the water. However, in remote areas or in developing countries the condition of the water supply is often uncertain. If there is any question about the quality of the water, drinking water should be boiled and people should not swim in areas where pathogens are known to be found.

Food-borne transmission

Food spoilage due to microbial growth is a well-recognised problem in the home as well as in the food industry. In general, people tend not to consume food that is obviously contaminated with microorganisms. We usually discard mouldy bread, rotten fruit and food that smells 'off'. However, food can be contaminated with some microorganisms and still be palatable. The handling, storage and preparation of food provide many opportunities for microorganisms to be deposited in or on the food, and for the organisms then to multiply. In this way, food can serve as an efficient vehicle for the transmission of disease.

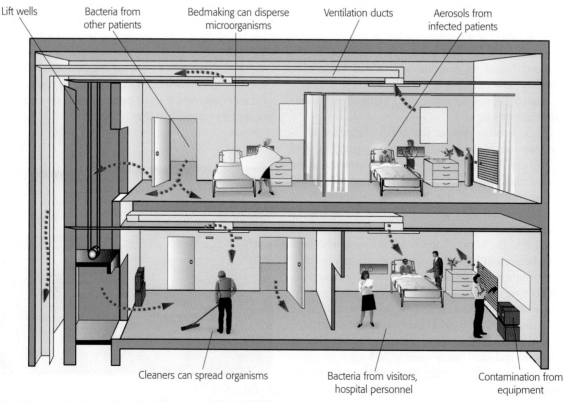

Figure 8.5

Air currents in a hospital

Some common modes of transmission of infections in a hospital setting.

Disease-producing microorganisms may be present in food at its source: for example, meat from animals infected with parasites such as tapeworms or *Toxoplasma*. Careful inspection of meat at abattoirs can usually detect helminth infections. Bacteria that cause diseases such as anthrax, brucellosis and listeriosis, as well as the rickettsia, *Coxiella burnetii* (responsible for Q fever), are also sometimes found in or on meat for human consumption. Thorough cooking destroys most pathogens, but the ingestion of raw or inadequately cooked products can cause disease.

Salmonella is commonly found on raw chicken and can be transmitted to humans if the chicken is not thoroughly cooked. It can also be transmitted by poor food-handling procedures from raw chicken to other foods such as salads. Health department regulations do not allow the handling of raw meats with the same utensils that are used for processed food that is eaten without further cooking (e.g. sliced meats). Pathogenic, toxin-producing strains of *Escherichia coli*, derived from humans or animals, may be present on raw meat or badly processed food (see Spotlight box, page 423). Endospores of *Clostridium perfringens* are ubiquitous in the environment and are not destroyed by cooking. They are often the cause of gastroenteritis characterised by stomach cramps due to the toxin produced (Case History 13.1).

In South-East Asia, raw fish is often contaminated with the larval stages of parasites such as flukes. Shellfish that are eaten raw (e.g. oysters) can transmit a variety of gastrointestinal infections.

Milk can be a major means of disease transmission. It may be contaminated with pathogenic organisms from the cow, such as *Listeria monocytogenes*, *Mycobacterium* species or *Brucella*. Adequate pasteurisation destroys most pathogens in milk.

The transmission of infectious diseases in contaminated food occurs most frequently when the organisms, mainly bacteria, are introduced into the food by poor hygiene and sanitation, or inadequate handling or storage procedures. The source of the contamination is frequently the food handlers, who may be shedding pathogens from their person or in their faeces. It is therefore essential that people involved in food preparation should wash their hands thoroughly. In institutions such as mental hospitals, day-care centres or nursing homes, outbreaks of food-borne infections such as hepatitis A can occur if the staff are not careful about personal hygiene. Once bacteria are present in food, they can multiply and reach the numbers needed for an infective dose, especially if the food is stored at room temperature or left in a warming oven. *Salmonella*, *Campylobacter* and *Shigella* are the most common bacterial causes of gastrointestinal infections.

Another common contaminant is *Staphylococcus aureus* (which usually comes from the nose or skin of a carrier). When allowed to multiply at room temperature before the food is eaten, some strains produce an enterotoxin that is heat-stable and resistant to stomach acid. The toxin does not alter the taste of the food but causes rapid, severe symptoms after ingestion.

TRANSMISSION BY VECTORS

Vectors are living agents, usually insects, that are responsible for the transmission of an infectious agent from one host to another. The major vectors are mosquitoes, fleas, ticks, lice, sandflies and other biting flies and bugs. We can distinguish between mechanical transmission and biological transmission.

Mechanical transmission

Mechanical transmission is the passive transport of microorganisms on the outside of the insect's body from a source of infection to a susceptible host, either directly or indirectly. The source may be rotten food, faeces, or a contaminated wound or dressing; the vector may be a household fly. **Direct mechanical transmission** might involve a fly alighting on the source and then going to a portal of entry such as an open sore, a wound or even eyes. **Indirect mechanical transmission** might involve an insect carrying the pathogen from the source and depositing it on food that is later consumed, or on a dressing or equipment which then comes into contact with a susceptible patient.

Biological transmission

Biological transmission occurs when an insect bites an infected host and ingests some blood or body fluid containing the pathogen. The pathogen then multiplies (or goes through a stage in its life cycle) inside the vector, resulting in an increased number of organisms being present in the vector. When the insect bites the next host, the pathogen may be present in regurgitated blood or in faeces that is deposited at the site of the bite, and is introduced into the body when the bite is scratched. In the case of malaria, the protozoa are present in the saliva of the mosquito and are injected into the bloodstream of the new host when the mosquito feeds.

Insect vectors are the means of transmission for many serious diseases including malaria, leishmaniasis and sleeping sickness, as well as the arboviral diseases, encephalitis, yellow fever, dengue fever and Ross River fever. Many of these are zoonoses (i.e. they infect animals as well as humans) and can only be transmitted from the animal reservoir to humans by a vector. Mosquitoes are the most important insect vectors. Vector-borne diseases are listed in Table 8.4.

The best method of control of vector-borne diseases is to interrupt the transmission by destroying the vectors or their habitats. Sometimes, the development of an area for farming or settlement interferes with the natural ecosystem and creates areas where the vector can breed, and so the disease may be introduced. Drainage of swamps and emptying of containers of stagnant water help to reduce mosquito breeding grounds. In Australia, the major arboviral diseases are Ross River fever, Murray Valley encephalitis, Barmah Forest fever and dengue fever (see Chapter 5, page 100 and Spotlight box Chapter 14, page 336). Control of the mosquito population and avoidance of mosquito bites are the most effective means of

Table 8.4

Some diseases transmitted by arthropod vectors

ORGANISM	DISEASE	VECTOR
Bacteria		
Yersinia pestis	*Plague	Flea
Borrelia spp.	Lyme disease	Tick
Rickettsia		
Rickettsia prowazekii	*Typhus	Louse
Rickettsia australis	Queensland tick typhus	Tick
Orientia tsutsugamushi	Scrub typhus	Mite
Protozoa		
Plasmodium spp.	*Malaria	Mosquito
Leishmania donovani	*Leishmaniasis (kala-azar)	Sandfly
Viruses		
Alphavirus	Ross River fever	Mosquito
Alphavirus	Barmah Forest fever	Mosquito
Flavivirus	Murray Valley encephalitis	Mosquito
Flavivirus	Dengue fever	Mosquito
Flavivirus	*Yellow fever	Mosquito

*Not endemic in Australia

preventing outbreaks of these diseases, for which no vaccines or antibiotics are available.

Epidemiology

Epidemiology is the study of the occurrence, spread and control of disease. An epidemiological study can be applied to all kinds of disease, including cancer, heart disease, drug addiction and mental illness, as well as infectious diseases. It involves the systematic collection and processing of information about all aspects of the disease: its **aetiology** (cause), distribution, method of transmission and various other factors that contribute to the spread of the disease or the susceptibility of the population. For infectious diseases, the causative agent is a microorganism.

Infectious diseases have always had a huge impact on the health of the population and they are still the major cause of morbidity and mortality in developing countries (see Chapter 1). Improvements in public health have come about in the last hundred years due largely to the work of doctors and scientists who investigated the natural history of various diseases, identified causes and developed methods of controlling their spread.

The science of epidemiology is generally regarded as having been founded by JOHN SNOW, an English physician who worked in London in the 1850s. He was intrigued by the fact that some of his patients contracted cholera while others did not. Although the causative agent of cholera was not known at that time, he suspected that it was being transmitted in water. His investigations showed that the inhabitants of London who received their water supply from the River Thames *downstream* from London (i.e. after the river had passed through the city and been polluted with all the sewage and wastes from the city) were much more likely to contract cholera than those who received water drawn from the Thames *before* it reached London. He concluded that the agent responsible for cholera was being excreted by people suffering from the disease into the sewage which was dumped in the river, contaminating the water used by other inhabitants.

His work was confirmed by ROBERT KOCH in Germany who was investigating an outbreak of cholera in Hamburg at about the same time. He noticed that, although there was a high incidence of cholera in Hamburg, the nearby town of Altona, which filtered the dirty river water through sand before use, was essentially free of disease. The work of these two scientists laid the basis for our modern ideas of 'common vehicle transmission' and water purification.

Snow's work illustrates the basic principles of modern epidemiology:

- careful observation
- accurate recording of quantitative data
- thorough analysis of all contributing factors (e.g. environmental exposure and susceptibility)
- development of recommendations for control based on valid data from the study.

Epidemiology refers both to the methods applied to the study of disease and to the knowledge derived from the studies. Epidemiological studies also incorporate data that may have been recorded for purposes other than treatment of the disease. Factors such as age, sex, socioeconomic group, ethnicity and nutritional state all impact on the susceptibility of the patient and the risk of infection occurring (see Chapter 7). They provide the data necessary for informed decision making about the control of disease through public health intervention strategies. Epidemiology includes:

- a description of the natural history of the disease – how the disease occurs and progresses in the human body (signs and symptoms)
- the development of methods of early diagnosis (laboratory tests) so that treatment can begin as soon as possible
- identification of risk factors in order to direct the treatment protocol or nursing management
- development of guidelines to control the incidence and spread of the disease.

It differs from clinical practice in that it focuses on the health of a group or community rather than an individual.

EPIDEMIOLOGICAL MEASUREMENTS

In today's society, people share many common sources of food and water and live or work in close proximity to each other. They also travel extensively and are exposed to a wide variety of microorganisms which they may pick up on their bodies and transport from one habitat to another, thus spreading disease. When there is an outbreak of disease, or sometimes even an isolated case, the epidemiologist is called in to determine the facts surrounding the incident.

An **outbreak of infection** is defined as the occurrence of a number of cases of the disease in excess of the number expected in a given time or place. During the investigation, the natural history of the disease is determined, the '**case definition**' is established (i.e. a description of the syndrome), questionnaires are distributed to patients to collect information about their lifestyle, risk factors, people they have been in contact with, food they have eaten and places they have visited, in order to pinpoint the source and method of transmission of the disease-causing microorganism. Food samples may be tested and patients' symptoms and clinical results collated. Statistics may be collected giving the levels of **morbidity** (serious illness) and **mortality** (death) from the disease.

As well as determining the cause and source of an infectious disease, epidemiologists also study the pattern of its occurrence.

The **incidence** of a disease is the number of *new* cases of the disease seen in a specific period of time. Incidence statistics are important in determining whether the number of new cases of the disease is increasing or decreasing; that is, whether the outbreak is being contained.

Attack rate is a measure of the cumulative incidence of a disease among a particular population at risk – for example, in an outbreak of food poisoning, the number of people who become ill out of the number exposed represents the attack rate.

Prevalence is the number of people who are infected with the disease at any one time. If a count is made of people suffering from the disease on a particular day, it would include both old and new cases. So, depending on the duration of the disease, a single case may be counted more than once. Thus, if prevalence studies are carried out once a week, but the disease lasts three weeks, then the same patient will contribute to the prevalence statistics each week (i.e. three times altogether). If only incidence statistics are collected, the patient will only be counted once. Incidence statistics reflect more accurately the occurrence and, therefore, the actual rate of transmission of the disease.

Seroprevalence is the number of people who are carrying antibodies to a particular disease at any time. The presence of antibodies in the blood gives information about a person's immune status or a present or past infection. The person is not necessarily infected or symptomatic. It can also indicate the number of people in a community who are immune to a particular disease (**herd immunity** see Chapter 14, page 320). In a disease such as AIDS, detection of antibodies to the human immunodeficiency virus (HIV) in the blood gives an indication of the prevalence of the infection in the community. People who are HIV-antibody-positive are infected, even though they may be largely asymptomatic. However, the incidence – that is, the number of new people testing positive – will indicate whether the spread of the disease is being contained.

The use of rates to measure the frequency of disease provides a scientific approach to a systematic study of the distribution of the disease and the determination of causal factors. It can give a measure of the 'burden of disease' in a particular society and its impact on public health. It is important to determine accurately which factors are associated with the occurrence and progression of the disease, so that appropriate control measures can be implemented.

IDENTIFICATION OF SOURCE AND CAUSALITY

To contain an outbreak of disease, it is essential that the causative agent be identified and its source located so that the chain of transmission can be broken. Sometimes, the source may be a single person who has entered the community and is infected with a particular disease which then spreads. This person is called the **index case**. The exact source can sometimes be determined by identifying the particular strain of the pathogen isolated from the index case and comparing it with the strains causing the disease in later cases.

Modern techniques of DNA analysis have contributed to scientists' ability to distinguish between different bacterial strains and different viral types. In Sydney in 1993, when it was alleged that transmission of the AIDS virus from patient to patient had occurred in a doctor's surgery, the claim was substantiated by viral typing, showing that all four patients had been infected with the same virus type as the original patient (i.e. the index case).

Nucleotide sequence analysis of the different DNA or

RNA samples is also used to identify the strain present in a clinical specimen. This technique was particularly useful in the identification of flying foxes as the natural reservoir of the new zoonotic viruses – Hendra virus, Menangle virus and bat lyssavirus (see Spotlight box, page 157).

Occasionally, the epidemiologist is confronted with a totally new disease, one caused by a previously unknown microorganism. The outbreak of an atypical pneumonia, severe acute respiratory syndrome (SARS), that occurred in March 2003, spread rapidly around the world and involved epidemiologists, infectious disease specialists and health professionals from many countries. The causative organism, a new coronavirus, SARS-CoV, was identified within two months and infection control guidelines developed. This rapid result was possible because of international cooperation and the availability of new technologies such as nucleic acid testing. SARS is highly infectious with most cases occurring in close contacts of the patients (family members and health-care workers). See Spotlight box, page 162. The original source of the virus is not known but is thought to be of animal origin.

Legionnaires' disease, which appeared in the United States in 1976, is another example of an epidemiological investigation which identified a previously unknown organism, *Legionella pneumophila* (see Spotlight box, page 167). In this case, it was necessary to find the reservoir for the causative agent (the cooling tower for the air conditioner), the mode of transmission (air currents) and the presence of a susceptible host (people around the hotel). Unlike SARS, Legionnaires' disease is not transmitted person to person.

When a number of factors are implicated a statistical approach to causality is needed. This involves the use of group data rather than individual data. The causal relationship may be direct or indirect, or there may be multiple factors that are not independent of each other. For example, although it was found that the *cause* of Legionnaires' disease was a new type of bacterium, the *risk* of becoming infected was dependent on the wind currents when the person was in the vicinity of the hotel cooling towers and the *severity* of the outcome was related to the state of health of the patient.

The ultimate determination of causality is reached through experimentation. The bacterium *Helicobacter pylori* was shown to be implicated as a cause of gastric ulcers when Barry Marshall swallowed a culture of the bacteria and developed the symptoms of the disease (see page 431).

CLASSIFICATION OF DISEASE

Epidemiologists classify diseases according to their incidence in our society. The incidence can be affected by seasonal variation or climatic changes. A disease is said to be **endemic** in a particular geographical region if a reservoir of the causative organisms is always present in that area and able to give rise to an outbreak of disease at any time. For example, the childhood diseases of measles, mumps and chickenpox are endemic in most parts of the world, but

may have seasonal variation. Most outbreaks of chickenpox occur in the spring. Rotavirus, which causes severe diarrhoea in infants, is usually seen in winter. Outbreaks of endemic diseases may be **sporadic**; that is, they may occur as unrelated isolated cases, anywhere in the country.

Epidemics occur when there is a sudden rapid rise in the incidence of a disease in a particular locality. This can be due to a number of factors. For example, an epidemic may occur when a new organism or strain of an organism is introduced into a population that is not immune, such as occurs with the regular outbreaks of influenza each winter. Travellers may carry organisms to areas where they were not previously found. The early settlers in Australia brought with them European diseases, such as smallpox and measles, which killed many of the Australian Aborigines who had not previously been exposed to them.

Between 1992 and 1994 there were several serious outbreaks of measles in Australia that were classed as epidemics. They occurred because, despite the availability of a vaccine, many people were not immune to measles partly because of lack of compliance with the recommended vaccination schedules (see Chapter 14 Spotlight box, page 321). Endemic diseases can become epidemics given the right conditions – for example, lack of immunity in a large proportion of the population of the community. Sometimes, epidemics are due to the emergence of a particularly virulent strain of the pathogen, such as occurs in some influenza epidemics.

A **pandemic** is a series of epidemics that occur when the disease spreads worldwide. Examples include the devastating influenza epidemic of 1918, which killed 21 million people worldwide, and the AIDS epidemic which has spread from Africa throughout the rest of the world.

SURVEILLANCE

Ongoing **surveillance** – that is, the collection and analysis of data on all aspects of the occurrence and spread of a disease – is an important aspect of epidemiology that is necessary for effective control of disease. Included in surveillance data are the laboratory results on the isolation and identification of the causative organisms, morbidity and mortality statistics, results of field investigations, and reports of adverse reactions to immunisation or exposure to chemical or biological hazards. Epidemiologists are also concerned with all the factors that determine a person's susceptibility to a particular disease. They collect information about age, sex, lifestyle, occupation and history of immunisation together with data about exposure to common vehicles (food, water) or sources of the infectious agent. These data can be analysed and used to predict the likelihood of future outbreaks of the disease.

Public health authorities are responsible for collecting and recording data on outbreaks of infectious diseases. In Australia a number of diseases are classified as *notifiable*. When a patient is diagnosed with a notifiable disease, the doctor or hospital involved is obliged to inform the appropriate health authority. In this way, it is possible to keep statistics on the incidence of disease, which assists health authorities to formulate policies to try to control the spread of infectious diseases.

Surveillance can be used to predict an outbreak of disease. Public health authorities use sentinel chicken flocks to monitor the appearance of antibodies to arboviruses such as Ross River virus, which, together with observations of mosquito populations, can give warning of potential outbreaks. This is discussed further in Chapter 14.

Epidemiology is the scientific discipline underlying much infection control work and is the science on which public health guidelines are based. Infectious diseases are one type of disease where intervention strategies of proven efficacy are available to treat and prevent the spread of those diseases. Among these strategies are immunisation programs, antibiotic therapy and prophylaxis, infection control programs in hospitals, and public health programs for infection control. The surveillance data from the community at large are used to develop health department policies and provide guidelines to prevent or contain the spread of infectious diseases.

LEVELS OF PREVENTION

Three levels of prevention are generally recognised:

- **Primary prevention** involves the maintenance of good health by good nutrition, the elimination of infection risks by good hygiene, and the provision of protection by vaccination.
- **Secondary prevention** refers to strategies such as the development of tests for early detection of infection, and screening programs.
- **Tertiary prevention** involves actions to prevent further complications of the disease or deterioration in health, such as secondary infections or transmission in health-care facilities. This is especially relevant to good nursing care.

EVIDENCE-BASED PRACTICE

This brief overview of epidemiology is included to provide students with some understanding of an important discipline that has applications in many areas of health. A knowledge of the principles of epidemiological investigation is of use in the critical evaluation of research papers and in the development of research projects to assist clinical practice.

There is an increasing trend towards '**evidence-based practice**' in all health-related areas. In other words, it is widely accepted that the development of new procedures or changes in protocols should be based on valid research that has evaluated the improvement to be gained in terms of clinical outcome, patient well-being, cost benefit and community health. Such research should embrace the principles of epidemiology and quantitative assessment of outcome. Anecdotal or qualitative description based on individual cases is not sufficient grounds for change in practice. Frequently, a study is inconclusive because the data collection is flawed or incomplete. An understanding of epidemiology and the use of quantitative methods will allow valid conclusions to be reached.

Retrospective studies can identify the source of an outbreak and the practices that contributed to transmission.

Prospective studies are used to evaluate the effect of a change in practice on infection rates.

Experienced clinicians often recognise deviations from normal occurrences – for example, an outbreak of infection or an increase in wound infection rates. A surveillance project, with data collected and analysed over a defined time period, allows them to determine whether it is a real or perceived variation, to investigate the cause and implement appropriate change.

When evaluating research findings, it is important to be able to detect bias in a study. Bias may occur in the selection of the sample group to be monitored, by not correctly identifying all confounders (i.e. factors that influence the outcome, such as underlying illnesses) or by selective collection of data. Determining risk factors requires prior knowledge of all the determinants of a particular disease. The move towards evidence-based practice in health care relies on epidemiological studies that involve good surveillance and quantitative data collection and analysis, to ensure that optimum care is given to patients. Good surveillance is therefore an essential part of clinical research.

- Communicable diseases are easily spread from one host to another.
- Non-communicable diseases are not usually spread during the normal course of activities. They may be opportunistic, require a vector or be caused by a toxin.

RESERVOIRS OF INFECTION

- For a disease to persist in a community, there has to be a permanent reservoir of the infectious agent. It may be human, animal or non-living.
- The source of an infection is the individual or object from which the infection is acquired.
- Human reservoirs include patients who have an acute, latent or chronic infectious disease.
- Normal flora of the body also act as a reservoir of infection.
- Diseases that occur in both animals and humans are called zoonoses.
- Transmission of the infectious agent from animal to human may be by direct contact with fur, feathers or body secretions, by the ingestion of cysts, or via the bite of an insect vector.
- Soil and water are major reservoirs of infectious agents.

PORTALS OF ENTRY

- Endogenous infections are caused by flora that are already present on the human body.
- Exogenous pathogens are microorganisms derived from a source outside the human body; they enter via a characteristic portal of entry.
- Many pathogens have a preferred portal of entry. It may be the skin, respiratory tract, GI tract or genitourinary system.
- Intact skin is a major barrier to the entry of pathogenic microorganisms.
- Puncture wounds, injuries, insect bites and the use of hypodermic syringes break the skin and facilitate the entry of microorganisms.
- Hospital-acquired infections may occur in surgical patients or patients subjected to procedures such as the use of central lines, IV lines and catheters.
- Microorganisms gain entry to the respiratory tract by adhering to the mucosal cells.
- The use of respiratory equipment creates conditions where microorganisms can be introduced directly into the respiratory tract.
- A major portal of entry for pathogens is the ingestion of contaminated food or drink.
- Urinary tract infections are very common in catheterised patients in hospital.
- The genital tract is the portal of entry of sexually transmitted diseases.

- Some microorganisms cross the placenta and infect the foetus *in utero*.
- The neonate is susceptible to infections acquired during passage through the birth canal.

PORTALS OF EXIT

- Microorganisms are continuously shed from the body.
- Health workers need to be aware of the ways in which pathogens are shed.
- Organisms such as viruses are expelled as fine aerosols by coughing and sneezing.
- Faeces contain normal flora as well as pathogens that may contaminate food and water.
- Microorganisms are shed on dead skin scales, as particles from dried crusts on wounds, and from skin lesions.
- Organisms responsible for sexually transmitted diseases are present in semen and vaginal secretions.
- Urine contains bacteria from urinary tract infections, as well as pathogens such as cytomegalovirus and *Leptospira*.
- Blood-borne pathogens such as HIV, and hepatitis B and C, are present in blood and body fluids.

TRANSMISSION OF MICROORGANISMS

- Transmission of microorganisms occurs horizontally from person to person or vertically from mother to baby.
- Transmission may be by direct or indirect contact, via a common vehicle such as air, water or food, or by insect vectors.

EPIDEMIOLOGY

- Epidemiology is the study of the occurrence, spread and control of disease.
- There is an outbreak of infection when the number of cases that occur is in excess of that expected in a given time or place.
- The index case is the person who is the primary source of the infection.
- The incidence of a disease is the number of new cases of the disease seen in a specific period of time.
- Prevalence is the number of people infected at any one time.
- Seroprevalence is the number of people carrying antibodies to a particular disease at any time.
- A disease is endemic if there is a constant reservoir of causative organisms in the area.
- Epidemics occur when there is a sudden rapid rise in the incidence of disease in a particular locality.
- A pandemic is a worldwide epidemic.
- Surveillance data are used to develop public health guidelines and infection control policies.

1. What is meant by a reservoir of infection?
2. Give examples of some of the major reservoirs of infection for human pathogens.
3. What is the difference between the source of an infection and the reservoir of infection?
4. Give some examples of fomites found in the hospital environment.
5. What is a zoonosis? Give examples.
6. Describe three diseases caused by members of the genus *Clostridium*.
7. What are the major non-living reservoirs for microorganisms?
8. What is the difference between endogenous and exogenous infections?
9. What is meant by a cutaneous infection? Give two examples.
10. Which diseases flourish in deep puncture wounds?
11. Which hospital procedures are likely to allow pathogens to enter the body via breaks in the skin?
12. Describe how microorganisms gain entry to the body via the respiratory tract.
13. What is pneumonia?
14. What are the risks to patients associated with the use of mechanical ventilation?
15. What is cystitis?
16. What are the major organisms that can cross the placenta?
17. How are pathogens shed from the human body?
18. Which diseases are likely to be transmitted in blood or blood products?
19. What is meant by vertical transmission?
20. What is the difference between direct contact and indirect contact?
21. What is meant by common vehicle transmission?
22. How can the spread of airborne microorganisms be controlled in the hospital?
23. Why is it important to use different utensils for handling raw and cooked food?
24. Why should milk be pasteurised?
25. Which insects can act as vectors for infectious disease?
26. What is the best method of controlling vector-borne diseases such as malaria?
27. What is the difference between the rates of morbidity and mortality?
28. What is meant by the index case?
29. What is meant by seroprevalence?
30. What is the difference between an epidemic and a pandemic?

TEST YOUR UNDERSTANDING

1. Why can a person who is suffering from a subclinical infection, or who is a chronic carrier, transmit the disease to another person?
2. Under what circumstances can the normal flora of the body cause an infection?
3. What is meant by the 'preferred portal of entry'?
4. Why is an intact skin so important?
5. How do microorganisms evade the hostile pH in the stomach in order to gain entry via the gastrointestinal route?
6. Why do patients with urinary catheters suffer from urinary tract infections?
7. What is meant by faecal-oral transmission?
8. How does epidemiology benefit the community?
9. What is the difference between incidence and prevalence statistics?
10. What is the value of carrying out surveillance programs?

Further reading

Halpin K, Young PL, Field H, Mackenzie JS 1999, Newly discovered viruses of flying foxes. *Veterinary Microbiology*; 68: 83–87.

Peiris JSM, YK Yuen, ADME Osterhaus & K Stohr 2003, Current Concepts: The Severe Acute Respiratory Syndrome. *New England Journal of Medicine*; 349(25): 2431–2441.

SARS reports in *Emerging Infectious Diseases* 10 (2): February 2004. www.cdc.gov/eid

Valanis B 1999, *Epidemiology in Health Care*, Connecticut, Appleton Lange.

Wang J-T & S-C Chang 2004, Severe acute respiratory syndrome. *Current Opinion in Infectious Diseases*; 17(2): 143–148.

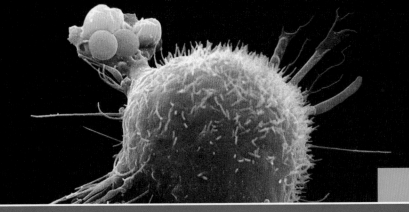

CHAPTER 9

The Body's Defence Systems

[CHAPTER FOCUS]

■ *What are the non-specific defences of the body?*

■ *How do the skin and mucous membranes protect the body against infection?*

■ *What cells act non-specifically to protect the body against foreign particles and microorganisms?*

■ *What is inflammation and what is its role in defence?*

■ *What are the characteristics of the acquired immune system?*

■ *What cells and tissues comprise the acquired immune system?*

■ *What is humoral immunity and what are the functions of antibodies?*

■ *What is cell-mediated immunity?*

■ *What are the principles of immunisation?*

■ *What disorders are associated with the failure or improper function of the immune system?*

Introduction

In Chapters 7 and 8 we looked at the relationship between microorganisms and the human host. Whether or not a person becomes infected by a certain microorganism depends on the balance between the attributes of the microbe that enable it to cause disease and the ability of the body to resist them. In this chapter we examine the ways in which the human body protects itself from infection. In Chapter 10 we look at some of the mechanisms that microorganisms possess that enable them to overcome or evade the body's defences and cause disease. The ability of the body to prevent infection occurring is called **resistance**, while a lack of resistance, or vulnerability to an infection, is called **susceptibility**.

Given the multitude of microorganisms present in our environment and on our bodies, it is rather miraculous that we are not continually suffering from some kind of infection. We owe this to a highly complex and efficient system of defences. Because we are exposed to a wide range of microbes that possess different characteristics and mechanisms for causing disease, the body needs a battery of different types of defences. The body's resistance to infection depends on two major groups of defences:

1. **Non-specific defences** act as the body's first line of defence and offer general protection against all potentially harmful agents, including pathogens (infectious agents) and foreign substances. These defences do not discriminate one agent from another, and act in a similar way each time the same agent enters (or attempts to enter) the body.
2. **Specific defences** are the body's second line of defence. They help to eliminate the pathogens that succeed in circumventing the non-specific defences and also protect the host against future attack by the same pathogen. These defences rely on the detection of the structural and chemical features of pathogens that mark them as distinct from the body's own cells.

Although the specific and non-specific defences are usually considered separately, it is important to recognise that they overlap and interact substantially with each other to protect the body. Some non-specific components aid in the production of specific responses, and many of the specific defence mechanisms direct or enhance the action of non-specific defences, especially the body's phagocytic cells (see pages 180–81). The specific defences, and some of the non-specific defences, comprise the body's **immune system**, the protective system that eliminates foreign microorganisms and substances and provides the body with long-term immunity to them.

Non-specific defences

The function of the non-specific defences (also called **non-specific immunity**, **innate immunity**, **natural immunity**) is to prevent the entry of pathogens and other foreign materials into the tissues of the body, or to destroy them quickly if they do manage to enter. These defences include the skin and mucous membrane barriers (and their secretions), certain cells, inflammation, various antimicrobial proteins and fever.

SKIN AND MUCOUS MEMBRANE BARRIERS

The body's first line of defence against invasion by microorganisms is the skin and the mucous membranes. These are very resilient physical barriers which protect against the entry of potentially pathogenic microorganisms and other foreign particles. The skin comprises two distinct layers, the epidermis and the dermis (see Figure 9.1). The epidermis is the outer layer and consists of multiple layers of tightly packed epithelial cells. The outermost of these cells contain the strong protein, **keratin**. Keratin is not affected by weak acids and bases and is resistant to bacterial enzymes and toxins. As long as the epidermis is unbroken, this tough layer represents a formidable barrier to most microorganisms. However, if the epidermis is damaged (e.g. in wounds) the skin and underlying tissues become much more susceptible to infection.

In the dermis there are sebaceous glands that secrete sebum, an oily substance containing fatty acids that lowers the pH of the skin and inhibits the growth of certain bacteria and fungi. There are also sweat glands. The high salt concentration in sweat inhibits many microorganisms, although the normal flora that live on the skin's secretions (e.g. some staphylococci) are tolerant to salt and low pH.

Intact mucous membranes provide physical barriers within the body. Mucosal membranes line all the body cavities that are open to the environment; that is, the digestive, respiratory, urinary and reproductive tracts, and the inner surface of the eyelids and outer surface of the eye. Mucous membranes comprise two distinct structures: a thin layer of tightly packed cells (sometimes only one cell thick) called the *epithelium*, and an underlying layer of tissue that provides support and nutrients for the epithelium. Although these surfaces suffer considerable wear and tear, the damaged cells are rapidly replaced and the integrity of the membrane quickly restored. Also, a film of sticky mucous secretion traps foreign particles and microorganisms that might enter the body via these routes. The mucus helps to prevent microbes from attaching to the epithelial surface and entering the tissues. Inside the nose there is a meshwork of tiny hairs that, together with mucus, traps inhaled particles. There are mechanisms (described below) which then move the mucus and entrapped particles out of the body.

The mucosal membranes are the sites of secretion or formation of a large variety of substances that contribute to defence. For example:

- **Lysozyme**. This enzyme breaks down the cell wall of many bacteria. It is found in saliva, sweat, tears, and nasal and vaginal secretions.
- **Acids**. The hydrochloric acid secreted in the stomach (pH 2) kills most microorganisms, and is a highly

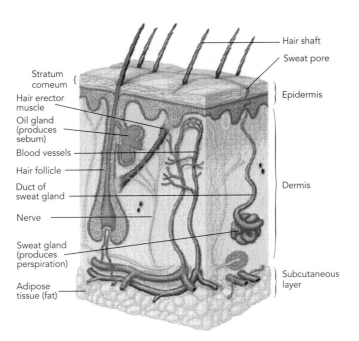

Figure 9.1

A section through skin
The top layers of the cells contain the tough protein called keratin.

effective protection against the enormous numbers of microbes that enter the body in food and beverages. The pH of the vagina in adult females is acidic (pH 4) which inhibits the growth of some harmful microbes.

- **Digestive enzymes and bile salts**. These substances, which are secreted into the gastrointestinal tract for digestion, also kill microorganisms and inactivate viruses.
- **Lactoferrin**. This substance inhibits the growth of some microorganisms by binding free iron, a necessary growth factor for them. It also impairs the motility and ability to form biofilms of some bacteria. It is found in a number of secretions, including saliva, milk and seminal fluid.
- **Spermine**. This is an antibacterial substance found in semen.
- **Defensins**. α- and β-defensins are small peptides that have killing activity against a broad range of microorganisms.

The movement of fluids over mucosal surfaces is a highly effective mechanism of the upper respiratory tract that eliminates many potential pathogens from the body. A vital non-specific defence mechanism is the ciliated epithelium (see Figure 9.2). The cilia move mucus and anything trapped in it upwards towards the throat, either to be expelled or swallowed, thus preventing it from entering the lower respiratory passages. This **mucociliary escalator** is enhanced by two other forms of movement: coughing and sneezing.

The movement of fluids over mucosal surfaces can also have a washing effect, helping to eliminate foreign particles (including microbes) from the body. Thus, tears wash particles from the eyes and the flow of urine in the urinary tract flushes the urethra. In fact, normal urine flow is one of the most important defences in the urinary tract, and people

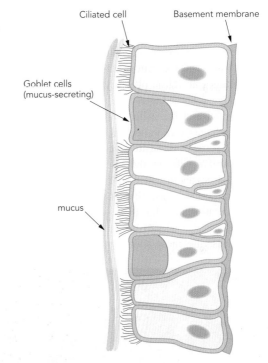

Figure 9.2

The mucociliary escalator
The cilia of the upper respiratory tract sweep mucus and any foreign material caught in it upwards away from the lungs.

with urinary obstruction often suffer urinary tract infection.

The skin and mucous membranes are highly effective barriers. However, sometimes microorganisms are able to break through these barriers, either because their integrity is disrupted by cuts, wounds or abrasions, or because the particular microbes possess special properties that enable them to bypass or penetrate these barriers. The thin epithelium of the mucous membranes is not as effective a barrier as the multiple layers of dead cells in skin, so microbes more often invade through mucous membranes than through skin. When microorganisms breach these barriers they are able to gain entry to the tissues. Fortunately, other non-specific mechanisms then come into play (described in the following sections).

However, the vital contribution that these barriers play should not be underestimated. This is clearly demonstrated in situations where some of these defences are disrupted or lost. For example, burns patients are highly susceptible to infection and this is one of the more common causes of death in badly burned patients.

NON-SPECIFIC CELLULAR DEFENCES

When microorganisms or foreign substances penetrate the skin or mucous membranes and enter the tissues, the body has certain cellular defences for protection. The most important of these are phagocytes and natural killer cells. The vital role played by phagocytes is reflected in the serious infections suffered by people with a deficiency in these cells.

Phagocytes

Phagocytes are body cells that actively ingest and digest foreign particles (see Figure 9.3). They also break down dead tissue cells and remove cellular debris from the tissues. The two major types of phagocytes in the body are the macrophages and the neutrophils.

Macrophages are large phagocytic cells derived from blood monocytes. Some travel around the body looking for foreign material and are called wandering macrophages. Other macrophages stay in specific tissues and organs of the body, and some of these are given different names – for example, Kupffer cells in the liver, microglia in nerve tissue and histiocytes in connective tissue (see Table 9.1). At sites of infection, extra blood monocytes can migrate from the circulation into the tissue where they mature into macrophages.

Neutrophils, the most abundant type of white blood

Table 9.1	
The monocyte/macrophage system of the human body	
ANATOMICAL SITE	CELLS
alveoli	macrophages
spleen	macrophages
blood	monocytes
lymph nodes	macrophages
brain	microglia
liver	Kupffer cells
connective tissue	histiocytes
bones	osteoclasts

cell, are highly phagocytic and actively motile cells. Neutrophils are also referred to as **polymorphonuclear leukocytes** (**PMNs**), **polymorphs** or **pus cells**. Neutrophils phagocytose foreign material in the bloodstream, but also migrate from the bloodstream into tissues in the early stages of infection and inflammation.

The process of phagocytosis involves four major phases (see Figure 9.4):

1. chemotaxis
2. attachment
3. ingestion
4. digestion.

Phagocytes are attracted to sites of damaged tissue or microbial invasion by chemicals released at the site. This attraction is called **chemotaxis**. A variety of chemical substances act as attractants, including substances released from damaged tissues and some components of microorganisms. These chemical attractants cause the phagocytes to move along an increasing concentration gradient of the attractant towards its source – the site of infection or tissue damage.

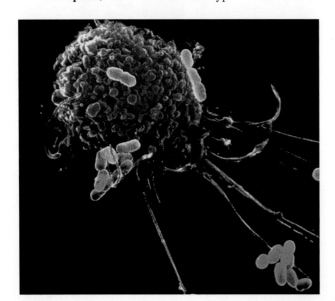

Figure 9.3

A scanning electron micrograph showing a macrophage engulfing bacteria

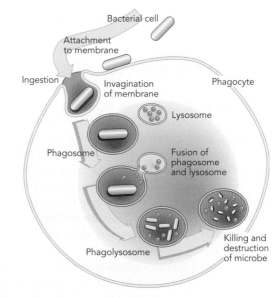

Figure 9.4

The mechanisms of phagocytosis
Phagocytosis of a bacterial cell, showing the major steps of attachment, ingestion and killing/destruction of the microbe.

The phagocyte must first be able to attach to the foreign particle or microorganism in order to ingest it. Attachment occurs via non-specific receptor sites on the surface of the phagocyte. There is a variety of such receptors on phagocytes, including an important group referred to as **Toll-like receptors** (TLRs). TLRs are found particularly on macrophages and dendritic cells, but also on other cell types including neutrophils, eosinophils and epithelial cells. TLRs recognise **pathogen associated molecular patterns** (PAMPs), which are types of molecules found on microorganisms but not on host cells. PAMPs include lipopolysaccharide, peptidoglycan and double-stranded RNA. Thus they allow phagocytes and some other cells to recognise microorganisms in a general way.

Some microorganisms have structures, such as polysaccharide capsules, that enable them to avoid being bound to the phagocyte surface (see Chapter 10). Host factors, particularly complement and antibodies (discussed later in this chapter), enhance the adherence of microorganisms to phagocytes, a process called *opsonisation*.

Phagocytes ingest microorganisms and foreign material by a process called **endocytosis**. The cytoplasm invaginates at the point where the particle is attached and then closes around it. Having been taken up, the particle is contained in a membrane-bound vacuole called a **phagosome** within the cytoplasm of the phagocyte.

Digestion of the foreign material is brought about by fusion of the phagosome with lysosomes, to form a **phagolysosome**. Inside the phagolysosome, the foreign material or microbe is exposed to a variety of digestive enzymes (e.g. proteases, lipases) which can break down the foreign material, as well as to a wide range of toxic substances such as hydrogen peroxide, nitric oxide, hydroxyl radicals, acids and defensins (small antimicrobial peptides). Some microbes, such as the bacteria that cause tuberculosis and Legionnaires' disease – which appear to be resistant to intracellular digestion – are thought to prevent the fusion of lysosomes with the phagosome. Other organisms, like the *Rickettsiae*, appear to avoid destruction by escaping from the phagosome before it merges with the lysosome. Since lysosomal enzymes are not released into the cytoplasm, the bacteria are not digested.

The importance of phagocytosis as a defence mechanism is clearly reflected by the number of microorganisms that have developed means of escaping the process. This is discussed more fully in Chapter 10.

Apart from their phagocytic activity macrophages also have an important regulatory role. Through the release of certain cytokines (see later in this chapter) they actively recruit other cells, particularly neutrophils, by attracting them to sites of infection.

A distinct group of cells called **dendritic cells** also has a type of phagocytic function. Dendritic cells are derived from the bone marrow and reside in skin and lymphoid tissues. The best known of them are the *Langerhans cells* in the skin. Dendritic cells and macrophages play a critical role in presenting antigen to T lymphocytes and hence in the initiation of specific immune responses. They are discussed in more detail later in this chapter (see 'Acquired Immune System').

Natural killer cells

Natural killer (NK) cells are a unique group of cells that are capable of destroying tumour cells and virus-infected cells. They are part of a distinct group of lymphoid cells called *large granular lymphocytes*. NK cells have a complex system of receptors that allows them to recognise changes on the surface of abnormal cells. The name 'natural killer' reflects the fact that they do not recognise specific cells or foreign substances, but are able to attack a variety of such targets. NK cells bring about killing of the target cell by the insertion of protein molecules, called **perforins**, into the cell membrane, creating a pore through which toxic substances can be injected into the cell.

NK cells can be stimulated by factors (called **cytokines**) released in specific immunity, and they then show greater killing activity (see 'Cell-mediated Immunity', page 201). They also release cytokines (e.g. interferon-γ) which activate macrophages. NK cells also have receptors for antibody (see 'Humoral Immunity', page 194) and so can also kill antibody-coated target cells.

INFLAMMATION

The **acute inflammatory response** is a non-specific defence that is the body's response to tissue injury. It occurs in response to any injury, including physical damage (e.g. cuts and abrasions), burns, radiation (e.g. sunburn) and chemical injury (e.g. acids), as well as to infection by microorganisms. Although the physiologic events are similar each time, the inflammatory response produced is usually appropriate to the cause and extent of the injury. Inflammatory conditions are named by adding the suffix *-itis* to the affected organ or tissue (e.g. conjunctivitis for inflammation of the conjunctiva of the eye, appendicitis for inflammation of the appendix).

The major function of inflammation is to clear the injured site of cellular debris and any foreign material or pathogens (if present), thereby preparing the area for repair processes. In the case of infection, it can also serve to localise the microorganisms, preventing their spread to adjacent areas. When effective, the inflammatory response eliminates any pathogen or foreign material, removes injured tissue components and enables tissue repair processes to occur.

The four main signs of acute inflammation are:

- redness
- heat
- swelling
- pain.

The major events of the inflammatory process are described below and summarised in Figure 9.5.

Vasodilation and increased vascular permeability

Once an injury has occurred, several events take place, leading to the activation or release of a variety of

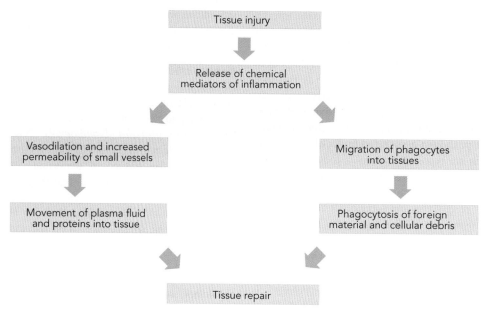

Figure 9.5

A summary of the events in acute inflammation

chemicals. These chemicals are responsible for the physiological events that occur in inflammation and are called the chemical mediators of inflammation. Derived from a variety of sources, the most important are histamine, kinins, prostaglandins, leukotrienes, tumour necrosis factor and complement. The sources and activities of inflammatory mediators are summarised in Figure 9.6. Many of these mediators cause dilation of the arterioles in the area of damage. This causes more blood to flow into the area, accounting for the redness and warmth of inflamed tissue.

Some mediators increase the permeability of local capillaries and post-capillary venules by causing retraction of the endothelial cells of these vessels. As a result, plasma fluid and proteins, such as clotting factors, complement and antibodies, are able to move from the bloodstream into the tissue spaces. This fluid is called an **exudate**. An accumulation of exudate in tissue causes **oedema**, or swelling. The pain that is usually associated with inflammation is due to compression of adjacent nerve endings by this swelling, as well as to the direct effects of some inflammatory mediators on pain receptors. Depending on the site of injury, swelling and pain may cause temporary loss of function of a body part (e.g. in a joint), and this is sometimes regarded as the fifth sign of acute inflammation.

The different chemical mediators of inflammation come from a variety of sources. **Histamine** is present in many different body cell types, especially in mast cells in connective tissue, and in basophils and platelets in the bloodstream. It is released when these cells are injured or stimulated, and it has a potent action on small blood vessels (arterioles and capillaries) causing them to dilate (see Figure 9.7) and increase their permeability to plasma fluid and proteins. **Antihistamines** are used to alleviate the redness and swelling prominent in such clinical conditions as hay fever and hives.

Kinins (bradykinin is the best known one) are small peptides present in blood and other body fluids in an inactive form (kallikrein). The kinin system is activated by tissue injury. Kinins cause vasodilation and increased vascular permeability as well as inducing pain.

Prostaglandins and **leukotrienes** are vasoactive mediators synthesised from a long-chain fatty acid called *arachidonic acid*, which is released from mast cell membranes. They cause dilation of post-capillary venules, increased vascular permeability and neutrophil chemotaxis. Prostaglandins also induce pain. Several of the leukotrienes cause sustained constriction of bronchioles, as occurs in asthma.

The importance of prostaglandins and leukotrienes as inflammatory agents is reflected in the action of some commonly used anti-inflammatory drugs. Aspirin, indomethacin and certain other non-steroidal anti-inflammatory agents act by blocking the synthesis of prostaglandins, as shown in Figure 9.8. Their analgesic (pain-reducing) effect is also due to inhibition of prostaglandin synthesis. Steroidal anti-inflammatory drugs are very potent partly because they block both prostaglandin and leukotriene synthesis.

The complement system amplifies many of the processes in acute inflammation. The activation and actions of this system of proteins are discussed on pages 186–87. Cytokines (see page 187), such as interleukin-1, interleukin-2 and tumour necrosis factor, also play an important role in acute inflammation. These are released by activated macrophages.

The purpose of local vasodilation and increased vascular permeability is to provide the injured site with a variety of blood-borne substances that assist in tissue repair. The plasma fluid that enters injured tissue contains oxygen and nutrients necessary for the repair process, as well as important proteins like antibodies, complement and clotting proteins. In some infections, the clotting proteins

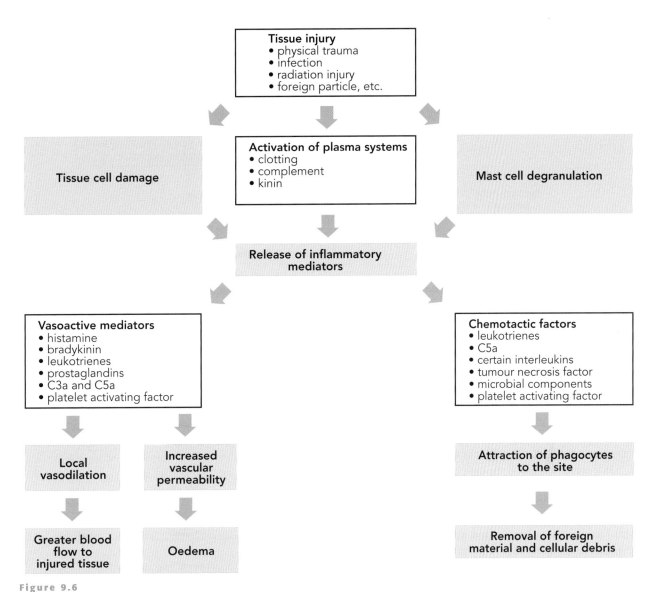

Figure 9.6

The sources and activities of the chemical mediators of acute inflammation

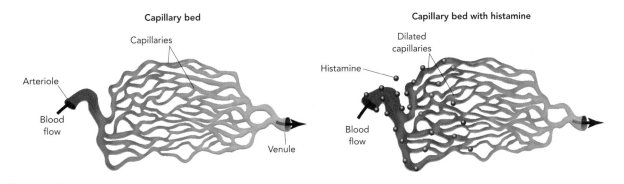

Figure 9.7

The dilating effect of histamine on arterioles and capillaries

form a fibrin barrier around the site to isolate the injured area and prevent the spread of bacteria or other harmful agents into surrounding tissues. As described later in this chapter, the antibodies and complement in plasma fluid are substances that help to eliminate foreign organisms.

Although inflammation is an important defence mecha-nism, there are situations where it can actually harm the body. For example, the swelling and pain associated with a disorder such as rheumatoid arthritis cause severe dis-comfort because an excessive degree of inflammation occurs. The role of inflammation in the production of disease is discussed later in this chapter.

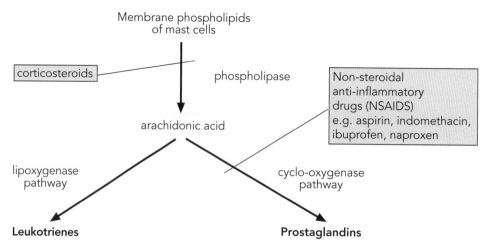

Figure 9.8

The synthesis of prostaglandins and leukotrienes and the actions of some anti-inflammatory drugs

Phagocyte migration

During inflammation there is an influx of phagocytic cells into the injured tissue. First, the neutrophils arrive and, later, the macrophages. Activated mediators from plasma and injured cells stimulate the release of extra neutrophils from the bone marrow into the blood and then their attraction to the site of injury. In severe infections, the number of neutrophils in the blood may increase four or five times within several hours. A significant increase in the number of white cells in blood is called **leukocytosis**; when neutrophils predominate it is called **neutrophilia**. Neutrophilia is a characteristic sign of severe bacterial infection.

Some of the inflammatory mediators, such as complement factors, prostaglandins and kinins, act as chemotactic agents for phagocytes, attracting them to the site of the injury. During inflammation, the blood flow in the region of the injury slows and neutrophils begin to stick to the inner walls of the capillaries. This phenomenon is known as **margination** (see Figure 9.9). Neutrophils stick to the endothelial cells of the capillaries because the endothelial cells exhibit specific adhesion molecules in response to inflammatory mediators. The neutrophils then squeeze between the endothelial cells of the capillary walls (a process called **diapedesis**) and move into the tissue spaces, where they can devour dead or damaged tissue cells and any foreign particles or microbes that are present.

Late in the inflammatory response, monocytes from the bloodstream enter the area, replacing the neutrophils, which leave or die *in situ*. **Monocytes** are only weakly phagocytic, but after entering the tissues they swell and develop large numbers of lysosomes to become mature, highly active macrophages. Macrophages are responsible for the final clearing of cell debris and foreign matter from the injured area so that the tissue can be repaired.

In sites of bacterial infection, pus may accumulate in the wound. **Pus** is a thick, creamy-coloured fluid comprising a mixture of dead and dying neutrophils, tissue debris and remaining pathogens. Neutrophils are the major component of pus because many die *in situ*, having expended themselves in voracious phagocytic activity. Pus

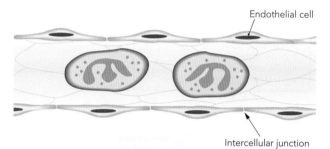

Phagocytes in blood vessels

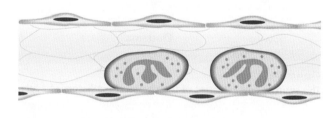

Margination (adherence of phagocytes to endothelial cells)

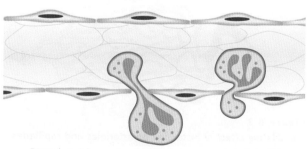

Diapedesis (phagocytes squeeze between endothelial cells) and phagocytes enter tissues

Figure 9.9

Margination and diapedesis of phagocytes

During inflammation, phagocytes stick to the insides of capillaries (margination) at the site of injury and then enter the tissue spaces by passing between the endothelial cells (diapedesis).

formation is typically induced by bacteria, but not by viruses. This can sometimes be helpful in distinguishing between bacterial and viral infections.

Certain bacteria (e.g. staphylococci, gonococci) are particularly strong attracters of neutrophils and are termed **pyogenic**, or pus-forming, bacteria. When the sac of pus is walled off by a layer of fibrin, an **abscess** is formed. This represents the body's attempt to localise the infection and the potentially damaging neutrophil enzymes and other toxic substances that are released from these cells as they die. The pus remains locked up in the abscess. Thus, physical drainage of abscesses is often necessary before healing can occur.

Repair

During the final stages of inflammation, tissue repair begins, but can only be completed if all microbes, other foreign material and damaged tissue cells have been effectively removed from the area. The most favourable outcome is the restoration of the tissue's original structure and physiologic function by **regeneration**, the proliferation of remaining cells by mitosis. This occurs if the destroyed tissue is capable of regeneration, if the damage is minor or if there are no other complications. If the tissue is incapable of regeneration (e.g. nerve tissue) or is extensively damaged or if the clean-up is incomplete (e.g. in abscess formation), the tissue is repaired by **scar tissue replacement**. Scar tissue is comprised mainly of collagen. It fills in the lesion but it does not have the physiological functions of the destroyed tissue.

Chronic inflammation

Chronic inflammation occurs if the acute inflammatory response is unsuccessful in eliminating the organisms or foreign material from the tissues. For example, if foreign objects (e.g. glass, dirt) and/or bacteria persist in a wound, the inflammatory response may continue beyond two weeks. In chronic inflammation, pus may be formed continuously, sometimes for months or even years. Large numbers of lymphocytes and macrophages are involved in chronic inflammation, in contrast to acute responses in which neutrophils predominate.

Chronic inflammation can also occur as a distinct process from the outset, in the absence of acute inflammation. Certain microbes, such as the bacteria that cause tuberculosis and leprosy, induce chronic inflammation because of their resistance to intracellular digestion by phagocytes. The persistence of these organisms continues to stimulate an inflammatory response. Other agents that typically evoke chronic inflammation are low-grade, persistent irritants such as talc, silica and asbestos. These substances persist in tissues but do not penetrate or spread.

A **granuloma** is a special kind of chronic inflammation produced in response to certain microorganisms, such as the bacteria that cause leprosy, tuberculosis and syphilis. Granulomas are formed in these infections because the macrophages are unable to eliminate the organisms. Granulomas typically consist of a mass of different types of cells arranged in fairly discrete layers, completely walled off (encapsulated) by fibrous deposits of collagen. At the centre of the granuloma are macrophages or 'epithelioid cells' (modified macrophages) clumped in a mass, or coalesced together to form multi-nucleated cells. Around these giant cells is a layer of epithelioid cells and then a layer of lymphocytes. This mass of cells represents the body's attempt to surround and isolate the foreign agent. Granulomas are sometimes given special names, such as 'gummas' in syphilis and 'tubercles' in tuberculosis.

In the past, surgical gloves were dusted with talc powder so that they would slip on easily, but it was found that particles of talc often entered the surgical field and caused granulomas to develop there after surgery. Gloves are now dusted with an absorbent starch to avoid this problem.

Fever

Inflammation is the local response to tissue damage. **Fever**, higher-than-normal body temperature, is a systemic response to infection and often accompanies severe or systemic inflammation. Body temperature is regulated by a cluster of neurons in the hypothalamus, considered to be the body's thermostat. Normally, the thermostat is set at approximately 37°C. Fever occurs when the set-point of the thermostat is raised to a higher temperature.

Pyrogens are chemical substances that produce fever. They are referred to as **exogenous pyrogens** if they come from outside the body, and **endogenous pyrogens** if they are formed inside the body. Exogenous pyrogens are, in the main, components of microorganisms, the best characterised being the lipopolysaccharide (endotoxin – see Chapter 10) of the cell wall of Gram-negative bacteria. Endogenous pyrogens are released from macrophages and neutrophils during inflammation or in response to the presence of exogenous pyrogens. The best known endogenous pyrogens are interleukin-1 (IL-1) and tumour necrosis factor (TNF). These are the substances that actually alter the set-point in the hypothalamus, whereas exogenous pyrogens act indirectly by causing their release. This is summarised in Figure 9.10.

The clinical approach to the management of fever has changed in recent years. In the past, **antipyretic** (fever-reducing) drugs and physical measures (e.g. tepid baths) were routinely used to reduce fever. Now, there are many who advocate allowing a slight to moderate fever to run its course. Although high fevers (above 40°C) are dangerous because of the possibility of thermal damage to nerve cells and convulsions, mild or moderate fever may have some benefit for the body. The rate of cell division of bacteria is slowed at temperatures above 37°C. Also, bacteria require iron and zinc for growth, but during fever the liver and spleen sequester these nutrients, making them less available. A small increase in body temperature may also increase the metabolic rate and activity of defence cells, such as T lymphocytes and phagocytes, and is also thought to speed up repair processes.

It is accepted, however, that high fever, or fever in patients with cardiovascular disease, seizures or respiratory

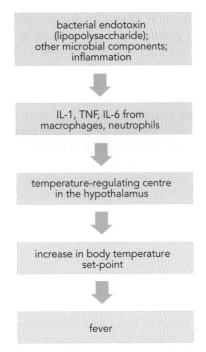

Figure 9.10

The production of fever

disorders, should be treated immediately. Antipyretic drugs such as aspirin appear to reduce fever by restoring the temperature set-point in the hypothalamus to normal.

ANTIMICROBIAL PROTEINS

Apart from the various protective chemicals mentioned earlier in this chapter, the body also has certain anti-microbial proteins that act non-specifically. The most important of these are the complement proteins, interferon and acute phase proteins.

Complement

The complement system, or simply **complement**, comprises a complex system of plasma proteins that are present in the blood in an inactive state. The major components of the system are designated as factors C1 through to C9 (C stands for complement), and factors B, D and properdin. It is an enzymatic cascade system, similar to the blood coagulation system. When it is activated, the complement system enhances the inflammatory response and is largely responsible for the destruction of foreign cells in the body. Its major functions are to:

- enhance phagocytosis
- produce inflammation
- directly lyse foreign cells.

Complement enhances the action of many non-specific and specific defences, and is in turn enhanced by some specific defences. Hence it is a major interface between the non-specific and specific defence systems.

Complement can be activated by one of three pathways (outlined in Figure 9.11). The **classical pathway** is initiated by the binding of antibodies to antigen. Complement proteins are activated and bound to a receptor on antibody molecules in a step called **complement fixation**. The **alternate (properdin) pathway** is initiated by an interaction between the plasma proteins, properdin and factors B and D, with the polysaccharides that are

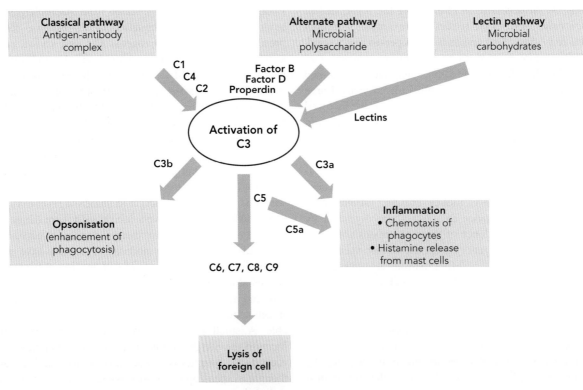

Figure 9.11

The pathways of complement activation and its biological activities

present in the cell walls of many microorganisms. The third pathway is the lectin pathway. Lectins are carbohydrate-binding proteins found in serum that are able to bind to a wide range of microorganisms. This complex causes activation of the complement system as shown in Figure 9.11. Together, these three pathways enable the complement system to clear or destroy a wide range of microorganisms and foreign molecules.

In the three pathways the complement proteins are activated in a particular sequence, with each protein activating the next one in the sequence. All pathways lead to the cleavage of C3 into two fragments (C3a and C3b). These fragments are responsible for the induction of three different processes which result in the destruction of foreign cells and substances. They are cytolysis (cell breakage), opsonisation (enhancement of phagocytosis) and inflammation.

The complement proteins are able to destroy foreign cells by damaging their cell membranes. This **cytolysis** is initiated by the C3b fragment and other components which activate the C5 to C9 sequence of reactions. The activated proteins produced from these reactions form a complex which is inserted into the foreign cell membrane (see Figure 9.12). This **membrane attack complex** acts as a trans-membrane channel which allows the leakage of water and electrolytes out of the cell and, ultimately, cytolysis. Complement-mediated cytolysis is important in protection against microorganisms, and is also the basis for other reactions, such as transfusion reaction following transfusion of incompatible blood, transplant rejection and some autoimmune diseases.

The C3b fragment can also bind covalently to the surface of microorganisms and then bind with specific C3b receptors on phagocytes. By binding to both the microbe and the phagocyte, the C3b effectively holds the microorganism against the surface of the phagocyte (see Figure 9.13), thereby promoting the phagocyte's ability to

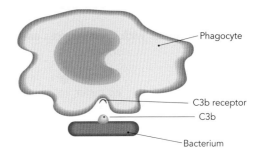

Figure 9.13

Opsonisation of a bacterial cell by complement

ingest the organism. This enhancement of phagocyte activity is termed **opsonisation** and C3b is called an **opsonin**.

C3a (the other cleavage product of C3) and C5a (the cleavage product of C5) are **anaphylatoxins**; that is, they bind to mast cells, basophils and platelets, triggering the release of histamine and other substances (see Figure 9.11). As mentioned earlier in this chapter, histamine and leukotrienes are major inducers of inflammation. C5a also contributes to inflammation by acting as a potent chemotactic factor, attracting phagocytes to the site of injury.

Acute phase proteins

Acute phase proteins are a group of plasma proteins that enhance resistance to infection, limit tissue damage due to infection, trauma, malignancy and so on, and promote tissue repair. Plasma levels of these proteins increase in response to infection, inflammation or tissue injury. One of the proteins, C-reactive protein, is measured in serum to indicate current disease activity in people with certain inflammatory conditions (e.g. rheumatoid arthritis).

CYTOKINES

Cytokines are a group of chemical substances that act as messengers within the immune system and between the immune system and other systems of the body. As a group, cytokines are involved in many facets of non-specific immunity, especially in inflammation and phagocyte chemotaxis and activation. As you will see, they also play a critical role in the development of specific immune responses by inducing cell activation and proliferation. Overall, these substances provide communication between cells and have a central role in regulating the immune system. In general, cytokines have multiple activities and sources and usually have different effects on different cell types. The major groups of cytokines are interleukins, interferons, colony stimulating factors, tumour necrosis factors and chemokines (see Table 9.2 for examples).

The term **interleukin** was initially used for cytokines that are released by leukocytes; however, it is now recognised that other cell types also produce some interleukins. There have been almost 30 different interleukins identified, referred to as interleukin-1 (IL-1), interleukin-2 (IL-2) and so on. Interleukins have numerous actions including cell activation, cell proliferation, cell differentiation and antiviral activity.

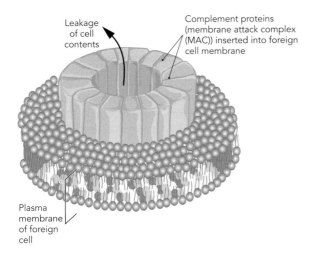

Figure 9.12

The membrane attack complex (MAC) of complement
Complement proteins are inserted into the membrane of the foreign cell, forming a pore through which the cell contents can leak out.

Table 9.2
Examples of cytokines with their sources and functions

CYTOKINE	SOURCE(S)	MAJOR FUNCTION(S)
Interleukin 1 (IL-1)	Macrophages, epithelial cells	Induction of fever; T cell activation; macrophage activation; induction of acute phase proteins
Interleukin 2 (IL-2)	T cells	Proliferation of T cells; activation of NK cells
Interleukin 4 (IL-4)	T cells, mast cells	B cell activation; differentiation of T_h cells into T_h2
Interleukin 9 (IL-9)	T cells	Stimulates T_h2 cells; enhances mast cell activity
Interleukin 10 (IL-10)	T cells, macrophages	Inhibits macrophage functions
Interleukin 12 (IL-12)	Macrophages, dendritic cells	Activates NK cells
Granulocyte-macrophage colony stimulating factor (GM-CSF)	T cells, macrophages	Increases production of granulocytes, macrophages and dendritic cells;
Tumour necrosis factor-α (TNF-α)	Macrophages, NK cells, T cells	Kills tumour cells; induces inflammation, endothelial cell activation
Tumour necrosis factor-β (TNF-β)	T cells, B cells	Kills tumour cells; endothelial cell activation
Interferon-α (IFN-α)	Leucocytes, dendritic cells	Induction of antiviral state in cells
Interferon-β (IFN-β)	Fibroblasts	Induction of antiviral state in cells
Interferon-γ (IFN-γ)	T cells, NK cells	Macrophage activation, NK cell activation, increased expression of MHC molecules

Interferons were first identified as antiviral proteins produced by virus-infected cells to help other cells resist infection. One of the important features of interferons is that they are *not virus-specific*; that is, interferon produced against a particular virus protects against a variety of other viruses. Three types of interferon, produced by different cell types, are now recognised. Virus-infected leukocytes produce **alpha interferon (IFN-α)**, whereas fibroblasts, epithelial cells, macrophages and possibly all body cells secrete **beta interferon (IFN-β)** when infected by viruses. IFN-α and IFN-β do not protect already infected cells but, when secreted from them, protect neighbouring cells from infection. They do this by binding to interferon receptors on neighbouring cells, causing them to produce intracellular antiviral proteins (see Figure 9.14).

The third type, **gamma interferon (IFN-γ)**, is not produced by virus-infected cells, but is secreted by activated lymphocytes and NK cells. As you will see later in this chapter, IFN-γ has an important role in the development of acquired immune responses by enhancing the actions of macrophages, neutrophils, natural killer cells and lymphocytes.

Colony stimulating factors (or growth factors) are cytokines that stimulate certain cells to divide and differentiate. Examples are GM-CSF (granulocyte-monocyte colony stimulating factor), which stimulates monocytes, dendritic cells and granulocytes, and G-CSF (granulocyte colony stimulating factor) which stimulates neutrophils.

Tumour necrosis factors are cytokines that kill tumour cells, but they may also have other functions such as regulation of immune responses, endothelial cell activation and induction of inflammation. The two main types are TNF-α and TNF-β.

Chemokines are cytokines that are responsible for the attraction of phagocytes to a site of injury – that is, they are chemotactic factors. Chemokines also activate certain leukocytes and control the migration and homing of lymphocytes in the body. More than 60 different chemokines have been identified.

Some cytokines that enhance immune responses are now used in the treatment of certain disease conditions. For example, IL-2 and IFN-γ have been used in the treatment of certain tumours. G-CSF has been used to increase the neutrophil numbers in some people (e.g. undergoing chemotherapy) who are deficient in these cells. IFN-α is now part of the standard treatment for chronic hepatitis B and C.

NORMAL MICROBIAL FLORA

The normal microbial flora of the human body are described in detail in Chapter 8. These organisms suppress the growth of potentially pathogenic bacteria and fungi by:

- competing for essential nutrients
- changing environmental conditions to be unfavourable to other microorganisms, but favourable to themselves (e.g. low pH created by *Lactobacilli* in the vagina)
- secreting toxic substances (e.g. colicins of *Escherichia coli*, which inhibit other microbes)
- forming bacterial layers over tissue surfaces (e.g. in the intestine).

The importance of the normal flora in preventing infection is clearly demonstrated when broad spectrum antibiotics are administered to a patient. In some cases, such drugs can reduce the normal flora and allow infection to occur. Thrush, caused by the yeast *Candida albicans*, is an infection of the oral cavity, or gastrointestinal or genital tracts, and often follows broad spectrum antibiotic therapy.

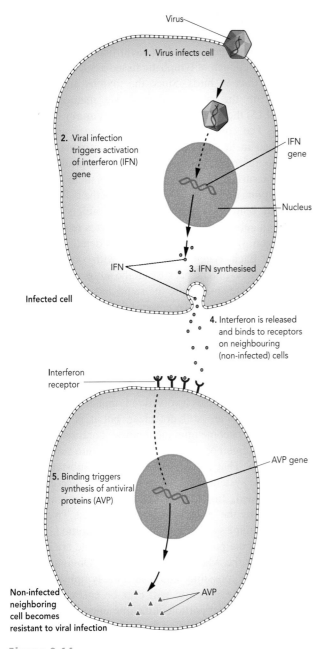

1. Virus infects cell

2. Viral infection triggers activation of interferon (IFN) gene

IFN gene

Nucleus

Infected cell

IFN

3. IFN synthesised

4. Interferon is released and binds to receptors on neighbouring (non-infected) cells

Interferon receptor

5. Binding triggers synthesis of antiviral proteins (AVP)

AVP gene

Non-infected neighboring cell becomes resistant to viral infection

AVP

Figure 9.14
The antiviral action of interferon

Specific body defences: the acquired immune system

The specific body defences, or **acquired immune system** (also called the **specific immune system** or **adaptive immune system**), is a functional system consisting of a variety of cells, especially lymphocytes and macrophages, and various organs such as the thymus gland and lymph nodes. It is the body's second line of defence and protects it from infection and from damage by foreign cells and substances that enter the body; it is also active against tumour cells. If it fails or is disabled, serious diseases such as cancer or life-threatening infections may result. **Immunity** is the capacity of the immune system (the acquired immune system plus some components of the

non-specific immune system) to successfully defend the body against a potentially infectious agent. **Immunology** is the study of the immune system and immunity.

CHARACTERISTICS OF THE ACQUIRED IMMUNE SYSTEM

The non-specific immune system is highly effective in quickly eliminating many microorganisms from the body, but some microbes find ways around these defences. When a microbe is able to evade the non-specific defences and persist in the tissues, the body reacts by producing a response specifically directed against the invading organism. This is the **immune response**. It is responsible for:

- identifying the antigens (foreign molecules) of the microbe
- producing a specific defence reaction to destroy the microbe
- providing memory, which enables the body to react more vigorously on subsequent exposures to the same microbe.

The immune response also amplifies the inflammatory response and provides a mechanism for the activation of the complement system.

A major principle of immunity is that, once a person has had an infectious disease, they are unlikely to contract the same disease again. The basis of this immunity was revealed in 1890, when Emil von Behring and Shibasaburo Kitasato demonstrated that animals that survive an infection have protective factors (now called *antibodies*) in their blood that protect them against future attacks by the same pathogen. It was further shown that serum from surviving animals, when injected into other animals, protected the recipients from the same infection. These and subsequent studies revealed some important characteristics of the acquired immune system:

- It is able to distinguish between host substances (self) and foreign substances (non-self) – that is, it *recognises* foreign substances.
- It is directed only against the particular pathogen or foreign substance that stimulated it – that is, it is *specific*.
- It recognises and mounts a more rapid and stronger response to a previously encountered pathogen – that is, it has *memory*.

THE DUAL NATURE OF THE ACQUIRED IMMUNE SYSTEM

In the 1960s it was found that, for some diseases, injection of antibody-containing serum did not protect recipients from the disease the donor had survived, but that injection of the donor's lymphocytes did provide immunity. Jacques Miller in London, and Noel Warner and Aleksander Szenberg (of the Walter and Eliza Hall Institute in Melbourne) determined that there are two different populations of lymphocytes, called **B lymphocytes** (or **B cells**) and **T lymphocytes** (or **T cells**). Each type is responsible for a different form of immunity.

Humoral immunity is immunity provided by **antibodies**, which are present in the body's 'humors' or fluids. The antibodies are produced and secreted by plasma cells (derived from B lymphocytes) and they then circulate in the blood and other body fluids. Antibodies are most effective against bacteria and their toxins, and against viruses *before* they enter host cells. They act by binding to the invading microbes or their products, leading to their inactivation, destruction or elimination by various means (see pages 199–201).

Because antibodies are unable to enter cells, another type of defence is needed to deal with intracellular pathogens. This is called **cell-mediated immunity**, or **cellular immunity**, because of the direct involvement of cells in the immune processes. In cell-mediated immunity, T lymphocytes act against target cells by directly killing the cells, or by releasing chemicals that enhance the inflammatory response and/or activate other defence cells to bring about destruction of the target cells. Cell-mediated immunity provides the major form of defence against viruses and bacteria that have invaded host cells, and also against fungi, other eucaryotic parasites and cancer cells.

Before describing the humoral and cell-mediated responses separately, we consider the cells involved in these two components of the immune response and the foreign substances that trigger their activity.

CELLS AND TISSUES OF THE ACQUIRED IMMUNE SYSTEM

Lymphocytes

The cells that are largely responsible for a specific immune response are the lymphocytes and macrophages. As stated above, the **B lymphocytes** are mainly responsible for humoral immunity and the **T lymphocytes** provide the cell-mediated immunity. These two types of lymphocytes interact with other defence cells to produce a specific immune response to a large variety of pathogenic microorganisms and other foreign substances and cells. A third type of lymphocyte, the NK cell, is described earlier in this chapter in relation to its role in non-specific immunity. NK cells also have a prominent role in acquired immunity, since they are activated by cytokines produced in a specific immune response.

Lymphocytes are the second most numerous type of white cell in blood, and their total number in the body is among the highest of all cell types. Like all blood cells, lymphocytes originate in the bone marrow. Immature lymphocytes are released from the marrow and mature into B cells or T cells depending on the site in the body where they undergo final maturation and become immunocompetent.

T cells are lymphocytes that migrate from the bone marrow to the thymus, and they undergo a maturation process brought about by hormones within the thymus (hence the term T cell). After puberty the thymus begins to regress in size and is progressively replaced by fatty tissue, but it continues to be responsible for T cell maturation

until late in life. B cells are believed to mature in the bone marrow itself (or in the liver in the foetus). B cells are so called because they were first identified in the 'bursa of Fabricius', a pouch of lymphatic tissue associated with the digestive tract in birds. Since the thymus and the bone marrow are the sites of lymphocyte maturation, (see Figure 9.15) they are referred to as the **primary lymphoid organs**. The collection of lymphoid organs and tissues (described in the next section) where immune reactions occur are referred to as the **secondary lymphoid organs**.

On the surface of mature lymphocytes there are numerous receptors of a single type that enable the cells to recognise and bind to a single, specific foreign substance. A foreign substance to which lymphocytes react is called an **antigen**. (Antigens are discussed in detail later in this chapter.) Each lymphocyte reacts with one particular antigen, and no others, because all the antigen receptors on the lymphocyte surface are the same and specific for that antigen. For example, receptors of one lymphocyte can recognise only the toxin of the tetanus-causing bacterium, whereas those of another lymphocyte might bind only to the cold virus. Generally, there will be populations of both T lymphocytes and B lymphocytes that recognise each type of antigen.

The exact processes involved in lymphocyte processing and maturation are still not clear, but it is known that lymphocytes become immunocompetent and specific for a particular antigen before actually coming into contact with that antigen. That is, the specific foreign substances that the immune system is able to recognise and respond to are predetermined. Importantly, they are predetermined by genes, not by the antigens that are contacted. This means that the immune system consists of precommitted lymphocytes for all the possible antigens that people are likely to contact over the whole of their lifetime. Obviously, only some of the possible antigens our lymphocytes are programmed to recognise will ever be encountered and, therefore, only a proportion of the immunocompetent cells present in the body will ever be utilised.

Mature lymphocytes that have not yet encountered their

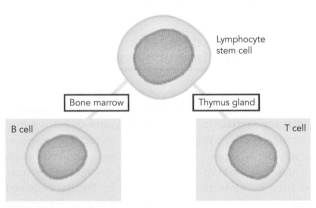

Figure 9.15

The maturation of lymphocytes
The maturation of immature lymphocytes occurs in the thymus and bone marrow, where they become antigen-specific T cells and B cells respectively.

specific antigen are referred to as **naive lymphocytes**. Some naive lymphocytes recirculate around the body, giving them maximum opportunity to contact their specific antigen. These lymphocytes move about freely between lymphoid organs and tissues, transported in the bloodstream and lymphatic system. Other naive lymphocytes remain in lymphoid organs and tissues (see section below on 'The Lymphatic System') where they lie in wait for their specific antigen to pass by.

T Lymphocyte subsets and their functions

Several different functional types of T cells are involved in the process of acquired immunity. T cells possess a number of different glycoproteins on their surface called CD, for clusters of differentiation. Two of these glycoproteins that distinguish between the major functional groups of T cells are the CD4 and CD8 markers. T cells that possess the CD4 marker, called **CD4 cells** or **T4 cells**, are primarily T helper cells, whereas T cells with the CD8 marker, the **CD8 cells** (or **T8 cells**), are cytotoxic T cells. Like B cells, T cells also have antigen receptors, although the nature of T cell receptors is different from that of B cell receptors.

T helper cells (T_h cells) play a central role in the immune response. Once activated by antigen, they release cytokines to help B cells and other T cells to respond to antigen (Figure 9.16). They can also release other cytokines that activate other cell types or induce inflammation. Two major types of T_h cells can be distinguished according to the types of cytokines they produce. The type 1 T helper cells (T_h1) release cytokines (IL-2 and IFN-γ) that help to activate other T cells and macrophages in cell-mediated immunity, whereas type 2 T helper cells (T_h2) release cytokines (IL-4 and IL-5) that are important in humoral immunity. Most antigens require the involvement of T_h cells for the activation of B cells and other T cells to occur. These are called **T dependent antigens**.

T_h cells are so important in the activation of other lymphocytes that, without them, the immune response to most antigens is severely diminished. This is starkly demonstrated in infections caused by the human immunodeficiency virus (HIV). The HIV attacks the T_h cell population, rendering the infected person incapable of mounting immune responses, and thus highly susceptible to infection and cancer.

Cytotoxic T cells (T_c cells) bind directly to and kill target cells. Activated cytotoxic T cells circulate in the bloodstream and lymphatic system in search of cells displaying the antigens they specifically recognise. They attack mainly virus-infected cells, but they are also involved in defence against intracellular bacteria and tumour cells.

Some T lymphocytes appear to have suppressor activity – that is, they down-regulate immune responses by releasing suppressor cytokines. T lymphocytes with suppressor activity may be involved in the winding down of the immune response after an antigen has been successfully eliminated. This would help to prevent uncontrolled or unnecessary immune system activity. Suppressor T cells may also be important in maintaining tolerance to some self-antigens (see page 211).

There do not appear to be functional subtypes of B lymphocytes.

The lymphatic system

The lymphatic system is a network of vessels, cells and specialised organs. Lymph is the fluid that is formed in tissues from blood components that enter the extracellular spaces. The lymph is drained from the tissues and carried in lymph capillaries that converge into larger vessels, ultimately returning the lymph to the bloodstream. On its way, the lymph is filtered through numerous lymph nodes. The **lymph nodes** are small, bean-shaped organs that tend to occur in clusters along lymphatic channels. Because lymph capillaries carry substances and pathogens absorbed from nearly all body tissues, immune cells in lymph nodes are in a strategic position to encounter antigens that have entered tissues.

The **secondary lymphoid organs** comprise the lymph

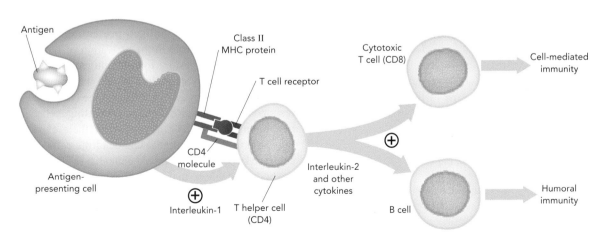

Figure 9.16

The central role of T helper cells in humoral and cell-mediated immunity

T helper cells are activated by antigen presented by an antigen-presenting cell; the activated T helper cells then release various cytokines which help to activate other T helper cells, cytotoxic T cells and B cells.

nodes as well as the spleen, tonsils and clusters of lymphoid cells in the gastrointestinal tract, respiratory tract and other mucosal surfaces. The clusters of lymphoid cells lining the mucosal surfaces are called gut-associated lymphoid tissue (GALT), bronchi-associated lymphoid tissue (BALT) and so on, or are collectively referred to as the mucosa-associated lymphoid tissue (MALT).

The lymphoid organs have a common structure that is a loose framework housing numerous lymphocytes and macrophages. They are strategically placed throughout the body to provide defence where it is likely to be needed (see Figure 9.17). For example, lymphocytes and macrophages in the tonsils act primarily against micro-organisms that invade the oral and nasal cavities, whereas the spleen acts as a filter to trap blood-borne antigens. Collections of lymphocytes underlying mucous membranes provide local defence at those sites.

The **thymus** is found in the upper thoracic region beneath the sternum (see Figure 9.18). Its size, proportional to the rest of the body, is greatest at birth. It continues to grow until puberty, after which it progressively shrinks to become largely replaced by fatty tissue in later adulthood. As mentioned earlier, immature lymphocytes

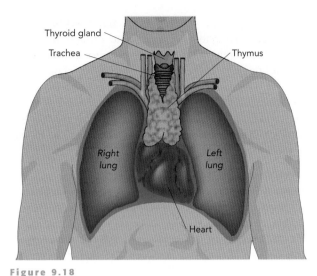

Thyroid gland
Trachea
Thymus
Right lung
Left lung
Heart

Figure 9.18

The thymus gland

develop into mature T cells under the influence of thymic hormones. The importance of the thymus gland is clearly demonstrated in babies born without a functional thymus (DiGeorge syndrome). These children are highly susceptible to infection – even common childhood infections like chickenpox can be very serious, and even fatal.

Some lymphocytes circulate continuously between the bloodstream and lymphoid organs. This enables the lymphocytes to come into contact with antigens present in different parts of the body, as well as with other lymphocytes and antigen-presenting cells.

To summarise: the acquired immune system's ability to identify and destroy foreign substances is based on the ability of its cells, the lymphocytes, to recognise and respond to foreign substances (antigens) in the body. Different types of lymphocytes interact with one another and with other cells to mount a concerted response specific to each antigen.

Antigen-presenting cells

While B and T lymphocytes are considered to be primarily responsible for immune responses, they cannot do this alone. They actually require the help of other cell types, known collectively as **antigen-presenting cells**. These cells play a critical role in the activation of lymphocytes. They do this by ingesting foreign antigen, processing the antigen by partially degrading it, and then presenting the antigen to lymphocytes in a form that the lymphocytes can respond to. The major antigen-presenting cells are the macrophages (we have already seen their capacity for ingestion of foreign antigen) and dendritic cells. Dendritic cells are bone-marrow-derived cells that reside throughout the body and whose major function is antigen presentation to lymphocytes.

Antigen-presenting cells form a sentinel network that is continually on the lookout for foreign antigens in the body, ingesting them, processing them and transporting them to lymphoid tissues for interaction with lymphocytes. Other cells in the body, such as B cells and epithelial cells, also have the capacity for antigen processing and presentation.

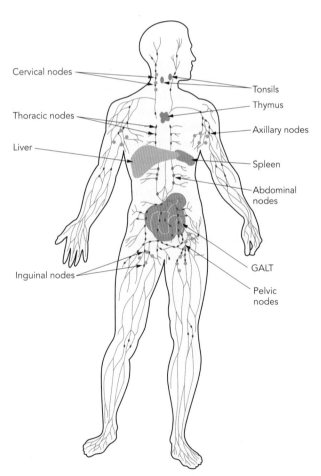

Cervical nodes
Thoracic nodes
Liver
Inguinal nodes
Tonsils
Thymus
Axillary nodes
Spleen
Abdominal nodes
GALT
Pelvic nodes

Figure 9.17

The components of the lymphatic system

The lymph vessels, lymph nodes, thymus, spleen, tonsils and aggregates of lymphocytes lining the small intestine (gut-associated lymphoid tissue, GALT), bronchi (BALT) and other musosal surfaces.

The mechanisms by which antigen-presenting cells process and present antigens to lymphocytes are described on pages 194–95.

ANTIGENS

The acquired immune system does not direct its activity against whole microorganisms, but instead focuses its actions against parts of them. The parts of microorganisms that are foreign (i.e. different from substances in the body) and that activate the acquired immune system are called **antigens**. The word 'antigen' is in fact a contraction of the term '*anti*body *gen*erating'. Most antigens are large, complex molecules (macromolecules) of the following types: proteins (and polypeptides), nucleic acids, some lipids and polysaccharides. Antigens are present on the surfaces of viruses, bacteria and other microorganisms, as well as on human, animal and plant cells.

Complete antigens and haptens

Complete antigens are foreign substances that stimulate specific T and B lymphocytes, inducing them to produce an immune response. Complete antigens are thus said to be **immunogenic** (or **antigenic**) – that is, capable of inducing an immune response. In general, proteins and macromolecules containing proteins (e.g. glycoproteins, lipoproteins) tend to be the strongest antigens. Microorganisms are strongly immunogenic because they possess many different antigens, many of which are proteins exposed on the cell surface.

In contrast, smaller molecules, such as peptides, nucleotides and saccharides, are generally not immunogenic, even if they are foreign. However, some of them become immunogenic if they become attached to the body's own proteins and the immune system recognises the combination as foreign. A small foreign molecule such as this is called a **hapten**. Although haptens cannot initiate an immune response on their own, they can react with antibodies or activated T cells produced against them. A good example of a hapten is penicillin, which can bind with a serum protein in some people and induce an immune response. In this case the immune response is manifested as an allergic reaction (see page 208).

Epitopes

Although antigens are foreign molecules of a certain minimum size, only a small part of the whole antigen molecule is immunogenic. This important part of the molecule is called the **epitope** (or **antigenic determinant**) and is the part to which free antibodies or activated B or T lymphocytes can bind.

Most naturally occurring antigens are very complex molecules and consist of a number of different epitopes (see Figure 9.19). Different epitopes are recognised by different lymphocytes; thus, a single, complex antigen may activate many different lymphocytes, stimulating the formation of many different kinds of antibodies. Large proteins often comprise hundreds of different epitopes, which is why these substances are so strongly immunogenic. In contrast, large molecules formed from many

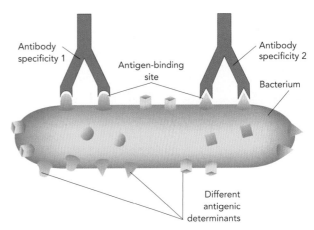

Figure 9.19

Different epitopes (antigenic determinants) on a bacterial cell

Bacteria generally have multiple epitopes on their surface, each one capable of stimulating a different antibody response.

identical repeating units, such as plastics, are often non-immunogenic. Such substances are ideal for making artificial body implants (e.g. bone replacements) because they are not recognised as foreign by the immune system, and therefore not rejected.

THE MAJOR HISTOCOMPATIBILITY COMPLEX

The **major histocompatibility complex** (**MHC**) is so named because of its importance in determining the compatibility of tissues when attempting to transplant an organ or tissue from one person to another. The MHC is a set of genes on chromosome 6 that code for a large number of proteins with a variety of functions in the body. Two groups of these proteins have a critical role in the immune system, and are referred to as class I MHC proteins and class II MHC proteins. As you will see in the following sections, these proteins are vital for certain cell-to-cell interactions that must occur for an immune response to be produced. MHC proteins are particularly abundant on the surface of leucocytes, and hence are also referred to as **human leucocyte antigen** (**HLA**) proteins. But they are also present on virtually all other cells of the body. Class I MHC proteins are found in the membranes of all nucleated cells, whereas class II MHC proteins are found only on B lymphocytes and antigen-presenting cells (see Figure 9.20).

Different individuals have different HLA proteins (unless they are genetically identical as in identical twins), although the more closely two people are related the more likely they will share some common HLA proteins. A difference in HLA proteins between donor and recipient is the basis for rejection of organ transplants. Thus, HLA proteins are our personal antigens, a mixture of those inherited from each of our parents.

Antigen processing by antigen-presenting cells involves the intracellular degradation of foreign proteins into small peptides and the combining of these peptides with MHC

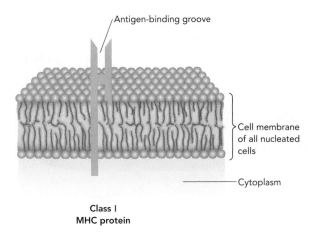

Class I
MHC protein

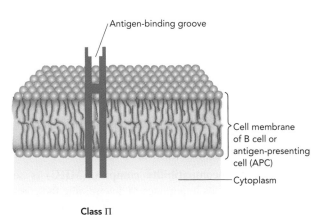

Class II
MHC protein

Figure 9.20

The two classes of MHC proteins involved in cell-to-cell interactions

proteins. Presentation involves the transport of this peptide-MHC protein complex to the surface of the antigen-presenting cell for display to lymphocytes (see Figure 9.21).

HUMORAL IMMUNITY

If foreign cells or antigens enter the body and evade the non-specific defences, they then encounter the cells and tissues of the lymphoid system.

Activation of B cells and formation of antibodies

Each naive B lymphocyte carries around 300 000 molecules of a specific antigen receptor (actually an antibody molecule) on its membrane. This is known as the **B cell receptor** (see Figure 9.22). Activation of a B lymphocyte is a multistage process involving antigen presenting cells, T_h cells, B cells and cytokines (see Figure 9.23):

1. The antigen is phagocytosed by an antigen-presenting cell (APC) and this APC then presents the antigen fragment together with an MHC II molecule to a T helper lymphocyte (T_h).
2. The T_h cell differentiates into a T_h2 cell following its binding to the presented antigen and MHC II molecule and due to secretion of IL-1 by the antigen-presenting cell.
3. Antigen is also bound to a specific B cell via its antibody receptors. This antigen is internalised and processed and the antigen fragment is then presented on the surface of the B cell together with an MHC II molecule. This is known as *clonal selection* (see below for further explanation).
4. The B cell presents the antigen fragment and MHC II molecule to the T_h2 cell which then secretes IL-4, resulting in the activation of the B cell.

Following the activation of B cells, there are two important processes:

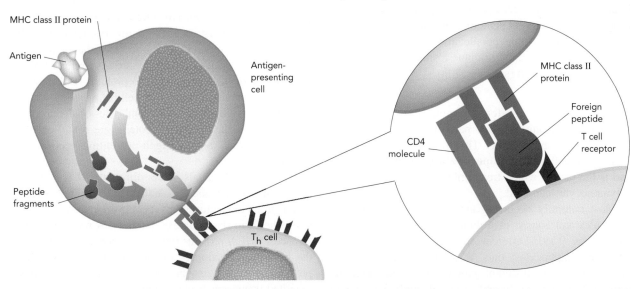

Figure 9.21

Antigen processing
Specialised antigen-presenting cells, such as macrophages, ingest antigens, process them and join them to a recognition molecule (called an MHC protein) so that lymphocytes can respond to the antigen.

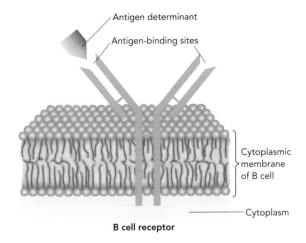

Antigen determinant

Antigen-binding sites

Cytoplasmic membrane of B cell

Cytoplasm

B cell receptor

a. The B cell receptor (an antigen receptor)

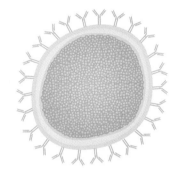

b. The B cell has hundreds of thousands of antigen receptors on its surface

Figure 9.22

The antigen receptor of B cells is an antibody molecule

- Proliferation of the B cells – to expand the number of cells capable of reacting to the particular antigen
- Differentiation of the cells in the expanded population – to obtain large numbers of clone cells (see below).

The activating event first stimulates the B cell to transform into a *blast cell*, which is an enlarged, highly active cell prepared for mitotic division. The blast cell multiplies through successive mitotic divisions to produce a large population of cells all bearing the same antigen receptors (Figure 9.24). This population of cells, all with the same specificity, is called a **clone**. Thus, it is the antigen that does the selecting in clonal selection by 'choosing' a lymphocyte with complementary receptors. This is the basis of the **clonal selection** theory, first proposed by the Australian immunologist Sir Frank Macfarlane Burnet in the 1950s. There are thought to be approximately 10^{11} different antibody receptors – that is, 10^{11} different B cell clones.

After multiplication, the clone cells differentiate into functional cells. Some of them become **plasma cells**, which are the cells responsible for synthesis and secretion of antibodies. Plasma cells are able to synthesise enormous amounts of antibody (as many as 10 million anti-

body molecules per hour!) for several days and then they die. Each antibody has the same antigen specificity as the receptor molecules on the surface of the parent B cell. The antibodies are secreted by the plasma cells into the blood and other body fluids, where they can bind to specific antigens and thus prepare them for destruction by other specific or non-specific mechanisms.

The clone cells that do not become plasma cells become long-lived **memory cells**, which persist in the body for months to years, and can react with the same antigen if it enters the body again at a later time. Memory cells respond to antigenic stimulation in the same way that the original parent B cell responded to antigen, again increasing the clone size, producing even more cells with the same specificity. The larger population of memory cells is more easily activated and therefore is able to respond more rapidly and more strongly compared to the group of cells in the original B cell population.

The events described so far in this section constitute the **primary immune response**; that is, the response of the acquired immune system the first time it is exposed to a particular antigen. Immediately after antigen challenge in a primary immune response there is characteristically a lag period of several days (sometimes longer) in which there is no observable increase in the specific antibody levels in blood (or serum). During this time there is much activity; the lag period is the time required for processing of antigen, for the small number of B cells specific for the antigen to be activated and proliferate, and for the newly formed cells to differentiate into plasma cells. Once antibodies start to be produced in large amounts, the specific serum antibody level begins to rise, peaking within several weeks; it then declines over the next few weeks to months (Figure 9.25).

If a person is exposed to the same antigen a second time, a **secondary immune response** occurs that is:

- faster
- stronger
- longer-lasting (Figure 9.25).

The secondary response is very different because the immune system has been primed to the antigen in the primary response. This priming produces large numbers of memory B lymphocytes. The increased numbers of specific memory lymphocytes and their easier triggering are responsible for this powerful secondary response. The advantage of this response is that it provides a quick and potent reaction on re-exposure. These memory cells provide what is commonly called **immunological memory**. This memory effect is the basis for giving boosters when using some vaccines. When a booster is given, even more memory cells are produced and the antibody levels in the blood can remain high for many years.

It should be stressed that the primary antibody response described above relates to the injection of non-living (and therefore non-replicating) antigen. In the case of infection or vaccination with a living organism, the antibody

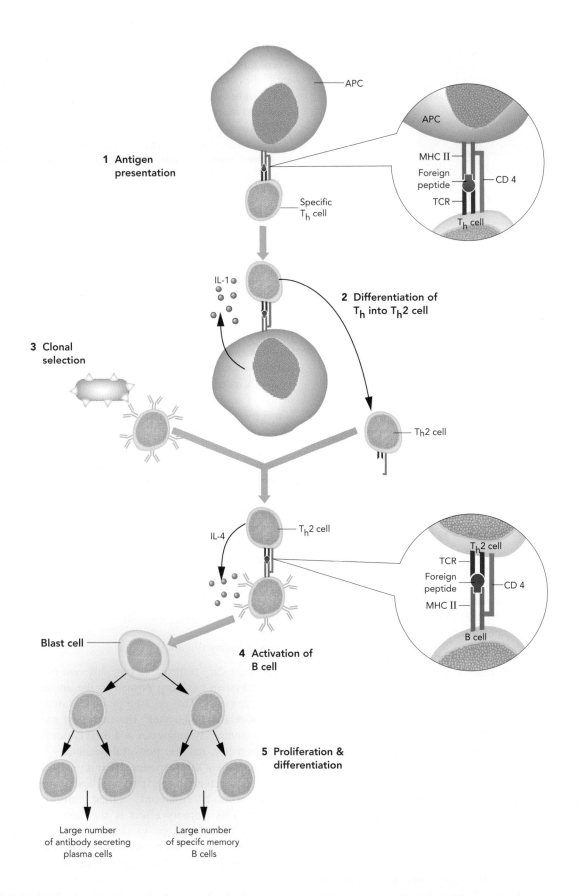

1 Antigen presentation

APC

Specific T$_h$ cell

APC
MHC II
Foreign peptide
CD 4
TCR
T$_h$ cell

IL-1

2 Differentiation of T$_h$ into T$_h$2 cell

3 Clonal selection

T$_h$2 cell

T$_h$2 cell

IL-4

T$_h$2 cell
TCR
Foreign peptide
CD 4
MHC II
B cell

Blast cell

4 Activation of B cell

5 Proliferation & differentiation

Large number of antibody secreting plasma cells

Large number of specifc memory B cells

Figure 9.23

The humoral immune response
Activation of a specific T$_h$ cell and a specific B cell by antigen leads to a large number of antibody secreting cells and memory cells.

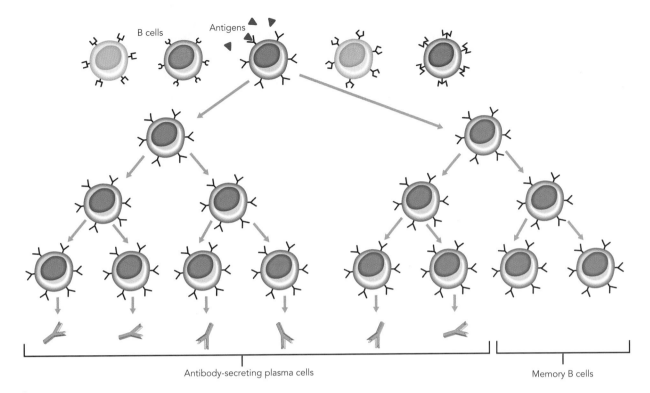

Figure 9.24

Clonal selection

There is a multitude of different lymphocyte populations in the body, each population being able to recognise a single antigen. When an antigen enters the body it virtually selects the clone that is specific to it. When activated by antigen, that small clone proliferates and then differentiates to produce a much larger clone, comprising antibody-secreting plasma cells and long-lived memory cells. All cells in this large clone are specific for the same antigen.

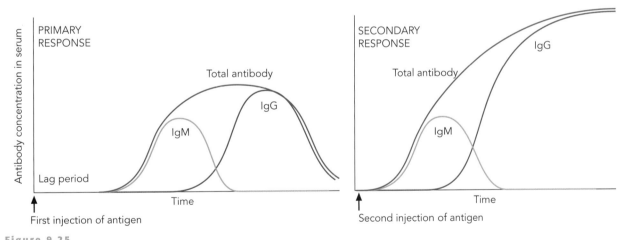

Figure 9.25

The primary and secondary antibody responses to injection of a non-replicating antigen
The secondary response is faster, larger and longer-lasting.

response is more like that of a combination of primary and secondary responses. The reason for this is that living organisms stimulate the immune system repeatedly as they replicate in the body. Effectively, it is the equivalent of having multiple boosters. Vaccines containing attenuated organisms (see page 205), which are alive and replicate but don't cause disease, stimulate the immune system in this way. Thus, infection or a single vaccination of attenuated organisms can provide long-term and sometimes lifelong immunity.

Basic antibody structure

Antibodies, also called **immunoglobulins**, are proteins found in blood and other body fluids, including lymph, urine, CSF and mucosal secretions. They constitute the **gammaglobulin** fraction of blood proteins. All antibodies in humans can be grouped into one of five immunoglobulin types (called isotypes, or classes), based on differences in their structure and function. We look at how these immunoglobulin classes differ in Table 9.3.

All antibody molecules have a basic structure consisting of four polypeptide chains linked together by disulphide bonds (Figure 9.26). Two of these chains are long and identical, and are called **heavy (H) chains**. The other two chains, the **light (L) chains**, are also identical but much shorter. The molecule has a Y-shaped structure, which can change to a T-shape because of a flexible hinge region that allows the arms of the molecule to change position. This is the basic, single antibody molecule or *monomer*.

As shown in Figure 9.26, the two 'arms' of the antibody molecule are called **antigen-binding fragments (Fab)**, and at the ends of the arms are grooves called the **antigen-binding sites**, which is where the molecule binds to its antigen. The remainder, or tail part, of the molecule is called the **crystallisable fragment (Fc)**. There are two antigen-binding sites per monomer. The high specificity of the antigen-binding sites for their antigens is similar to that of the active site of enzymes for their substrates.

The binding sites are complementary to the antigen. These binding sites have to be different for different antigens, and are part of what is called the *variable (V) region* of the molecule. The specific sequence of the amino acids in the variable region determines the antigen specificity of the antibody. The other end of the molecule is the *constant (C) region*, where the amino acid sequence is the same (or very similar) in all antibodies of the same class. The Fc fragment, which is part of the C-region, is involved in binding to other molecules, such as complement, and cells of the immune system.

Antibody classes

Five major immunoglobulin classes have been identified in humans and are designated IgD, IgM, IgG, IgA and IgE,

on the basis of differences in the C-region of their heavy chains. 'Ig' stands for immunoglobulin, followed by a letter designating the different types of heavy chains. As illustrated in Figure 9.27, IgG, IgD and IgE have the single, basic Y-shaped structure and therefore exist as monomers. IgA exists as either a monomer or dimer (two linked monomers). IgM is made from five linked monomers.

Each class of antibody has a different biological function. For example, IgM is the first type of antibody that is produced after primary antigenic stimulation, and lasts for only a short time (weeks to months) in body fluids. IgG is the most abundant antibody in blood and is the type that persists for months to years after antigenic stimulation (see Figure 9.25), thus providing long-term protection. It is the only antibody class that is able to cross the placental barrier from mother to foetus.

IgA is found primarily in the mucus that covers the body's mucosal surfaces. In these secretions it exists as a dimer and has an extra component, called a secretory piece, which makes it resistant to proteolytic digestion by enzymes in these fluids. IgA plays a major role in preventing pathogens from gaining entry into the body by stopping them from crossing the mucosal epithelium. IgA aggregates antigens and keeps them in the secretions; when the secretions are expelled so, too, are the antigens.

The monomeric forms of IgM and IgD are membrane proteins present on the surface of B lymphocytes where they act as antigen receptors. IgE antibodies are involved in immunity to worm infections of the intestinal tract, and also in allergic reactions. These and other characteristics unique to each of the immunoglobulin classes are summarised in Table 9.3.

The basis of antibody diversity

It is thought that the acquired immune system of a person can make antibodies to millions of different antigens. Given the number of possible antigens in the world that the body might contact, this would seem to be necessary if the immune system is to protect us against most microorganisms. Since antibodies, like all proteins, are coded

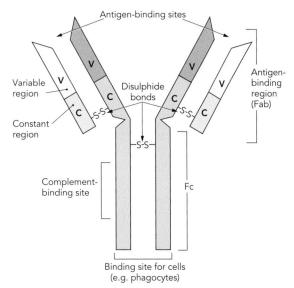

Figure 9.26

The basic structure of an antibody molecule
The four polypeptide chains (two heavy and two light) are joined together by disulphide bonds. In each chain there is a variable region (V) and a constant region (C). Antigen binding occurs in the variable region of the antigen-binding fragment (Fab). The molecule binds the complement proteins and binds to a phagocyte via parts of the Fc region.

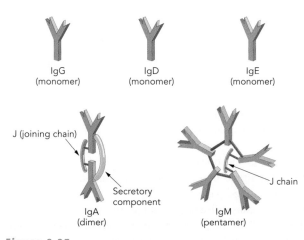

Figure 9.27

The structures of the five classes of human immunoglobulins

Table 9.3

The biological properties of human immunoglobulins

	IgG	IgM	IgA	IgE	IgD
Bind to antigen	yes	yes	yes	yes	yes
Cross the placenta (protects foetus)	yes	no	no	no	no
Trigger complement system	yes	yes	no	no	no
Fix to mast cells and basophils (involved in allergic reactions)	no	no	no	yes	no
Bind to phagocytic cells (enhances phagocyte activity)	yes	no	sometimes	no	no

for by genes, it might be expected that an individual will have millions of genes just for antibodies. However, this cannot be the case, since humans are thought to have only about 100 000 genes for all the proteins that the body's cells must make. There are believed to be only about 600 genes for antibodies.

The critical question that vexed immunologists for many years was how so few genes could produce so many different antibody proteins. The answer began to unfold in the 1970s when it was shown that the genes that code for antibodies are not present as such in embryonic cells. Instead of containing a complete set of antibody genes, cells contain sets of mini-genes that act as 'building blocks' for antibody genes. Antibody diversity comes from the shuffling and combining of these gene segments in different ways by each B cell as it becomes immuno-competent. The information of these reassembled genes is then expressed as the surface receptors of B cells, and in the antibodies later released by their clone members. The light and heavy chains are manufactured separately and then joined to form the antibody molecule.

This has been likened to using a child's building block set – the set contains a small number of different blocks, but they can be used to build numerous different objects. It is estimated that the diversity in the light and heavy chains allows for almost two million different antibody genes.

However, the random mixing of gene segments to make antibody genes, plus the diversity that results from different combinations of H- and L-chains account for only part of the huge number of antibody specificities. The joining process adds even more diversity. The enzymes that combine the gene segments add random DNA bases to the segments as they are being joined.

As a result of gene shuffling and mutation on a large scale, the lymphoid system is thought to be capable of producing millions of different clones of lymphocytes. And according to the clonal selection theory:

- each mature lymphocyte is preprogrammed
- each mature lymphocyte can respond to one antigen only
- each clone of specific lymphocytes is selected and expanded only when the appropriate antigen enters the body.

Because the total lymphocyte population must express such a large number of different specificities, it follows that there can only be a relatively small number of lymphocytes (perhaps a few hundred) that have the same specificity before first contact with the antigen. A considerable part of the lag period in the antibody response is spent increasing this small number of cells to a larger population, capable of producing large amounts of antibody.

Activities and functions of antibodies

The basic function of antibody molecules is to bind specifically with their antigens and form **antigen-antibody** (or **immune**) **complexes**. Once they have bound to antigen, antibodies help to bring about removal of the antigen from the body in a number of different ways:

- opsonisation
- complement fixation
- neutralisation
- agglutination or precipitation.

Different actions of antibodies are necessary for different types of antigens. These functions are summarised in Figure 9.28.

Antibodies can **opsonise** antigens in a similar way to complement (Figure 9.29). Microorganisms or other particles, when coated with opsonising antibody, become more readily recognised and ingested by phagocytes. Opsonising antibodies are particularly important in defence against microbes that have capsules or other structures that enable them to avoid being ingested by phagocytes (see Chapter 10).

Antibody attachment followed by **complement fixation** (or activation) is an important defence against foreign cells, such as bacteria and cancer cells. When antibodies bind to cellular targets, complement-binding sites are exposed on the Fc fragments of the antibody molecules. This triggers complement activation which leads to the insertion of complement proteins (the membrane attack complex) into the plasma membrane of the foreign cell, creating holes in the membrane and resulting in cell lysis.

Neutralisation is a process in which antibodies bind to and block specific attachment sites on viruses or bacterial

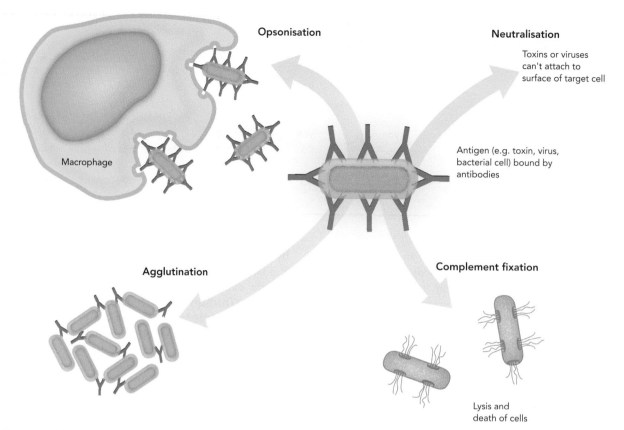

Figure 9.28

The functions of antibodies

Antibodies have different functions depending on the class of the antibody and the nature of the antigen. Once bound to antigen, antibodies can enhance the phagocytosis of particulate antigens (called opsonisation), aggregate particulate antigens (called agglutination), coat toxins and viruses (called neutralisation) or, in conjunction with the complement system, cause lysis and death of foreign cells.

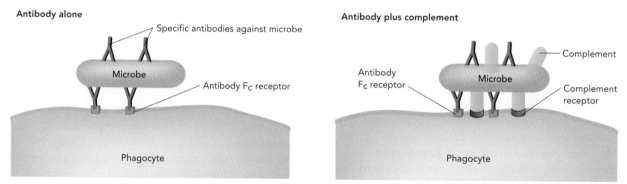

Figure 9.29

Opsonisation of microorganisms

Adherence of microbes to phagocytes can be facilitated by (a) antibodies, or (b) antibodies together with complement. The mechanisms are similar to opsonisation with complement alone (illustrated in Figure 9.13).

exotoxins (toxic substances secreted by bacteria, see Chapter 10). As a result of being coated by antibody, the virus or toxin is prevented from binding to receptor sites on tissue cells, thus preventing invasion or injury. The antigen–antibody complexes are eventually destroyed by phagocytes. **Antitoxin** is the name given to antibodies that neutralise bacterial toxins.

Because an antibody molecule has two or more antigen-binding sites, it can bind to the same epitope on different antigen molecules. In this way, antibodies can cross-link

antigens to form large lattices (see Figure 9.28). When cell-bound antigens are cross-linked, clumping of the foreign cells occurs, and this is called **agglutination**. IgM, with (theoretically) ten antigen-binding sites (see Figure 9.27), is a very potent agglutinating antibody. Examples of this type of reaction occur with bacterial cells and with foreign red cells when mismatched blood is transfused.

In **precipitation**, soluble molecules (instead of cells) are cross-linked into large complexes which then precipitate out of solution. The protective benefits of these reactions are that agglutinated bacteria and precipitated foreign molecules are much more easily identified and captured by phagocytes.

The Fc part of the antibody molecule is also functional. Once antigen is bound, areas of the Fc fragment become activated and can bind to receptors on some host defence cells, including macrophages, neutrophils, mast cells and NK cells. In opsonisation, the antibody binds to the foreign cell or particle via its binding sites, and then the Fc part of the antibody binds to the surface of neutrophils or macrophages, effectively binding the antigen to these phagocytes. Some antibodies have receptors for the fixing (activating) of complement. IgE antibodies bind specifically to mast cells and basophils and, when antigen is bound, they cause the release of allergic mediators such as histamine (see pages 208–11). Since NK cells have receptors for antibodies, foreign cells coated with antibody are readily recognised and destroyed by NK cells.

CELL-MEDIATED (CELLULAR) IMMUNITY

Usually, at the same time that B cells are responding to an antigen, a clone of specific T cells is similarly activated. The cell-mediated immune response involves the activation, differentiation and actions of T cells, and the actions of chemical mediators produced by them. This arm of the acquired immune system is designed to recognise body cells that have viruses or bacteria residing or growing within them. It also provides defence against tumour cells, fungi and parasites (helminths and protozoa).

In cell-mediated immunity, the stimulus for clonal selection and T lymphocyte activation, proliferation and differentiation is the binding of foreign antigen. The T cell receptor (Figure 9.30) is not an antibody, but consists of two transmembrane polypeptide chains (α and β). T cells are unable to recognise free antigens carried in blood or lymph; but work carried out by Australian Nobel laureate Peter Doherty showed that they do recognise and respond to processed fragments of foreign antigens displayed with MHC proteins, on surfaces of the body's own cells. T cell activation therefore requires a simultaneous recognition of non-self (the antigen) and self (an MHC protein). As described earlier, the MHC protein brings the antigen fragment to the surface of the antigen-containing cell, to which a T cell can bind and respond.

A cell that is infected by a virus or intracellular bacterium usually displays microbial antigen fragments in conjunction with class I MHC proteins on its surface. If a T_h cell with receptors for that antigen contact the infected cell, the antigen-class I MHC protein combination causes the T_h cell to differentiate into a $T_h 1$ cell, which then secretes IL-2 and IFN-γ. These two cytokines enable cytotoxic T cells to be activated (see Figure 9.31) by the antigen on the infected cell. The CD8 molecule on cytotoxic T cells in fact binds to part of the class I MHC protein.

Once the cytotoxic T cell (T_c) is activated, it enlarges and proliferates to form more T_c cells and memory T cells of the same antigen specificity. The new T_c cell population targets and kills cells infected by the specific microbe by

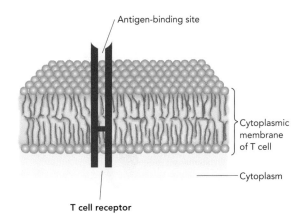

Figure 9.30

The T cell receptor
A surface molecule composed of two polypeptide chains (α and β) that form the antigen binding site.

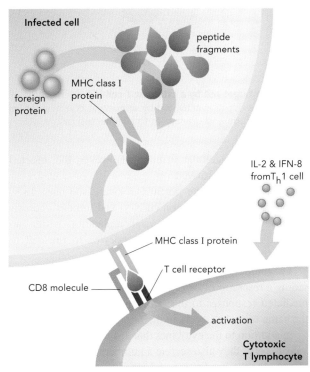

Figure 9.31

Activation of cytotoxic T cells
Cytotoxic T cells are activated by antigen in combination with a class I MHC protein on an infected cell.

two mechanisms. The T_c cell binds tightly to the target cell and then releases molecules of a protein called **perforin**, which are inserted into the plasma membrane of the target cell (see Figure 9.32). The proteins form a pore in the cell membrane through which enzymes, called *granzymes*, can be injected into the target cell. These granzymes cause the target cell to commence a process of programmed cell death, called **apoptosis**, in which the cell begins to kill itself from within. Additionally, the perforin pore disrupts the integrity of the cell membrane, which also leads to cell death. By killing the infected cells, virus (or bacterial) replication is disrupted and the microbe can then be

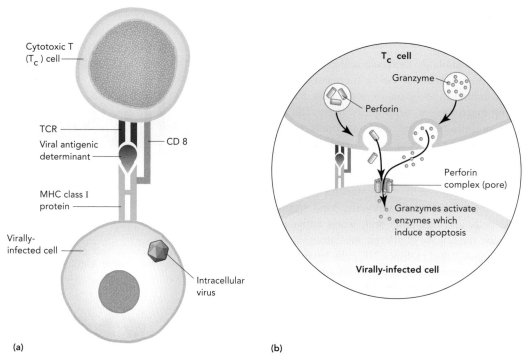

(a)   (b)

Figure 9.32

Killing of a target cell by a cytotoxic T cell (T$_c$)

(a) Cytotoxic T cell is activated by antigen in combination with a class I MHC protein on an infected cell; (b) Cytotoxic T cell releases perforin and granzymes to kill infected cell.

exposed to extracellular defences. However, the infected host cell is also destroyed.

T$_c$ cells also secrete potent cytokines (see page 187), including gamma interferon (IFN-γ) and tumour necrosis factor (TNF), which limit viral replication inside an infected cell and also attract phagocytes to the cell to destroy it.

The memory T cells persist for a long time, thereby providing a reservoir of cells that can mediate secondary cell-mediated responses to the same antigen if reinfection by the same microbe occurs in the future.

In addition to the cytokines that T$_h$1 cells secrete to activate T$_c$ cells, they also secrete a number of other cytokines to enhance the production and activity of other cell types involved in cell mediated immunity (see Figure 9.33). These include TNF-β which activates neutrophils, GM-CSF which activates macrophages and increases production of macrophages and dendritic cells, and IL-3 which increases production of macrophages and granulocytes. IL-2 and IFN-γ not only activate T$_c$ cells, but also NK cells.

ACTIVE VERSUS PASSIVE IMMUNITY

Specific immunity can be acquired either actively or passively (see Figure 9.34). **Active immunity** is the immunity developed when the acquired immune system responds to microorganisms or other foreign substances that enter or are introduced into the body. Active immunity is *naturally acquired* during microbial infections, and *artificially acquired* as a result of vaccination (see pages 204–6). Generally, active immunity is long-lasting, often for a lifetime, especially when naturally acquired.

Passive immunity is the immunity resulting from the transfer of premade antibodies (or immune cells) from an immune person (or animal) to a non-immune person. The recipient becomes immune, but only for a short time (up to several months) until the transferred antibodies (or cells) are naturally degraded in the body. The immunity is short-lived because the immune system of the recipient is not stimulated.

Passive immunity can also be naturally or artificially acquired. Passive immunity is conferred naturally on a foetus as the mother's antibodies pass across the placenta into the foetal circulation. Antibodies are also transferred to an infant in colostrum and breast milk. These antibodies protect the foetus and then the young infant for several months after birth against the wide variety of microbes to which the mother is immune. In the meantime, the baby's own immune system is maturing.

Passive immunity is artificially conferred when a person is injected with antibodies from an immune human or, rarely, from an immune animal. **Normal immunoglobulin** is an immunoglobulin preparation extracted from the pooled serum of large numbers of blood donors. Each batch of this serum contains a mixture of antibodies that offers protection against a broad range of common infectious diseases. It is generally used to prevent diseases such as rubella and hepatitis A in people who have recently been exposed to these viruses. It is also sometimes used to replace antibodies in immunodeficient patients.

Specific immunoglobulin (SIG), on the other hand, is a specific antibody preparation obtained from the serum

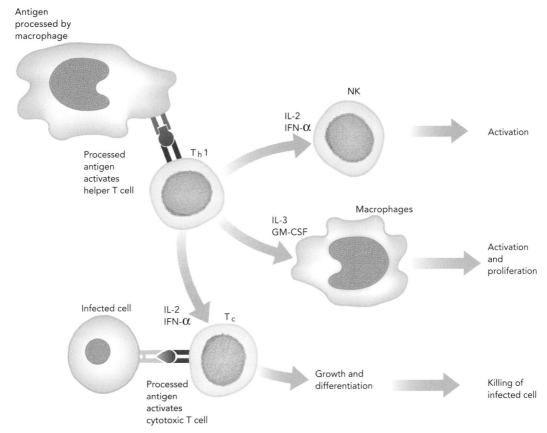

Figure 9.33
Cell-mediated immunity
T cells are activated by antigen-presenting cells and/or infected cells and can perform a variety of functions, depending on their type.

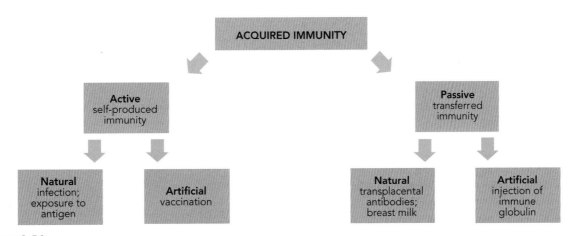

Figure 9.34
The different types of acquired (specific) immunity

of people who are convalescing and in a hyperimmune state after an infection. Specific immunoglobulins are usually prepared against such diseases as pertussis, tetanus and hepatitis B. For example, a health worker who is accidentally exposed to hepatitis B virus by a needle-stick injury is given hepatitis B immunoglobulin in an attempt to prevent establishment of infection. These preparations are preferable to normal immunoglobulin because they contain higher titres of specific antibodies against these potentially more serious diseases. The injected antibodies provide immediate protection, but their effect is short-lived.

TUMOUR IMMUNOLOGY

Cancer is one of the leading causes of death in industrialised countries. The term **tumour** refers to a swelling due to a new growth of cells. Development of a tumour involves a series of genetic changes in a group of cells, usually over a period of years, which ultimately lead to the cells replicating in an uncontrolled manner. Tumour cells are genetically unstable so, during tumour growth, genetic variants of the original cells usually develop. The term **cancer** refers to a tumour that is **malignant**, meaning that it has certain properties. These properties include a rapid growth rate, a lack of cell differentiation and normal tissue organisation, and a tendency to metastasise (spread to other tissues).

The transformation of a normal cell into a tumour cell can be caused by a wide range of factors that are termed **carcinogens** (cancer-promoting factors):

- virus infection – e.g. genital wart viruses in cervical cancer; hepatitis B and C viruses in liver cancer
- bacterial infection – e.g. *Helicobacter pylori* infection and stomach cancer
- radiation – e.g. UV radiation in skin cancer; X-rays
- chemicals – e.g. cigarette smoke.

Tumours can also result from spontaneous mutation in a normal cell. Furthermore, specific genes called **oncogenes** have been identified in normal cells which, when activated in certain conditions, lead to malignant transformation of the cell.

It is generally accepted that tumour cells are usually recognised by the immune system and eliminated as they arise. Thus, if a tumour does develop it means that the tumour cells have somehow avoided or escaped from these body defences. The term **immune surveillance** was coined by MacFarlane Burnet in the 1960s to suggest that the immune system does seek out and destroy tumour cells. The modern usage of this term not only recognises the role of the immune system in tumour destruction, but also acknowledges that tumours are not passive targets – they are able to escape from, and even disable, the immune system in some circumstances.

Destruction of tumour cells by the immune system necessarily depends on the cells being recognised as foreign. Some tumours have been found to have 'foreign' chemical groupings on their surface and these are called **tumour-associated antigens** (TAAs). In the main, these tumour-associated antigens appear to be altered self-antigens. Many of the non-specific and specific defences that we discuss in this chapter are thought to be involved in tumour cell destruction. In particular, NK cells, macrophages, granulocytes, cytotoxic T cells and specific antibody in conjunction with complement have the capacity to eliminate cells that are considered foreign.

With all these defences, how is it that some tumours escape? There are several potential ways by which tumours escape the body's defences. Some tumours appear to lack TAAs and hence are not recognised as foreign. Other tumours have TAAs that are only weakly immunogenic, and thus induce a poor immune response. As stated earlier, tumours tend to be genetically unstable and can lose or change their antigens over time, making the immune response to the original antigens ineffective. Many tumours have been shown to produce immunosup-

pressive cytokines – for example IL-10. Some tumours surround themselves with a layer of collagen or fibrin. Because these are normal body proteins the tumours are invisible to the immune system. In some cases, antibodies produced against the tumour cells do not kill the cells, but instead act as blocking factors. That is, they bind to the tumour cells, forming a coat around them, and thereby prevent other defences from attacking the tumour.

Currently, relatively little is known about these mechanisms, but a huge amount of scientific work is being done to understand them better and to determine how the immune system can be enhanced to deal more effectively with tumours.

IMMUNISATION

Immunisation (also termed **vaccination**) is a procedure that aims to induce specific immunity in a person by artificial means. It involves exposing a person to material that is antigenic (able to stimulate the immune system) but not pathogenic (without causing disease). The discovery of vaccination just over 200 years ago by EDWARD JENNER (see Figure 9.35) was one of the farthest reaching and most important developments in medical science. It profoundly reduced the prevalence and impact of a number of infectious diseases that were once common and often deadly. Vaccines for viral diseases are particularly important because of the lack of effective treatment for many of these diseases. In this section, we examine the nature of vaccines and aspects of their usage.

Types of vaccines

In natural, acquired immunity, an infectious agent stimulates specific B and T lymphocytes and creates clones of memory cells which can give lifelong immunity. In immunisation, the objective is to generate the same response with a modified version of the microbe or its components. A safe and effective vaccine should mimic the natural protective response but not cause the infection; it should

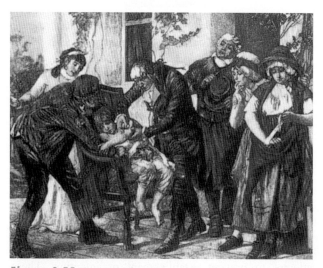

Figure 9.35

Jenner inoculating a child
Source: The Granger Collection

have long-lasting effects and be easy to administer. Most vaccine preparations comprise one of the following:

- killed, whole bacterial cells or inactivated viruses
- live, attenuated bacteria or viruses
- inactivated bacterial toxins
- parts of bacterial cells or viruses.

The common types of vaccines in use are listed in Table 9.4.

Killed vaccines are prepared by cultivating large numbers of the required bacterium or virus and treating them with formalin, radiation or some other agent that kills them but does not destroy their immunogenicity. The vaccine contains whole, killed organisms. The vaccines for hepatitis A and inactivated polio vaccines are of this type. Because the microbe does not multiply in the host and, therefore, does not strongly stimulate the immune system, killed vaccines often require several boosters to be effective.

A number of vaccines are prepared from live, attenuated microbes. **Attenuation** is any process that substantially reduces or (preferably) eliminates the virulence of microorganisms (i.e. their ability to cause disease) while still keeping them alive. It can be achieved by growing the organism in unusual conditions or by manipulating its genes in a way that eliminates its virulence factors. For example, the vaccine for tuberculosis (the BCG – Bacille Calmette et Guerin) was obtained by Calmette and Guerin after more than ten years of sub-culturing the agent of bovine tuberculosis on an artificial culture medium. Vaccines for measles, mumps and rubella, and the oral polio (Sabin) vaccine contain live, non-virulent viruses.

The advantages of attenuated vaccines are that viable microorganisms can multiply and produce mild or sub-clinical infection, which will induce long-lasting immunity. Many attenuated vaccines provide lifelong immunity without the need for boosters. The major disadvantages of using live vaccines are the inherent risk that the organism might mutate back to a virulent strain (see Spotlight box, page 321) and the possibility that they may cause full-blown disease in people whose immune system is compromised (see next section). However, live vaccines, where available, are generally preferred to killed types because of their greater efficacy.

For protection against diseases that are due primarily to the actions of a bacterial exotoxin (see Chapter 10), immunity to the toxin is often more useful than immunity to the whole bacterium. A special type of vaccine is the **toxoid**, which consists of a bacterial exotoxin that has been inactivated so that it no longer causes disease, but is still antigenic. Toxoids elicit the production of **antitoxins** – antibodies that, in the event of real infection, neutralise the toxin and prevent it from causing disease. Examples of toxoids are the highly effective vaccines for diphtheria and tetanus, two of the components of the triple antigen vaccine for children.

If the exact antigenic determinants that stimulate good immunity are known, it may be possible to produce a vaccine based on that particular part of a microorganism. These are called **subunit vaccines**. Examples of subunit antigens are the capsular polysaccharides of *Haemophilus influenzae* (Hib vaccine), pneumococcus and meningococcus, and the surface antigen of hepatitis B virus and influenza viruses.

The immunogenic components of some subunit vaccines are prepared by genetic engineering techniques. In this process, the gene for the synthesis of the protective antigenic determinant (epitope) is introduced into a bacterium or yeast cell. These microbes are grown in large numbers and the antigen harvested for use in the vaccine. The hepatitis B vaccine is a subunit vaccine prepared in this way. A list of the major vaccines in use in Australia is provided in Chapter 14.

Subunit and toxoid vaccines are non-living and thus need several boosters to produce strong, effective immunity.

An additional, major advantage of immunisation is the establishment of **herd immunity** in the population. Herd immunity is based on the principle that individuals who are immune to an infectious disease will not be carriers of the organism, reducing the occurrence of that microbe and, therefore, the number of susceptible people who will encounter it. In other words, mass immunisation confers indirect protection on the whole population, including the non-immune. Herd immunity helps to avert epidemics. This is discussed more fully in Chapter 14.

Side effects of vaccines

Before vaccines are licensed they must undergo stringent trials in experimental animals and humans. However,

---

Table 9.4

Types of vaccines in common use

TYPE OF VACCINE	DISEASE
Killed bacteria	Cholera
	Typhoid
Inactivated viruses	Influenza
	Rabies
	Polio (Salk)
Live, attenuated bacteria	Tuberculosis
Toxoids (inactivated toxins)	Tetanus
	Diphtheria
Attenuated virus	Measles
	Polio (Sabin)
	Mumps
	Rubella
Microbial subunit	*Haemophilus* infections, Pneumococcal infections, Meningococcal infections (polysaccharides)
	Hepatitis B (viral surface antigen)
	Whooping cough (acellular)

most vaccines can cause minor adverse effects. The most common of these are local hypersensitivity reactions (redness and swelling) at the injection site, pain and fever. For certain vaccines there are rare, but more severe complications; for example:

- encephalitis following measles vaccine (although the incidence of this is much lower than following infection)
- acute neurological complications following pertussis vaccine (although the incidence of this is much lower than following infection)
- vaccine-associated paralytic poliomyelitis associated with the live, attenuated polio vaccine
- systemic allergic reactions (anaphylaxis) following several vaccines, such as measles, mumps, rubella and influenza vaccine.

Health professionals involved in giving vaccinations should be aware of the possible risks, but also aware that the risk of contracting the disease could be far more serious (see Chapter 14). Extreme caution must be exercised in giving live vaccines (a) to the immunocompromised, because even low-virulence organisms can produce disease in such people, and (b) to pregnant women, because of possible risk to the foetus.

Disorders of the immune system

There are certain situations where the immune system fails or functions inappropriately. When it fails, the individual becomes more susceptible to infectious diseases and sometimes cancer, and when it functions inappropriately it can cause disease and sometimes damage to the body. These disorders of the immune system can be classified as immunodeficiency, hypersensitivity or autoimmune disease, although some conditions are a combination of two or more of these.

IMMUNODEFICIENCY

Immunodeficiency includes both inborn and acquired conditions in which the production or function of lymphocytes, phagocytes or complement is abnormal. These are the key components of the immune system, and a person with a defect in one or more of them is said to be **immuno-compromised**, or **immunodeficient** if seriously immuno-compromised. **Primary immunodeficiency** is generally due to the improper foetal development of one or more of these components. **Secondary immunodeficiency** results from damage to otherwise normal components and may be due to infection, cancer, malnutrition or the use of drugs and other therapies that suppress the immune system.

Primary immunodeficiency

Selected primary immunodeficiencies are listed in Table 9.5. Phagocytes, lymphocytes and complement are the key components of the immune system, so a defect in any one of them will lead to impaired ability to resist infection and/or cancer. The two most serious primary immunodeficiency diseases are (a) congenital thymic hypoplasia or aplasia, caused by a failure of the thymus to develop fully, resulting in a deficiency in T cells, and (b) severe combined immunodeficiency disease (SCID) in which lymphocyte precursors in the bone marrow fail to develop properly, resulting in a marked deficiency in both B and T cells. Since T cells are required for the proper functioning of both humoral and cell-mediated immunity,

Table 9.5
Selected primary immunodeficiency diseases

DISEASE	NATURE OF DEFECT
Defects in B lymphocytes	
• X-linked infantile agammaglobulinaemia (Bruton's disease)	Pre-B cells do not mature – no circulating B cells
• acquired hypogammaglobulinaemia	B cells respond to antigen but do not secrete antibody
• selective IgA deficiency	IgA is synthesised but not released
Defects in T lymphocytes	
• congenital thymic aplasia (DiGeorge syndrome)	Improper development of the thymus gland – few T cells
Defects in both T and B lymphocytes	
• severe combined immunodeficiency	Stem cell defect resulting in T and B cell deficiency
• Nezelof's syndrome	Thymic hypoplasia and T and B cell deficiency
Defects in phagocytes	
• chronic granulomatous disease	Phagocyte enzyme deficiency
Defects in complement	
• complement defect	Deficiency in any component of complement

individuals afflicted with either condition have little or no protection against infection. Even normally minor infections can be fatal.

X-linked (Bruton's) agammaglobulinaemia is a primary immunodeficiency caused by incomplete maturation of B lymphocytes. Children (usually boys) with this disorder suffer repeatedly from infections such as pneumonia, otitis media, meningitis and septicaemia.

Different types of immunodeficiency will result in increased susceptibility to different types of pathogenic microorganisms. In general, a T cell deficiency will mainly increase susceptibility to viruses, intracellular bacteria and other intracellular parasites like the malaria protozoan and fungi, since it is the T cell that attacks infected host cells. A selective deficiency in B cells or antibodies, on the other hand, will greatly increase a person's susceptibility to most bacterial infections and, to a lesser extent, viruses. A deficiency in both cell types, as occurs in SCID, will make the individual highly susceptible to all pathogenic microbes and even to organisms with low virulence.

Complement mainly attacks foreign cells in extracellular fluids, so a deficiency in any one of the complement proteins will increase the risk of bacterial infections. A defect in macrophage activity will greatly impair defences against bacteria, and defence against viruses will also be affected, but to a lesser extent.

Secondary immunodeficiency

There are numerous potential causes of secondary immunodeficiency. Any condition or agent that causes a suppression or malfunction of the bone marrow or lymphoid organs may cause a secondary immunodeficiency. For example, in leukaemia, a massive number of cancer cells are produced in the bone marrow, preventing the normal production of white cells. In Hodgkin's disease, the immune system is suppressed because of the growth of tumour cells in the lymph nodes.

Treatments for certain diseases can also cause immunodeficiency. For example, the cytotoxic drugs and radiation therapy used in the treatment of cancer suppress white cell production in the bone marrow. Corticosteroids, used to reduce inflammation in certain diseases, can reduce the number of leukocytes in the blood. Immunosuppressive drugs are used to prevent rejection of organ transplants, but they also make the patient more susceptible to infection.

The most obvious and devastating of the secondary immunodeficiencies is the **acquired immunodeficiency syndrome (AIDS)**, caused by the human immunodeficiency virus (HIV). The HIV severely damages the immune system by infecting and destroying T helper cells (this is described more fully in Chapter 19). A large variety of other microbes, including the measles virus, mumps virus, *Mycobacterium leprae* (leprosy) and the protozoa that cause malaria, cause less severe suppression of the immune system.

The common predisposing factors that can lead to secondary immunodeficiency are summarised in Table 9.6.

In addition to these secondary immunodeficiency diseases, non-specific defences can be impaired in certain situations. These are not regarded as immunodeficiency disorders because the defences affected are not strictly part of the immune system, but nevertheless they increase the risk of infection. For example, broad spectrum antibiotics can temporarily lower the body's non-specific defences by

---

Table 9.6
Examples of factors that cause secondary immunodeficiency

FACTOR	EFFECT ON BODY DEFENCES
Some tumours	
• leukaemia	Production of dysfunctional bone marrow cells
• Hodgkin's disease	Disease of lymph nodes
Tumour therapy	
• cytotoxic drugs	Suppression of white cell production
• radiotherapy	Suppression of white cell production
Malnutrition	
• protein deficiency	Poor lymphoid organ development, low antibody and complement concentrations, low lymphocyte numbers
Immunosuppressive therapy	
• in transplant patients	Suppression of lymphocyte function
Anti-inflammatory therapy	
• corticosteroids	Reduction of white cell production, impairment of lymphocyte function and antibody and cytokine production
Infection	
• human immunodeficiency virus	Destruction of T helper lymphocytes

reducing the normal flora of the body. When the skin barrier is disrupted by burns, surgical wounds or other trauma, infection becomes more likely. A urinary catheter predisposes a person to urinary tract infection because of the loss of the flushing action of urine over the urethral surface, and impairment of mucociliary activity in the airways as a result of cigarette smoking is an important factor in some types of lower respiratory infection.

HYPERSENSITIVITY

Hypersensitivity is an overreaction of the immune system to an antigen it has previously encountered. There are different types of hypersensitivity reactions, which may be classified according to whether antibodies or T cells are the principal elements involved. The British immunologists PHILLIP GELL and ROBIN COOMBS categorised them into four types. The first three types in their scheme are due primarily to the action of antibodies, and the fourth type is due to the action of T cells. Some disorders are actually a combination of more than one type.

Type I: Immediate hypersensitivity

Immediate hypersensitivity, or allergic reaction, such as hay fever and hives, affects around 25% of people and appears to be increasing in incidence in Australia and other countries with a Western lifestyle. **Allergy** occurs within minutes to several hours after a sensitised, susceptible person comes into contact with a foreign antigen. The term **allergen** is used to distinguish this type of antigen, which has the potential to elicit this type of reaction. Typical allergens include pollens, dust mites, fungal spores, certain foods, and some antibiotics and other drugs (see Figure 9.36).

The predisposition for allergies is associated mainly with the production of IgE antibodies to the allergens; that is, allergic people produce IgE antibodies after exposure to allergens, whereas non-allergic people produce another class of antibody (mainly IgG) to the same antigens. The precise reason why only some people produce IgE antibodies to these antigens is not known. This predisposition for allergy is at least partly due to genetic factors, since a person with two parents who suffer from allergies is much more likely to also suffer from them than a person who has only one allergic parent or no allergic parents.

There is also some evidence that environmental factors may play a role. It is argued by some scientists that childhood exposure to a large variety of antigens is protective and that such people are less likely to develop allergies. Children who are less exposed to antigens are more likely to develop allergies later in life. This hypothesis has been used to explain the increasing incidence of allergies in Western populations (see Figure 9.37).

The basis of immediate (Type I) hypersensitivity is the production of the IgE class of antibodies after initial exposure to the allergen. If this class of antibody is produced, the person becomes sensitised to the allergen, whereas the production of any other class of antibody to the allergen does not sensitise the person. The IgE molecules have a

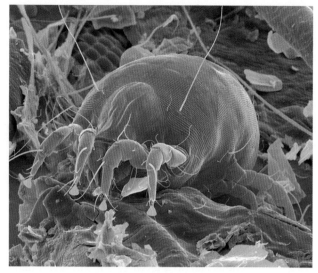

(a)

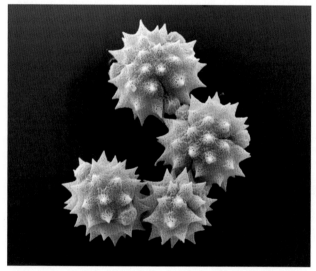

(b)

Figure 9.36
Common allergens
(a) dust mite; (b) daisy pollen.

special affinity for mast cells and basophils and attach to these cells via their Fc fragments. The sensitised cells may remain in the tissues for years. On subsequent exposure to the allergen, the allergen molecules cross-link the IgE antibodies attached to mast cells or basophils. This stimulates the cells to degranulate, releasing histamine and other inflammatory chemicals (e.g. kinins and proteases) that rapidly induce an inflammatory response (Figure 9.38). Activation of these cells also induces them to synthesise other powerful inflammatory mediators, particularly the prostaglandins and leukotrienes.

Eosinophils also play an important role in allergic reactions. They accumulate in tissues where allergic reactions are occurring and contribute to the process by secreting additional inflammatory mediators, especially leukotrienes.

Most allergic reactions are local, occurring typically

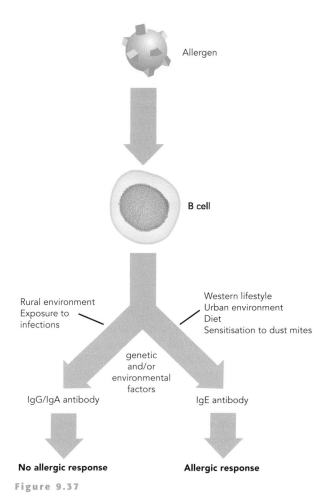

Figure 9.37

The basis of an allergic response

where the allergen enters the body. Thus, most involve the skin, the respiratory passages or the gastrointestinal tract, because of binding of allergen to local mast cells. Because the mediators cause dilation and increased permeability of blood vessels, local reactions are usually characterised by redness and swelling. Other familiar signs and symptoms, such as a runny nose, watery eyes and itching, reddened skin (hives), are related to inflammation in the specific tissues affected. When the allergen is airborne and inhaled, symptoms of asthma may appear as a result of bronchiolar smooth muscle contraction, which constricts the bronchioles, restricting air flow. Excessive mucus production further constricts the airways. When the allergen is ingested (e.g. in food), gastrointestinal hypersensitivity may occur (cramping, vomiting or diarrhoea) and sometimes a skin rash.

Table 9.7 details some common allergic reactions.

Fortunately, systemic allergic reactions, referred to as **anaphylaxis**, are far less common than local allergy. Anaphylaxis typically occurs when the allergen enters the blood and circulates through the body, as may happen with bee stings. It may also follow injection or ingestion of a foreign substance, such as penicillin or other drugs, in a susceptible individual. Anyone who has had any adverse reaction to penicillin, such as hives or throat or chest constriction, should not be given the drug again.

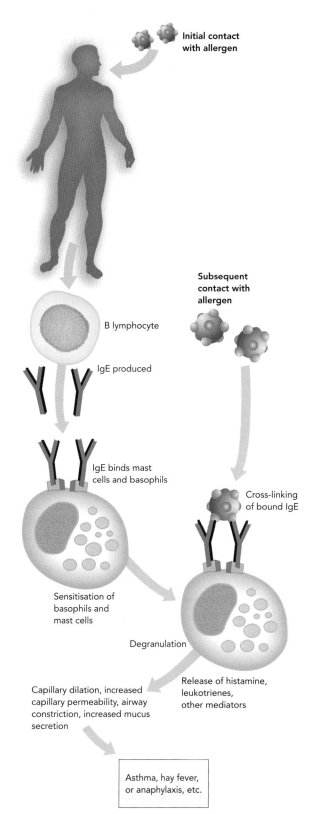

Figure 9.38

The mechanisms of allergy
Following first contact with an allergen, B lymphocytes are stimulated to produce IgE antibodies. These antibodies bind to mast cells and basophils, via their Fc region, thereby sensitising those cells. On subsequent contact with the allergen, it is bound to the sensitised cells, causing release of various inflammatory mediators which cause allergic reactions.

Table 9.7

Common allergic reactions mediated by IgE

SYNDROME	TYPICAL ALLERGENS	ROUTE OF ENTRY	CLINICAL MANIFESTATIONS
Wheal and flare	Insect bites	Subcutaneous	Redness; oedema; itching
Hay fever (allergic rhinitis)	Pollens Dust-mite faeces	Inhaled	Oedema of nasal mucosa Irritation of nasal mucosa
Asthma	Pollens Dust-mite faeces	Inhaled	Bronchial constriction; increased mucus production; inflammation of airways
Food allergy	Shellfish Milk Eggs Peanuts	Ingested	Vomiting; diarrhoea; urticaria (hives); anaphylaxis
Systemic anaphylaxis	Penicillin Bee venom	Intravenous (directly or following rapid absorption)	Oedema; circulatory collapse; death

The mechanism of anaphylaxis is essentially the same as that of local responses but, when mast cells and basophils are degranulated throughout the body, the generalised inflammatory response can be life-threatening. The sudden vasodilation may cause lowered blood pressure, circulatory collapse and physiological shock and, together with constriction of bronchiolar smooth muscle, can cause death within minutes. This serious form is called **anaphylactic shock**.

Type II: Cytotoxic hypersensitivity

Cytotoxic hypersensitivity results from the binding of antibodies to antigens on the surface of a cell, followed by complement activation and lysis of the target cell. The cell may be a foreign cell or a cell of the person's own body that is mistakenly recognised as foreign. In addition, complement activation leads to the formation of the anaphylatoxins C3a and C5a (see page 187) which stimulate mast cells to degranulate, leading to an inflammatory response. Examples of this type of hypersensitivity include reactions following transfusion of the wrong blood type, and a disease referred to as haemolytic disease of the newborn (or erythroblastosis foetalis). In both these cases, red cells are recognised as foreign, and antibodies in conjunction with complement cause lysis of the cells. In the case of transfusion reaction, red cells with foreign ABO or Rh antigens are present in the donor blood. In haemolytic disease of the newborn, the baby's Rh positive (D-antigen) red cells are destroyed by maternal anti-D antibodies of the IgG class, which are able to cross the placenta.

Cytotoxic (Type II) reaction is a major cause of damage in many autoimmune diseases (see below).

Type III: Immune complex hypersensitivity

Immune complex hypersensitivity results when antigen-antibody complexes are formed and are not cleared quickly from the body. In contrast to type II hypersensitivity reactions, type III reactions involve antigens that are not cell-associated. Normally, immune complexes are engulfed and destroyed by phagocytes, but if the complexes persist or are being formed continuously, this type of hypersensitivity occurs. If the number of circulating complexes is large, they may be deposited in the basement membranes in certain sites, such as the kidneys, lungs, joints, and blood vessels of the skin. The complexes activate complement and an inflammatory reaction occurs that can damage local tissues (Figure 9.39).

Acute glomerulonephritis is an example of an immune complex disease in which the complexes are deposited on the basement membrane of kidney glomeruli. Certain skin rashes result from the deposition of immune complexes in the basement membrane of surface blood vessels. Rheumatoid arthritis is due to a combination of immune complex hypersensitivity and autoimmune disease.

Type IV: Delayed type hypersensitivity

Delayed type hypersensitivity reactions (also called **cell-mediated hypersensitivity**) are mediated by T cells and take a day or more to appear after the introduction of antigen, compared to the few minutes or hours in antibody-mediated hypersensitivity reactions. The mechanism involved is basically that of a cell-mediated immune response. A subgroup of sensitised T cells, sometimes called **delayed type hypersensitivity T cells**, when stimulated by antigen, secrete cytokines which activate macrophages and cause inflammatory reactions such as eczema, oedema and granuloma formation. A massive infiltration of macrophages and lymphocytes often occurs. This reaction represents a normal cell-mediated response in which host tissue cells are unfortunately damaged.

The *Mantoux test* for assessing immunity to tuberculosis depends on a delayed hypersensitivity reaction. When protein antigens of the tuberculosis bacterium are inoculated intradermally (just under the skin), a small, hard inflammatory reaction occurs two to three days later if the person has been previously sensitised to the antigen. Contact dermatitis is another example of delayed type hypersensitivity. Contact dermatitis may occur when a hapten (incomplete antigen) present in a chemical product binds to a body protein (usually a skin protein) and then induces a cell-mediated response, manifested as a delayed hypersensitivity reaction. Chemicals containing haptens

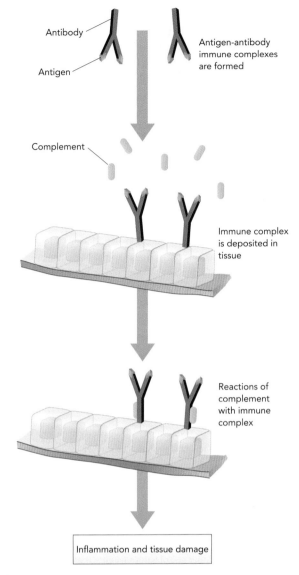

Antibody

Antigen

Antigen-antibody immune complexes are formed

Complement

Immune complex is deposited in tissue

Reactions of complement with immune complex

Inflammation and tissue damage

Figure 9.39

The mechanism of immune complex hypersensitivity
Immune complexes that are not rapidly removed by phagocytes are deposited in tissues where complement activation causes inflammation and tissue damage.

that may induce contact dermatitis include some cosmetics, metals, soaps and dyes.

AUTOIMMUNE DISEASES

For the immune system to operate effectively it must be able to react to foreign antigens and at the same time not react to the body's own (self) antigens. The non-responsiveness to self-antigens is called **tolerance**. Occasionally, the immune system loses its ability to distinguish self from non-self; that is, it loses its tolerance to one or more self-antigens. When this happens, the body produces antibodies (**autoantibodies**) and sensitised T cells against its own tissues. Studies have shown that self-reactive lymphocytes are actually part of the normal cell repertoire and that only in certain situations do some of these cause damage. If the damage is significant and disease results, it is called an **autoimmune disease** (see Table 9.8).

In most cases, it is not known what precipitates autoimmunity but genetic factors, environmental factors, sex, age and some infections are known to influence its incidence. In some disorders, the body's own cells are thought to appear 'foreign' because they are distorted or altered in some way. Autoimmune haemolytic anaemia is a condition in which red cells are destroyed by autoantibodies in conjunction with complement. In this disease, an alteration to the surface composition of red cells (often for unknown reasons) causes the immune system to recognise them as foreign and produce antibodies to these antigens. The factor that causes the surface of the red cells to be altered is often unknown, although some viruses and drugs have been shown to be involved in some instances.

In rheumatoid arthritis, an altered antibody molecule (an IgG) is thought to be the basis of the disease. First, the IgG to some unknown antigen is formed within a joint. Then, also for unknown reasons, this IgG becomes altered and eventually appears sufficiently foreign to stimulate an immune response in the form of antibodies (usually IgM). This anti-IgG antibody can be found in serum and is called the **rheumatoid factor**. The immune complexes formed by the binding of IgM to the altered IgG antibodies activate complement, leading to chronic inflammation

Table 9.8

Examples of autoimmune diseases

DISEASE	TARGET OF THE AUTOANTIBODY
Autoimmune haemolytic anaemia	Red blood cells
Idiopathic thrombocytopenic purpura	Platelets
Grave's disease	TSH receptor on thyroid cells
Rheumatic fever	Cardiac muscle
Myasthenia gravis	Acetylcholine receptor at the neuromuscular junction
Goodpasture's syndrome	Basement membrane in kidney and lungs
Systemic lupus erythematosis	Nucleic acid, red blood cells, platelets, etc.
Insulin-dependent diabetes mellitus	Pancreatic beta cells
Rheumatoid arthritis	Antibodies, connective tissue

and joint damage. This disorder is thus a combination of autoimmune disease and immune complex hypersensitivity.

Antibodies made against a foreign antigen sometimes cross-react with a self-antigen that has a similar structure and composition. For instance, antibodies produced during a streptococcal throat infection have been found to cross-react with components of heart muscle, causing inflamma-tion and damage to the heart muscle and valves. This rare autoimmune sequela of streptococcal sore throat is called rheumatic fever (see Chapter 19). It affects only a small percentage of people, those with the genetic makeup to produce the cross-reacting antibodies.

In many autoimmune diseases the self-antigens that are the target of attack have not been clearly identified.

SUMMARY

- The ability of the body to prevent infection is called resistance.
- Lack of resistance, or vulnerability to an infection, is called susceptibility.
- The body's resistance to infection depends on non-specific defences (the body's first line of defence) and specific defences (the body's second line of defence).
- The specific defences and some of the non-specific defences comprise the body's immune system.

NON-SPECIFIC DEFENCES

- The function of the non-specific defences is to prevent the entry of pathogens into the body, or to destroy them quickly if they do manage to enter.
- The body's first lines of defence against invasion by micro-organisms are the skin and the mucous membranes.
- Phagocytes are body cells that actively ingest and digest foreign particles and remove cellular debris from the tissues. The two main types of phagocytes are the macrophages and the neutrophils.
- The process of phagocytosis involves four main phases: chemotaxis, attachment, ingestion and digestion.
- Phagocytes are attracted to sites of damaged tissue or microbial invasion by chemicals released in a process called chemotaxis.
- Natural killer (NK) cells are a unique group of cells that are capable of destroying cancer cells and virus-infected cells.
- NK cells kill the target cell by insertion of perforins into the cell membrane, creating a pore through which toxic substances can be injected into the target cell.
- The acute inflammatory response is a non-specific defence that is the body's response to tissue injury.
- The major function of inflammation is to clear the injured site of cellular debris and foreign material, thereby preparing the area for repair processes.
- Inflammation also serves to localise microorganisms, preventing their spread to adjacent areas.
- The four main signs of acute inflammation are redness, heat, swelling and pain.
- The chemicals responsible for the physiological events that occur in inflammation are called the chemical mediators of inflammation.
- The most important mediators of inflammation are histamine, kinins, prostaglandins, leukotrienes, tumour necrosis factor and complement.

- Aspirin, indomethacin and other non-steroidal anti-inflammatory agents act by inhibiting the synthesis of prostaglandins.
- Steroidal anti-inflammatory drugs block both prostaglandin and leukotriene synthesis.
- Chronic inflammation occurs if the acute inflammatory response is unsuccessful in eliminating the organisms or foreign material from the tissues.
- Chronic inflammation can occur as a distinct process from the outset due to infection by microbes that are resistant to intracellular digestion by phagocytes or due to the presence of foreign materials that are typically low-grade, persistent irritants such as talc, silica and asbestos.
- Fever represents a systemic response to invading microorganisms and often accompanies severe or systemic inflammation. It occurs when the set-point of the body's thermostat is raised to a higher temperature.
- The complement system is a complex system of plasma proteins that normally circulate in an inactive state. When activated, complement can enhance phagocytosis, produce inflammation and directly lyse foreign cells.
- Acute phase proteins are plasma proteins that enhance resistance to infection, limit tissue damage and promote repair.
- Cytokines are chemical substances that act as messengers between cells in the immune system.
- The major groups of cytokines are interleukins, interferons, colony stimulating factors, tumour necrosis factors and chemokines.
- The normal microbial flora of the body suppress the growth of potential pathogens by competing for essential nutrients, secreting toxic substances and forming bacterial layers over tissue surfaces.

SPECIFIC BODY DEFENCES

- The specific body defences (acquired immune system) consist of a variety of cells, especially lymphocytes and macrophages, and various organs.
- When a microbe is able to persist in the tissues, the body reacts by producing a specific immune response.
- The immune response is able to recognise foreign substances, is specific and has memory.
- There are two major populations of lymphocytes: the B lymphocytes (B cells) and T lymphocytes (T cells).
- B cells are mainly responsible for humoral immunity and T cells provide cell-mediated immunity.

- T cells undergo a maturation process under the direction of thymic hormones.
- B cells mature in the bone marrow.
- On the surface of mature lymphocytes there are receptors of a single type, which enable the cells to recognise and bind to a specific antigen.
- The two main populations of T cells involved in the process of cellular immunity are (a) effector cells (called cytotoxic T cells) and (b) regulatory cells (called helper T cells).
- T cells that possess the CD4 marker (CD4 cells or T4 cells) are the T helper cells; T cells with the CD8 marker (CD8 cells or T8 cells) are cytotoxic T cells.
- T helper cells play a central role in the immune response. Once activated by antigen they release cytokines to help B cells and other T cells to respond to antigen.
- Cytotoxic T cells bind directly to and kill target cells. They attack virus– or bacteria-infected cells and tumour cells.
- Antigen-presenting cells play a critical role in activating lymphocytes by presenting processed antigen to them.
- The major antigen-presenting cells are macrophages and dendritic cells.
- The lymphatic system is a network of lymph vessels, cells and specialised organs.
- Immune cells in lymph nodes are in a strategic position to encounter antigens that have entered tissues.
- The secondary lymphoid organs comprise the lymph nodes, spleen, tonsils and clusters of lymphoid cells in mucosal surfaces.

Antigens

- Antigens are present on the surfaces of microorganisms and human and animal cells.
- The major histocompatibility complex (MHC) codes for class I and class II MHC proteins which are vital for cell-to-cell interactions in immune reactions.
- MHC proteins are also called HLA proteins; they are important in organ transplantation.

Humoral immunity

- Macrophages or dendritic cells are usually the first cells to recognise antigen. They act as antigen-presenting cells because they engulf and process antigen for presentation to lymphocytes.
- Each mature B lymphocyte carries molecules of specific antibody (the antigen receptor) on its surface and is activated when an antigen binds to this receptor.
- Following activation, B cells proliferate to expand the number of cells capable of reacting to the particular antigen and then differentiate into plasma cells or long-lived memory B cells.
- Antibodies are secreted by the plasma cells into body fluids.
- The primary immune response is the response of the acquired immune system the first time it is exposed to a particular antigen.
- A secondary immune response occurs if a person is exposed to the same antigen for a second time; this response is faster, stronger and longer-lasting.
- Antibodies (or immunoglobulins) are protective proteins found in blood and other body fluids.

- Five major immunoglobulin classes exist in humans: IgD, IgM, IgG, IgA and IgE.
- The basic function of antibody molecules is to bind specifically with their antigens and form antigen-antibody (or immune) complexes.
- Microorganisms or other particles, when coated with opsonising antibody, become more readily recognised and ingested by phagocytes.
- Antibody attachment, followed by complement fixation, can lead to lysis of foreign cells such as bacteria and cancer cells.
- Neutralisation is a process in which antibodies bind to and block specific attachment sites on viruses or bacterial toxins.

Cell-mediated (cellular) immunity

- The cell-mediated immune response involves the activation, differentiation and actions of different types of T cells.
- When T helper cells are activated by exposure to specific antigen, they secrete a variety of different cytokines.
- Cytotoxic T cells directly attack and kill target cells, especially virus-infected cells.

Active versus passive immunity

- Active immunity is developed when the acquired immune system responds to microorganisms or other foreign substances entering the body.
- Active immunity is naturally acquired during microbial infections, and artificially acquired as a result of vaccination.
- Passive immunity results from the transfer of premade antibodies (or immune cells) from an immune person (or animal) to a non-immune person. The recipient becomes immune, but only for a short time.
- Passive immunity is conferred naturally on a foetus as the mother's antibodies pass across the placenta into the foetal circulation; they are also transferred via colostrum and breast milk.

Immunisation

- Active immunity may be conferred artificially by immunisation (vaccination).
- Most vaccine preparations comprise one of the following: killed, whole microorganisms; live, attenuated microorganisms; inactivated bacterial toxins (toxoids); parts of bacterial cells or viruses.
- Herd immunity is based on the principle that individuals who are immune to an infectious disease will not be carriers of the organism, thus reducing the occurrence of that microbe and the number of susceptible people who will encounter it.

DISORDERS OF THE IMMUNE SYSTEM

- Immunodeficiency includes both inborn and acquired conditions in which the production or function of lymphocytes, phagocytes or complement is abnormal.
- Primary immunodeficiency is due to improper foetal development of one or more of these components.
- Any agent that causes a suppression or malfunction of the bone marrow or lymphoid organs may cause a secondary immunodeficiency.
- The most serious infectious secondary immunodeficiency is

- the acquired immune deficiency syndrome (AIDS), caused by the human immunodeficiency virus (HIV).
- Hypersensitivity is an overreaction of the immune system to an antigen it has previously encountered.
- An immediate hypersensitivity (type I immediate hypersensitivity) or allergy, occurs within minutes to several hours after a sensitised, susceptible person comes into contact with the foreign antigen to which they are allergic.
- IgE molecules have a special affinity for mast cells and basophils and attach to these cells. On subsequent exposure to allergen, the allergen molecules cross-link the IgE antibodies, stimulating the cells to degranulate, releasing histamine and other inflammatory chemicals that induce an inflammatory response.
- Systemic reactions, referred to as anaphylaxis, occur when the allergen enters the blood and circulates through the body.
- Type II cytotoxic hypersensitivity results from the binding of antibodies to antigens on the surface of a cell, followed by complement activation and lysis of the target cell.
- Type III immune complex hypersensitivity results when antigen-antibody complexes are formed and are not cleared quickly from the body by phagocytes. If circulating complexes are deposited on the basement membranes of certain tissues, the complexes activate complement and an inflammatory reaction occurs that can damage the tissues.
- Type IV delayed type hypersensitivity reactions are mediated by T cells and take a day or more to appear after contact with the antigen.
- Occasionally, the immune system loses its ability to distinguish self from non-self; that is, it loses its tolerance to one or more self-antigens.
- When the body produces autoantibodies and sensitised T lymphocytes against its own tissues, disease can result, called an autoimmune disease.

STUDY QUESTIONS

1. What are the major differences between the non-specific and specific defences of the body?
2. What factors make intact skin such an effective barrier against infection?
3. Describe the functions of mucus in preventing infection.
4. What is the mucociliary escalator and what is its function?
5. What are the major phagocytic cells of the body and what are their functions?
6. Describe the process of phagocytosis.
7. What are the major events in acute inflammation, and what are their functions?
8. What are chemical mediators of inflammation?
9. What is pus and what is its significance?
10. Explain the physiological basis of fever.
11. What is complement and what are its functions?
12. Describe the types and activities of interferon.
13. Define the terms: immune system, acquired immune system, immune response.
14. What are the three important characteristics of the acquired immune system?
15. What are the major differences between humoral immunity and cell-mediated immunity?
16. List the primary and secondary lymphoid organs in humans.
17. Distinguish between an antigen, a hapten and an epitope.
18. Describe the functions of plasma cells.
19. Describe the functions of memory cells.
20. Draw a graph showing the major differences between a primary and secondary immune response.
21. Draw a basic antibody molecule showing its antigen-binding sites.
22. What is an antitoxin?
23. Distinguish between gammaglobulin and specific immune globulin.
24. List the major types of T lymphocytes and describe their functions.
25. What is meant by the term 'immunodeficiency'?

26. Give two examples of secondary immunodeficiency.
27. What is meant by the term 'hypersensitivity'?

TEST YOUR UNDERSTANDING

1. Why are regular booster doses needed for some vaccines but not for others?
2. Explain the principle behind the clonal selection theory.
3. A 25-year-old nurse pricks herself with a needle after using it to collect blood from a patient with hepatitis B. She has not been vaccinated against hepatitis B. What prophylactic treatment should she receive, and why?
4. Describe four conditions that would directly reduce a person's non-specific immunity and the effects each of these conditions would have.
5. What is opsonisation? Why is opsonisation important in the defence against microorganisms like *Streptococcus pneumoniae*?

Further reading

Banchereau J & RM Steinman 1998, 'Dendritic cells and the control of immunity', *Nature* 392, p. 245. (This article summarises the important roles of dendritic cells in the immune system.)

Beutler B 2004, 'Innate immunity: an overview', *Molecular Immunology* 40, p. 845. (Reviews the major components of the innate immune system.)

Borish LC & JW Steinke 2003, 'Cytokines and chemokines', *Journal of Allergy and Clinical Immunology* 111, p. S460. (A detailed description of the action of cytokines.)

Chaplin DD 2003, 'Overview of the immune response', *Journal of Allergy and Clinical Immunology* 111, p. S442. (Reviews the functions and the interactions of the major components of the acquired immune system.)

Delves PJ & IM Roitt 2000, 'The immune system', *New England Journal of Medicine* 343, p. 37. (A well written overview of the immune system including innate immune responses.)

Holgate ST 2000, 'Allergic disorders', *British Medical Journal*

320, p. 231. (A review of the underlying mechanisms of allergy and the ways in which allergic reactions may be prevented.)

Janeway CA 1993, 'How the immune system recognises invaders', *Scientific American* 269, p. 41. (A detailed explanation of the basis of antibody diversity.)

Minchinton RM, H Liley & DP Eisen 2004, 'The body as a fortress: innate immune surveillance', *Vox Sanguinis* 87, p. S30. (A review of the innate immune system.)

National Health & Medical Research Council 2003, *The Australian Immunisation Handbook*, 8th edn, Australian Government Department of Health and Ageing. (Provides comprehensive information about vaccines and immunisation procedures as recommended by Australian health authorities.)

Whiteside TL 2003, 'Immune responses to malignancies', *Journal of Allergy and Clinical Immunology* III, p. S677. (Describes the role of the immune system in defence against tumours.)

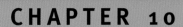

CHAPTER 10

Pathogenic Mechanisms and Evasion Strategies of Microorganisms

- *How do microorganisms cause disease?*

- *What substances do microorganisms produce that enable them to cause disease?*

- *How do microorganisms damage human cells?*

- *How do pathogenic microorganisms evade the defence systems of the body?*

Introduction

Chapter 9 describes the ways in which the human body protects itself against infection and other types of diseases. In this chapter we look at the other end of the balance between infection and health (see Figure 10.1). In order to cause disease, pathogenic microorganisms have to possess properties that enable them to bypass or overcome the host's defences.

As described in Chapter 7, the ability of an organism to cause disease is referred to as its **pathogenicity**. The factors that contribute to an organism's ability to cause disease are called **virulence factors**. The virulence factors of many organisms are either unclear or not known, but for some they are well defined. We examine some of these factors in this chapter.

It should be recognised, as outlined in Chapter 7, that some microorganisms (true pathogens) are able to cause disease in normal hosts, whereas others can only cause disease in hosts whose defences have been compromised in some way (called opportunistic pathogens). The true pathogens have attributes or virulence factors that enable them to cause disease despite the presence of normal defences. It should also be recognised that disease is a complex process which can be due to the activities of the microorganism alone, to the response of the body to infection, or to a combination of both. For example, *Clostridium tetani* causes tetanus by releasing a specific substance that has toxic effects on nerve cells. The symptoms of rheumatic fever, on the other hand, are essentially due to a damaging immune response initiated by *Streptococcus pyogenes*. The pathophysiology of bacterial meningitis appears to be due to focal tissue damage caused by the bacteria as well as the inflammation in the brain tissue induced by the infection.

Most microorganisms enter the human body by way of a mucous membrane or a break in the skin. The routes by which microbes usually enter the body, called portals of entry, are detailed in Chapter 8. In order to establish themselves, most microbes must first adhere to specific tissues within the host. Once inside the body, pathogenic microorganisms may cause damage to the host, and hence disease, in a variety of ways. This usually involves the invasion of tissues and cells and/or the release of substances that cause cell damage or cellular dysfunction. Some microbes have to enter cells to damage them whereas others can cause damage from outside the cell.

As described in Chapter 7, some pathogens enter the lymphatic or circulatory systems and spread to other parts of the body where further foci of infection may be established. In other diseases, the organisms remain localised at or near their site of entry, but cause damage at remote sites by secreting toxic substances which are transported in body fluids to other parts of the body.

Adherence

Adherence is the process by which microorganisms attach to host tissues. Some non-pathogens (e.g. some normal flora organisms) adhere to tissues in a specific way. Adherence is also an important step in the disease process of many pathogenic organisms, particularly those that enter the body via mucous membranes. If, after entering the body, the microorganism is quickly swept away (e.g. as a result of coughing, sneezing or urination), it will be unable to cause infection. Often adherence involves a specific interaction between surface components of a microorganism and surface receptors on host cells. For example, fibronectin, a protein found on the surface of many human cells, is the receptor to which *Streptococcus pyogenes* and some other Gram-positive bacteria attach when colonising the upper respiratory tract.

In some cases, this specific interaction helps to explain why a certain organism can only infect a particular host species and even a particular cell type in that species. It is this specificity that largely determines the potential sites of infection of a given microorganism. This is especially true for viruses, which tend to infect a single type of cell or, at most, a limited number of cell types.

The substances or structures on the surfaces of microorganisms that enable them to attach to cell surfaces are

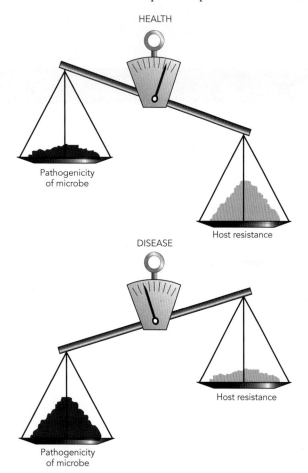

HEALTH

Pathogenicity
of microbe

Host resistance

DISEASE

Host resistance

Pathogenicity
of microbe

Figure 10.1

The balance between disease and health

When the resistance of the host is greater than the pathogenicity of the microbe, the host remains healthy; when the pathogenicity of the microbe is greater than the resistance of the host, disease occurs.

called **adhesins**. The adhesins of some bacteria are specific attachment structures called *pili*, or *fimbriae*, hairlike appendages extending from the cell surface (see Chapter 4). The tip of the pilus (sing.) attaches to specific molecules on the host cell surface. Strains of *Escherichia coli* that cause urinary tract infections have attachment pili that enable them to establish infection in the bladder and kidneys. The piliated strains are much more commonly associated with urinary tract infections than the non-piliated strains; that is, the piliated strains are more virulent. Other strains of *E. coli* that cause diarrhoea adhere specifically to epithelial cells of the small intestine by way of pili (different to those for the urinary tract).

Similarly, pathogenic strains of *Neisseria gonorrhoeae*, the cause of gonorrhoea, have pili which allow them to attach to epithelial cells in the urogenital tract, whereas non-piliated strains of this organism rarely cause disease.

Some bacteria adhere to surfaces by secreting sticky substances. These substances are usually polymers of polysaccharides that form a meshwork of fibrils extending from the cell surface. This type of adhesin is called a **glycocalyx** (or slime layer) (see Figure 10.2). Some bacteria use polysaccharide secretions to form multilayer communities on surfaces, called **biofilms**. Biofilms may contain a single microorganism, but usually there is more than one species involved. The polysaccharide slime cements the bacteria together and to the surface. Dental plaque begins as a bacterial biofilm. *Streptococcus mutans*, one of the organisms responsible for tooth decay, has a glycocalyx composed of the polysaccharide, glucan. The organism attaches to the tooth surface by this sticky layer and, by colonising this site and producing acids, contributes to plaque formation (see Figure 10.3).

Biofilms can also form on medical devices, such as replacement heart valves, endotracheal tubes, central venous catheters and possibly in chronically infected wounds. When involved in infection, bacterial biofilms can be a real problem. They can adhere strongly to surfaces and be difficult to remove. Also the bacteria in biofilm infections are protected from host defences because the glycocalyx forms a physical barrier that defence cells have difficulty in penetrating. Furthermore, the bacteria are much less susceptible to antibiotic therapy because of the diffusion barrier created by the layer of polysaccharide.

Adherence is also important in the pathogenesis of bacterial meningitis. To cause meningitis, bacteria must enter the central nervous system from the bloodstream, and to do this they have to cross the highly specialised capillaries that comprise the blood-brain barrier. Although the exact way in which bacteria cross this barrier is not clear, it is thought that polysaccharide capsules may play a critical role in the attachment of the bacteria to the endothelial cells of the capillaries. Indeed, pathogenic strains of the three important causes of acute bacterial meningitis – *Neisseria meningitidis*, *Haemophilus influenzae* and *Streptococcus pneumoniae* – are all encapsulated.

Viruses attach to specific membrane receptors on the cells they infect. Some have specialised attachment structures like tail fibres (as in bacteriophages) or envelope spikes (see Chapter 5). Generally, the presence of a particular receptor on the membrane of a cell is the key determinant of whether a particular virus can infect that cell or not. For example, the human immunodeficiency virus (HIV) preferentially infects cells that possess a glycoprotein called the CD4 receptor on their surfaces (see Chapter 19). This receptor is found mainly on T helper lymphocytes, which are therefore the major targets for this virus. Many parasitic helminths fasten to host tissues by way of suckers or hooks (see Chapter 6). Similarly, the

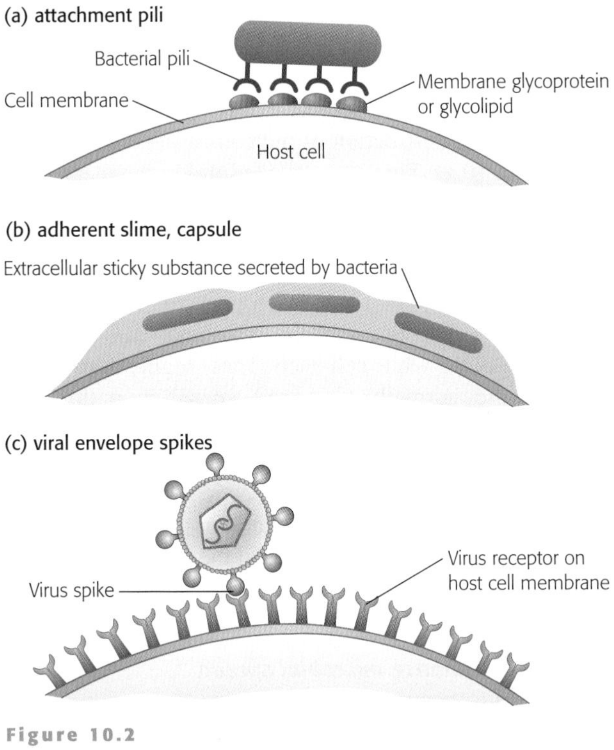

(a) attachment pili

Bacterial pili

Cell membrane

Membrane glycoprotein or glycolipid

Host cell

(b) adherent slime, capsule

Extracellular sticky substance secreted by bacteria

(c) viral envelope spikes

Virus spike

Virus receptor on host cell membrane

Figure 10.2

Mechanisms of adherence of pathogenic microorganisms

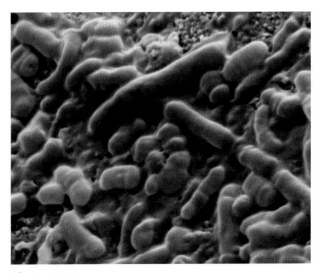

Figure 10.3

Micrograph of dental plaque

protozoan *Giardia intestinalis* attaches to epithelial cells lining the intestine via an adhesive disc.

Toxins

Toxins are substances produced by some microorganisms that interfere with the normal functioning of host cells or tissues. They do this either by directly damaging cells or tissues or by altering normal cellular processes. Not all microorganisms produce toxins, but the production and release of toxins are, for some, the most important determinants of their ability to damage tissues and thus cause disease. A loss of their ability to produce toxins results in their loss of pathogenicity. We know most about bacterial toxins, but still only understand in detail the action of some of them. Some species of protozoa, fungi and helminths also produce toxins. Viruses do not produce toxins but cause cell damage by other means.

Bacterial toxins are classically divided into two broad groups:

1. **Exotoxins** are toxins secreted into the environment in which the bacteria are growing (e.g. host tissues, food, soil, water).
2. **Endotoxins** are toxins that form part of the outer membrane of Gram-negative bacteria; they are not actively secreted but are released when the bacterial cell is damaged or lysed.

EXOTOXINS

Exotoxins are heat-labile proteins that are usually released as the organism grows, although in some spore-forming bacteria, like the clostridia, toxin release occurs as a by-product of spore formation. While many different forms of toxins exist, there is a general structure to which a number conform. This is a *two-subunit* structure: one subunit is responsible for initial binding of the toxin to the target cell and its entry into the cell; and the other subunit is responsible for the inhibition or alteration of some cellular function.

Some bacteria produce a single exotoxin, and the major manifestations of the disease are due to the action of that toxin. Others produce many toxins, which have a number of different effects on the host. The more common exotoxin-producing bacteria are listed in Table 10.1. Some exotoxins are extremely potent and include some of the strongest poisons known. One gram of botulinum toxin, for example, is sufficient to kill 10 million people, and 300 grams would be enough to kill the entire population of the world! The tetanus and *Shigella* toxins are also very potent.

Most bacteria secrete their toxins while growing in the host. But some, like *Clostridium botulinum* and *Staphylococcus aureus*, secrete their toxins into food and the preformed toxin is ingested when a person eats the contaminated food. To produce disease these organisms don't need to grow inside the host. In fact, they don't survive well in the body even when ingested. Since the toxin is responsible for disease, and not the growth of the organism

itself, this type of disease is often referred to as an **intoxication**, rather than infection.

Bacterial exotoxins vary greatly in their degree of specificity. Some affect a wide range of cells and tissues. Others have specific targets and are sometimes grouped and named according to the tissues they primarily affect. The major groups are **neurotoxins**, which act predominantly on nervous tissue, and **enterotoxins**, which act specifically on the small intestine. The term **toxaemia** refers to the presence of toxins in the bloodstream.

For a clear understanding of how exotoxins produce disease, it is most appropriate to examine them in terms of their mode of action; that is, what the toxins actually do to damage the host tissues or interfere with normal processes.

Toxins that break down cells

A large number of exotoxins act by damaging host cell membranes, resulting in lysis and death of the cells. Some of these toxins are phospholipases, like the α-toxin of *Clostridium perfringens*, a cause of gas gangrene. Phospholipase enzymes lyse cells by hydrolysing the phospholipid lecithin (phosphatidylcholine), a common component of mammalian cell membranes. Other lytic toxins damage host cell membranes by inserting themselves into the cell membrane, creating pores or channels. The membrane becomes more permeable to water and, because of the higher solute concentration of the cytoplasm compared to the environment, water rushes into the cell, causing it to swell and rupture. The α-toxin of *Staphylococcus aureus* and the streptolysin-O of *Streptococcus pyogenes* are examples of pore-forming toxins.

Many phospholipase and pore-forming types of toxins damage red blood cells and are therefore referred to as **haemolysins**, although they can break down other cells as well. When bacteria that secrete haemolysins are grown on culture media containing blood (e.g. sheep blood agar), distinct zones of red cell clearing can be seen around the bacterial colonies. The soluble exotoxins diffuse into the agar and cause destruction of red cells around the colony (see Figure 10.4). This property is useful in the identification of some bacteria.

Some bacteria, such as *S. aureus* and *S. pyogenes*, secrete toxins called **leukocidins** that kill phagocytic leukocytes (neutrophils and macrophages). These leukocidins induce the release of the lysosomal enzymes into the cytosol of the white cell itself. These highly destructive enzymes are normally packaged up safely within the lysosomal membrane but, once released into the cytosol, cause lethal damage to the cell by breaking down cellular components. Destruction of phagocytic white cells in this way increases the ability of leukocidin-producing organisms to survive and persist longer in the body. In addition, release of the lysosomal enzymes from dead phagocytes can cause further damage to the surrounding tissue.

Toxins that enhance microbial spread or survival in tissues

Many bacteria secrete enzymes that break down tissues. These enzymes increase the *invasiveness* of bacteria by

Table 10.1
Examples of diseases caused by exotoxins

ORGANISM AND DISEASE	EXOTOXIN	ACTION OF TOXIN	SYMPTOMS PRODUCED
Bacillus anthracis (anthrax)	cytotoxin	Increases vascular permeability	Pulmonary oedema
Bordetella pertussis (whooping cough)	pertussis toxin	Damages respiratory mucosal cells	Paroxysmal cough
Clostridium botulinum (botulism)	neurotoxin	Blocks acetylcholine release at neuromuscular junctions	Flaccid paralysis
Clostridium perfringens (gas gangrene, food poisoning)	α-toxin enterotoxin	Lysis of various cell types Causes excessive loss of fluid and electrolytes from intestinal cells	Tissue destruction Diarrhoea
Clostridium tetani (tetanus)	tetanus toxin	Interferes with transmission in inhibitory interneurones	Severe muscle spasm
Corynebacterium diphtheriae (diphtheria)	diphtheria toxin	Damages many cell types by stopping protein synthesis	Damage to throat, heart, and nerve tissue
Entamoeba histolytica (amoebic dysentery)	enterotoxin	Lysis of epithelial cells lining the colon	Bloody, mucoid diarrhoea
Escherichia coli (gastroenteritis)	enterotoxin	Causes loss of fluid and electrolytes from intestinal cells	Diarrhoea
Listeria monocytogenes (listeriosis)	listeriolysin	Lysis of many cell types	Tissue damage, loss of red cells and white cells
Pseudomonas aeruginosa (various infections)	exotoxin A	Inhibits protein synthesis in cells	Tissue damage
Shigella dysenteriae (dysentery)	shiga toxin	Inhibits protein synthesis in many cell types	Bloody diarrhoea
Staphylococcus aureus (various infections)	α-toxin leukocidin enterotoxin exfoliatin TSST-1	Lysis of red and white cells Kills white cells Stimulates intestinal cells Unclear Stimulates T cells to release cytokines	Infection and abscess Infection and abscess Vomiting, diarrhoea Scalded skin syndrome Toxic shock syndrome
Streptococcus pyogenes (scarlet fever and other infections)	pyrogenic exotoxin streptolysin O and S	Vasodilation of skin capillaries Lysis of red and white cells	Diffuse rash and fever Tissue damage
Vibrio cholerae (cholera)	cholera toxin	Causes severe loss of fluid and electrolytes from intestinal cells	Profuse diarrhoea

breaking down substances that would otherwise impede their spread through tissues. **Hyaluronidases** are produced by many bacteria, including staphylococci, streptococci and clostridia. These enzymes break down hyaluronic acid, a component of the ground substance of virtually all connective tissue, making the tissue less viscous and easier to penetrate. **Collagenases** are enzymes that break down collagen, the tough fibres that give strength and a supporting network to connective tissues. *C. perfringens* and some helminths (worms) are examples of organisms that secrete collagenases.

Skin is a highly protective coating against microbial infection, due mainly to the presence of the relatively indigestible protein called *keratin*. However, the fungi that cause tinea (ringworm) are able to infect skin because they secrete a keratin-degrading enzyme, or **keratinase**. Some organisms (e.g. *Vibrio cholerae*) secrete a **mucinase** which digests a glycoprotein in mucus, thereby enhancing their ability to colonise mucous membranes.

The body's defence against local infection sometimes involves the deposition of a layer of fibrin around the infected site. This is designed to wall off the infection, preventing the spread of microorganisms into adjacent tissue. **Kinases** are a group of enzymes produced by certain bacteria that help them to dissolve fibrin clots and hence break through this barrier. **Streptokinase** is produced by some streptococci, including *S. pyogenes*, and **staphylokinase** is produced by *S. aureus*. Streptokinase is in fact used therapeutically as a thrombolytic agent that breaks down blood clots in patients with thromboses (see Spotlight box, page 222).

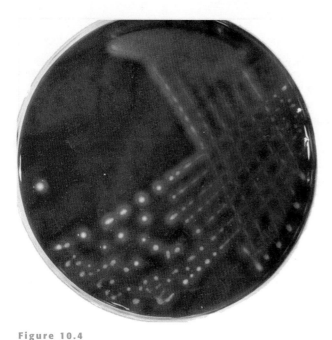

Figure 10.4
Bacterial haemolysis
Clearing or complete haemolysis of blood in the agar caused by colonies of *Streptococcus pyogenes*.

Coagulase is an enzyme produced by some staphylococci that has almost the opposite effect to kinases. This enzyme coagulates fibrinogen to form a deposit of fibrin material around the bacterial cells, and this is thought to offer them some protection against host phagocytic cells. The pathogenicity of staphylococci depends largely on their ability to produce coagulase. Some coagulase-negative staphylococci are pathogenic, but generally they are less frequently associated with disease than the coagulase-positive species.

SPOTLIGHT ON
Streptokinase

Streptokinase is an enzyme produced by some streptococci that breaks down fibrin clots by converting plasminogen into the proteolytic enzyme, plasmin. Streptokinase assists the bacteria to spread and produce disease, but a therapeutic use for the enzyme has been uncovered.

Because of its action in breaking down thrombi (blood clots), streptokinase is used in patients with disorders where clots may develop and obstruct vital blood vessels. Its use is thus indicated in patients with acute myocardial infarction, pulmonary embolism or arterial thrombosis.

Streptokinase, however, is a foreign protein and so a patient may develop some immunity to the substance. For this reason, it may not be effective in patients who have previously been administered with the substance or who have recently had a streptococcal infection. Its use is contraindicated in people with an existing or recent haemorrhagic (bleeding) disorder.

Toxins that interfere with cellular functions

There are several toxins that enter cells and alter the cell's metabolism in some way. The toxin of *Corynebacterium diphtheriae* is one of the best understood of all bacterial toxins. The toxin first binds to a receptor on the host cell membrane and then enters the cell by an endocytotic process. The toxin blocks protein synthesis by inactivating elongation factor 2, an enzyme necessary for the growth of the polypeptide chain in translation. The cell dies because it can no longer synthesise proteins. The pathogenicity of *C. diphtheriae* is entirely due to this toxin; strains that do not have the gene for toxin production are non-pathogenic.

Although *C. diphtheriae* remains localised in the throat during the infection, the secreted toxin is absorbed and enters the bloodstream. The actions of the toxin in the throat cause considerable damage to mucosal cells, resulting in a membrane (called a pseudomembrane) over the mucosal surface, consisting of fibrin, bacteria and inflammatory cells. When the larynx is involved, a life-threatening obstruction of the airway can occur (see Chapter 17). The action of diphtheria toxin on other organs, especially the heart, can result in irregular heartbeat, coma and death.

The exotoxin A of *Pseudomonas aeruginosa* appears to have a similar action on protein synthesis to that of diphtheria toxin.

The enterotoxin of *Vibrio cholerae*, the causative agent of cholera, is an exotoxin that alters the regulatory control in cells, rather than directly damaging them. Cholera toxin binds specifically to intestinal epithelial cells. It then enters the cell and causes increased and uncontrolled production of cyclic AMP, the mediator of a number of regulatory systems in cells. The increased levels of cyclic AMP cause unregulated secretion of chloride and bicarbonate ions from the epithelial cells lining the intestine. This change in ionic balance results in a massive outflow of water from the cells into the lumen of the intestine, manifested as a profuse diarrhoea (see Figure 10.5).

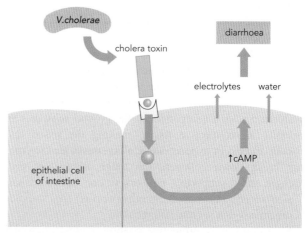

Figure 10.5
The mode of action of cholera toxin
The toxin increases cyclic AMP production in epithelial cells of the intestine. This results in an outflow of water and ions from these cells, producing diarrhoea.

The loss of water can be so great that cholera victims may die from extreme dehydration if their fluids and electrolytes are not replaced. The toxins of enteropathogenic *Escherichia coli* and *Salmonella* are believed to have a similar action.

Toxins that affect the nervous system

The neurotoxins of the anaerobic bacteria *Clostridium tetani* and *Clostridium botulinum* are two of the most potent toxins known. *Clostridium tetani* usually grows in deep, necrotic puncture wounds where anaerobic conditions exist. The bacterium itself does not spread far from the initial site of infection, but the exotoxin that it secretes travels to the central nervous system to cause severe neuromuscular dysfunction.

Cl. tetani is a good example of an organism that produces only a single toxin. The toxin, called *tetanospasmin*, binds to the surface of nerve cells, is internalised and then transported to the spinal cord, where it becomes fixed to nerve synapses. It interferes specifically with synaptic transmission in inhibitory interneurones, creating an imbalance in the excitatory and inhibitory transmissions to motor neurones. This causes an excessive stimulation of muscles, resulting in an uncontrolled, rigid muscle contraction, or spastic paralysis. Different muscles may be affected, such as the powerful masseter muscles of the jaw, resulting in the classic condition of tetanus known as *lockjaw*. Often, back muscles are affected, causing arching of the back and sometimes even crushing of spinal processes in severe cases (see Figure 20.7, page 494).

Botulism occurs when the preformed toxin of *Cl. botulinum* is ingested in contaminated food. The organism itself normally causes no problem if ingested because it is unable to compete successfully with the normal gut flora. Botulism is therefore usually an intoxication, caused by toxins produced outside the body, rather than an infectious disease. The botulinum toxin is resistant to gastrointestinal digestion. After ingestion it crosses the gut wall and ultimately localises at neuromuscular junctions.

Infant botulism is different in that growth of the clostridia and production of botulinum toxin occur in the colon. In this disease the clostridia are able to grow and produce toxin because the infant colon has a poorly developed microbial flora which is unable to inhibit the pathogen.

In contrast to tetanus toxin, botulinum toxin acts on peripheral nerve endings. At neuromuscular junctions the toxin binds to presynaptic terminal membranes and inhibits the release of acetylcholine, preventing transmission of impulses from the nerve cell to the muscle cell, and hence markedly reducing muscle contraction (see Figure 10.6). This flaccid paralysis in botulism can lead to the death of the patient due to dysfunction of the respiratory muscles and respiratory failure.

Some strains of *Staphylococcus aureus* can produce enterotoxins in foods they contaminate. After the toxins are ingested they are absorbed in the intestine and then stimulate neural receptors that activate the vomiting centre in the central nervous system. Projectile vomiting can result.

TOXOIDS AND ANTITOXINS

Exotoxins are proteins and, as such, are usually antigenic; that is, they are capable of stimulating the production of antitoxins by the immune system (see Chapter 9). An **antitoxin** is a specific antibody produced against a toxin; it is able to bind to the toxin and neutralise it, thereby preventing it from binding to its target cell or tissue. Exotoxins are thus effective immunogens, but of course cannot be used in their natural form in vaccines. Fortunately, many exotoxins can be modified by heat or chemicals, such as formaldehyde or phenol, to remove their toxicity but still retain their ability to elicit an immune response.

Toxins modified in this way are called **toxoids** and are used in vaccines to stimulate immunity without causing disease. Toxoids are particularly useful in vaccines when the toxin is the major (or only) virulence factor of the organism. Toxoids for diphtheria and tetanus are used in the combined diphtheria-pertussis-tetanus (DPT) vaccine.

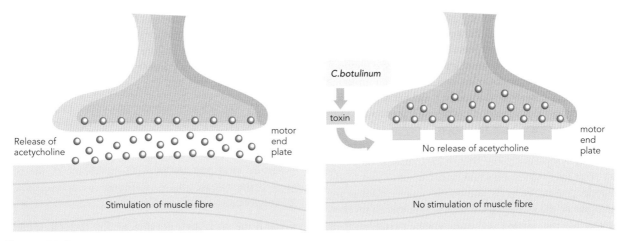

Figure 10.6

The mode of action of botulinum toxin
The toxin blocks the release of acetylcholine at the neuromuscular junction, causing a flaccid paralysis.

It is interesting to note that in some diseases, such as tetanus, so little toxin is required to produce the symptoms of disease that the person's immune system may not be sufficiently stimulated by the toxin to produce antibodies. That is, the clinical disease does not confer immunity, and a person who survives clinical tetanus may not subsequently be immune to the disease unless actively immunised.

The treatment of diseases caused by exotoxin-producing bacteria sometimes involves the use of antitoxins to neutralise the toxin already in the body. Antitoxins are usually derived from the serum of immune humans or animals. They are particularly important for diseases such as tetanus and botulism, which can have a rapidly fatal outcome. Injection of specific antitoxin (also called **specific immunoglobulin**) is aimed at immediate neutralisation of the toxin before it is able to bind to target cells.

Without antitoxin, patients may die because their immune system does not have sufficient time to make the required antibodies. Thorough excision and cleansing of the wound and appropriate antibiotic therapy are important for the elimination of tetanus organisms from the wound, but are of secondary importance to antitoxin therapy. Antibiotics are not necessary in botulism at all, since the organism does not survive inside the body.

ENDOTOXINS

Endotoxins are the lipopolysaccharides (LPS) of the cell walls of Gram-negative bacteria. As described in Chapter 4, the outer membrane of the Gram-negative cell wall contains LPS. The exact composition of LPS varies from genus to genus and species to species. The lipid A portion of LPS is the actively toxic component. Being a part of the bacterial cell wall, endotoxins only exert their effect once the cell wall breaks down. During infection, small amounts of LPS may be sloughed off as cells grow or may be released as older bacterial cells die. Death of bacteria and release of endotoxin can be greatly accelerated once phagocytes begin to digest them or antibiotics that kill the bacteria are administered. Thus, in some cases, antibiotics may initially increase LPS release and thus cause a worsening of symptoms in the short term.

Other major differences between exotoxins and endotoxins are that the latter are generally less toxic, relatively heat-stable and cannot be made into toxoids (see previous section). Although endotoxins can induce an immune response, they cannot be treated in a similar way to exotoxins to render them non-toxic while still preserving their ability to induce antibody formation.

Endotoxin, regardless of its source, produces similar signs and symptoms in the host. It can cause a variety of host responses, many of which involve some part of the immune system. Fever is one of the more common and important of the symptoms. Endotoxin produces fever by stimulating the release of endogenous pyrogens from mononuclear phagocytes. Currently, the best known of these pyrogens are the cytokines interleukin-1 (IL-1) and tumour necrosis factor (TNF) (see Chapter 9). These act on the temperature-regulating centre in the hypothalamus to reset the body temperature set-point (or thermostat) to a higher level, resulting in an increase in body temperature. Other possible responses of the host to endotoxin include muscle weakness, generalised aches, diarrhoea and malaise.

Large amounts of endotoxin may be released during systemic infection caused by Gram-negative bacteria such as *E. coli*, *Neisseria meningitidis* and *Pseudomonas aeruginosa*. This can have severe effects on the body. **Endotoxic** (or **septic**) **shock**, the shock caused by large amounts of endotoxin, is frequently fatal. In this situation, endotoxin is believed to induce the release of cytokines from a variety of cells, including monocytes, macrophages and lymphocytes. The systemic release of large amounts of cytokines causes damage to blood capillaries and alters their permeability characteristics. Large amounts of fluid leak into the tissues, causing a severe drop in blood pressure, resulting in shock. The complement system is activated (see Chapter 9) causing further inflammation.

Septic shock due to Gram-positive bacteria and other organisms is thought to be caused by a similar triggering of cytokine release from host cells.

Endotoxin may also cause a non-specific activation of blood-coagulation mechanisms, resulting in the blockage of small vessels by thrombi in organs such as the kidney, brain and lungs. Tissue necrosis in the blood-deprived areas of these organs (infarction) may then occur. This potentially fatal disorder is referred to as **disseminated intravascular coagulation**. In rare cases of *N. meningitidis* infection, infarction of adrenal glands can occur (called the Waterhouse-Friderichsen syndrome – see Chapter 20), leading to a rapid death.

Invasion of cells

Viruses typically cause disease by invading and damaging host cells. As explained in Chapter 5, viruses are obligate intracellular parasites and are able to replicate only inside their specific target cells. Once inside the cell a virus can cause changes to the cell, called **cytopathic effects** (CPE). Different viruses cause different CPE in cells, and some of these can be observed by microscopic examination of the viruses grown in tissue culture (see Figure 10.7). Some viruses kill the cells they infect and are said to be *cytocidal*. They can do this by:

- diverting the cell's metabolic processes and stopping the synthesis of proteins or other macromolecules
- causing the release of lysosomal enzymes into the cytoplasm of the cell
- inserting viral proteins into the membrane of the cell during the release phase, resulting in rupture of the membrane and cell lysis.

Even if the virus does not directly kill the cell, it takes control of the regulatory mechanisms of the cell and produces viral proteins and nucleic acids, causing the cell to become dysfunctional. Some non-cytocidal viruses cause

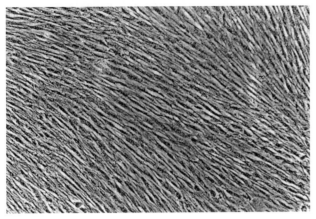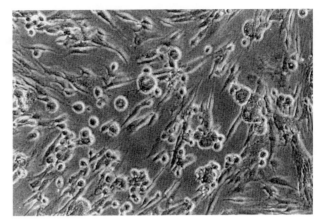

Figure 10.7

Cytopathic effects caused by viruses
(a) Uninfected fibroblasts; and (b) the same cells after being infected with herpes virus.

CPE characterised by the formation of inclusion bodies within the cell, such as the Negri bodies found in the brain cells of humans and animals infected with the rabies virus. These inclusion bodies are granules of unassembled viral components or deposits of viral remnants.

Other viruses cause host cells to fuse with each other, producing multi-nucleated 'giant cells' (e.g. measles virus and respiratory syncytial virus). Eventually, the accumulated damage to the cell results in its death. However, some viruses, like the herpes simplex viruses, do not kill the cell; instead they remain dormant inside the cell for long periods, sometimes for life. These highly adapted parasites cause minimal damage to the nerve cells they infect, allowing them to remain there for years. Sometimes the viruses are reactivated many years later and cause symptomatic disease (e.g. the herpes zoster virus and shingles).

Another important effect is the viral transformation of normal cells into cancer cells. This is discussed in the following section.

A few other organisms, apart from viruses, also invade cells and damage them. For example, *Chlamydia* are bacteria that are obligate intracellular parasites. They enter epithelial cells and multiply quickly, lysing these cells within a couple of days. *Rickettsia* are also obligate intracellular bacteria which can invade many types of mammalian cells, especially vascular endothelium. They grow slowly in these cells, eventually breaking them open to release large numbers of organisms. *Plasmodium* spp., the causative agents of malaria, typically go through cycles of red blood cell invasion, multiplication, lysis of the red cells with release of large numbers of the merozoite form into the bloodstream, and then infection of many more red cells.

Cellular transformation into tumour cells

Some viruses cause disease by transforming host cells into tumour cells. Transformed cells differ markedly from normal cells in a number of ways. Typically, they have an altered morphology and do not have an ordered pattern of growth. Instead, they divide in an unregulated manner and form random aggregations of dysfunctional cells. These cells are not responsive to normal growth-regulating factors. Some human papillomaviruses (e.g. HPV 1, 2, 3 and 10) cause cutaneous warts, which are benign tumours. Other viruses are believed to be involved in malignant tumours, such as HPV types 16, 18, 31 and 33 in cervical cancer, and hepatitis B and C viruses in hepatocellular carcinoma.

Transformation of cells is brought about by the incorporation of viral nucleic acid into the host cell genome, which is then replicated along with the cell's DNA. The tumour-causing viruses and their relationship to oncogenes are described in Chapter 5.

Other mechanisms of pathogenesis

Microorganisms can cause disease in a variety of other ways. Sometimes, the clinical features of a disease arise from the physiological responses of the host to infection. For example, the major disease symptoms may be due to an abnormal response of the immune system. If the invading organism causes the host's immune response to be 'overreactive', then tissue damage may occur. This overreactivity of the immune system is referred to as **hypersensitivity**, and is the basis of many important diseases. For example, many pathogenic helminths release waste products during infection that induce allergic reactions. The bases of hypersensitivity reactions are described in Chapter 9. Examples of hypersensitivity reactions induced by microorganisms are listed in Table 10.2.

Another way in which microorganisms can cause damage is by inducing autoimmunity. If microbes can confuse the immune system so that self-tissues appear foreign to it, then the immune system may attack those tissues and produce an autoimmune disease. Some strains of *Streptococcus pyogenes* have antigens that cross-react with heart muscle and can cause a type of autoimmune disease called rheumatic fever (see Chapter 19).

Some microorganisms produce substances that non-specifically and indiscriminately activate large numbers of

Table 10.2

Hypersensitivity reactions induced by microorganisms

TYPE OF HYPERSENSITIVITY INDUCED	EXAMPLES
Allergy/anaphylaxis	Some helminths, e.g. *Ascaris*
Cytotoxic hypersensitivity	Hepatitis B
Immune complex disease	Malaria
	Acute glomerulonephritis (*Streptococcus pyogenes*)
	Syphilis
	Allergic alveolitis
Cell-mediated hypersensitivity	Tuberculosis
	Leprosy
	Tertiary syphilis
	Viral rashes

T cells. These substances are called **superantigens**. The activation of large numbers of T cells is believed to result in a massive release of cytokines (including interleukin-1 and tumour necrosis factor) that can cause injury to host tissues and septic shock, as well as suppressing normal immune responses. Enterotoxins of some strains of *Staphylococcus aureus*, the toxic shock syndrome toxin-1 (TSST-1) of other strains of *Staphylococcus aureus* and some exotoxins of *Streptococcus pyogenes* are examples of superantigens.

Microorganisms may also cause tissue damage by physical means. For example, a mass of *Ascaris* worms in the intestinal tract may cause obstruction. The larvae of a number of pathogenic helminths cause damage by blocking the flow of blood in small vessels, thus reducing the amount of oxygen and other nutrients to the adjacent tissues. In some diseases, other narrow, tubular structures such as lymph vessels may be obstructed, such as occurs in elephantiasis, caused by the nematode *Wuchereira*.

Clostridium perfringens, the major cause of gas gangrene, produces gas in the tissues where it is growing. The gas causes compression of the tissue and blood vessels in the area. The resultant lack of oxygen in the site allows further growth of this anaerobic bacterium, causing more tissue necrosis. These physical effects may then be aggravated by the body's inflammatory response to infection, in particular the exudation of fluid from the blood into the injured tissue. This fluid may compress the tissue further, causing more damage.

Evasion strategies

When a microorganism invades the body it usually faces a hostile response from the host. The human body has developed numerous mechanisms by which it defends itself against microbial invasion and these are mobilised when organisms gain entry. However, many microbes are known to possess special structures or attributes that protect them from the host's defences. Although these microbial countermeasures do not directly cause tissue damage, some are nevertheless largely responsible for the organism's pathogenicity, or capacity to cause disease.

ESCAPE FROM PHAGOCYTES

Phagocytes are vital components of the body's defence system. They are responsible for scouring the body's tissues, searching for foreign substances and microbes, which they then engulf and destroy. Their critical role in defence is described in Chapter 9. Many microorganisms have developed ways of escaping phagocytosis by blocking or avoiding some part of the phagocytic process. Indeed, the large variety of ways that microbes have developed to avoid being phagocytosed reflects the importance of phagocytosis in defending the body.

You will recall from Chapter 9 that phagocytosis involves:

1. attraction (chemotaxis) of phagocytes to the site of infection
2. binding of the phagocyte to the microbe, followed by ingestion and containment of it within a membrane-bound vesicle called a phagosome
3. fusion of lysosomes with the phagosome to form a phagolysosome
4. destruction of the microbe by a variety of toxic substances and degradative lysosomal enzymes.

Avoidance of, or interference with, one of these steps can allow a microbe to escape destruction by these cells.

A few bacteria, such as *Bordetella pertussis*, the cause of whooping cough, produce factors that inhibit leucocyte chemotaxis. Some organisms possess capsules or a surface slime layer (see Chapter 4) which prevents the phagocytes from ingesting them. The chemical composition of these structures prevents binding of the phagocyte. *Streptococcus pneumoniae* appears to lack any major virulence factor other than its capsule, but this enables it to avoid being ingested by alveolar macrophages, and thus to survive and multiply in the lungs. Mutant strains of the organism that do not have a capsule are unable to cause disease.

Other organisms that rely on an antiphagocytic capsule for pathogenicity include *Haemophilus influenzae*, *Neisseria meningitidis*, *Yersinia pestis* and *Cryptococcus neoformans*, the yeast that causes meningitis.

Host immunity to these organisms is based on the production of specific anti-capsular antibodies, which opsonise the bacteria and permit the phagocytes to engulf them (see Chapter 9). Instead of a capsule, *Streptococcus pyogenes* has a cell wall component, termed an M-protein, which helps it to avoid ingestion by phagocytes by interfering with complement-mediated opsonisation (see Chapter 9).

Some microorganisms allow themselves to be ingested by phagocytes but have developed ways of surviving inside them. Not only does this allow them to avoid destruction, but the phagocytes provide them with a place to hide and multiply and may even help them to spread through the body. Some organisms, like *Listeria monocytogenes* and *Mycobacterium leprae*, appear to avoid being digested by exiting the phagosome and entering the cytoplasm of the phagocyte. This is a privileged site since lysosomes do not normally release their enzymes and toxins into the cytoplasm.

Other organisms, like *Mycobacterium tuberculosis* and *Legionella pneumophila*, avoid intracellular digestion by inhibiting the fusion of lysosomes with the phagosome. The protozoan, *Toxoplasma gondii*, actively attaches to macrophages, inducing its own phagocytosis. It then prevents lysosomal fusion and multiplies within the cell, eventually killing it. *Staphylococcus aureus* resists intracellular killing by producing the enzyme **catalase**, which breaks down hydrogen peroxide, one of the substances phagocytes produce to kill microbes.

Still other organisms, like the protozoa *Leishmania*, are innately resistant to lysosomal enzymes and can survive in the phagolysosome. Such organisms probably have resistant cell surface structures and/or secrete substances that inhibit the lysosomal enzymes.

The most aggressive strategy is to kill the phagocyte. As stated earlier in this chapter, certain bacteria, such as staphylococci and streptococci, secrete toxins called leukocidins, which kill phagocytes as well as other cells.

CONCEALMENT

Some microorganisms evade the host defences by hiding, usually inside cells or in other so-called 'privileged sites', where defence cells do not normally circulate. If a microorganism can remain inside a cell, without any sign of its antigens on the surface of the cell, it will be invisible to defence cells. Even if specific immune responses are induced before the organism invades the cells, once inside, the antibodies or activated immune cells would be ineffective against these hidden enemies. Fortunately, in most cases, antigens of the microbe are displayed on the cell surface after it infects the cell. This allows components of the immune system (especially cytotoxic T cells and natural killer cells – see Chapter 9) to recognise the infected cells and destroy them, thereby exposing the microbes to other immune factors.

In latent viral infections, however, the viruses inhibit the display of their antigens on the infected cell surface. The herpes simplex and varicella zoster viruses can remain in this way in sensory neurones for years, sometimes for a lifetime, despite the presence of specific immunity. Retroviruses, like the human immunodeficiency virus (HIV), are also thought to remain hidden in lymphoid cells or macrophages by first having their RNA transcribed into DNA and then having this integrated into the cell's DNA. Again, as long as there is no display of viral antigens on the surface of the cell, the virus remains undetected.

The cytomegalovirus protects itself from natural killer cells by displaying an imitation of host self-recognition antigens on the surface of the host cells it infects. Malaria parasites spend some of their time inside liver cells (see Chapter 19). During this latent period they avoid presenting a target for the immune system.

Other privileged sites include those areas of the body where complement, antibodies and lymphocyte activity are low. A good example is the central nervous system (CNS). Complement and antibody levels are very low in cerebrospinal fluid (CSF), and there are few white cells. Even though white cells may enter the CNS during infection, their activity appears to be limited by the lack of opsonic antibodies and complement proteins. Other such privileged sites include the joints and testes.

Some microorganisms are able to create their own privileged sites. Hydatid disease is caused by *Echinococcus granulosus*, a tiny tapeworm that can infect the liver, lung or brain. This parasite evades host defences by forming and residing within thin-walled capsules that resemble small bladders (see Figure 10.8). The worms can survive inside these fluid-filled cysts, even if there are protective antibodies in the blood of the patient. A connective tissue coating of host origin around the cyst prevents it from being attacked by host defences.

The blood fluke, *Schistosoma*, conceals itself by becoming coated with plasma glycoproteins and glycolipids. These host substances are not recognised as foreign and the worm escapes detection. *Toxoplasma gondii* forms cysts within macrophages of the nervous system and

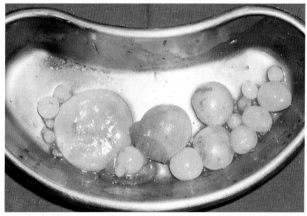

Figure 10.8

Hydatid cysts
Hydatid cysts are thin, fluid-filled sacs produced by the tapeworm *Echinococcus granulosus*. The worms hide from the body's defences by residing inside cysts.

lungs. Within these cysts the protozoan avoids stimulating the immune system.

ANTIGENIC VARIATION

Antigenic variation is a phenomenon in which some bacteria, viruses and protozoa repeatedly or progressively change their cell surface components, or antigens. If the microbe changes the antigens to which immune responses have been developed, it will be unaffected by any immunity directed at those original antigens. Microorganisms contain numerous antigens, but immunity to only some of these is protective. That is, the strategy of changing antigens to escape host defences depends on changes being made to critical antigens against which protective immune responses are directed. Antigenic variation can occur during the course of infection, enabling the organism to persist longer, or it may occur as the organism spreads through the community, allowing it to reinfect the same individual over time (see Figure 10.9). The ways in which microbial antigens can be changed are antigenic drift, antigenic shift and gene switching.

Antigenic drift is the term used for repeated minor mutations in the genes that code for antigens of microorganisms. The antigens are sufficiently critical, and the mutations change them sufficiently, to reduce the effectiveness of prior immunological memory, allowing the organism to cause infection again, despite immunity in the host to a prior infection. The influenza virus is the classic example of this. The tendency for influenza to occur repeatedly in a population and in an individual is due partly to the ability of influenza viruses to undergo antigenic drift. The influenza viruses have two surface glycoprotein antigens (the haemagglutinin and neuraminidase 'spikes') to which neutralising antibodies are formed. Antigenic drift can occur when minor mutations in DNA result in small changes in the amino acid sequence of these antigens. If the changes occur in areas where antibodies bind to the antigen, the virus is not susceptible to antibodies produced in previous infections. The cold viruses (rhinoviruses) have a similar ability.

We can thus have the flu or a cold year after year, partly because of antigenic changes to the viruses that cause them.

The HIV is also capable of antigenic drift, while it is infecting a person. This is thought to occur partly because the infection persists for so long, and partly because the viral reverse transcriptase is prone to making mistakes in transcribing RNA into DNA. This antigenic drift may be part of the reason why the immune system is so ineffective in controlling this infection.

Antigenic shift is displayed by the influenza A virus. When two different strains of this virus infect the same cell, a recombination of the genes that code for the surface glycoproteins can occur. This results in a new strain, different to previous strains, which can spread through a population because of the lack of protective antibodies in the population. Major pandemics of influenza in 1957, 1968 and 1977 are thought to have been due to the sudden appearance of a new strain of influenza A, as a result of antigenic shift.

Another form of antigenic variation results from the ability of some microorganisms to switch the genes (gene switching) that code for certain surface antigens. The best known example of this occurs in the protozoa that cause African sleeping sickness, the *Trypanosoma*. These organisms are covered with a thick coat made of proteins called 'variable surface glycoproteins'. These protozoa carry genes for hundreds of distinct surface glycoproteins, but only one is expressed at any given time. Periodic switching of these genes (e.g. at weekly intervals) during the course of infection results in new antigenic forms being produced during infection. By the time antibodies are made to a given antigenic type, the gene may have been switched and a new antigenic type has appeared.

Some bacteria are also thought to be capable of switching their surface antigens, such as *Neisseria gonorrhoeae* and species of *Brucella*.

IMMUNOSUPPRESSION

A number of microorganisms cause a depletion or reduction in the defences of the host. As a consequence, the

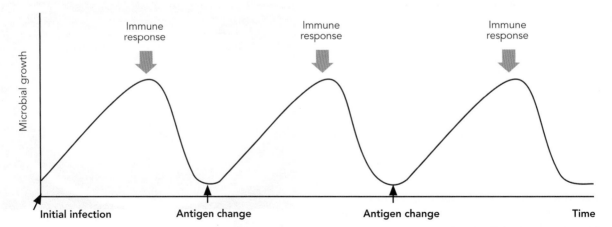

Figure 10.9

Antigenic variation

By repeatedly changing its critical antigens, an organism is not affected by prior immune responses to it, thereby evading the host's immune system.

immune response to the antigens of the microbe (and sometimes other unrelated antigens) may be depressed, resulting in little or no antibody production or cellular immunity (see Chapter 9) to these antigens. The human immunodeficiency virus (HIV) is the most dramatic of microbial immunosuppressors, in fact deriving its name from this activity.

The HIV suppresses the immune system in a number of ways. Much of it is believed to be due to infection, killing and depletion of T4 lymphocytes, which play a central role in immune responses. This greatly reduces the host's ability to produce adequate amounts of antibody, activated T cells or cytokines (see Chapter 9). However, the virus is also believed to cause damage to the immune system in other ways, including:

- prevention of T4 cells responding to antigens by blocking the cell receptor sites
- infection of lymph nodes, leading to their damage or destruction
- infection of other protective cells bearing the CD4 receptor, particularly macrophages and glial cells in the brain
- the initiation of autoimmune responses to T4 cells and other cells bearing the CD4 receptor.

The end result of this immunosuppression is that patients in the terminal stages of HIV infection are incapable of mounting an immune response to many infections and cancers that are normally readily dealt with by the immune system. AIDS patients may then die from one of these secondary diseases.

Other microbes do not have such a dramatic and devastating effect on the immune system, but can cause immunosuppression nevertheless. For example, *Staphylococcus aureus* seems to interfere with immune defences by secreting toxins that are potent T cell mitogens (stimulators). These cause an uncontrolled and excessive activation of T lymphocytes, thus diverting the immune system to unproductive activity. Other microbes, such as the Epstein-Barr virus, may cause a similar diversion of the immune system by polyclonal activation of B lymphocytes, with the production of large amounts of irrelevant antibodies.

Some organisms release substances that interfere with immunologically important molecules. For instance, many pathogenic strains of *Neisseria gonorrhoeae*, *Streptococcus pneumoniae* and *Haemophilus influenzae* secrete a protease that cleaves the IgA molecule, the major antibody type in mucosal secretions. This presumably facilitates the persistence of these bacteria on mucous membranes even if specific antibodies of this class are produced. Strains of *Pseudomonas* secrete enzymes that inactivate components of the complement system. This is thought to inhibit the critical role that complement plays in opsonising (enhancing the phagocytosis of) foreign particles (see Chapter 9).

NON-INDUCTION OF AN IMMUNE RESPONSE

There is an intriguing group of diseases called *transmissible spongiform encephalopathies*, or *prion* diseases, that result from an accumulation of an abnormal form of a protein in brain cells (see Chapter 20). They are neurodegenerative diseases and are nearly always fatal. Some of these diseases can be transmitted from person to person (Creutzfeldt-Jakob disease and kuru) or from animal to person (bovine spongiform encephalopathy in cows to variant Creutzfeldt-Jakob disease in humans) by transfer of the abnormal protein. One of the many unusual features of these diseases is that they do not induce any perceptible inflammation or immune response. These abnormal proteins can therefore persist and induce the production of more abnormal proteins in the body without any intervention of the immune system.

The almost 100% mortality is presumably due to the non-induction of an immune response and hence the inability of the immune system to remove the proteins from the body. Fortunately, there are only a small number of these diseases (that we know of) and they are presently in very low incidence in the world.

It appears that many microorganisms have mechanisms that inhibit the defence systems of the host in some way. Even a temporary suppression of host factors can give the microbe enough advantage to enable its establishment and growth in the body.

- The ability of an organism to cause disease is referred to as its pathogenicity.
- The factors that contribute to an organism's ability to cause disease are called virulence factors.

ADHERENCE

- Adherence is an important step in the pathogenicity of many organisms.
- The substances or structures on the surfaces of micro-organisms that enable them to attach to cell surfaces are called adhesins.
- Viruses attach to specific membrane receptors on the cells they infect.
- Many parasitic helminths fasten to host tissues by means of suckers or hooks.

TOXINS

- Toxins are substances produced by some microorganisms that interfere with the normal functioning of host cells or tissues.
- Exotoxins are heat-labile proteins that are usually released as the organism grows.
- Exotoxins include some of the strongest poisons known (e.g. the botulinum toxin).
- A number of exotoxins act by damaging host cell membranes, resulting in lysis and death of the cells.
- An antitoxin is an antibody that is able to bind to a toxin and neutralise it, thereby preventing it from binding to its target cell or tissue.
- Many exotoxins can be chemically modified to remove their toxicity, while still retaining their ability to elicit an immune response. Toxins modified in this way are called toxoids, and can be used in vaccines.
- Endotoxins are the lipopolysaccharides (LPS) of the cell walls of Gram-negative bacteria.
- Endotoxin, regardless of its source, produces similar signs and symptoms in the host.
- Fever is one of the more common symptoms induced by endotoxin.
- Endotoxic (septic) shock is caused by the release of large amounts of endotoxin.

INVASION OF CELLS

- Viruses typically cause disease by invading and damaging host cells.
- Viruses cause changes to the cell that are called cytopathic effects (CPE).

CELLULAR TRANSFORMATION INTO TUMOUR CELLS

- Some viruses cause disease by transforming host cells into tumour cells.
- Some viruses are believed to be involved in malignant tumours, such as HPV types 16, 18, 31 and 33 in cervical cancer, and hepatitis B and C viruses in hepatocellular carcinoma.

OTHER MECHANISMS OF PATHOGENESIS

- Superantigens produced by some microbes indiscriminately activate T cells to release cytokines that cause tissue injury.
- Some microorganisms cause tissue damage by physical means (e.g. a mass of worms in the intestinal tract may cause obstruction).

EVASION STRATEGIES

- Some organisms possess capsules or a surface slime layer which prevents phagocytes from ingesting them.
- Some microorganisms have developed ways of surviving inside phagocytes.
- Some microorganisms evade the host defences by hiding inside cells, or in 'privileged sites' where defence cells do not normally circulate.
- Antigenic variation is a phenomenon in which micro-organisms repeatedly or progressively change their cell surface antigens, enabling them to evade the immune system.
- Several microorganisms cause a depletion or reduction in the host's defences, resulting in little or no immunity to their antigens.
- The group of diseases called transmissible spongiform encephalopathies (e.g. Creutzfeldt-Jakob disease) does not induce an immune response.

STUDY QUESTIONS

1. What are virulence factors?
2. By what routes do most microorganisms enter the body?
3. What are adhesins? Give two examples.
4. How do viruses attach to the cells they infect?
5. Define the terms 'endotoxin', 'enterotoxin' and 'neurotoxin'.
6. How do microorganisms break down the cell membranes of humans?
7. What are leukocidins and how do they operate?
8. What is coagulase and how does it increase the pathogenicity of staphylococci?
9. Describe how the tetanus and botulinum toxins cause disease.
10. Define the terms 'toxoid' and 'antitoxin'.
11. What is an endotoxin?
12. What is septic shock?
13. What are cytopathic effects?
14. How do viruses kill host cells?
15. Describe the ways by which microorganisms avoid being ingested by phagocytes.
16. How can microorganisms hide from the immune system?
17. What is meant by the terms 'antigenic variation' and 'antigenic drift'?
18. What is thought to be the main way in which the human immunodeficiency virus causes immunosuppression in the host?
19. How could an IgA protease assist microorganisms to cause disease?

TEST YOUR UNDERSTANDING

1. Describe the differences between exotoxins and endotoxins.
2. Why must many pathogenic microbes have specific mechanisms for adherence to tissues?
3. In a patient with tetanus, why is the administration of specific immune globulin more important than antibiotics?
4. Explain why the administration of antibiotics to a patient with an infection caused by Gram-negative bacteria can initially cause a worsening of symptoms.

Further reading

Casadevall A & L Pirofski 1999, 'Host-pathogen interactions: Redefining the basic concepts of virulence and pathogenicity', *Infection and Immunity* 67(8), pp. 3703–13. (Reviews the concepts of microbial virulence and pathogenicity.)

Edwards, R & KG Harding 2004, 'Bacteria & wound healing', *Current Opinion in Infectious Diseases* 17, pp. 91–96. (Discusses wound colonisation and infection from the point of view of wound healing.)

Ewald PW 1993, 'The evolution of virulence', *Scientific American* 268(4), pp. 56–62. (A discussion of microbial pathogenicity from an evolutionary viewpoint. It contends that the pathogenicity of microorganisms could be controlled if evolutionary pressures were controlled.)

Mims CA, A Nash & J Stephen 2001, *MIM's Pathogenesis of Infectious Disease*, 5th edn, San Diego: Academic Press. (Details the mechanisms by which microbes cause disease.)

Salyers AA & DD Whitt 2002, *Bacterial Pathogenesis: A Molecular Approach*, 2nd edn, Washington DC: ASM Press. (This comprehensive text focuses on the mechanisms of infectious diseases and how the host responds to them.)

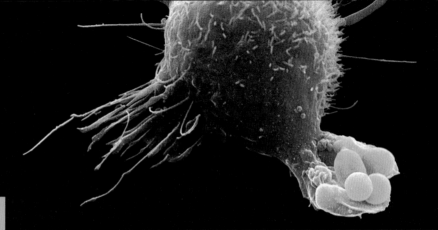

Control of Microbial Growth

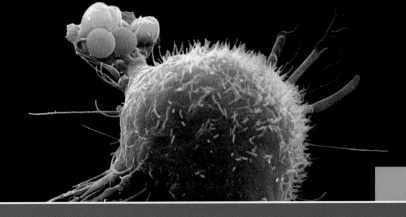

CHAPTER 11

Principles of Sterilisation and Disinfection

[CHAPTER FOCUS]

- ■ *What are the basic principles used for the effective control of microbial growth?*

- ■ *What are the main methods used to destroy or inactivate microorganisms?*

- ■ *Why are thorough cleaning procedures an important part of disinfection and sterilisation procedures?*

- ■ *What determines the method of sterilisation to be used?*

- ■ *How are chemical disinfectants used?*

Introduction

Microorganisms are an integral part of our environment. They play an essential role in agriculture, in food production, in industry, in the recycling of nutrients by the decomposition of organic material and as part of the normal body flora. However, they are also responsible for food spoilage and the contamination of water supplies and are the causative agents of disease in plants and animals. To avoid the harm that microorganisms can cause, it is essential to have methods of controlling their growth and transmission.

The most appropriate method of control to be used in a given situation depends not only on the type of microorganisms that are present, but also on the location – for example, in the home, in a health-care facility, in an operating room, in a laboratory, on surgical instruments or in pharmaceutical products.

In the home or community environment, it is usually sufficient to use cleaning agents and occasional chemical disinfectants to reduce the number of microorganisms to an acceptable level. In a health-care setting, however, standards of cleaning and disinfection need to be much higher because of the type of microorganisms that are present and the susceptibility of the patients to infection. Any equipment that is used for invasive procedures must be sterile. Equipment that comes into contact with a patient's mucosa or non-intact skin needs to be, as a minimum, high level disinfected but preferably sterilised. **Sterility** is defined as the complete absence of any kind of living organism.

The CDNA publication *Infection Control Guidelines for the prevention of transmission of infectious diseases in the health care setting 2004* describes the chemicals and methods of disinfection and sterilisation that are to be used in health-care facilities. It is important for health professionals, especially nurses, to understand how these processes work, their limitations and how and when to use them safely. It is also essential to recognise situations that have a high risk of transmission of infection, and to identify those patients who are particularly susceptible so that appropriate methods of control are used.

Infection control procedures for the prevention of cross-infection are described in more detail in Chapter 13. In this chapter we focus on the physical and chemical methods used to control microbial growth.

Traditional methods of control

PRESERVATION OF FOOD

Humans have always needed to devise ways to prevent food spoilage and to preserve food for the winter months. Methods such as drying or curing (smoking) of meat and fish have been used for centuries. In areas where salt was available, meat and fish were salted in large barrels; other foods were pickled in vinegar. Vegetable seeds, such as beans and lentils, were dried. We now know that these methods create conditions of low water content, high osmotic pressure or low pH, all of which are unfavourable for the growth of bacteria.

The use of heat to destroy bacteria and preserve food arose from the work of Louis Pasteur in the 19th century (see Chapter 1). Pasteur was responsible for showing that food spoilage was due to microorganisms already present in the food and that these could be destroyed by the application of heat. Provided the food was in a container that prevented the re-entry of microbes, the food would remain unspoiled. The technique he developed, which now bears his name (**pasteurisation**), does not kill *all* microbes but it does kill most of the ones that produce organic acids (mainly the lactic acid bacteria) and cause souring of wine and milk.

Pasteur's work was of enormous economic importance to the wine industry in France in the 19th century. When applied to milk, the method was found not only to prevent spoilage by lactic acid bacteria, but also to destroy certain pathogens such as those responsible for tuberculosis. *Mycobacterium bovis* causes TB in dairy cattle and can easily be transmitted to humans in unpasteurised milk.

The early explorers, sailing for months or years around the world, took food that had been heated and stored in sealed containers. They knew it preserved the food, even though they did not understand the mechanism responsible for spoilage. The use of heat to destroy microorganisms is still one of the most efficient and reliable methods available today.

PREVENTION OF DISEASE

For centuries people have been aware of the seriousness of infections and infectious diseases (see Chapter 1) and have tried various methods to cure them or prevent their spread. During the plague in Europe in the Middle Ages, people burnt the bodies and clothes of those who had died and burnt sulphur and aromatic plants in their houses to try to 'purify the air'.

The middle of the 19th century saw the first attempts at disinfection, or the use of chemicals to destroy microorganisms. JOSEPH LISTER, a Scottish surgeon, was one of the first to use chemicals to prevent the death of patients from infection, especially following surgery (see Chapters 1, 13). IGNAZ SEMMELWEIS, a Hungarian physician working in Vienna, introduced handwashing in a solution of chlorinated lime for all nurses and physicians (see Chapters 1, 13). The methods used by Lister and Semmelweis involved very crude, corrosive chemicals. Modern antiseptics and disinfectants are more effective. Florence Nightingale advocated cleanliness and hygiene and introduced measures into the field hospitals in the Crimea that dramatically reduced the number of infections.

'Germ' control

Different methods of control or destruction of microorganisms are required for different situations. In the community, good hygiene practices such as keeping homes and buildings clean and well ventilated, the provision of a safe, clean water supply and the correct disposal of waste and sewage, will create a healthy environment. In our modern society there is now a strong focus on household cleaners and disinfectants – often with little understanding of the correct use and application of the chemicals involved. There is a risk that overuse of antimicrobial agents in domestic settings could lead to the emergence of resistant strains of microorganisms.

The terms commonly used to describe the destruction or control of microorganisms are listed in Table 11.1.

Pattern of microbial death

The control of microbial growth can be achieved in a number of ways:

- by killing all the organisms (sterilisation)
- by reducing the number of microbes to an 'acceptable level' (disinfection)
- by preventing the organisms from gaining access to a susceptible site
- by exposing them to conditions that inhibit their growth.

The methods used to control microorganisms damage their structure and interfere with their ability to reproduce. Nucleic acids, which contain the genetic information, are essential for reproduction and so agents that damage or destroy nucleic acid will prevent cell replication. If the proteins are altered or denatured, cell function is impaired. Damage to the wall or membrane, which play an integral role in maintaining the structure and internal environment of the cell, will allow the cell contents to leak out, resulting in the death of the cell.

RATE OF DEATH

When a microbial population is exposed to a killing (biocidal) agent, the pattern of death obeys certain laws. In general, each microbial cell has to come into actual contact with the biocidal agent. Thus, in order to be effective, the biocidal agent must have sufficient time to penetrate throughout the whole population of cells. This means that, under specified conditions, a certain number of microbes will be killed in a certain period of time; for example, 90% may be killed in one minute. After these cells are killed, it will take another minute for the killing agent to come into contact with 90% of the remaining live cells. So 90% will be killed in the next minute, and so on. This is called an *exponential killing curve* (see Figure 11.1). If the rate of death is plotted logarithmically it is a straight line.

Obviously, the more microorganisms that are present initially, the longer it will take to destroy them all. It is therefore essential that any process is continued for a sufficient period of time to ensure the death of all

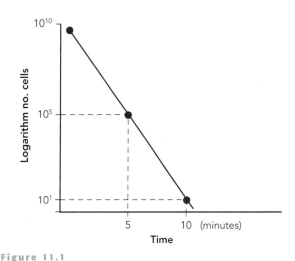

Figure 11.1

Killing curve: logarithmic plot of the rate of microbial death versus time

Table 11.1

Terms used in the destruction or control of microorganisms

TERM	DEFINITION
• Antiseptic	A type of chemical disinfectant, suitable for use on skin or living tissue, used to kill or remove harmful microorganisms without damaging the tissue.
• Biocidal agent	An agent that is capable of killing microorganisms.
• Decontamination	The removal of possibly harmful microorganisms from an object by cleaning or disinfecting.
• Disinfectant	A chemical substance normally used for the disinfection of inanimate objects.
• Disinfection	The destruction, removal or reduction in numbers of harmful microorganisms to an acceptable level. Usually kills vegetative bacteria, not endospores or viruses.
• Germicide	Any agent capable of killing microorganisms (germs).
• Pasteurisation	A method developed to preserve milk and other liquids without altering their taste or quality. Destroys bacteria responsible for spoilage and some pathogens, but not all microorganisms.
• Sanitisation	Thorough cleaning of an object or utensil to remove most microorganisms. Does not imply use of disinfectant.
• Sterile	Free of all living organisms, unable to reproduce.
• Sterilisation	The complete destruction or removal of all microorganisms, including endospores.
• Sterility assurance level	The probability of a viable microorganism being present on an item after sterilisation.

organisms. Most procedures are standardised and recommend that articles are treated for a specified period of time to ensure that all organisms present are destroyed. For example, hospital-based sterilisation processes have been designed to achieve a level of safety in the order of a one-in-a-million chance of an organism surviving the process. Failure to follow instructions and to allow the article to be in contact with the biocidal agent for the correct period of time may jeopardise the efficiency of the killing procedure.

Several other factors can affect the rate of killing of microbes by heat or chemicals. A major factor is the type of microorganisms that may be present. Some chemicals have a different action depending on whether the bacterium is Gram-negative or Gram-positive. Some bacteria, such as the pseudomonads and the mycobacteria, are particularly resistant to chemical disinfectants.

Mycobacterium tuberculosis is killed by relatively mild heat treatment (the temperature used in pasteurisation is 63°C for 30 minutes). On the other hand, bacterial endospores have been shown to survive for several hours at 100°C, requiring the higher temperature of 121°C for 15 minutes to kill them.

Cysts of the protozoan *Giardia* are resistant to chlorine, which is used for water purification.

The phase of growth of the microorganisms also has a direct effect on the efficiency of the killing process. In general, when cells are dividing rapidly they are very susceptible to chemical damage, whereas cells in stationary phase are more resistant and many of them form highly resistant cysts or endospores.

CONCENTRATION OF BIOCIDAL AGENT

For chemical inactivation of microorganisms to take place, there has to be a sufficient number of molecules of the chemical present to interact with each microbial cell. Thus, any chemically based sterilisation process, disinfectant or antiseptic solution must be used at an adequate concentration to ensure that all microbes are killed. The manufacturer's instructions usually specify the optimum concentration to be used to ensure that the chemical will be effective. A weaker or stronger solution may compromise the effectiveness of the treatment.

In summary, a disinfection or sterilisation process relies on three critical factors to be effective:

1. an appropriate biocidal agent
2. effective contact of the agent with all surfaces to be treated
3. sufficient exposure (this may be in terms of the length of time of exposure and/or the concentration of the biocidal agent).

Cleaning, disinfection and sterilisation of reusable equipment

RISK LEVEL

When contaminated medical equipment is to be reused, the processes of cleaning, disinfection and sterilisation are of the utmost importance in preventing the transmission of infection. Staff should be specially trained and the procedures outlined in Australian Standards AS/NZS 4187 and AS/NZS 4815 should be followed. The level of cleaning, disinfection and sterilisation required for instruments and equipment depends on the risk (*critical, semi-critical* or *non-critical*) associated with the body site where it will be used. See Table 11.2 and Chapter 13.

The highest risk (critical) is associated with equipment that penetrates the skin or mucous membranes during surgery or during the insertion of devices such as catheters or intravenous lines. These procedures allow direct access for microbes to susceptible sites. Solutions for intravenous (IV) infusion must also be sterile. An added risk factor is that these procedures are often performed on seriously ill patients (e.g. in intensive care) who usually have other contributing conditions that make them particularly susceptible to infection. Any item of equipment that falls into the high-risk category must be sterile and the highest level of aseptic technique must be followed.

Equipment that comes into contact with the patient's skin or mucosal surfaces, but does not necessarily breach them, should also be sterile whenever possible (semi-critical risk). This includes equipment such as flexible endoscopes and respiratory equipment which require special methods of cleaning and sterilisation (see Spotlight box, opposite).

A non-critical level of risk is associated with equipment that only comes into contact with intact skin. X-ray equip-

Table 11.2	
Requirements for sterilisation and disinfection of equipment	
Sterile (*critical site*)	• All equipment that penetrates the skin or mucous membranes: surgical instruments, needles (syringes), IV and urinary catheters, endoscopes • All invasive devices, implants • All solutions that are administered parenterally • All objects that contact a break in the skin or mucosal surfaces: dressings, swabs • Surgical gowns, drapes and gloves
Sterile or high-level disinfection (after cleaning) (*semi-critical site*)	• Equipment that comes into contact with patients' skin or intact mucosa but does not penetrate: X-ray machines, bedpans, thermometers
Cleaning (*non-critical site*)	• Equipment that does not pose significant risk to the patient from contact: beds, sinks, eating utensils

Some types of equipment are very specialised and difficult to clean and reprocess. They include flexible fibreoptic scopes, some respiratory equipment and diagnostic ultrasound probes. When these instruments are contaminated with body fluids and microorganisms they must be properly cleaned and reprocessed before they can be used again in a critical site. Since most of them cannot withstand heat or some chemicals, alternative methods must be used.

Endoscopes

Flexible scopes should be immersed in water and enzymatic detergent immediately after use to prevent any organic matter drying out. They should be cleaned and reprocessed as soon as possible to minimise the risk of microbial growth.

Scopes consist of multiple small channels that must be cleaned carefully. When available, sterilisation by low temperature hydrogen peroxide plasma (HPP) or peracetic acid (PAA) is suitable. An alternative is high-level disinfection with glutaraldehyde.

Reprocessing should be done by trained health workers following the guidelines published by the Gastroenterological Society of Australia (GESA) and the Gastroenterological Nurses College of Australia (GENCA).

Respiratory equipment

The use of specialised respiratory and resuscitation equipment has the potential to introduce organisms directly into a patient's airways. Transmission of infection can occur patient to patient via the equipment used in operating rooms, high dependency units and accident and emergency departments. Aerosol transmission can also occur with respiratory and anaesthetic apparatus.

Protective filters should be incorporated in the breathing circuit. Ventilators and resuscitation equipment used in high dependency units should be thermally disinfected or sterilised. Components that cannot be disinfected should be discarded.

ment, trolleys, beds and other furniture carry a low risk of cross-infection and adequate cleaning is usually sufficient. Some pieces of equipment are very large or have parts that are damaged by heat, so are difficult to sterilise.

It is necessary to assess the risk category carefully to determine the best method of cleaning and disinfection to be used.

SINGLE-USE EQUIPMENT

Many items are labelled 'single use only' and these *must not be reprocessed*. **Any single-use article or instrument that has penetrated the skin, mucous membrane or tissue must be discarded immediately after use.**

STORAGE OF EQUIPMENT

Sterilised equipment should be stored correctly, away from moisture and dust. It has a finite shelf life and expiry dates should be checked before use and the equipment re-processed if necessary. The wrappings of packages must remain intact and free from moisture, otherwise bacteria may penetrate and the contents cannot be considered to be sterile.

Cleaning instruments and equipment

One of the most important aspects of the control of microbial growth is cleaning. Bacteria thrive in moist organic matter such as tissue, blood, body fluids, soiled linen and dressings, food and garbage. Before any disinfecting or sterilising procedures are carried out on equipment or utensils, they must be freed of organic material, grease and dirt as these provide a protective barrier for the microorganisms and prevent the penetration of the biocidal agent. Organic matter may react with some chemical disinfectants, rendering the disinfection process less effective. If an item cannot be cleaned effectively, sterilisation may be compromised.

Detailed procedures for cleaning of reusable instruments and equipment can be found in the Australian Standards AS/NZS 4187 and AS/NZS 4815. Standard Precautions, including protective clothing and gloves, should always be followed (see Chapter 13).

Flexible endoscopes are particularly difficult to clean so it is recommended they be immersed in water and enzymatic detergent immediately after use so that any organic matter present does not dry out and harden, making it difficult to remove.

Washing of equipment with hot water and detergent does not kill all bacteria, but it does reduce their numbers to a level where disinfection and sterilisation procedures are usually effective. Ultrasonic cleaning is useful for complicated instruments with parts that are difficult to reach with standard cleaning techniques. This method involves placing the equipment in a solution of detergent and water which is subjected to high-frequency sound waves. The action of the sound waves dislodges dirt, blood and tissue from inaccessible parts of the instrument.

Environmental cleaning

In hospitals, the cleaning of wards, bathrooms, floors and equipment is an important part of infection control (see Chapter 13). The equipment used for cleaning should be kept dry when not in use to prevent the growth of bacteria. Very often, a damp, contaminated mop head can be responsible for spreading pathogens around the hospital. Cleaning also helps to maintain medical equipment in good condition. In general, the use of disinfectants for routine cleaning tasks is not necessary.

A description of the correct cleaning procedures to be followed for the fixtures and equipment in a hospital is usually contained in the hospital's infection control manual. Terminal cleaning of a room that has contained an infectious patient may require the use of a disinfectant. Guidelines for the decontamination and/or sterilisation of the equipment, bedding and other objects from an infectious area are usually provided in each hospital manual.

Sterilisation

Sterilisation is the complete destruction or removal of all living organisms from an object with an acceptably low probability of an organism surviving the process. For medical equipment, the required level of sterility assurance is one-in-a-million. Achievement of this level of sterility assurance relies on the initial reduction in the number of microbes by thorough cleaning. In practical terms, an object is considered to be either sterile or non-sterile

Several methods can be used to sterilise an object (Table 11.3). They include physical methods that make use of heat or radiation, mechanical methods such as filtration (used for air and fluids) and chemical methods that use ethylene oxide, hydrogen peroxide or peracetic acid. The method employed depends on the nature of the object to be sterilised, the type of facility where it will be used and the subsequent use to which the object will be put.

HEAT

Heat is the most widely used of all methods of sterilisation. It is cheap, efficient and easily controlled. Dry heat kills microorganisms by inactivation of cell components by oxidation, whereas moist heat destroys microorganisms mainly by denaturation of essential cellular proteins. Microorganisms vary in their susceptibility to heat. To establish suitable protocols to be followed to render an

---

SPOTLIGHT ON
Prions

Prions are infectious agents that are highly resistant to hydrolysis by proteolytic enzymes (in the digestive tract) and to conventional methods of sterilisation and disinfection. They are the cause of a range of rare but fatal neurodegenerative disorders called *transmissible spongiform encephalopathies* (TSEs). Among these, classic Creutzfeldt-Jakob disease (cCJD) is most common. CJD manifests itself in a range of neurological symptoms. No specific antibody response is detectable and definitive diagnosis depends on post-mortem examination of brain tissue, which exhibits distinctive spongiform degeneration, astrocytosis and accumulation of amyloid filaments. About 85% of CJD cases occur sporadically; about 10% of cases occur in people with a family disorder and a small percentage are acquired.

Iatrogenic (medically acquired) cases of cCJD have occurred in Australia in patients treated with contaminated hormone preparations (prepared from pooled pituitary glands from cadavers) or who have been infected via contaminated dura mater or corneal transplants.

A new form of CJD, variant CJD (vCJD), appeared in Britain in the 1990s, linked to the consumption of beef products made from cattle suffering from BSE (bovine spongiform encephalopathy), or 'mad cow disease'. The infectious agent of vCJD, the abnormal prion protein Prp^{SC}, has been detected in human tonsillar tissue and it is thought that this abnormal protein may be distributed more widely in human tissue in vCJD than in patients with CJD. In the UK, procedures such as tonsillectomy, appendectomy, and lymph node and gastrointestinal biopsy have a high risk of contamination of instruments with vCJD.

So far, no cases of vCJD have been detected in Australia but the government has banned blood dona-

tions from people who spent more than six months in Britain between 1980 and 1996.

In the health-care setting there are concerns about the possible risks of iatrogenic transmission of CJD from high-risk patients via contaminated surgical instruments, organ and tissue donation or blood transfusion. High-risk patients include those exhibiting neurological symptoms of CJD, those with familial or genetic predisposition and recipients of contaminated transplant organs or hormone injections. In Australia, medical records can identify people who are high-risk because of hormone preparations, but there is no way of knowing how many other people are silently incubating the disease. For this reason, health authorities are instituting precautions to prevent the spread of CJD.

The CDNA Guidelines (2004) deal specifically with the procedures that should be used for patients with known or suspected cCJD and related diseases. Body tissues that are considered to carry the highest infection risk are brain, spinal cord, eye, retina and optic nerve, pituitary gland and dura mater tissue. The infectious agent is resistant to normal sterilisation and disinfection so surgery lists should be arranged to minimise the risk of transmission. Where possible, disposable instruments and equipment should be used for patients categorised as higher risk and for lower risk patients requiring procedures involving high infectivity body tissues. After use, disposable instruments and equipment must be incinerated. In cases where a diagnosis is uncertain or in other special cases as outlined in the CDNA Guidelines (2004), instruments may be subjected to special methods of reprocessing such as steam sterilisation at 134°C for 18 minutes, or soaking in IN NaOH for one hour at room temperature followed by steam sterilisation.

- See Chapter 20 for a discussion of transmissible spongiform encephalopathies.

Table 11.3

Methods of sterilisation

METHOD	ADVANTAGES/DISADVANTAGES
Steam steriliser Steam under pressure 121°C 15 mins	Requires special equipment; reliable, inexpensive to run; kills all microbes; *not* suitable for heat-sensitive objects or solutions.
Dry heat 180°C more than 1 hour (or 160°C for 120 minutes)	Inexpensive, slow; not suitable for heat-sensitive materials.
Incineration	Total destruction of contaminated articles.
Ionising radiation (gamma)	Requires access to commercial cobalt-60 source; good for prepackaged materials.
Filtration	Used for sterilising heat-sensitive solutions; awkward to handle; difficult to monitor efficiency.
Ethylene oxide gas	Useful for heat-sensitive materials, disposable plastics; requires special facility in sterilising department; gas is toxic; flammable equipment; must be well aired before use; difficult to monitor efficiency.
Hydrogen peroxide	Low temperature 'plasma' sterilisation; requires special unit. Suitable for delicate instruments; fast, non-toxic; not suitable for cellulose, paper or fabric.
Peracetic acid	Low temperature; commercial equipment; kills most organisms.

object sterile, it is useful to determine the type of organisms that are likely to be present so as to ensure that the methods employed are sufficient to kill all the organisms. It is also essential to monitor the outcome regularly.

The **thermal death point (TDP)** is defined as the lowest temperature at which all the microorganisms in a liquid suspension will be killed in 10 minutes. As mentioned earlier, the time required to kill all the microorganisms will depend on the number of microorganisms present, or the level of contamination. We can therefore define another value, the **thermal death time (TDT)**, which is the minimum time it takes to kill all the organisms in a liquid culture at a given temperature.

It is useful to determine these values for situations where the objects to be sterilised would be affected by prolonged exposure to excessive heat. They are especially relevant in the food industry, in the preparation of canned food for example, in order to preserve the quality of the product. In the laboratory, these values are important in the preparation of culture media or other sterile solutions, where some of the essential ingredients might be broken down by extended exposure to high temperatures.

MOIST HEAT STERILISATION: USE OF STEAM UNDER PRESSURE

In the hospital setting, patients are protected from infection by the use of sterile equipment, instruments, dressings and IV solutions. To ensure these objects are sterile, they must be subjected to a reliable procedure that can be closely monitored. The most reliable method is *moist heat sterilisation*, which uses a machine called a steam steriliser. This process is able to kill endospores as well as vegetative bacterial cells and viruses.

Although boiling is used to kill microorganisms, it is *not* an accepted method of sterilisation. Some organisms can withstand the temperature of boiling water (100°C at normal atmospheric pressure) for long periods. To achieve sterility, it is necessary to use higher temperatures. These can be reached by increasing the pressure in the sterilising chamber so that the temperature at which the water boils (i.e. the temperature of the steam) is raised. The higher the pressure, the higher the temperature that can be reached.

For example, when steam from boiling water is placed under a pressure of 1 atmosphere (or 15 pounds per square inch, psi) in excess of normal atmospheric pressure (i.e. twice atmospheric pressure), the temperature of the steam is increased to 121°C. At three times atmospheric pressure, the temperature reaches 134°C. A temperature of 121°C is sufficient to kill all microorganisms, including endospores, in 15 minutes. At 134°C, the time required for sterilisation is reduced to 3 minutes.

It is important to note that these times are measured from the time when steam penetrates to all parts of the object to be sterilised. This is especially important when thick or bulky items are being treated.

Steam sterilisers vary in size from small bench-top models, used in medical and dental surgeries, to large, fully automated commercial models used in hospitals and industry.

A steam steriliser generally consists of a double-walled or jacketed chamber made of thick steel. Steam is circulated through the outer jacket and then supplied under pressure to the closed inner chamber (see Figure 11.2). Both the inner chamber and the airtight doors are constructed to withstand the pressures and temperatures generated.

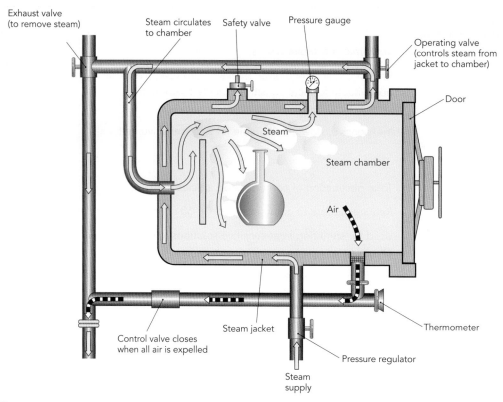

Figure 11.2

Diagram of steam steriliser
Steam enters and forces air out through an opening on the bottom of the chamber. When all air is expelled the control valve is closed by the higher temperature of the steam. As the pressure is increased the temperature of the steam is raised.

For sterilisation to be effective, steam must be able to contact every part of the object to be sterilised (and thus every microorganism that is present). To ensure the correct temperature is reached and all surfaces of the items can be contacted, all the air must be eliminated from the load and the chamber and replaced with steam. The most effective method of air removal is achieved by the use of a mechanical pump to suck all the air out of the chamber and the load. A steriliser that uses this type of air removal is often referred to as a 'prevacuum' steriliser.

Older models of steam sterilisers may use passive methods of air removal, such as gravity, to remove the air from the chamber and load. This method of air removal is less efficient and reliable air removal from complex medical devices cannot be guaranteed.

There are four main stages in the sterilising cycle.

1. Removal of air, admission of steam and heating of the chamber to the selected sterilising temperature.
2. Sterilisation time, which includes:
   (a) *penetration time*, the time taken for the least accessible part of the load to reach operating temperature;
   (b) *holding time*, including a safety factor, which is the minimum time required for the whole load to be maintained at operating conditions in order to reach the level of sterility assurance required.

> *Example*
> **Steam at 121°C**
> recommended holding time   15 mins
> **Steam at 134°C**
> recommended holding time   3 mins
> (Penetration time must be established at the time of validation and added to the holding time.)

3. Removal of steam and drying of the load.
4. Restoration of atmospheric conditions by admission of filtered air.

Equipment to be sterilised must be wrapped in a suitable material such as paper or fabric, which allows penetration of steam and maintains sterility after removal from the steriliser. Aluminium foil does not allow steam to penetrate and should not be used. Special chemical indicators and tapes that change colour when the desired temperature is reached are placed in the middle of a wrapped package and should change colour evenly if the heat has penetrated uniformly. The load should be allowed to dry inside the autoclave before being exposed to the outside air. This is to prevent bacteria from passing through the wet wrappings and contaminating the inside of the package. Liquids should be placed in loosely stoppered flasks and allowed to cool below 100°C before being removed from the chamber, to avoid explosions due to superheating.

When properly used and maintained, a steam steriliser is a very efficient method of sterilisation. It should be regularly calibrated and maintained by trained, competent personnel. The steriliser must be performance-tested and the sterilisation process routinely monitored every cycle, according to the requirements of AS/NZS 4187 to ensure that the steriliser is functioning correctly and reaching the required temperatures and pressures for the required amount of time.

At the end of a sterilisation cycle, the process record must be checked to ensure that sterilisation parameters were achieved. Packages must be visually inspected for the correct colour change of the chemical indicator and for any damage to the packaging, and there should be no visible wetness. Any moisture that comes into contact with the outside of a package, or remains on the packaging after the sterilisation process, allows the passage of microorganisms through the packaging and may cause contamination of the contents. The wrapping of the package must remain intact, or the contents cannot be considered sterile. Sterilised equipment has a finite shelf life and staff should check the expiry date before use and reprocess the equipment if necessary.

DRY HEAT STERILISATION

To sterilise using dry heat, a temperature of 180°C for 60 minutes is required. Dry heat sterilisers are only suitable for sterilising equipment that is not harmed by long exposure to high temperatures. Glass and some metal objects can be sterilised in this way. Fabrics and wrapping materials cannot usually withstand these temperatures. Reusable equipment must be packaged in heatproof containers (metal or glass).

The time required to heat the oven, in addition to the sterilising time, makes this method less practical than a steam steriliser. The high temperature required is also a major limitation, although the dry atmosphere is preferable for some metal instruments as it does not cause corrosion.

INCINERATION

Incineration of contaminated material is another method of destroying the microorganisms present in biological materials, contaminated waste, soiled dressings and disposable equipment. It is also used to sterilise the inoculating loops that are used to handle microorganisms in the laboratory. The platinum wire of the loop is heated to red hot, allowed to cool and then used to transfer organisms in a sterile manner.

RADIATION

Ionising radiation can damage or kill microorganisms by causing disruption to the structure of the DNA chains. Most vegetative bacteria are easily killed but bacterial endospores and many viruses (e.g. HIV) are highly resistant. Gamma rays from a radioactive cobalt-60 source are used industrially to sterilise much of the disposable equip-

ment used in hospitals, such as prepackaged dressing packs, needles, syringes, suture material, catheters and prostheses. Because gamma rays can penetrate materials, a product can be packaged first and then sterilised.

It is a useful method for heat-sensitive organic material such as pharmaceutical products for injection – anaesthetics, therapeutic drugs, hormones, vaccines and antibiotics. Not all materials can be sterilised by this method without causing changes to their composition. Because of the highly dangerous nature of the radiation, this type of sterilisation treatment is carried out at a specially designed commercial facility.

Microwave radiation consists of electromagnetic radiation that interacts with molecules such as water, producing heat. Although microwaves are capable of killing most microorganisms, including endospores, the uneven distribution of heat means that they are unsuitable for use as a controlled method of sterilisation.

FILTRATION

Filtration involves the removal of microorganisms from liquids or gases by passage through a filter with pores small enough to retain microorganisms. Filters are used to sterilise materials that cannot be sterilised by other methods. Many of the aqueous solutions used for procedures such as surgical irrigation, peritoneal dialysis, intravenous therapy or total parenteral nutrition of hospitalised patients contain substances that are adversely affected by high temperatures. Some pharmaceutical preparations such as ophthalmic solutions, drugs and vitamins, and biological materials such as blood, serum and some culture media used in microbiology laboratories are also sensitive to high temperatures. They can be sterilised by filtration through specially designed membrane filters (see Figure 11.3). These are made of nitrocellulose and manufactured in a range of specific pore sizes capable of retaining different-sized particles (Table 11.4).

It is more difficult to control sterility with filtration, as the equipment can be awkward to use and the efficiency of the filtration process is difficult to assess.

ETHYLENE OXIDE GAS STERILISATION

Ethylene oxide gas is a useful sterilising agent for articles made of rubber or other heat-sensitive components. It is an odourless, highly toxic, flammable gas that explodes when mixed with oxygen. The gas is effective against all microorganisms, as it inactivates proteins by combining with sulfhydryl groups.

It is teratogenic, mutagenic and carcinogenic, and exposure causes irritation to the eyes and respiratory tract, nausea and dizziness. For these reasons, the method is confined to industrial facilities or the central sterilising units of large hospitals. Careful control of the conditions is necessary, as time, temperature, humidity and gas concentration all affect the efficiency of the sterilisation.

Items sterilised in this way must be aerated with filtered air for up to 12 hours to remove residual toxic gas. Staff handling ethylene oxide need to be aware of its toxicity

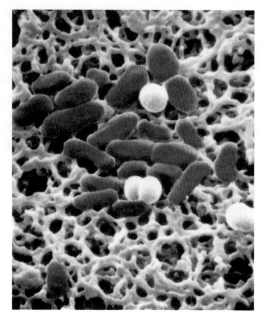

Figure 11.3

Membrane filters

Scanning electron micrograph showing rod-shaped *Serratia marcescens* and round *Staphylococcus epidermidis* cells trapped on the surface of a 0.22-μm Millipore membrane filter. Membrane pore size may be selected so as to allow viruses, but not bacteria, to pass through, or to prevent both from passing.

Table 11.4

Pore sizes of membrane filters

PORE SIZE	FILTRATION USE
Less than 0.025 μm (ultrafilter)	Required to ensure removal of all bacteria, viruses and mycoplasmas.
0.22 μm	Allows passage of all viruses and molecules. Retains bacteria.
0.45 μm	Allows a few bacteria through. Retains yeasts, protozoa, blood cells.
1.2 μm	Allows viruses and most bacteria through. Retains yeasts.

and of the occupational health and safety guidelines for its use. If articles are not adequately aerated, patients can suffer from hypersensitivity reactions when the article touches the skin.

The method is difficult to monitor, requiring the use of spore strips (specimens of endospores of *Bacillus subtilis*), which should be exposed during each sterilising cycle. The time required for aeration, and for assessing whether the spores have been killed, makes this a rather slow method of sterilisation; it is not suitable for reusable equipment that cannot be out of use for two days. It has good powers of penetration, however, and is most useful for sterilising delicate equipment that would be damaged by heat or liquids.

LOW-TEMPERATURE HYDROGEN PEROXIDE PLASMA STERILISATION (HPP)

Hydrogen peroxide vapour is used as a low-temperature sterilant suitable for heat- and moisture-sensitive equipment (e.g. electronic equipment, fibreoptic cables, camera heads). It is designed to replace ethylene oxide and is suitable for use in hospital central sterilising departments.

The commercially available system (Sterrad™) uses hydrogen peroxide which is vapourised and exposed to radio waves, giving rise to gaseous plasma (a mixture of high-energy species of hydrogen peroxide, H_2O_2). This acts as an oxidising sterilant and is active against a wide variety of microorganisms including viruses, bacterial endospores and mycobacteria. The products of the process are non-toxic (water and oxygen).The system uses low temperatures (around 45°C), the cycle is rapid (75 minutes) and no venting time is required.

The process is suitable for sterilising medical devices made from stainless steel and most plastics, but should not be used for cellulose materials, which absorb liquids. The presence of organic material on instruments can compromise efficiency, and equipment with a narrow lumen may require the use of a booster to ensure penetration of the plasma into the tube.

PERACETIC ACID STERILISATION (PAA)

This system uses 0.2% buffered peracetic acid solution at low temperatures (50–55°C) to sterilise a wide range of instruments in about 30 minutes. This system is largely being used to replace glutaraldehyde for the processing of flexible endoscopes and other temperature-sensitive devices capable of being immersed in a liquid. Peracetic acid is an oxidising agent and can be corrosive to instruments immersed in it. The Steris™ system is a commercial process that eliminates the corrosive property. It involves an automatic cycle and the products are non-toxic.

As this method of sterilisation uses a liquid chemical, items are not dry at the completion of the cycle and must be used immediately to ensure sterility is maintained. Peracetic acid is active against vegetative bacteria and endospores, fungi, viruses and mycobacteria.

Disinfection

Disinfection is a process that kills or inactivates large numbers of microorganisms, but does not sterilise. Disinfecting methods must be able to reduce the number of microbes present to an 'acceptable level'. The definition of an 'acceptable level' in the clinical environment depends on the purpose for which the article is to be used. Current European standards make very clear distinctions between the level of disinfection expected for a variety of non-critical and semi-critical patient-care equipment. For example, the level of disinfection required for an item such as a bedpan is less than that expected for an item of respiratory equipment because of the intended use of that item and the level of risk associated with infection transmission by use of that item.

An article that has been **disinfected** has usually been treated in one of the ways described below. Methods include the use of heat, radiation and various chemical agents that destroy microorganisms. See Table 11.5

As mentioned earlier, all articles to be disinfected should first be thoroughly cleaned. The presence of organic matter, grease or dirt interferes with the ability of the disinfecting agent to penetrate, contact and inactivate the microorganisms present.

Sanitisation is a poorly defined term. It usually means that an article has been cleaned, although it is used in some contexts to imply that the article is 'germ-free'. It does *not* usually mean that an object has been exposed to a disinfecting procedure, and health workers should not assume that an article that is 'sanitised' has been treated with a disinfectant.

PHYSICAL METHODS OF DISINFECTION

Heat

Heat is a very useful method of disinfection as it penetrates readily and is easier to control than most chemical disinfectants. Boiling water (100°C for 5 minutes) kills most microorganisms except for endospores and some viruses. As such, it is an inexpensive and reliable method of decontaminating many articles and utensils. However, the simple use of boiling water as a method of disinfection is no longer acceptable in health-care facilities. To be effective, the process must be controlled and so the old-fashioned boiling-water 'sterilisers' are considered obsolete.

Thermal disinfection in health-care facilities is now achieved by the use of automated washer-disinfectors that meet stringent international standards. These machines must be calibrated, maintained and routinely monitored to ensure that disinfection is being achieved. Standard AS/NZS 4187 gives the correct time and temperature combinations required to achieve thermal disinfection of medical equipment.

It is important to remember that thermal disinfection is *not* a method of sterilisation and should not be used as the only process for instruments that breach the body's defences (such as dental instruments, surgical equipment, vaginal speculae, etc.). As explained above, these should be sterilised in a steam steriliser.

Many organisms are killed by exposure to temperatures below 100°C. A temperature of 63°C for 30 minutes is the standard method of **pasteurisation** and destroys most pathogens likely to be present in food or milk, without causing deterioration in the quality of the food. Another method (flash pasteurisation) involves passing milk through a tube heated to 72°C, holding it there for 15 seconds and then cooling it quickly. Various heat treatments to preserve food have been developed. One involves the **ultra-high temperature process**, **UHT**, in which the milk is heated to 140°C for less than 5 seconds and then cooled rapidly back to 74°C.

Ultraviolet radiation

Many microorganisms are killed or damaged by exposure to short-wave ultraviolet (UV) light. UV light does not penetrate into liquids or through paper or even through a layer of dust. However, it is useful for killing bacteria on clean surfaces and for disinfecting limited air spaces such as microbiological safety cabinets. The amount of UV radiation received depends on the time of exposure and the distance the object is placed from the UV source (see Figure 11.4), the amount of radiation absorbed being inversely proportional to the square of the distance of the object from the source.

Sunlight is a significant source of UV light, especially in Australia, and the exposure of articles to sunshine significantly reduces their microbial population. Exposure of contaminated wounds or ulcers to sunshine is an old-fashioned but sometimes effective treatment.

Table 11.5 **Methods of disinfection**	
METHOD	USE
Heat	
Controlled temperature	Instruments
Automated washers	
100°C boiling water	Food
63°C pasteurisation	Food, milk products
Radiation	
Short wave UV	Surfaces, air spaces
Filtration	Air in safety cabinets, operating theatres, isolation units.
Chemicals	Surfaces, equipment. Decontamination of skin, blood spills, handwashing.

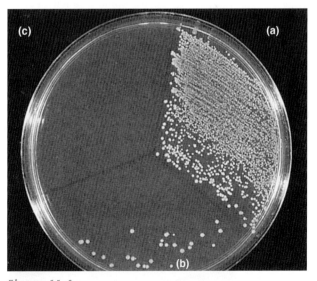

Figure 11.4

Effect of UV radiation on the growth of bacteria on a plate
Effect on bacterial growth of different times of exposure to UV light (280 nm, d = 15 cm): (a) control, no exposure; (b) one minute; (c) five minutes.

Ultraviolet light is absorbed by the DNA of the cell and causes the strands of nucleic acid to break, interfering with DNA and cell replication.

FILTRATION

Microorganisms can also be removed from air by the use of special high-efficiency particulate air filters (HEPA). Some laboratory work involves the use of hazardous materials, such as infectious microorganisms or contaminated objects, and these can be handled safely in specially designed laminar flow cabinets that provide protection from dangerous aerosols (Figure 11.5). Air is drawn into the cabinet away from the worker and filtered before leaving the cabinet. This method does not sterilise the air, but significantly reduces the number of organisms that are present in the exhaust and released into the atmosphere.

Filters are used in ventilation systems to clean the air entering operating theatres, burns wards, isolation units and high dependency wards. They can also be used on exhaust systems in isolation units to trap pathogens that might be released from infectious patients. The filters should be changed regularly and decontaminated before disposal.

CHEMICAL DISINFECTANTS AND ANTISEPTICS

A large number of chemicals are able to kill or inactivate microorganisms. However, not all of them can be safely used as disinfectants, usually because they are too toxic or corrosive. The widespread use of chemical disinfectants in hospitals for routine cleaning has been largely replaced by the use of neutral detergent. However, disinfectant chemicals are still used to clean contaminated articles or surfaces, to kill microorganisms present in accidental spills of potentially infected body fluids, and as antiseptics for disinfecting skin and tissue. Surface disinfectants are regulated by the Therapeutic Goods Administration (TGA). The list of solutions that should be used for cleaning or disinfecting various areas under certain prescribed conditions is usually contained in the infection control manual for each hospital.

It is important that health workers in the hospital environment understand the processes involved and are aware of the importance of following manufacturer's instructions and using the correct concentration of chemicals and exposure times to achieve the desired result (see page 237).

When using chemical disinfectants, care must be taken to ensure that every part of the article to be disinfected comes into contact with the disinfecting solution. The article must be free of dirt, grease, blood or any other organic material that might reduce the activity of the chemical. The solution must be used at the correct concentration to ensure there are sufficient molecules of the disinfectant present to kill all the microorganisms.

Some chemical disinfectants are unstable, especially in dilute solution, and so should always be used as freshly prepared solutions. It is also essential that the articles are immersed for a sufficient period of time, as the killing curve for chemical disinfection is similar to that for all sterilising and disinfecting methods (see Figure 11.1).

Not all chemical disinfectants are equally useful. A major factor in their use is cost, as well as their stability, ability to penetrate, and residual activity on surfaces. The advantages and disadvantages of some disinfectants are listed in Table 11.6.

Some chemicals (e.g. alcohol) react very rapidly, but do not penetrate well into microbial cells in the absence of water. Others, like the hypochlorites, also act rapidly but are corrosive at high concentrations. Some chemicals are more active against one type of microorganism than another.

Other factors that need to be taken into account when developing adequate procedures include the fact that some chemicals interact with (i.e. are neutralised by) the salts present in hard water, or with the plastics of which the containers or the articles to be disinfected are made.

PHENOLIC DISINFECTANTS

One of the earliest disinfectants used by Lister was the phenol, carbolic acid. Carbolic acid has a very powerful odour, is quite corrosive and has been replaced by derivatives of phenol with more acceptable properties. Phenols are active against a wide range of bacteria, including mycobacteria, but they do not kill endospores. They exert their effect by disruption of the cell membrane, denaturation of proteins and inactivation of enzymes, leading to cell death. Phenolic disinfectants are still widely used as they remain active in the presence of organic material (e.g. pus, faeces, or other body substances) and they are inexpensive, stable and relatively non-toxic. However, they are slightly corrosive and should not be used on skin or tissue. Their strong odour makes them unsuitable for use on surfaces that come into contact with food.

The most commonly used phenolic disinfectant is **o-cresol**, which is the main ingredient in a number of commercial brands of disinfectants. A 1–2% solution of this 'clear' phenol is used for terminal cleaning of contaminated environments and high-risk areas and for decontamination of equipment.

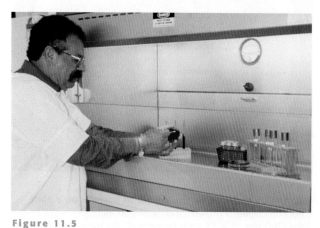

Figure 11.5
Biological safety cabinet

Table 11.6
Chemical disinfectants

DISINFECTANT	USE	ADVANTAGES/DISADVANTAGES
Phenolics	Environmental surfaces	Economical; not affected by organic material; unpleasant odour.
Chlorine (as sodium hypochlorite)	Environmental uses: • decontamination of blood spills • terminal cleaning • treatment of swimming pools • purification of drinking water	Inexpensive; active against viruses, spores, TB, bacteria; high concentrations are corrosive; unstable, inactivated by organic material.
Chlorhexidine	Skin, handwash, surgical scrub	Non-toxic, antibacterial, good residual activity; not active against viruses, endospores.
Povidone-iodine (iodophore)	Skin, preparation for surgery	Active against viruses, endospores; causes stains.
Alcohol 70% ethyl or isopropyl alcohol	Skin decontamination before injections Alcohol wipes for equipment	Inexpensive; active against bacteria and fungi; flammable.
Quaternary ammonium compounds	Preservative in pharmaceutical preparations	Stable, non-toxic; effective against most microbes; easily contaminated with *Pseudomonas*.

Hexachlorophene is a phenol derivative that was once widely used as an antibacterial agent in soaps, lotions and surgical scrubs, and in various cosmetic and hygiene products. It has a bacteriostatic action and is effective against Gram-positive staphylococci and streptococci. Hexachlorophene emulsion was once used routinely to bathe babies in hospital nurseries in order to prevent staphylococcal infections. However, it has been shown to have toxic effects after excessive use, causing neurological damage, and so its use has been largely discontinued.

Halogens

The halogens – iodine and chlorine – are very effective antimicrobial agents. **Chlorine**, in the form of **sodium hypochlorite (bleach)**, is an effective disinfectant that is active against a range of microorganisms. Chlorine kills bacteria and viruses and is active against the blood-borne viruses, HBV and HIV. It is relatively inexpensive and readily available for domestic use (swimming pools, bathroom cleaners, soaking baby's bottles and nappies). The chlorine released in aqueous solutions of sodium hypochlorite is a potent oxidising agent. However, because it is an oxidising agent it is inactivated by any organic material that may be present. It is therefore important to clean articles thoroughly before treating them with hypochlorite solutions.

The compound breaks down gradually, especially in sunlight, so fresh solutions should be used. A number of commercial preparations are available and the concentration of available chlorine varies among manufacturers. It is therefore necessary to check the strength of the solution used (usually stated as percentage of available chlorine)

and to ensure that the correct dilution is made. If the solution is too weak, the disinfecting action will not occur. However, chlorine is corrosive and care must be taken that the solution used is not too strong, especially if it comes into contact with skin or utensils used for babies.

Chlorine is used at a concentration of 10 000 ppm (parts per million) or 1% for decontamination of spillages of blood or body fluids. At this strength it is quite corrosive. It is sometimes replaced by sodium dichloroisocyanurate, a solid chlorine-releasing agent that is less corrosive. It comes in tablet or powder form and can be added as a solid to blood spills. It is advisable to wear gloves when handling these chemicals and to avoid inhaling the vapour.

For environmental decontamination, such as terminal cleaning of a room that has accommodated an infectious patient, or for the disinfection of contaminated equipment, chlorine is used at 1000 ppm or 0.1%. Chlorine is widely used to purify drinking water and in swimming pools, at a concentration of 1–5 ppm. **Chloramines** are organic chlorine-containing compounds that release chlorine slowly over a period of time. They are used to purify household water supplies as they do not have the unpleasant taste and odour sometimes associated with the chlorination of water.

Alcohol

Ethyl alcohol and **isopropyl alcohol** are effective antibacterial chemicals. Alcohols affect the cells by dissolving the lipids in the bacterial cell wall and membranes. They are most effective when mixed with water (usually 70% alcohol/water) as the water helps the alcohol to penetrate the cell. The alcohol/water preparation is also effective in the denaturation of proteins. Alcohols are used mainly to disinfect clean surfaces such as trolleys and thermometers, as alcohol wipes, and as a skin disinfectant before injections are given. The presence of organic material interferes with their action.

They are often used in combination with other antiseptics such as chlorhexidine in alcohol rubs for the quick disinfection of the hands, the main advantage being the ease of evaporation which removes the need for rinsing or drying.

Glutaraldehyde

Glutaraldehyde is a non-corrosive chemical that can act as a sterilising agent when used at high concentrations and for sufficient exposure time. However, it is more commonly used at lower concentrations and for shorter periods of time as a high-level disinfectant. It appears to exert its effect by disrupting the structure of the microbial proteins. It is a broad spectrum antimicrobial chemical that can kill vegetative cells in a few minutes and endospores within a few hours.

Glutaraldehyde can be used on delicate heat-sensitive instruments such as flexible endoscopes. It can retain its potency even in the presence of organic material. However, it acts as a fixative that hardens organic material and thus creates a protective barrier for the micro-organisms against contact with the agent. As with any disinfection or sterilisation process, equipment should be cleansed of grease and dirt before immersion in glutaraldehyde solutions.

Glutaraldehyde is somewhat unstable, especially at alkaline pH and high temperatures, so solutions may retain their activity for only a couple of weeks or for a certain number of uses.

Glutaraldehyde is toxic and allergenic and equipment treated with it must be thoroughly rinsed in sterile water before use. There is increasing concern about its toxic properties – contact with glutaraldehyde solutions, aerosols and vapours can cause irritation to the skin, eyes and the mucous membranes lining the nose, throat and lungs, as well as producing headaches and nausea. People working with glutaraldehyde can become sensitised to the chemical and develop allergic reactions. Worksafe Australia recommends a threshold exposure limit of 0.2 ppm (0.7 mg/m^3) for short-term exposure. Gloves should always be worn when handling glutaraldehyde and it must be used only in an area with local exhaust ventilation, but preferably in a closed containment system such as an automated endoscope reprocessor (AER).

It is not recommended for routine cleaning or disinfection. It should only be used when no other method of reprocessing is suitable.

Triclosan

Triclosan is a diphenyl compound used as a broad spectrum antibacterial. It is used as a preservative in the pharmaceutical industry and in hand and body wash preparations for laboratories and medical/surgical units. It has recently received a lot of publicity because of its inclusion in antimicrobial household products. There is no evidence that antibacterials are necessary in a healthy household and there is some concern that their use may lead to the selection of resistant organisms.

Quaternary ammonium compounds (QUATS)

These compounds are cationic detergents with a strong bactericidal action, due to the positive charge on the molecule. They are also effective against many fungi, some protozoa and enveloped viruses, but they do not affect endospores. They are thought to act by damaging the cell membrane. The main advantage of QUATS is that they are relatively stable, non-toxic, odourless and tasteless. However, some organisms – such as certain species of *Pseudomonas* – thrive in aqueous QUAT solutions. Because of the ease of contamination with *Pseudomonas*, which is a serious opportunistic pathogen, QUATS are no longer widely used in hospitals.

Two of the most common substances in use are benzyl alkalonium chloride, which is used as a preservative in eye drops, and cetyl pyridinium chloride, which is used extensively in oral preparations such as antibacterial lozenges and mouthwashes.

SKIN DISINFECTANTS – ANTISEPTICS

Specially formulated chemical disinfectants that are sufficiently mild to be used on skin, mucous membranes and exposed tissues are called **antiseptics**. Handwashing with antiseptic solutions is recommended as routine practice before carrying out medical and nursing procedures. Most antiseptics marketed in Australia are either registered medicines or listable medicines (e.g. tea tree oil) and require a registration number on the label. The label claims are important and should be followed. The Therapeutic Goods Administration (TGA) is responsible for regulating skin disinfectants and antiseptics.

Chlorhexidine

Chlorhexidine is a very effective antibacterial agent, widely used as an antiseptic for disinfection of skin and mucous membranes. A number of commercial preparations are available containing chlorhexidine in combination with various soaps or detergent, as alcohol rubs or in skin lotions (various preparations of Hibitane®).

It has an immediate, cumulative and residual action on skin bacteria, especially Gram-positive bacteria, where it acts by attacking the plasma membrane. It does not affect mycobacteria or endospores and *Pseudomonas* spp. are able to survive in aqueous solutions. It is effective against fungi and some viruses, including HIV. One of the main advantages of chlorhexidine is its low toxicity and its ability to persist on the skin for extended periods. This residual activity makes it useful in hospitals for hand disinfection and as a surgical scrub.

Povidone-iodine

Iodine is an effective antimicrobial compound and is generally used in an **iodophor**, which is a combination of the organic molecule, **povidone**, and iodine. The advantage of iodophors is that the iodine is released slowly, producing good residual antiseptic activity on the skin. Povidone-iodine, when combined with detergent, is an effective antiseptic surgical scrub and is used for disinfecting wounds. It has a broad spectrum of antimicrobial activity, including endospores, and is active against *Clostridium perfringens* (the causative agent of gangrene). For this reason it is widely used for skin disinfection pre-operatively, before a surgical incision is made.

The disadvantage is that it can produce hypersensitivity reactions and causes (temporary) discolouration of the skin. Solutions must be checked as *Pseudomonas* is able to grow in iodophor solutions.

Natural remedies – essential oils

Several essential oils, particularly **tea tree oil**, have gained widespread popularity as antimicrobial agents. A limited number of studies have been done on their effectiveness against various microorganisms. For household use they should be used in accordance with the manufacturer's instructions to ensure they meet the claims for efficacy and to avoid undesirable side effects.

Other methods of microbial control

OXIDISING AGENTS

Some oxidising agents are also used to destroy bacteria; for example, **hydrogen peroxide** can act as an antiseptic and weak solutions are used for cleaning deep puncture wounds. Hydrogen peroxide is used in low-temperature plasma sterilising units. **Benzoyl peroxide** is used to treat infections in anaerobic wounds and is also an ingredient in cosmetic preparations for the treatment of acne.

REFRIGERATION, FREEZING, DRYING

These methods are discussed here for completeness, but they are *not* methods of killing microorganisms. They are used mainly for control of microbial growth. Cold temperatures, such as are found in a domestic refrigerator (4°C), slow down the rate of cell division of most microorganisms but do not kill them. The rate of food spoilage can be slowed by refrigeration but, when the food is removed and warmed to room temperature, the microorganisms will continue to multiply.

Freezing is a more effective method of food preservation, but it does not kill microorganisms either. The rate of growth is negligible, so the food does not spoil. Some microbial cells may be destroyed by the formation of ice crystals, which disrupt the cell membranes, especially if repeated freezing and thawing occurs, but freezing does *not* cause significant death of microbes. In fact, a standard method for the preservation of bacterial cultures is rapid freezing in liquid nitrogen at –70°C.

Drying preserves food by reducing moisture but does not necessarily kill the organisms present; nor does the process of freeze-drying (**lyophilisation**) which involves the removal of water under vacuum from a frozen solution. Freeze-drying is also used to preserve microorganisms, which remain viable for long periods (months to years) at room temperature as a lyophilised powder.

CHEMICAL PRESERVATIVES

Chemicals are used as preservatives in food because they inhibit microbial metabolism or growth. Organic acids such as sorbic acid and benzoic acid inhibit the growth of mould at low pH. **Calcium propionate** is used as a fungal inhibitor in bread. The benzoic acid derivatives, methyl paraben and propylparaben, are used as preservatives in cosmetics and shampoos.

SUMMARY

- Microorganisms are present everywhere in the environment but only some cause disease.
- Different methods of control are required for different situations and different types of organisms.

TRADITIONAL METHODS

- Food can be preserved by physical methods such as drying, heating, pickling and salting.
- Joseph Lister was the first to use chemical disinfection to prevent infections following surgery.
- Ignaz Semmelweis observed that pathogens could be transmitted on unwashed hands.

PATTERN OF MICROBIAL DEATH

- Damage to any of the structural or functional components of a cell will result in its death.

- The rate of death of a population of microorganisms follows an exponential curve.

CLEANING, DISINFECTION AND STERILISATION

- The highest risk of transmission of infection is associated with equipment that penetrates the skin or mucous membranes.
- The removal of organic matter, dirt and grease is essential before carrying out disinfection or sterilisation procedures.

STERILISATION

- Sterilisation involves the complete destruction or removal of all living organisms from an object.
- Physical methods of sterilisation use heat or radiation; mechanical methods use filtration; chemical methods use glutaraldehyde, or ethylene oxide, or hydrogen peroxide.

- Dry heat kills by oxidation. Moist heat kills by denaturation.
- The cheapest and most effective method of sterilisation uses moist heat (steam under pressure). The efficiency of the steriliser should be monitored regularly.
- Heat-resistant metal and glass can be sterilised in a hot oven at 180°C for 60 minutes.
- Incineration is used for the complete destruction of contaminated articles.
- Ionising radiation kills microorganisms by disrupting the DNA chains.
- Filtration is used to sterilise heat-sensitive substances.
- Ethylene oxide gas is used to sterilise prepackaged disposable equipment.
- Low-temperature plasma sterilisation uses hydrogen peroxide.

DISINFECTION

- Disinfection involves the removal or destruction of microorganisms to an 'acceptable level'.

- Glutaraldehyde is used to disinfect delicate heat-sensitive instruments to a high level.
- Antiseptics are chemical disinfectants that are mild enough to use on skin.
- Methods of disinfection include boiling at 100°C, pasteurisation, UV radiation, filtration and the use of chemicals.
- Some examples of chemical disinfectants are phenols, halogens (iodine and chlorine), chlorhexidine, alcohol and QUATS.
- Every part of the article to be disinfected must come into contact with the disinfecting solution.

OTHER METHODS OF MICROBIAL CONTROL

- Other methods of control include refrigeration, freezing, drying and the use of chemical preservatives or oxidising agents.

STUDY QUESTIONS

1. What are some traditional methods of food preservation?
2. What is pasteurisation?
3. Who was the first doctor to use chemical disinfectants in surgery?
4. What contribution did Ignaz Semmelweis make to medicine?
5. What two factors determine the efficiency of the disinfecting process?
6. Why do instruments need to be cleaned before being treated with disinfectant?
7. What is the difference between sterilisation and disinfection?
8. What are the advantages of moist heat sterilisation?
9. How do you check whether a steriliser is functioning properly? Why is this important?
10. How do gamma rays have a sterilising effect?
11. When is filtration used to sterilise solutions?
12. What are the disadvantages of sterilisation with ethylene oxide?
13. Why is glutaraldehyde only recommended for use in special circumstances? What are those circumstances?
14. What is an antiseptic?
15. When is ultraviolet radiation used?
16. Why is hexachlorophene no longer used to bathe babies?
17. What are the advantages and disadvantages of phenolic disinfectants?
18. What antiseptics are the most effective for skin disinfection?
19. What disinfectant is used to decontaminate blood spills?
20. How is drinking water purified?
21. When is it appropriate to use alcohol as a disinfectant?
22. What is a major disadvantage of QUATS?
23. What happens to bacteria when they are stored in the refrigerator or freezer?
24. List two chemicals that are used as preservatives.

TEST YOUR UNDERSTANDING

1. Explain what you understand by the term 'killing curve' when applied to sterilising or disinfecting procedures.
2. How do you decide whether equipment needs to be sterilised or disinfected?
3. Why is boiling instruments at 100°C not considered to be a method of sterilisation?
4. How can hazardous substances or infectious microorganisms be safely handled in the laboratory?
5. Why is chlorine used extensively for disinfection?
6. Why is it important not to reuse disposable equipment?

References

AS/NZS 4187 (2003) *Cleaning, disinfecting and sterilising reusable medical and surgical instruments and equipment, and maintenance of associated environments in health care facilities.*

AS/NZS 4815 (2001) *Office-based health care facilities not involved in complex patient procedures and processes – Cleaning, disinfecting and sterilising reusable medical and surgical instruments and equipment.*

Communicable Diseases Network Australia (CDNA) 2004, *Infection Control Guidelines for the prevention of transmission of infectious diseases in the health care setting*, Canberra, Australian Government Publishing Service.

Gardner JF & M Peel 1998, *Introduction to Sterilization, Disinfection and Infection Control*, 3rd edn, Sydney: Churchill Livingstone.

Cowan AE et al 1999, *Infection Control in Endoscopy*, 4th edn published jointly by the Gastroenterological Society of Australia (GESA) and the Gastroenterological Nurses College of Australia (GENCA).

National Occupational Health and Safety Commission 1991, *Workplace Control of Hazardous Substances: National Model Regulations and National Code of Practice*, Canberra: Australian Government Publishing Service.

CHAPTER 12

Control of Infection: Antimicrobial Therapy

[CHAPTER FOCUS]

- Describe the discovery and development of antimicrobial drugs.

- What are the principles underlying the effective use of antimicrobial drugs?

- How do antimicrobials kill, or inhibit the growth of, microbial cells?

- What guidelines are advised when prescribing antimicrobial drugs?

- How do microorganisms become resistant to antimicrobial drugs?

- What are the consequences of the development of resistance to antimicrobial drugs?

- What strategies can be used to minimise the spread of resistant microorganisms?

- What are the responsibilities of the nurse in the administration of antimicrobial therapy?

Introduction

By the end of the 19th century the work of Robert Koch and other scientists had resulted in the isolation and identification of the bacteria responsible for many of the known infectious diseases, and various physical or chemical methods that killed or inactivated microorganisms were being used to control the spread of infection (see Chapter 11). However, the chemical disinfectants used to kill bacteria on skin, wounds and tissues were relatively non-specific in their action and the treatment of infectious diseases still relied mainly on supportive methods that alleviated the symptoms. So, in spite of these advances, at the beginning of the 20th century one-third of all children still died from an infectious disease before the age of five.

For centuries, extracts from plants and herbs have been used to treat illness. We now know that some of these preparations contain valuable therapeutic drugs. For example: aspirin was first extracted from the bark of the willow tree; morphine is derived from the seeds of the opium poppy; quinine, used against malaria, comes from the bark of the chinchona tree; and digitalis, used in the treatment of heart disease, was first extracted from foxglove leaves.

Ancient Chinese culture has traditionally used combinations of herbs to treat illness. The mouldy soybean preparation that was placed on infected wounds probably contained small amounts of an antibiotic such as penicillin. Plant extracts were used in a variety of ways – as medicinal teas, as inhalants, or as poultices placed on wounds or inflammation. Many of these treatments were successful but the mechanism by which they effected a 'cure' was, and still is, largely unknown. These alternative remedies are becoming increasingly popular in Australia.

(Any product for which therapeutic claims are made must be entered in the Australian Register of Therapeutic Goods (ARTG) before it can be supplied in Australia.)

THE MAGIC BULLET

The idea of finding a chemical that could specifically kill the microbe responsible for an infection without damaging the host cells (i.e. a 'magic bullet') was proposed by the chemist PAUL EHRLICH in 1908. It was known that arsenic was toxic to many bacteria, but it was also toxic to humans. Ehrlich set about trying to synthesise an organic compound containing arsenic that would retain the antimicrobial properties but would be less toxic to humans. The compound he prepared was called *salvarsan* and was found to be effective against spirochaetes, in particular the bacterium responsible for syphilis, *Treponema pallidum*.

Ehrlich's work opened up a whole new approach to the treatment of disease. Chemists tried to repeat his success with salvarsan by synthesising various chemical compounds, but most of them were found to be too toxic for human use. However, the new science of chemotherapy had been created.

Chemotherapy involves the introduction of a specific chemical compound, or drug, into the body in order to elicit a particular desired response, preferably without causing harm to the patient. It includes the use of drugs to kill or inhibit microorganisms as well as drugs used to treat other diseases such as cancer.

SULFA DRUGS

Inspired by Ehrlich's synthesis of salvarsan, another chemist, GERHARD DOMAGK in Germany, tested a dye called prontosil for its ability to kill streptococci. He found that it was active in animal tissues, where it was converted to a compound called **sulfanilamide**, a potent inhibitor of bacterial replication. The discovery of sulfanilamide led to the synthesis of a large number of similar drugs, collectively named **sulfonamides**, or **sulfa drugs**. These sulfa drugs exhibit activity against a variety of pathogens. However, many organisms have developed resistance to them and they frequently cause side effects such as skin rashes.

There are now few specific indications for the clinical use of sulfonamides alone. They are used mainly in combination for the treatment and prophylaxis of *Pneumocystis carinii* pneumonia and malaria and for the topical treatment of severe burns.

THE DISCOVERY OF ANTIBIOTICS

A breakthrough in the treatment of infections came with the discovery of antibiotics. In 1928, at about the same time the sulfa drugs were being developed, an English doctor, ALEXANDER FLEMING noticed that the growth of *Staphylococcus aureus* on an agar plate had been inhibited by a common blue/green mould. He correctly deduced that the mould had produced a chemical that diffused through the agar and killed the bacteria. He called the chemical **penicillin** from the name of the mould *Penicillium*. Surprisingly, he did not realise the therapeutic value of his discovery and it was not until 1940 that interest in the compound as a treatment for serious infections was revived.

Its development was due largely to an Australian physician, HOWARD FLOREY, who was working at Oxford and became interested in penicillin as a chemotherapeutic agent. In collaboration with the chemist ERNST CHAIN, he was largely responsible for the project that resulted in the isolation and purification of penicillin and the clinical trials that were necessary to establish it as a 'miracle cure'. With the backing of the US government, they undertook the production of large quantities of penicillin that were used successfully to treat infections in wounded soldiers in World War II.

The dramatic results obtained with penicillin encouraged scientists to look for other microorganisms that produced substances that might also have antimicrobial activity.

The term **antibiotic** is used to describe a compound *produced by a microorganism that in small amounts can kill or inhibit another microorganism*. Antibiotics are natural products of various microorganisms, including fungi, actinomycetes and bacteria, many of which are found in soil. More than half the antibiotics in use are produced by different species of filamentous soil bacteria belonging to the genus *Streptomyces*. See Figure 12.1. Although many antimicrobials are derived from natural sources, a number of them have been chemically modified in order to improve their antimicrobial properties and are, therefore, called 'semi-synthetic'.

Antimicrobial drugs

SELECTIVE TOXICITY

The principle of **selective toxicity** is fundamental to the successful development, production and use of any chemotherapeutic agent. It requires the drug to be able to kill or inhibit the microorganism responsible for the disease without causing damage to the host cells. It is relatively easy to find chemicals that can kill microorganisms – it is not so easy to find one that can do so without harming the human host. In order to find a suitable drug it is necessary to identify a reaction or structure that is unique to the target microorganism but which does not occur in, or is not essential to, the host cell. The drug must be able to alter or damage the microorganism in such a way as to either prevent replication, or cause the death of the microbial cell. The principle of selective toxicity, therefore, exploits any differences in structure or metabolism between the microbial cell and the host cell.

Procaryotic (bacterial) cells have a number of characteristics that are unique and provide possible sites of attack. It is more difficult to identify points of difference in eucaryotic microorganisms, because they have more structural and functional similarities to human cells. Viral replication involves taking over the host cell, so any compound that interferes with viral replication is also likely to

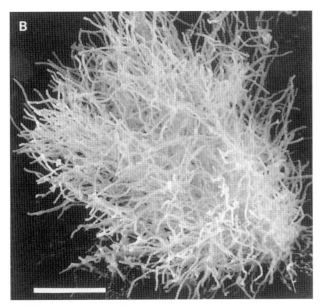

Figure 12.1

Scanning electron micrograph of a *Streptomyces* sp. which produces the antibiotic actinomycin, showing aerial mycelium with straight chains of spores

damage the host cell. Sometimes, a drug will be considered to be selectively toxic because of the greater affinity of the drug for the microbial enzyme than for the host cell enzyme.

ANTIMICROBIAL THERAPY

So far we have described the discovery of two different kinds of compounds that affect microbial growth. Antibiotics such as penicillin are naturally occurring substances, whereas the sulfa drugs are completely synthetic. Attempts by scientists to find effective antimicrobial agents have resulted in the production of a range of naturally occurring, synthetic and semi-synthetic drugs, with varying activity against the different types of microorganisms.

The term **antimicrobial** is used to describe a compound that is able to kill, or inhibit the growth of, a microorganism. Strictly speaking, antibiotics are a particular type of naturally occurring antimicrobial compound, but in practice the terms 'antibiotic' and 'antimicrobial' are used interchangeably. Thus, an 'antibiotic sensitivity test', performed in a diagnostic microbiology laboratory, should correctly be called an 'antimicrobial sensitivity test' because it tests the sensitivity of a particular microorganism to a range of compounds, some of which are naturally occurring, but some of which may be chemically modified antibiotics, semi-synthetic (e.g. amoxycillin) or completely synthetic (e.g. sulfa drugs and quinolones).

We can further separate antimicrobial drugs into groups depending on the type of organism they are active against. Thus, antibacterials are active against bacteria, antivirals against viruses, antifungals against fungi and antiprotozoals against protozoa. The reason that drugs tend to be active against only one type of organism (e.g. antibacterials do not kill viruses) is related to its mechanism of action. To selectively kill or inhibit the microorganism, the drug must attack or interfere with a structure or a step in a metabolic or replicative process that is unique to the organism and preferably not present in the host cell. Since different types of microorganisms have different cellular components and metabolic processes, the drugs that are most effective against one type of organism may not affect another type.

Compounds that are active against a number of different microorganisms are called **broad spectrum antimicrobial agents**, while those with a limited range of activity are called **narrow spectrum antimicrobial agents**. Some agents are able to kill microorganisms and are identified by the addition of the suffix *-cidal*; for example, penicillin is **bactericidal**. Others inhibit the replication of the organism without killing it and have the ending *-static*; for example, tetracycline is **bacteriostatic**.

These properties are also related to the drug's mechanism of action. In general, drugs that are bactericidal result in irreversible damage to a cell (e.g. the formation of an unstable cell wall) so that the cell is no longer viable. In contrast, agents that are bacteriostatic interfere with metabolism or the synthesis of a compound such as an enzyme protein, which prevents replication but does not necessarily cause the death of the cell. Their effect is thus reversed once they are removed from the cell. Even though they do not kill the cell, bacteriostatic agents are useful because they prevent further replication of the pathogen and allow the immune system time to mount its defences against the infection.

When possible it is preferable to use a bactericidal agent, especially for immunocompromised patients whose own defences are not able to complete the task of eliminating the pathogens from the body.

One of the major problems associated with the use of antimicrobials is the development of resistance to the antimicrobial drug. This can take many forms and is discussed later in this chapter.

Therapeutic Guidelines – Antibiotic, published by Therapeutic Guidelines Ltd, lists the antimicrobial drugs that are approved for use in Australia and describes in detail recommendations for the management of infections in various body systems. Students should be aware of the nomenclature used for drugs. The **generic name** is the chemical name of the compound. Different drug companies may market the same compound under different names – the **trade name**.

Antibacterial drugs

Procaryotic organisms (bacteria) are free-living single-celled organisms with several unique characteristics which distinguish them from their host cells.

There are four main target sites for selective antibacterial action (see Figure 12.2):

1. synthesis of the bacterial cell wall
2. protein synthesis
3. nucleic acid synthesis
4. function of the bacterial cell membrane.

COMPOUNDS THAT AFFECT THE CELL WALL

The integrity of the cell wall of a bacterium is essential to maintain its shape and provide structural support for the cell. Animal cells are enclosed only by a membrane so the bacterial cell wall is a very suitable target for antimicrobial action. Peptidoglycan, a major component of the bacterial wall is unique to bacteria and thus provides an ideal target for selective attack. A number of antibacterials have been found that exert their action by interfering with the synthesis of peptidoglycan. One of the most important of these is **penicillin**, which belongs to a group of antibacterials known collectively as **beta-lactams**. Beta-lactam antibacterials derive their name from the four-membered beta-lactam ring which is present in all these compounds (see Figure 12.3).

Resistance to these compounds is frequently associated with the production of an enzyme, beta-lactamase, which breaks open this ring and destroys the antibacterial compound. Other members of the beta-lactam group are the cephalosporins, carbapenems and monobactams (see Figure 12.4 and Table 12.2).

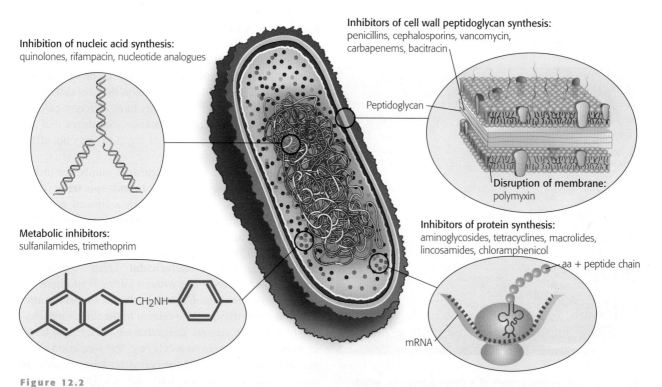

Figure 12.2

A summary of the major modes of action of antibacterial drugs
This illustration shows these actions as they might affect a highly diagrammatic representation of a bacterial cell.

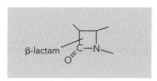

Figure 12.3

The beta-lactam ring

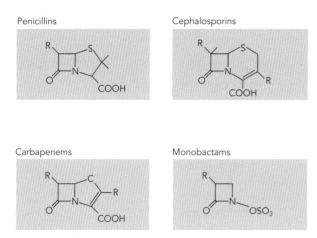

Figure 12.4

Comparison of the structures of the beta-lactam inhibitors of cell wall synthesis

Different drugs in each class are synthesised by the substitution of different chemical groups for the R-side chain.

The beta-lactams inhibit cell wall synthesis by combining with the transpeptidase enzyme responsible for cross-linking of the peptidoglycan chains. Thus, these drugs are mainly active against growing cells, preventing the formation of a rigid cell wall structure. This results in a cell without a protective support layer, making it vulnerable to cell lysis (i.e. a bactericidal effect).

Beta-lactam drugs are particularly useful because they affect the synthesis of a structure unique to bacteria and are thus of low toxicity to humans. A small number of people develop an allergy to them; this may be due to the formation of a conjugate of the beta-lactam ring with scrum proteins, which elicits an inflammatory immune response, or to impurities in the product. People who are truly allergic to penicillin are usually also allergic to most other beta-lactam antibacterials (see Spotlight box at right).

Penicillins

Penicillin is isolated from the mould *Penicillium chrysogenum* and occurs naturally in a number of closely related forms. These include penicillin G (benzyl penicillin), which is extremely effective but readily inactivated by the low pH encountered in the stomach. It is usually administered intramuscularly or intravenously as the sodium or potassium salt. Another commonly used natural penicillin, phenoxymethylpenicillin (penicillin V), is acid-stable and can be taken orally, although it is not well absorbed and is excreted rapidly.

Research has been directed at developing semi-synthetic penicillins in an effort to overcome the problems

SPOTLIGHT ON
Penicillin and anaphylactic shock

Anaphylaxis due to the parenteral administration of penicillin is a rare but life-threatening occurrence. It has an incidence of about 1 in 2000 of all patients receiving penicillin and a mortality of 1 in 50 000. Prompt administration of adrenaline (epinephrine) by intramuscular injection is essential.

An allergic (hypersensitivity) reaction to penicillin is a genetically determined reaction associated with the individual's immune system. In some people, exposure to the drug elicits an allergic immune response. The penicillin molecule is broken down and reacts with certain tissue proteins to form a complex that stimulates the immune system to produce IgE antibodies. The antibodies attach to the surface of mast cells and basophils which are distributed throughout the body. These cells are then 'sensitised'. If the patient is exposed to penicillin again, the sensitised cells rapidly release histamine and other active substances that cause anaphylactic reactions ranging from urticaria (rashes), hives and laryngeal oedema to bronchoconstriction and hypotension. The most severe form of anaphylaxis is described as anaphylactic shock and can be fatal.

A number of patients report being 'allergic' to penicillin, having reactions that may include symptoms such as a skin rash, but the anaphylactic response is the only major contraindication to its use. It is possible to ascertain whether a patient is hypersensitive to penicillin by the use of a skin test. A positive reaction to the injection of the penicillin complex occurs in 10–15 minutes.

Patients who are hypersensitive to penicillin also exhibit a reaction to the semi-synthetic penicillins as well as to other antimicrobials that have a beta-lactam ring (e.g. the cephalosporins). Usually, vancomycin is used instead of penicillin. However, it must be administered by slow intravenous infusion (see Case History 12.1, page 271).

Nursing management

It is essential that all patients be asked whether they have a history of allergy to penicillin before the drug is administered. If patients are unclear about their history or have no memory of having had the drug before, then special precautions must be taken. It is essential that adrenaline (epinephrine) is available when penicillin (or any drug) is administered parenterally. Nurses should check the 'use by' date on the ampoule to ensure the adrenaline is still current.

If penicillin is administered orally, the nurse should observe the patient for any signs of rash, difficulty in breathing, etc.

Note: Antihistamines and corticosteroids are *not* effective treatment for penicillin-induced anaphylaxis.

Table 12.1

The penicillins

PENICILLIN	ROUTE OF ADMINISTRATION	SPECTRUM OF ANTIBACTERIAL ACTIVITY
Natural penicillins		
Benzyl penicillin (Penicillin G)	IV, IM	Streptococci, pneumococci, meningococci
Phenoxymethyl penicillin (Penicillin V)	Oral	Gram-positives, esp. streptococci
Semi-synthetic penicillins		
Ampicillin Amoxycillin Amoxycillin + clavulanate (Augmentin®)	Oral, IM, IV	As for penicillin G plus *E. coli*, *Haemophilus influenzae*
Dicloxacillin Flucloxacillin	Oral, IM, IV	Mostly staphylococci
Ticarcillin Ticarcillin + clavulanate (Timentin®)	IM, IV	Pseudomonads
Piperacillin Piperacillin + tazobactam	IM, IV	Pseudomonads Gram-negatives

Note: Methicillin is no longer widely used because of nephrotoxicity.

associated with the naturally occurring compounds – problems such as susceptibility to gastric acid, lack of water solubility, rapid excretion (= short retention) time, narrow spectrum of activity, susceptibility to beta-lactamase enzymes and the development of resistance.

Table 12.1 lists the major penicillins in use. The naturally occurring penicillins are active mainly against Gram-positive organisms, whereas the newer, semi-synthetic compounds have a broader spectrum of activity. For example, ampicillin, amoxycillin, piperacillin and ticarcillin are also active against Gram-negative organisms. Penicillins that are resistant to breakdown by beta-lactamases include methicillin, flucloxacillin and dicloxacillin.

Clavulanic acid (a naturally occurring compound extracted from a streptomycete), sulbactam and tazobactam inhibit the beta-lactamase enzymes produced by a number of bacteria. They do not have significant antibacterial activity on their own but, when clavulanate is combined with amoxycillin in Augmentin®, or with ticarcillin in Timentin®, their spectrum of activity is extended.

Cephalosporins

Cephalosporins are produced by a species of the marine fungus *Cephalosporium*. They also inhibit synthesis of the peptidoglycan of the cell wall and have a similar structure to the penicillins, containing a beta-lactam ring (Figure 12.5). They are more active against Gram-negative organisms than the penicillins and chemical modification

Cephalosporins have the basic chemical structure illustrated here

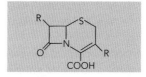

Figure 12.5

Cephalosporins

of the side chains of the cephalosporin nucleus has given rise to a series of compounds with increased antibacterial activity, known as second, third and fourth generation cephalosporins (see Table 12.2). These are now widely used for the treatment of all types of infections in hospitals, the choice of drug being determined by its mode of administration and spectrum of activity and its ability to be absorbed and penetrate to the site of infection.

Carbapenems

Carbapenems are synthetic beta-lactam compounds with a wide spectrum of activity and are stable against a wide range of beta-lactamases. **Imipenem** is rapidly broken down in the kidney but high concentrations of the drug can be achieved in the urine and serum if it is administered in combination with the enzyme inhibitor, cilastin. Imipenem causes neurological side effects such as convulsions and is being replaced by **meropenem**, which is not metabolised by the renal cells. Ertapenem is a newer drug with similar

Table 12.2

Some cephalosporins and their derivatives

CEPHALOSPORIN	ROUTE OF ADMINISTRATION
First generation – moderate spectrum	
Cephalothin	IM, IV
Cephalexin	Oral
Cephazolin	IM, IV
Second generation – moderate spectrum	
Cefaclor	Oral
Cefuroxime	Oral
Cephamandole	IM, IV
Cefoxitin	IM, IV
Cefotetan	IM, IV
Third generation – broad spectrum	
Cefotaxime	IM, IV
Ceftriaxone	IM, IV
Fourth generation – extended spectrum	
Cefepime	IM, IV
Cefpirome	IM, IV
Ceftazidime	IM, IV

properties to imipenem but with a long half-life so that it need be administered only once daily. Carbapenems are available only for parenteral use so are generally restricted to the specific treatment of pathogenic bacteria that are resistant to other antibiotics.

Monobactams

Monobactams are active mainly against aerobic Gram-negative bacteria (except *Pseudomonas*). Because anaerobes and Gram-positive organisms are resistant, monobactams may be used in combination with other antibiotics. They are useful for urinary tract infections, septicaemia and gonorrhoea and are not inactivated by Gram-negative beta-lactamase enzymes. They may be used for the treatment of Gram-negative infections in patients who cannot tolerate aminoglycosides because of impaired renal function.

Other cell wall inhibitors

The glycopeptides, **vancomycin** and **teicoplanin**, are large molecules that interfere with cell wall synthesis by binding to the growing peptide chains that are part of the peptidoglycan molecule, thus preventing further synthesis of the cell wall. Because of their size, these compounds cannot penetrate the Gram-negative outer membrane and so they are active mainly against Gram-positive organisms (exceptions are the *Flavobacteria* and some *Neisseria* spp.).

Vancomycin is poorly absorbed from the intestine. It *must* be administered by slow intravenous infusion over 1–2 hours in order to prevent histamine release and the 'red man syndrome' which can lead to cardiac arrest (see Case History 12.1, page 271). The drug is important as a

last resort treatment for methicillin-resistant staphylococcal infections (MRSA), but there is an increasing number of reports of the isolation of strains of MRSA with reduced sensitivity to vancomycin (called VISA or GISA – vancomycin/glycopeptide intermediate *Staphylococcus aureus*). The emergence of vancomycin-resistant enterococci (VRE) is also of concern, especially among seriously ill patients in high dependency areas (see Spotlight box, page 280). It should be used only in situations where other drugs are not effective.

INHIBITORS OF PROTEIN SYNTHESIS

The mechanism of protein synthesis is essentially the same in eucaryotic and procaryotic organisms. However, there are slight differences in the relative sizes and binding properties of the ribosomes in the two types of cell that permit some degree of selective toxicity. Antibacterials that inhibit protein synthesis act by interfering either with the translation of the messenger RNA into protein, or with the binding of the mRNA to the ribosomes. Because the 70S ribosomes in bacterial cells are smaller and less dense than the 80S eucaryotic host cell ribosomes, drugs that target the 70S ribosomes are able to affect the bacterial cells adversely, while not binding significantly to the host ribosomes. However, eucaryotic mitochondria also contain 70S ribosomes, so drugs that inhibit protein synthesis in bacteria can also affect the mitochondria of the host cells.

A number of different groups of antimicrobials affect protein synthesis in bacterial cells. They include the aminoglycosides, the tetracyclines and the macrolides, as well as lincosamides, chloramphenicol and fusidic acid. Compounds that inhibit the synthesis of protein in the cell may be bactericidal or bacteriostatic.

Aminoglycosides

This family of antibacterial agents contains a number of useful drugs, including streptomycin, gentamicin, tobramycin, amikacin and neomycin (see Table 12.3). They are most useful in the treatment of sepsis due to Gram-negative aerobes and *Mycobacterium tuberculosis*. Their action is bactericidal as they cause misreading of the messenger RNA, leading to substitution of the wrong amino acid into the peptide chain, thus forming an inactive protein. They are often used for their synergistic effect in combination with another drug to enhance the therapeutic effect. For example, penicillin or ampicillin may be used in combination with gentamicin. The penicillins open up the cell wall, allowing greater penetration by the gentamicin.

Aminoglycosides are not absorbed from the intestine so are administered intramuscularly or intravenously for systemic infections, and must be monitored carefully for toxic side effects. These include **ototoxicity** (vertigo and deafness) and **nephrotoxicity** (kidney damage). They should be used cautiously in patients with impaired renal function.

Gentamicin is the aminoglycoside of choice in hospitals

Table 12.3

Aminoglycosides

AMINOGLYCOSIDE	ROUTE OF ADMINISTRATION	SPECTRUM OF ACTIVITY
Gentamicin	IM, IV	Gram-negative, may be used
Tobramycin	IM, IV	with penicillins
Amikacin	IM, IV	
Streptomycin	IM, IV	TB in combination with other drugs
Neomycin	Topical or oral for	Gram-positive, coliforms
Kanamycin	'gut sterilisation'	

for the treatment of hospital-acquired infections, especially Gram-negative coliforms and *Pseudomonas* infections.

Amikacin is resistant to inactivation by enzymes but is expensive so it is reserved for use with organisms resistant to other aminoglycosides.

Streptomycin, isolated from *Streptomyces griseus*, was one of the earliest aminoglycosides identified and was used extensively in the treatment of tuberculosis. It is now rarely used due to its toxicity and the fact that resistance to streptomycin developed rapidly.

Neomycin is very toxic but is poorly absorbed so is useful mainly in topical preparations.

Tetracyclines

Tetracyclines are a group of broad spectrum bacteriostatic agents that have been isolated from the members of the genus *Streptomyces*. They are bacteriostatic, inhibiting protein synthesis by preventing the attachment of amino acids to ribosomes. They have a broad spectrum of activity against both Gram-negative and Gram-positive organisms, intracellular chlamydiae and rickettsiae, mycoplasmas and spirochaetes, as well as some non-tuberculous myco-bacteria and protozoa. They are useful in the treatment of non-specific urethritis (NSU) since they are active against both *Neisseria gonorrhoea* and *Chlamydia*.

Tetracyclines are used in the treatment of pelvic inflam-matory disease, periodontal disease, brucellosis, plague, cholera, Lyme disease and community-acquired pneu-monia, and for prophylaxis against all strains of malaria where endemic strains are resistant to other common anti-malarial drugs.

Tetracyclines can be administered orally and modifica-tion of the side chains (see Figure 12.6) has produced a number of useful compounds that are better absorbed and have longer retention times in the body than the parent compound. Side effects of the tetracyclines are due mainly to their broad spectrum of activity which can cause sup-pression of the normal flora, leading to a superinfection or overgrowth of undesirable organisms such as *Candida albicans* (thrush).

Tetracyclines should not be given to pregnant women as they may affect liver function, or to young children as they deposit in developing teeth, causing permanent yellow discolouration, and may interfere with bone formation. Resistance to tetracyclines develops easily,

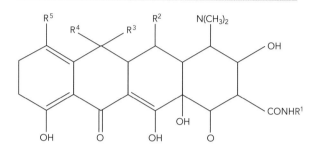

TETRACYCLINE STRUCTURE

	R^1	R^2	R^3	R^4	R^5
Tetracycline	H	H	CH_3	OH	H
Chlortetracycline	H	H	CH_3	OH	Cl
Oxytetracycline	H	OH	CH_3	OH	H
Doxycycline	H	OH	CH_3	H	H
Minocycline	H	H	H	H	$H(CH_3)_2$

Figure 12.6

Tetracycline structure
Tetracyclines are complex molecules consisting of four rings with five different sites for substitution. This gives rise to a family of molecules which differ more in their pharmacologi-cal properties than spectrum of activity.

and their widespread use in animal feeds has been thought to contribute to the transfer of resistant strains of bacteria to humans.

Doxycycline is the preferred tetracycline in most situa-tions, as it can be administered once daily. It can irritate the oesophagus so patients should be instructed to wash it down with water and remain upright for 30 minutes after taking it. It can also be used safely for long periods in low doses for the treatment of acne.

Macrolides

The **macrolides** are a group of antibacterials with a complex structure containing a macrocyclic (14-membered) lactone ring (see Figure 12.7).

The best known is **erythromycin** which is used exten-sively as an alternative drug for people who are allergic to penicillin. Its action is bacteriostatic, binding to 50S ribo-somes and preventing the release of transfer RNA (tRNA) after peptide bond formation. It has a wide spectrum of

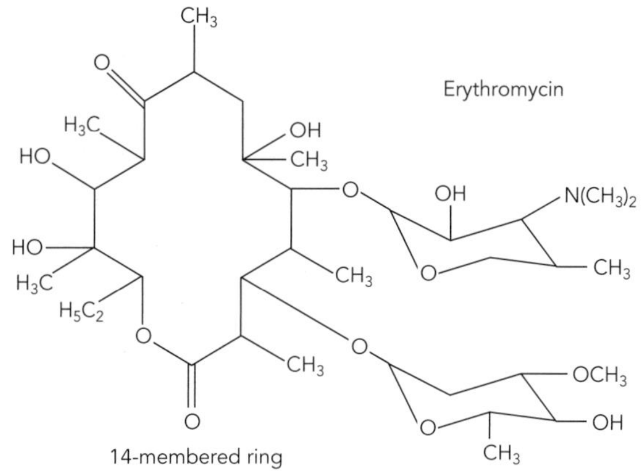

Figure 12.7

Structure of the macrolide antibiotic, erythromycin

activity against Gram-positive and Gram-negative cocci, but is not active against Gram-negative rods except *Campylobacter* spp. It is the drug of choice against *Legionella pneumophila* (Legionnaires' disease) and *Bordetella pertussis* (whooping cough). It is also active against *Mycoplasma* and *Chlamydia*. It is not affected by beta-lactamases and has been used extensively for streptococcal infections, especially in children, as it can be administered orally in a pleasant syrup. However, some resistance has been reported in both streptococci and staphylococci. Clinically, it is used for a variety of community-acquired respiratory infections, tonsillitis, bronchitis and pneumonia, as well as for non-specific urethritis.

Newer macrolides are **azithromycin**, **roxithromycin** and **clarithromycin**. They have better absorption and a longer shelf life than erythromycin. Clarithromycin has a similar spectrum of activity to erythromycin but is also active against *Mycobacterium avium intracellulare*, an opportunistic infection seen in immunocompromised patients. Azithromycin is excreted very slowly and is effective in single doses for chlamydial infections such as trachoma.

Lincosamides

Lincomycin and its chlorinated derivative, **clindamycin**, have been widely used in hospitals against Gram-positive aerobes and most anaerobes (*Clostridium* spp. and *Bacteroides*), especially for patients who are allergic to penicillin. They inhibit protein synthesis by binding to the 50S ribosomal subunit and inhibiting peptide bond formation. They penetrate tissue well and are particularly useful for bone and joint infections. However, a major side effect is the occurrence of antimicrobial-associated diarrhoea – in particular, pseudomembranous colitis caused by *Clostridium difficile* which is resistant to these drugs (see Chapter 18, page 425). Although other antibiotics have also been shown to give rise to this condition, it is particularly frequent following treatment with lincomycin or clindamycin and so their use has been restricted. Clindamycin is used for treatment of streptococcal toxic shock syndrome as it appears to interfere with superantigen production (see pages 225–26).

Chloramphenicol

Chloramphenicol is a simple compound (Figure 12.8) and has a wide spectrum of activity against both Gram-positive and Gram-negative organisms. It was originally isolated from *Streptomyces* but is now synthesised chemically because of its simple structure. It is bacteriostatic, inhibiting protein synthesis by binding to the 50S ribosomal subunit and preventing peptide bond formation by the enzyme peptidyl transferase. However, it is also able to bind to human mitochondrial 50S ribosomes, which may explain its toxicity to bone marrow.

Toxicity to chloramphenicol is of two types. The first is a reversible suppression of the bone marrow. The other is a rare type of toxicity (1 in 30 000) involving suppression of red blood cell synthesis in the bone marrow, leading to irreversible aplastic anaemia. The drug is metabolised in the liver, combining with glucuronic acid to be excreted via the kidneys in an inactive form. It is particularly toxic to neonates because they have immature liver enzyme systems. Because of its toxicity, the use of chloramphenicol has been limited to topical eye preparations. It is sometimes used to treat typhoid fever and, since it penetrates readily into the CSF, can be used for the treatment of some forms of bacterial meningitis.

Fusidic acid

Fusidic acid is a bacteriostatic agent that inhibits protein synthesis by complexing with the growing peptide chain. It is active against Gram-positive cocci and is useful in the treatment of staphylococcal infections that are resistant to the beta-lactams, or in patients allergic to penicillin. Resistance to fusidic acid develops easily so it should always be given in combination with other drugs (e.g. rifampicin).

INHIBITORS OF NUCLEIC ACID SYNTHESIS

Antibacterials that interfere with nucleic acid synthesis can do so either by inhibiting the synthesis of the nucleotide precursors or by inhibiting DNA or RNA replication.

Sulfonamides

The sulfonamides are a group of synthetic chemical compounds with antibacterial properties. The most commonly used compounds are structural analogues of para-aminobenzoic acid (PABA). They exert their action by competing with PABA in the synthetic pathway of tetrahydrofolic acid (THFA), a compound

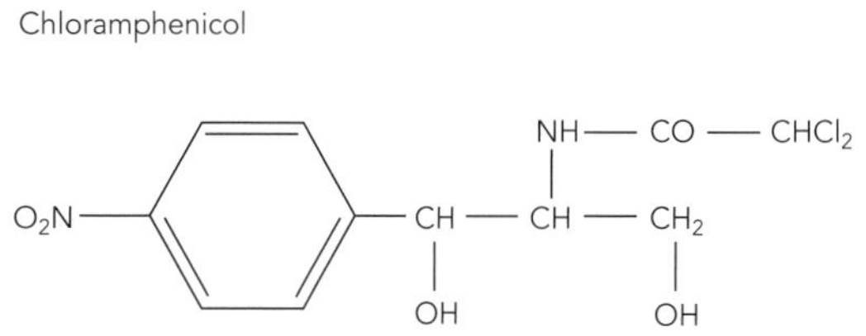

Figure 12.8

Structure of chloramphenicol

that is a precursor of the purines and pyrimidines required for nucleic acid synthesis (see Figure 12.9). The basis for the selective toxicity of the sulfonamide drugs is the fact that most bacteria have a pathway of synthesis of THFA, whereas humans are unable to synthesise folic acid and so have a requirement for it in their diet. Drugs that interfere with its synthesis will therefore not affect human cells.

Sulfonamides are broad spectrum bacteriostatic agents active against both Gram-positive and Gram-negative organisms. They can be administered orally and have had widespread use in the past for urinary tract infections, but their use has been associated with significant side effects. Sulfonamides, particularly in the elderly, can cause exfoliative dermatitis and may (rarely) be the cause of a fatal bone marrow suppression.

Trimethoprim is an analogue of the pyrimidine bases and competes for the enzyme dihydrofolate reductase, which converts dihydrofolic acid to tetrahydrofolic acid (see Figure 12.9). Although the enzyme is also present in human cells, the selective toxicity of the drug depends on the far greater affinity of trimethoprim for the bacterial enzyme than for the human enzyme. **Cotrimoxazole**, which combines sulfamethoxazole with trimethoprim, is no longer widely recommended for use. Trimethoprim alone is effective in the treatment of urinary tract infections. The current *Therapeutic Guidelines – Antibiotic* recommends that the combined preparation be restricted to clinical conditions where it is the treatment of choice – for example, *Pneumocystis jiroveci* prophylaxis and pneumonia in AIDS or other immunocompromised patients, *Listeria monocytogenes*, *Salmonella typhi* and *Nocardia* infections.

Trimethoprim alone or in combination with sulfamethoxazole may cause nausea.

Quinolones

Quinolones are a group of synthetic chemical agents that inhibit the activity of the enzyme, DNA gyrase, which is responsible for the coiling of the bacterial chromosome. Their action is specific to the bacterial enzyme and so is selectively toxic. The compounds in use are analogues of

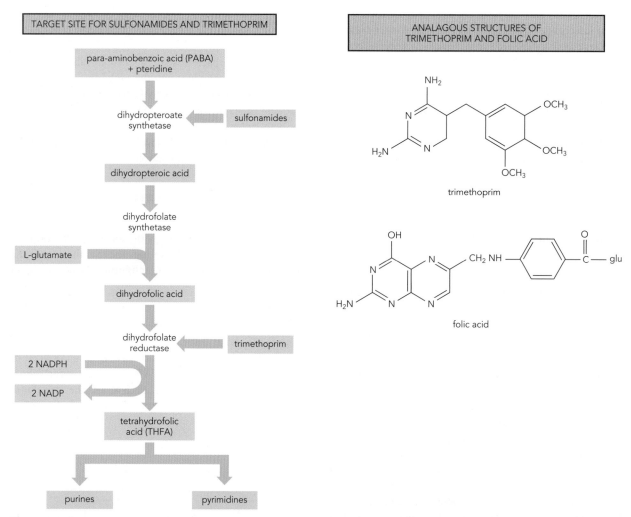

Figure 12.9

Mechanism of inhibition by sulfa drugs
Sulfonamides and trimethoprim inhibit in series the steps in the synthesis of tetrahydrofolic acid by interacting with key enzymes in the pathway.

nalidixic acid and have a broad antibacterial activity. They can be administered orally, reach good serum concentrations and are well distributed in the body.

Norfloxacin is used to treat urinary and gastro-intestinal infections. **Ciprofloxacin** and **enoxacin** have a wide range of activity against Gram-negative bacteria. **Moxifloxacin** and **gatifloxacin** are extended spectrum fluoroquinolones, effective against Gram-positive bacteria such as those causing pneumonia. Their advantage is that they can be administered orally or parenterally once daily.

Side effects of quinolones include nausea, photosensitivity and neurological disturbances. Convulsions have been reported, especially in patients with a history of epilepsy or other predisposing factors to seizures. They should be used in lower doses in patients with impaired renal function. They have been shown to damage the joints of immature animals so should not be used in children or pregnant women.

Rifamycins

Rifampicin and rifabutin are members of the family of **rifamycins**. They are bactericidal and affect the cell by binding to the enzyme, RNA polymerase, and blocking the synthesis of mRNA. The basis of their selective toxicity is the greater affinity of the drug for the bacterial enzyme than for the human RNA polymerase. Resistance develops rapidly so they should always be used in combination with other drugs.

Rifampicin is used against Gram-positive organisms (staphylococci) and mycobacterial infections (e.g. tuberculosis). Rifabutin is used mainly in the treatment of *Mycobacterium avium intracellulare* in HIV patients. They can be administered orally and reach high concentrations in serum and saliva. They are metabolised in the liver and excreted in body secretions (tears, urine, saliva), which are coloured red by the drug. Side effects include thrombocytopenia, renal failure and hepatitis.

They interact with a number of other drugs including anticoagulants, corticosteroids and hypoglycaemic agents. They also interfere with oral contraceptives and patients should be advised to use other methods of contraception while taking the drug and for 4–8 weeks after.

Nitroimidazoles

Metronidazole (Flagyl®) and **tinidazole** have a wide spectrum of activity against most obligate anaerobic Gram-positive and Gram-negative bacteria as well as intestinal protozoa including *Giardia lamblia*, *Entamoeba histolytica* and *Trichomonas vaginalis*. There are some side effects associated with their use, such as nausea and alcohol intolerance. Patients should be counselled to avoid alcohol during the course of the treatment.

INHIBITORS OF CELL MEMBRANE FUNCTION

The cytoplasmic membrane is a selectively permeable barrier surrounding the cytoplasm of all cells. The **polymyxins** are cyclic polypeptides which act as cationic detergents and disrupt the phospholipid bilayer of the membrane. They are especially active against Gram-negative bacteria such as *Pseudomonas aeruginosa*. They are not readily absorbed if administered orally and are toxic, causing nephrotoxicity and ototoxicity. They are used in topical preparations and occasionally for parenteral treatment of bacteria resistant to all other antibiotics.

ANTIMYCOBACTERIAL DRUGS

Patients with tuberculosis are managed by specialist doctors and require an extended course of antimicrobial drugs. The most commonly used drugs are combinations of **isoniazid**, **ethambutol**, **rifampicin** and **pyrazinamide** (see Chapter 17). A number of side effects are associated with these drugs. Compliance with the regime is of the utmost importance as drug resistance occurs easily.

Antifungal drugs

Many common fungal infections are caused by dermatophytes that attack cutaneous or mucocutaneous areas of the body. They include the various forms of tinea (e.g. ringworm, athlete's foot) and, in general, are only mild infections that can be treated by the application of topical antifungal preparations. In recent years, the number of opportunistic fungal infections occurring in immuno-compromised patients has increased (see Chapter 6). These infections are potentially life-threatening and require the use of systemic antifungal drugs.

Fungal cells are eucaryotic and it is difficult to identify points of selective toxicity. The main target is the synthesis or functioning of the fungal cell membrane which, unlike bacteria, contains sterols. **Azoles** and **polyenes** are the main compounds used for this purpose.

Azoles

The **azole** group of antifungal drugs includes **bifonazole, clotrimazole, econazole, miconazole, itraconazole, ketoconazole** and **fluconazole**. They inhibit the enzymes involved in sterol biosynthesis, the basis of selective toxicity being the greater affinity of the drug for the fungal enzyme than for the human enzyme. They are mainly used topically for dermatophyte infections and mucocutaneous candidiasis.

Fluconazole penetrates well into tissues, including the central nervous system, and can be used to treat vaginal candidiasis or as prophylaxis (and treatment) against cryptococcal meningitis in HIV-positive patients.

Voriconazole is a newer antifungal agent with a wider spectrum of activity than fluconazole. It may be used to treat invasive *Aspergillus* infections, and serious infections with *Candida*, *Scedosporium* and *Fusarium* spp.

Polyenes

The **polyene antibiotics**, which include **amphotericin B**, **nystatin** and **terbinafine**, act by combining with ergosterol, a major sterol component of the fungal cell membrane, thereby causing leakage of cell contents and cell death. These compounds are quite toxic to humans as they also bind, although less readily, to the cholesterol in human cell membranes.

TREATMENT OF FUNGAL INFECTIONS

Treatment of fungal infections is difficult because of the lack of solubility, the toxicity and the poor absorption of most of the available drugs. Cutaneous mycoses such as tinea and thrush are treated mainly with topical preparations. Although quite toxic systemically, nystatin is poorly absorbed and so is useful for topical application.

Some subcutaneous infections are very persistent and need to be treated with a systemic drug such as **griseofulvin**. This can be administered orally and appears to act specifically by binding to newly formed keratin present in cutaneous cells and inhibiting mitotic division. It must be used for a long time for best effect and has a number of drug interactions and toxic side effects so it is now rarely used in clinical practice.

Chronic mucocutaneous candidiasis is the most common fungal infection in immunosuppressed patients, followed by infections caused by the yeast *Cryptococcus neoformans*. Severe cryptococcal pneumonia and meningitis are now uncommon in Australian AIDS patients because of the widespread use of HAART (highly active antiretroviral therapy) and prophylactic antifungal agents.

Systemic fungal infections are difficult to treat because of the toxicity of most antifungal drugs. Amphotericin B is probably the main antifungal drug used for serious systemic infections while awaiting cultural diagnosis of the causative agent. Amphotericin B must be administered intravenously and is toxic, especially to the kidneys, but alternative formats involving liposomal preparations are less toxic and allow greater doses to be given.

Fluconazole can be taken orally, is better absorbed and is widely used as a treatment for sensitive systemic yeast infections (*Candida* and *Cryptococcus*). **Flucytosine** may occasionally be used orally or parenterally in combination with amphotericin against *Cryptococcus neoformans*. High levels of the drug are associated with bone marrow toxicity. **Caspofungin** is useful in the treatment of invasive *Aspergillus*.

Better antifungal drugs are needed, especially as there are increasing numbers of immunocompromised patients susceptible to opportunistic fungal infections.

Antiparasitic drugs

A number of parasitic infections, caused by protozoa and helminths (worms), have complicated life cycles and it is difficult to find drugs that are selectively toxic against them.

Infections due to intestinal protozoa such as *Giardia* and *Entamoeba histolytica* can be treated with metronidazole or tinidazole. These drugs are effective against gastrointestinal infections because, although somewhat toxic, they are poorly absorbed from the intestine. Other protozoal diseases such as toxoplasmosis or diarrhoea due to *Cryptosporidium* or *Microsporidium* do not usually require treatment unless the patient is immunocompromised.

Malaria is one of the most important of the protozoal infections. There are four species of the protozoan *Plasmodium*. Derivatives of quinine have been used for years to treat malaria, but quinine itself is now considered too toxic for general use.

Chloroquine is the main drug used to treat clinical attacks of malaria where the malarial strain is still susceptible to chloroquine. Strains of *Plasmodium falciparum* resistant to chloroquine have developed in many areas of the world and some of these are also resistant to **mefloquine** which may be recommended by some countries as prophylaxis against malaria infection. It is believed that this has contributed to the rapid emergence of resistance to this drug. Some people experience side effects from mefloquine so it is being used less for both prophylaxis and treatment. **Quinine** is very toxic and is used only if the infection is due to a resistant strain. **Primaquine** is used to eliminate *P. vivax* and *P. ovale* from the liver once the clinical attack is controlled in order to prevent relapses, which may occur for up to five years after the initial attack.

Prophylactic chemotherapy for travellers to endemic areas in South-East Asia usually involves the use of **doxycycline**. It is important that travellers to malarial areas consult their local health department or travel advisory clinic or the WHO website <www.who.int/ith> for advice on appropriate antimalarial prophylaxis.

Antihelminthic drugs are discussed in Chapter 6.

Antiviral drugs

A large number of diseases that afflict humans are caused by viruses. However, because viruses replicate inside the host cell, few antiviral compounds have been found which can kill or inactivate viruses without being severely toxic to the host. Instead, research has focused with considerable success on the development of vaccines against serious viral diseases. The advent of the human immunodeficiency virus, HIV, which attacks the immune system itself and therefore makes the development of a vaccine particularly difficult, has encouraged the search for antiviral compounds.

For an antiviral drug to be selectively toxic, it must target some point in the cycle of viral replication. This could be, for example, the specific attachment site of the virus to the host cell, or the mechanism of viral uncoating and replication, or a specific viral enzyme synthesised under the direction of the viral genes and required for viral replication. In fact, a number of specific viral enzymes have been identified and these have been used as targets for antiviral drugs.

There are a number of difficulties associated with effective antiviral therapy. Many of the drugs that inhibit the viral enzymes also inhibit (but with a much lower affinity for) the host cell enzymes, so side effects are common. Most available antiviral drugs are **virustatic** – that is, they inhibit viral replication (and relieve the disease symptoms) but they do not eliminate the virus from the body. This is of particular importance in immunosuppressed individuals whose immune system may not be able to attack the virus. Latent (non-replicating) viruses are not affected, so any reservoir of viruses in the body is preserved and can be reactivated later.

Mutations occur frequently during viral replication, giving rise to altered viral proteins with different antigenic properties, so antibodies formed in response to the initial infection may not inactivate the virus. This is important in infections with HIV. Mutation may also produce enzymes with altered substrate specificity so that the antiviral drugs are no longer effective and the virus becomes resistant to the drug.

NUCLEOSIDE ANALOGUES

The most successful antiviral drugs are analogues of the purine and pyrimidine bases, which are the building blocks of RNA and DNA. Antiviral drugs are listed in Table 12.4.

Herpes

One of the most effective compounds is **aciclovir** which is an analogue of the nucleoside guanosine. It is active against the herpes simplex virus (HSV) types I and II, and varicella zoster virus (VZV – shingles). HSV and VZV contain a virally encoded enzyme, thymidine kinase, which is able to phosphorylate aciclovir to the active monophosphate; this is then converted to aciclovir triphosphate and incorporated instead of thymine into the growing chains of viral DNA, where it prevents further elongation. Thymidine kinase is not present in human cells, which means that aciclovir is incorporated only into the DNA of virally infected cells, and so is relatively non-toxic even in high doses.

Aciclovir is used for primary herpes simplex (HSV) infections (oral, genital and conjunctival) as well as the prevention of recurrent genital HSV. An important use is in suspected cases of herpes encephalitis. It is used mainly in topical applications for HSV or by intravenous infusion as it is not well absorbed, but in severe cases it can be taken orally. For systemic infections in immunocompromised patients or for severe cases of *Varicella zoster* in adults, **famciclovir** and **valaciclovir** are used.

Cytomegalovirus (CMV)

Ganciclovir is also a nucleoside analogue of guanosine, but is active against cytomegalovirus as well as HSV and VZV. The mechanism of inhibition is similar to aciclovir, but the drug is more toxic so its use is limited to serious cases of CMV, such as CMV retinitis in AIDS patients. Neutropenia occurs in 25% of patients together with some degree of renal impairment. It is not well absorbed when taken orally.

Valganciclovir is absorbed well when taken orally and is hydrolysed in the body to ganciclovir. **Foscarnet** is a pyrophosphate nucleotide derivative that does not require phosphorylation by host or viral enzymes. It has been used

Table 12.4 **Antiviral drugs**	
VIRUS OR DISEASE	ANTIVIRAL DRUG
HSV Herpes simplex	Aciclovir, idoxuridine (topical) Fanciclovir, valaciclovir (oral)
VZV Varicella zoster	Aciclovir (topical)
CMV Cytomegalovirus	Ganciclovir Valganciclovir Foscarnet
HIV AIDS	**Nucleoside analogue reverse transcriptase inhibitors** • Zidovudine (AZT) • Dideoxycytosine (ddC) • Dideoxyinosine (ddI) • Lamivudine (3TC) • Stavudine (d4T) **Non-nucleoside reverse transcriptase inhibitors** • Nevirapine • Delavirdine • Efavirenz **Protease inhibitors** • Indinavir • Amprenavir • Nelfinavir • Ritonavir • Saquinavir
RSV Respiratory syncytial virus	Ribavarin
Influenza A Influenza A and B	Amantadine Zanamivir Oseltamavir
Hairy cell leukemia Chronic hepatitis B, C	Interferon Interferon, ribavarin, zidovudine

as an alternative to ganciclovir for CMV infections as well as for herpes and varicella zoster.

Ribavarin

Ribavarin is a broad spectrum antiviral compound which has a potentiating effect when used with other antivirals, especially nucleoside analogues. Its main use is in combination with interferon for hepatitis C and for severe cases of respiratory syncytial virus (RSV) infection in hospitalised children.

ANTIRETROVIRAL DRUGS

Retroviruses are a particular group of viruses responsible for a number of serious diseases including adult T cell leukaemia and AIDS. They have also been linked to the development of cancers in various animal species. In the search for suitable drugs to treat infections caused by these viruses, scientists have been able to make use of the viruses' unique method of replication (see Figure 5.6, page 93). Retroviruses contain RNA and the first step in the replicative process involves the synthesis of DNA from the RNA genome by a specific viral enzyme, an RNA-dependent DNA polymerase called **reverse transcriptase**. The DNA 'provirus' is then inserted into the host cell DNA and subsequently directs the synthesis of new viral RNA and protein.

Nucleoside analogue reverse transcriptase inhibitors

The reverse transcriptase enzyme, which does not occur in human cells, provides a target for antiviral drugs. Various analogues of the nucleosides that are used to synthesise DNA have been tested for their ability to bind to the enzyme, reverse transcriptase. Of these, zidovudine (AZT), an analogue of thymine, was the first to be licensed for the treatment of HIV infection. However, although the drug has a high affinity for viral reverse transcriptase, it is also incorporated to some extent into host cell DNA by human DNA polymerase. This leads to occasional depression of bone marrow function and may cause inhibition of mitochondrial DNA synthesis, leading to myopathy. Unpleasant side effects of treatment include nausea, myalgia and headaches.

Other analogues that have been used include DDI (dideoxyinosine), DDC (dideoxycytosine), 3TC (lamivudine) and d4T (stavudine). All the analogues block the transcription of viral RNA into DNA by combining with and inhibiting the enzyme, reverse transcriptase, leading to termination of the synthesis of the DNA chain. The action of these drugs is virustatic – that is, when the drug is removed, viral replication can resume.

Non-nucleoside inhibitors

The newest class of antiretroviral agents are the non-nucleoside reverse transcriptase inhibitors (NNRTIs). They stop HIV production by binding directly onto reverse transcriptase, preventing the conversion of RNA to DNA. Although they act at the same site as the nucleoside analogues, they exert their effect in a completely different way. They include nevirapine, delavirdine and efavirenz.

Protease inhibitors

Protease inhibitors are a group of compounds that act on HIV protease and interfere with the correct formation of viral proteins, thus reducing viral replication and the spread of the virus to uninfected cells. They include indinavir, amprenavir, nelfinavir, ritonavir and saquinavir.

Combination therapy

Current retroviral treatment for patients who are HIV-positive consists of triple-combination therapy or HAART (highly active antiretroviral therapy) – two nucleoside reverse transcriptase inhibitors together with a protease inhibitor or one drug from each group. Combination therapy reduces the risk of development of resistance to each drug. It has been shown to increase the CD_4 cell count, decrease HIV-RNA, reduce vertical transmission (mother to baby) and improve survival rates.

ANTI-INFLUENZA DRUGS

Amantadine is a cyclic amine that is active against influenza A but not influenza B. When used to treat influenza it is most effective if given within the first 48 hours after symptoms develop. During influenza epidemics, it can be administered to susceptible people who have not been vaccinated, thus reducing the risk of illness. However, the development of drug resistance is common and it is no longer widely used.

Oseltamivir and **zanamivir** are new drugs that are active against both influenza A and B. They inhibit the action of neuraminidase, an enzyme in the spikes of the virus that is essential for the release of new viral particles from infected cells. They have been shown to reduce the duration and intensity of symptoms by one or two days but should be administered within 48 hours of onset of symptoms.

INTERFERONS

Interferons are a family of small glycoprotein molecules produced by some mammalian cells, such as lymphocytes, fibroblasts and macrophages, in response to viral infection. The interferons are cell or species specific, not virus specific, and are cytokines, involved in cell growth and the regulation of immune reactions.

Three classes have been identified – alpha(α), beta(β) and gamma(γ). Gamma(γ)-interferon is a lymphokine produced by activated T cells in response to viral infection; α- and β-interferons are produced by many cell types. Virus-infected cells produce interferons that diffuse to neighbouring uninfected cells, where they induce the production of proteins that block translation of viral RNA to viral protein, thus preventing further viral replication (see Figure 9.14).

Interferons have now been produced commercially by genetic engineering. Alpha-interferon (IFN-a) is being used in the treatment of chronic hepatitis B and C. Studies of results of interferon treatment of chronic hepatitis C patients showed that, after an initial response rate of 50%, half the patients relapsed, so the overall response to treatment was 25%. Careful selection of patients for therapy – that is, patients without contributing conditions (e.g. cirrhosis) – may improve the response rate. Side effects of the therapy include fever, malaise, headache and myalgia; bone marrow depression may also occur. Improved results for treatment of hepatitis C are being obtained with combination therapy of interferon and ribavirin.

Therapeutic use of antimicrobial drugs

Many infections that were once considered life-threatening can now be successfully treated with antimicrobial drugs. This is particularly true of bacterial infections. The selection of drugs is wide and several factors need to be considered before a particular drug is prescribed. The approach taken by the medical practitioner to the treatment of infection may vary, depending on whether the patient is in the community or is hospitalised. The time and cost involved in carrying out a definitive microbiological identification is usually not warranted for most patients in the community so the doctor may prescribe empirically. However, doctors should be aware of the emergence of antibiotic resistance in common bacterial infections caused by *Streptococcus pneumoniae* and *Staphylococcus aureus*, which make infections with these organisms unresponsive to standard antibiotic therapies.

In hospital, patients are often sicker, they may have contributing illnesses and there is also a greater likelihood of the infection being due to a resistant organism, especially if the patient has been in hospital for more than three days. In these cases, it is usual to collect a specimen, send it to the laboratory for identification and determination of antibiotic sensitivities, and start **empirical (best guess) therapy** while waiting for the results (see below, page 266).

ANTIMICROBIAL SENSITIVITY TESTS

Specimens taken for microbiological detection and organism identification are sent to the laboratory and the predominant organism in the sample (hopefully the one responsible for the infection) is isolated and identified using methods described in Chapters 15. In order to decide on the best antibiotic treatment for a particular infection it is necessary to determine the antibiotic sensitivity of the clinical isolate to the available antimicrobial drugs.

The choice of drug is dictated by several factors including the **site** of infection, the infecting **organism**(s), the antimicrobial **sensitivity** pattern of the particular strain of the organism isolated and the available **route** of administration of the antibiotic. For example, although penicillin is effective against actively growing cells of many Gram-positive bacteria, a number of strains of these bacteria have developed mechanisms to resist its action (e.g. beta-lactamase enzymes). To select the most effective antimicrobial drug, it is necessary to test the actual strain of the organism that is causing the infection against different concentrations of a range of possible antimicrobial agents.

There are two main methods for carrying out sensitivity tests in the laboratory: disk diffusion tests and the minimum inhibitory concentration (MIC) test. In both methods, an appropriate specimen is obtained from the patient and cultured on a suitable medium to obtain single colonies. Cells from the colonies are suspended in nutrient medium and tested for susceptibility to a range of antimicrobials. The site of the infection, together with the provisional diagnosis, determines which antimicrobials are tested first. The choice is also based on the susceptibility pattern of the isolates usually encountered in the particular laboratory, especially for hospital-acquired infections.

Disk diffusion test

The bacteria to be tested are spread uniformly at a known concentration on an agar plate and disks impregnated with defined amounts of various antibiotics are placed on the plate. The drug diffuses into the agar and inhibits the growth of sensitive organisms in a zone around the disk. The **zone of inhibition**, or clear area (in mm) around the disk, represents the sensitivity of the organism to the drug being tested (see Figure 12.10). The amount of drug in each disk is related to its achievable serum concentration. The diameter of the zone of inhibition is a measure of the sensitivity of the organism to the drug but, as it is influenced by the ease of diffusion (solubility) of the drug in the agar, it is considered a qualitative method. If no clear zone is apparent or there is a reduced zone of growth inhibition compared to a published standard, the organism is considered and reported to be resistant to the drug being tested.

Minimum inhibitory concentration test

The **minimum inhibitory concentration (MIC) test** is a semi-quantitative procedure that measures the concentration of an antimicrobial required to inhibit the growth of a standardised inoculum. This can be done by broth dilution in a series of tubes, each containing different concentrations of drug but with a standardised number of organisms. The method measures the lowest drug concentration (MIC) that will inhibit visible growth. It is a laborious method and has been replaced by the E-test, a commercially available method to determine MICs (see Figure 12.11).

(Many automated systems use an MIC method but read the growth densities automatically and print out a report of their findings in a few hours. These methods are used in large laboratories where a large number of samples are tested each day.)

The results of antimicrobial sensitivity testing can vary from one laboratory to another unless standardised control cultures and testing media are used.

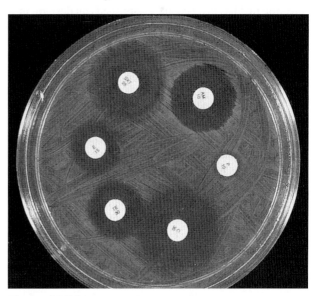

Figure 12.10

Disk diffusion test
The diameter of the clear zone around each disk represents the sensitivity of the test organism to the antibacterial drug in the disk. If there is no clearing, the organism is considered resistant to the drugs at that concentration.

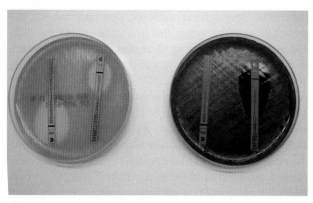

Figure 12.11

Measurement of minimum inhibitory concentration (MIC) using E-test

Calibrated strips with increasing concentrations of antibiotic impregnated into the strip are placed on a plate inoculated with the bacterium to be tested. Visual inspection of the concentration of antibiotic present in the clear zone of inhibition gives the minimum concentration of antibiotic which inhibits growth of the bacterium.

(a) Measurement of growth of *Pseudomonas aeruginosa* in the presence of gentamicin (left) and ciprofloxacin (right).

(b) Measurement of growth of *Enterococcus* in the presence of penicillin (left) and vancomycin (right). The bacterium is resistant to penicillin.

TREATMENT OF BACTERIAL INFECTIONS

In an ideal situation it would be preferable to delay treatment until sensitivity tests had been carried out but, in practice, by the time the patient shows obvious signs of infection (see Chapter 7) they require treatment as soon as possible. Waiting two or more days for definitive laboratory tests to be carried out before prescribing treatment may well jeopardise the health (or life) of the patient. An infection that has just become established can develop into fulminating sepsis in hours (e.g. meningococcal septicaemia). Balanced against this is the risk of the development of antibiotic-resistant microbial strains or selection of antibiotic-resistant bacteria due to overprescribing of antibiotics.

Usually, the medical practitioner makes a provisional diagnosis, prescribes medication based on the 'best guess' principle and then reviews the prescription when the results of the pathology tests are available. It is important that, whenever possible, clinical specimens are collected from the patient *before* any drug therapy is commenced; otherwise, the drug may kill or inhibit the microorganisms present and incorrect or inconclusive results may be obtained. An appropriate clinical sample of blood, sputum, pus, urine, faeces, CSF or tissue is usually collected. It should be adequate in amount, collected in an aseptic manner, correctly labelled and transported to the laboratory as soon as possible. (See Chapter 15 for methods of specimen collection.)

Empirical therapy

In deciding which drug to prescribe while awaiting results, the doctor takes into account such factors as:

- *the site of the body where the infection is located.* This will often indicate the types of organisms most likely to be present and the most effective drug to be used.
- *whether the infection was acquired in the hospital or community.* Many hospital organisms are resistant to antibiotics and the hospital will have developed a prescribing policy to address this problem. This often involves the use of two or more antibiotics at the same time.
- *the age of the patient.* Some drugs are more toxic for children. Some infections are more serious in children and require immediate effective therapy (e.g. meningitis caused by *Haemophilus influenzae* type b).
- *other contributing factors* such as the immune status of the patient, renal impairment, liver function, etc.

Prescribing principles

Once the causative organism has been identified, the empirical therapy can be modified if necessary. Sometimes, the appropriate drug is selected on the basis of clinical experience. However, it is more usual with hospital-acquired infections to carry out an antimicrobial sensitivity test, as described above, to determine the sensitivity of the pathogen to the range of antimicrobial agents available. It is essential to carry out sensitivity testing when:

- the organism is of a type that is frequently resistant to drug therapy (e.g. hospital-acquired Gram-negative rods)
- the infection is life-threatening (e.g. meningitis, septicaemia)
- bactericidal drugs are preferred (e.g. for immuno-compromised patients or in infective endocarditis).

When the doctor has the results of the laboratory tests, there are still a number of factors to be taken into account in order to select the most appropriate therapeutic agent.

- Absorption – the drug must be able to reach the part of the body where the infection is located. Thus, if the drug is to be given orally, it must be unchanged by gastric acid, be absorbed from the intestine and be able to be transported in the bloodstream to the site of infection. Some drugs must be given by intravenous infusion because of their poor absorption from the intestine and so are only suitable for use in a hospital or health facility (see Figure 12.12).
- The drug must be able to reach the target tissue. For example, if the infection is in the meninges, a drug must be selected that can cross the blood-brain barrier (although this is sometimes easier when the meninges are inflamed). The drug used to treat a urinary tract infection must be excreted in an active form via the kidneys and must be able to reach a high enough concentration in the urine to kill the microorganisms present in the bladder.
- Some drugs are not suitable for young children or women during pregnancy and lactation. For example,

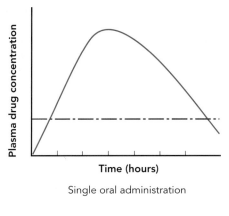

Single oral administration

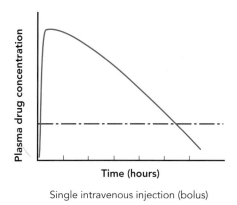

Single intravenous injection (bolus)

—·—·—·· MEC—minimum effective concentration

Figure 12.12

Comparison of plasma drug concentrations after different methods of administration

tetracycline has been shown to bind to calcium and deposit in developing teeth, causing permanent brown staining. It may also interfere with bone development in the foetus. Fluconazole may cause foetal damage.

Other medical conditions that may need to be taken into account include the status of the immune system and the integrity of organ function in the patient. For example, immunocompromised patients should be prescribed bactericidal drugs whenever possible, as their immune system is not able to eliminate the microorganisms left after treatment with a bacteriostatic drug. Infective endocarditis is best treated with a bactericidal drug, as macrophages are unable to penetrate to the site of the infection to destroy residual bacteria.

Metabolism and elimination of drugs depends on hepatic and renal function. Patients with some degree of renal impairment are not able to excrete drugs effectively via the kidneys. This means that high concentrations of the drug may develop in the bloodstream and thus the prescribed dose needs to be lower. Drugs that affect the kidneys (e.g. the aminoglycosides) are not usually prescribed for patients who already have impaired renal function.

Other factors usually taken into account when selecting the most suitable drug are the likelihood of development of resistance, the risk of interactions between the drug and any other medication being taken by the patient and, importantly, the cost of the drug.

Combined therapy

In hospitals it is common for two drugs to be prescribed simultaneously for the treatment of seriously ill patients when the cause of the infection is uncertain, or when delay while awaiting the results of conclusive sensitivity tests may be detrimental to the patient. One advantage of using more than one drug is the efficient treatment of mixed infections. The emergence of resistance can theoretically be retarded by the use of two drugs with different mechanisms of action.

Sometimes, the action of an antimicrobial is potentiated (enhanced) in the presence of another drug or antimicrobial. **Synergism** is the term used to describe the enhancement of one drug in the presence of another. For example, penicillin may be prescribed as well as an aminoglycoside. Penicillin damages the cell wall, allowing better penetration of the aminoglycoside. In systemic fungal infections such as candidiasis or cryptococcosis, amphotericin is used to weaken the cell membrane, allowing uptake of flucytosine.

Some infections respond better to the use of two or more drugs. Enterococcal endocarditis responds to a combination of penicillin or ampicillin, plus gentamicin, vancomycin or streptomycin. Tuberculosis is routinely treated with isoniazid, ethambutol and rifampicin in order to inhibit the development of resistant strains.

Some commercial preparations contain two drugs; for example, cotrimoxazole (Bactrim®, Septrin®) contains sulphamethoxazole and trimethoprim, two drugs which sequentially block the pathway of folate synthesis. Augmentin® contains amoxycillin plus the beta-lactamase inhibitor, clavulanic acid, which prevents inactivation of the amoxycillin.

However, there are some disadvantages to the use of combined therapy. There may be **antagonism** when a reaction occurs between the drugs being used, or when one drug interferes with the action of the other. If bacteriostatic and bactericidal drugs are administered simultaneously, the action of both may be affected. For example, tetracycline is bacteriostatic, inhibiting protein synthesis and cell replication. Penicillin is bactericidal and is active mainly against dividing cells. If they are used in combination, the tetracycline inhibits cell division and so the bactericidal action of the penicillin is considerably diminished. Some antimicrobials affect the efficacy of other kinds of drugs. Rifampicin stimulates the metabolism (and therefore removal from the body) of oral contraceptives, anticoagulants and corticosteroids.

PHARMACOKINETICS

The prescribed dosage must be such that an effective concentration of the drug is achieved at the site of infection. Ideally, the concentration of the antimicrobial agent in the blood or tissues should be maintained above the minimal inhibitory concentration (MIC). The rate of elimination of the drug from the body can be described in terms of **half-life** – that is, the time required for the concentration of the drug in the bloodstream to fall to half its maximum level. The number of times the drug needs to be administered each day will depend on the rate at which the drug is broken down or eliminated from the body.

It is also necessary to take into account the therapeutic index of the drug. The **therapeutic index** is the ratio of the effective concentration of the drug required to kill the pathogen to the concentration that would be a lethal dose for the host. The smaller the number, the more selectively toxic the drug will be and the less risk there will be of toxic side effects.

PROPHYLAXIS

Prophylaxis involves the administration of an antimicrobial drug before there is any evidence of infection, under conditions where the risks of an infection developing are considered to be very high. The risk of a patient acquiring an infection has to be weighed against factors such as cost, the toxicity of the drug and the risk of superinfection (i.e. an overgrowth by opportunistic pathogens).

Prophylaxis may be considered necessary for some surgical procedures, especially where prosthetic devices are involved. In general, prophylaxis is not so essential if the patient is immunocompetent. However, it is recommended for patients who are undergoing abdominal surgery or who are susceptible to infection for other reasons. For example, patients who suffer from rheumatic heart disease involving damage to the heart valves are usually prescribed penicillin following dental surgery. This is to reduce the risk of infection by viridans streptococci which may enter the bloodstream and infect the damaged valves, causing endocarditis.

Pregnant women colonised with group B streptococci are given intra-partem antibiotics to reduce the risk of neonatal infection.

LIMITATIONS OF ANTIMICROBIAL THERAPY

There are a number of problems associated with the use of antimicrobials.

- The suppression or elimination of normal flora can lead to an overgrowth of opportunists such as *Candida albicans* or *Clostridium difficile.*
- The occurrence of adverse side effects such as hypersensitivity, ototoxicity, nephrotoxicity and bone marrow suppression. Like all drugs most antimicrobials have some side effects and the nature of the side effects must be weighed against the benefits available from their use. The most important of these adverse effects are listed in Table 12.5.
- The emergence of strains of pathogens that are resistant to currently available antimicrobial drugs.

Development of resistance to antimicrobial drugs

The first antibiotic (penicillin) was introduced in the 1940s. In the 'Golden Age' from 1950–70 most of the drugs described above were developed and used therapeutically. However, since then no new classes of antimicrobial drugs have been discovered. Any 'new' drugs are mainly chemical derivatives of existing drugs. One of the major challenges confronting medical practice today is

---

Table 12.5
Some serious adverse effects of antimicrobial therapy

DRUG	ADVERSE EFFECT
Antibacterials	
• Aminoglycosides	Ototoxicity (deafness) and nephrotoxicity (renal impairment).
• Chloramphenicol	Bone marrow depression – aplastic anaemia.
• Penicillin (and other beta-lactams)	Hypersensitivity occurs in some people. Occasionally fatal.
• Fluoroquinolones	Nausea, photosensitivity, neurological disturbances.
• Sulfonamides	Hypersensitivity, skin rashes, agranulocytosis.
• Tetracyclines	Combine with calcium in developing bones and teeth, cause permanent discolouration of teeth.
• Vancomycin	Ototoxicity, nephrotoxicity. Local inflammation – phlebitis. Must be given by slow infusion to avoid histamine release.
Antivirals	
• Zidovudine	Bone marrow depression, anaemia, nausea, headaches, skin rashes.
Antifungals	
• Amphotericin	Nephrotoxic.

the number of microorganisms that are resistant to currently available antimicrobial agents. Strains of *Staphylococcus aureus* resistant to penicillin were isolated in 1944, only a couple of years after its introduction, and strains resistant to a number of antimicrobials (e.g. MRSA) are now common in most hospitals. See Spotlight box, page 278.

This is not surprising given that the bacterial mutation rate is $1:10^7$ cell divisions. When a mutation occurs that confers resistance, then, in the presence of the antimicrobial drug, sensitive cells will be killed and resistant cells will multiply (see Figure 12.13).

Prior to the introduction of penicillin, most hospital infections were caused by Gram-positive staphylococci and streptococci. Very few were due to Gram-negative organisms. However, in the late 1970s and 1980s, due to the selective pressure of antimicrobial use, infections with Gram-negative organisms became more common. Gram-negative bacteria resistant to the broad spectrum cephalosporins emerged. These bacteria produce enzymes described as 'extended spectrum beta-lactamases' (ESBLs) because of their ability to destroy the beta-lactam antibacterials.

Some microorganisms (e.g. *Pseudomonas*) have cellular characteristics that give them a natural resistance to many antimicrobial drugs. But the main problem facing clinicians is that, since antimicrobial drugs have been used therapeutically, an increasing number of microorganisms have acquired resistance to drugs they were previously sensitive to. Worldwide, there has been the development of multiple-drug-resistant strains of organisms such as *Mycobacterium tuberculosis*, *Neisseria gonorrhoeae*, *Staphylococcus aureus*, *Streptococcus pneumoniae*, *Klebsiella*, *E. coli* and *Enterococcus* species.

Bacteria may develop resistance to antimicrobial drugs in any of the following ways:

- By the production of enzymes that are able to destroy or inactivate the drug. For example, the beta-lactamase enzyme produced by many organisms breaks open the beta-lactam ring in the penicillin or cephalosporin

molecule, destroying its structure and preventing the drug from binding to its target, which is the enzyme involved in the synthesis of peptidoglycan.
- By a change in membrane permeability that results in the drug being unable to penetrate through the membrane into the cell. This may be due to a change in structural protein, a decrease in pore size or an alteration in the transport system.
- The rate of efflux of the drug from the cell may be increased so that the drug is not able to attain a sufficiently high concentration inside the cell to cause inhibition. This is the basis of resistance to drugs such as the tetracyclines, which inhibit protein synthesis on the ribosomes inside the cell.
- By an alteration in the binding sites for the drug in the bacterial cell. Most drugs bind to a specific site in the cell and exert their effect by interfering with enzyme activity or protein synthesis. If the structure of the binding site is altered, the drug is no longer able to bind and so is unable to have any effect on the cell and the cell becomes resistant. Some penicillin-resistant bacteria (e.g. *Streptococcus pneumoniae*) have altered penicillin-binding proteins, so that penicillin is no longer active against them. Alterations to the specific sites on the bacterial ribosome prevent the action of the aminoglycosides and erythromycin which inhibit protein synthesis.
- Some drugs, such as the sulfonamides, exert their effect by inhibiting reactions in essential metabolic pathways. One way in which bacteria develop resistance to these drugs is by the production of other enzymes that have no affinity for the drug and can synthesise the required compounds via an alternate pathway.

The development of these resistance mechanisms involves a change in the genetic properties (DNA) of the cell. This can occur as the result of a spontaneous mutation. Subsequent exposure of the cell population to an antimicrobial drug then exerts a selective pressure, killing sensitive organisms and allowing the resistant mutants to multiply, see Figure 12.13. This may occur during a

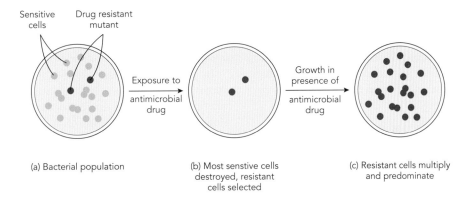

Figure 12.13

Effect of exposure to antimicrobial drugs
If the concentration of drug is not sufficient to kill *all* cells, the resistant mutant cells are selected and can multiply.

prolonged course of antimicrobial therapy. It can also occur when a patient does not complete the full course of a prescribed drug. Resistant mutants will also be selected under these conditions, although the level of drug resistance (i.e. the concentration of drug required to kill the cells) may not be quite as high. Without the selective pressure applied by the use of antimicrobial drugs, the population of cells would remain sensitive. The overuse or misuse of antimicrobial drugs can therefore contribute to the development of resistant strains of microorganisms.

TRANSFER OF RESISTANCE

Another mechanism whereby the cell can become resistant is by the transfer of resistance genes from resistant to susceptible strains of closely related genera. This is usually mediated by plasmids during conjugation (see Chapter 4). The initial appearance of resistance in susceptible bacteria is usually due to a mutation in only one gene. However, the level of resistance can be increased if the bacteria acquire additional resistant genes or R-factors from other bacteria.

It is now recognised that an important method of spread of resistance is the conjugative transfer of resistance factors on plasmids, not only within species but also between closely related genera. Thus, if a patient who is carrying a sensitive strain of *E. coli* acquires a multi-resistant strain of, say, *Shigella*, the resistance genes may be transferred in the intestine from the related genus *Shigella* to *E. coli*. The patient then harbours and excretes a strain of multi-resistant *Shigella* as well as multi-resistant *E. coli*, even though the original *E. coli* strain in the patient has not been exposed to any antimicrobial drugs.

Often the genes for resistance to a number of different antimicrobials are located beside each other on a **transposon**, so the transfer of a plasmid will also transfer multiple resistance genes. The increase in resistance in hospital isolates of Gram-negative bacteria is thought to be largely due to the transfer of resistance factors in this manner. In addition, it is thought that the extensive use of antimicrobials in animal feed may contribute to an increase in the numbers of resistant organisms in animal products which can then be transferred to humans in food or by contact with the animal.

Cross-resistance refers to the situation where an organism that has developed a mechanism of resistance to one drug will also be resistant to related drugs. For example, an organism that produces a beta-lactamase enzyme may be resistant to both penicillin and cephalosporin, even though it may have been exposed to only one of the drugs. The enzyme inactivates the drug in both cases by destroying the beta-lactam ring.

DRUG RESISTANCE IN HOSPITALS

The high usage of antimicrobial drugs in hospitals, especially in high dependency (intensive care) units, provides an atmosphere in which resistant organisms can flourish. Resistant strains of *Pseudomonas aeruginosa*, *Acinetobacter baumanni*, *Klebsiella* and vancomycin-resistant *Enterobacter* (VRE) are often implicated in ventilator-assisted pneumonia (VAP). Attention to infection control procedures, especially handwashing, is essential to prevent the spread of resistant organisms to other patients in the hospital (see Chapter 13).

Strategies being devised to control the spread of infections and to limit the rate of development of antimicrobial resistance include:

* hospital policies for prescribing antimicrobials
* the use of narrow spectrum antimicrobials whenever possible
* restrictions on the use of vancomycin
* improved surveillance to determine resistance patterns of hospital organisms
* infection control procedures to prevent the spread of hospital-acquired infections
* the introduction of vaccines against bacterial infections; for example, the vaccine against *Haemophilus influenzae* type b (Hib) has significantly reduced the incidence of meningitis (see page 319). It is hoped that the introduction of the pneumococcal vaccine will reduce the incidence of invasive *Streptococcus pneumoniae* infections.

ANTIMICROBIAL RESISTANCE IN THE COMMUNITY

The availability of drugs to treat even minor infections has led to an overuse of antibacterial drugs, especially in the community. Viruses are responsible for many respiratory tract infections, including the common cold, influenza, RSV, viral pneumonia and viral gastroenteritis. These infections do not respond to treatment with antibacterial drugs, and the prescribing of such drugs for illnesses that are primarily viral in nature is one of the contributing factors to the widespread development of resistance in bacteria.

If the patient's population of normal flora is exposed to an antibacterial drug, a few mutant cells resistant to the drug are likely to arise and they will flourish in an environment where other cells that normally compete for nutrients have been destroyed, see Figure 12.13. If this happens, the patient may acquire a population of resistant bacteria, even though the original infection was due to a virus. The use of antibacterials is indicated only when secondary bacterial infections occur following a viral infection of the respiratory tract.

It is important to note that *it is not the person who becomes resistant to the antimicrobial – it is the bacteria.*

In the past, resistant strains of organisms such as *Staphylococcus aureus* were mainly limited to hospitals where high usage of antibiotics encouraged their selection. However, resistant strains of a number of important pathogens are increasingly being isolated in the community. Research is needed to identify the source of these strains and to implement policies to limit their spread.

The occurrence of resistant strains in the community may be a reflection of early discharge policies, in that patients may take the hospital strains out into the community when they leave hospital. It may also be due to high levels of prescribing in the community. A particular problem is the increase in resistant strains of *Streptococcus pneumoniae*, which is a common cause of community-acquired pneumonia (CAP) and otitis media (middle ear infections). This problem has been partly addressed with the development of pneumococcal vaccines (see Chapter 14).

A number of strains of methicillin-resistant *Staphylococcus aureus* (MRSA) have been isolated from remote communities in Western Australia. These are referred to as WA-MRSA and are distinct from other strains of MRSA because they tend not to be multiply resistant. Worldwide, the occurrence in the community of multi-resistant strains of pathogens such as *Neisseria gonorrhoea* and *Mycobacterium tuberculosis* presents a serious public health problem.

The World Health Organization has recently called for a global strategy to overcome the problem of increasing resistance to antimicrobial drugs. In Australia the National Health and Medical Research Council (NHMRC) has set up an expert advisory group to provide continuing advice on antimicrobial resistance and related matters.

THE SEARCH FOR NEW ANTIMICROBIALS

Although there has been a rapid increase in resistance in recent years, the rate of development of new antimicrobial drugs has decreased. Most antimicrobials are developed by major drug companies who claim that the cost of development, clinical trials, marketing and surveillance of new drugs is prohibitive. In developed countries, there is an insistence on 'zero risk' for any new drug, which means that the clinical trials need to be very extensive (and costly). Unfortunately, drugs soon become obsolete if resistance develops rapidly.

To deal with the dwindling supply of antimicrobials, authorities are advocating more attention to appropriate prescribing practices and increased infection control measures to limit the spread of resistant organisms within the hospital environment.

Alternative medicines

The use of alternative and traditional medicines is widespread in developing countries and is becoming increasingly popular in Western societies. There is an assumption that 'natural' remedies are better and safer. However, these medicines are largely unregulated and sold over the counter without prescription and there may be no medical advice given or follow-up of patients. There have been questions about the quality of products and reports of people using inappropriate medication for their condition or taking too large a dose.

Some therapies such as acupuncture have proven benefits and products containing the Chinese herb, *Artemisia annua*, are effective against malaria. The World Health Organization (WHO) has recently issued guidelines to help health authorities to provide information to the mass media that will facilitate proper use of these medicines

available at <http://www.who.int/mediacentre/news/releases/2004>. In Australia, the Therapeutic Goods Administration (TGA) regulates all medicines for which there are therapeutic claims. These include prescription medicines, over-the-counter medicines and complementary medicines. Complementary medicines, also known as traditional or alternative medicines, include vitamins, minerals, nutritional supplements, herbal remedies, aromatherapy and homeopathic products.

Any product for which therapeutic claims are made must be entered in the Australian Register of Therapeutic Goods (ARTG) before the product can be supplied in Australia.

It is important that patients inform their doctor about any 'natural' medication they are taking. For example *Ginkgo biloba* is a popular herb used to prevent vascular disease but can cause excessive bleeding during surgery.

Implications for nursing practice

Nurses are the health professionals who have most patient contact. Although the microbiologist identifies the organism causing an infection and the doctor prescribes the appropriate antimicrobial, it is usually the nursing staff who are responsible for administering the medication and monitoring the outcome. All health professionals need to be aware of the importance of handwashing to prevent the spread of infection. This section examines the nurse's role in the treatment of infections.

CASE HISTORY 12.1
Drug administration

A patient in a Sydney hospital suffered a cardiac arrest and died after receiving a 'bolus' injection of vancomycin to treat a *Staphylococcus aureus* infection.

A number of common antimicrobials can cause serious, even fatal, reactions if they are administered by the wrong method. The administration of a bolus injection can cause reactions such as phlebitis (inflammation), histamine release and even cardiac arrest. The drugs that have been shown to have this effect are vancomycin, quinine, lincosamide and macrolides such as erythromycin.

These drugs must be given by slow intravenous infusion, usually over 30 minutes or longer, to avoid local high concentrations. Because phlebitis is also a problem, they are usually given via a centrally placed line.

Nursing management
Most antimicrobial therapy is administered by nursing staff. It is therefore essential that they read carefully all the literature provided by the manufacturer and follow instructions for the correct usage of the drugs. Hospital microbiologists and pharmacists also provide advice on correct procedures.

SPECIMEN COLLECTION

The careful collection of specimens for analysis by the microbiology laboratory is essential for correct identification of the pathogen and determination of antimicrobial sensitivities. Whenever possible the specimen should be collected *before* any antimicrobial therapy is commenced. An appropriate specimen is collected in a sterile container, using aseptic technique, labelled and transported to the laboratory as soon as possible. Information such as provisional diagnosis, type of sample, site of infection (or sample site), date and time of collection should be included on the request form, together with any other information that might assist the microbiologist such as travel history, previous illnesses, current medications (especially antimicrobial therapy) and vaccination status.

INTERPRETATION OF REPORTS

Nurses need to be familiar with the terms used in microbiology and be able to interpret the reports. Frequently, results are telephoned from the laboratory and the nurse must be able to record results accurately. The nurse is in a position to check that the treatment and medication the patient is receiving is in accord with the diagnostic results. It is important to be aware of the use of generic and trade names for drugs and ensure that the correct drug is used.

ADMINISTRATION OF ANTIMICROBIAL THERAPY

This is usually carried out by the nursing staff and, as for any drug, it is important that they are aware of the correct procedures. Before administering any drug, the nurse should take a patient history of allergies (especially to penicillin). The manufacturer's directions accompanying the antimicrobial drug should be read carefully to ensure that the administration of the drug is by the correct route, at the correct time and that any special precautions are followed. The nurse should check the package for such information as:

- expiry date
- method of reconstitution
- storage condition
- contraindications for use
- method of administration – oral or parenteral.

Oral administration

For maximum efficacy, the drug should be maintained at a constant level in the blood or tissues throughout the 24-hour period. For this reason, oral doses are generally given at regular intervals throughout the day, depending on the excretion rate of the drug. Sometimes, this needs to be monitored by taking blood samples at regular time intervals to measure the drug level. Other factors may need to

be taken into account. The rate of absorption of the drug may be affected by the type of tablet or capsule, the particle size of the drug powder, and the presence or absence of food in the intestine. Some drugs, such as tetracycline, bind to antacids or the calcium in milk and are then poorly absorbed.

Side effects such as nausea can be minimised by the administration of the drug with food. Instructions for administration either before, or with food, are therefore important. Sometimes, other adverse reactions can occur; for example, metronidazole (Flagyl®) produces alcohol intolerance.

Patients should be educated about the correct way of taking their medication, the need to take it at regular intervals, and the importance of finishing the prescribed course of the antimicrobial so that the drug level is maintained for a sufficient time to kill all the organisms. It is desirable to explain that the relief or disappearance of clinical symptoms does not mean that all the pathogens have been eliminated from the body, and that the full course of the drug should be taken to prevent a recurrence of the disease.

Parenteral administration

The correct procedure for administration should be ascertained (intravenous or intramuscular), and calculations for reconstitution or dilution of the preparation checked by another member of staff. Usually, the drugs are given by slow IV infusion over a period of time. This is important in the case of a number of drugs where a bolus (single injection) can cause histamine release or vasodilation (flushing) and may even lead to cardiac arrest (see Case History 12.1 on page 271).

Monitoring the outcome

After parenteral administration of antimicrobials (especially penicillin) patients should be closely monitored for any adverse reactions, such as local inflammation or difficulty in breathing. Hypersensitivity reactions causing anaphylaxis can occur in patients who are allergic to penicillin and may require the use of resuscitation equipment and injection of adrenaline (see Spotlight box, page 255).

As with all drugs, the effect of the antimicrobial therapy should be monitored over a period of time and the patient observed for signs of improvement or any side effects (e.g. rashes, ringing in the ears). Suppression of the normal flora may cause an overgrowth of opportunistic organisms such as *Candida albicans*, causing thrush, or *Clostridium difficile*, causing diarrhoea. Some drugs may build up to toxic levels if renal function is impaired, so blood levels in these patients need to be monitored. Careful taking of patient history is important, as factors such as age, weight and hepatic and renal functions affect the action of the drug.

SUMMARY

- The idea of finding a chemical to kill the specific microbe responsible for an infection without damaging the host cells (i.e. a 'magic bullet') was proposed by the chemist Paul Ehrlich in 1908.
- The first successful antimicrobials were the chemically synthesised sulfonamides, or sulfa drugs.
- An antibiotic is a chemical, produced by a microorganism, that in small amounts can kill or inhibit another microorganism. Some antibiotics are chemically modified to improve their antimicrobial properties and are called 'semi-synthetic'.

ANTIMICROBIAL DRUGS

- Selective toxicity is the ability of a drug to kill or inhibit the microorganism responsible for the disease without damaging the host cells.
- Antimicrobials are compounds that can kill or inhibit the growth of a microorganism. They include antibacterial, antifungal, antiprotozoal and antiviral drugs.
- Compounds that are active against several different types of microorganisms are broad spectrum drugs; those with a limited range of activity are narrow spectrum drugs.
- Drugs that kill microorganisms have names ending in -cidal, while those that inhibit replication end in -static.

ANTIBACTERIAL DRUGS

- The main target sites for antibacterial action are the synthesis of the bacterial cell wall, protein synthesis, nucleic acid synthesis and the function of the bacterial cell membrane.
- Peptidoglycan is a compound unique to the bacterial cell wall and therefore provides an ideal target for selective toxicity.
- The beta-lactam antibacterials inhibit cell wall synthesis by combining with the enzyme responsible for cross-linking of the peptidoglycan chains. They include the penicillins, cephalosporins, carbapenems and monobactams.
- The production of the enzyme, beta-lactamase, which destroys these antibacterials, is a major mechanism of resistance.
- Other cell wall inhibitors include the glycopeptides, vancomycin and teicoplan, which interfere with cell wall synthesis by binding to the growing peptide chains of the peptidoglycan molecule.
- Compounds that inhibit the synthesis of protein include the aminoglycosides, the tetracyclines and the macrolides, as well as chloramphenicol, clindamycin and fusidic acid.
- Antimicrobials may inhibit the synthesis of nucleotide precursors, or DNA or RNA replication. They include the sulphonamides, quinolones and rifampicin.
- Metronidazole (Flagyl®) is active against anaerobic bacteria as well as some intestinal protozoa.
- Polymyxins are cyclic polypeptides which act as cationic detergents and disrupt the phospholipid bilayer of the membrane.

ANTIFUNGAL DRUGS

- The main target of antifungal drugs is the synthesis or function of the fungal cell membrane. They include the imidazoles, which inhibit the enzymes involved in sterol biosynthesis, and the polyene antibiotics, amphotericin B and nystatin.
- Cutaneous mycoses such as tinea and thrush are treated mainly with topical preparations containing miconazole, clotrimazole or nystatin.
- Increasing numbers of immunocompromised patients are susceptible to opportunistic fungal infections.

ANTIPARASITIC DRUGS

- Various quinine derivatives are used for the treatment of malaria.
- Prophylactic malaria chemotherapy involves the use of chloroquine or doxycycline.

ANTIVIRAL DRUGS

- For an antiviral drug to be selectively toxic, it must target a unique point in the cycle of viral replication.
- The most successful antiviral drugs are chemically synthesised analogues of the purine and pyrimidine bases.
- Antiretroviral drugs target a specific viral enzyme, called reverse transcriptase.
- The action of these drugs is virustatic (i.e. when the drug is removed, viral replication can resume).
- Interferons are a family of small glycoprotein molecules produced by many kinds of mammalian cells in response to viral infection.

THERAPEUTIC USE OF ANTIMICROBIAL DRUGS

- To select the most effective antimicrobial to use, the actual strain of the organism causing the infection is tested against a range of possible antimicrobial agents. Two methods are disk diffusion tests, and the minimum inhibitory concentration (MIC) test.
- The use of antimicrobial drugs can lead to suppression of the normal flora, the occurrence of various adverse side effects and the emergence of resistant strains of pathogens.
- Usually, doctors prescribe on the 'best guess' principle and then review the prescription if and when the results of the pathology tests are available.
- The prescribed dosage aims to achieve an effective concentration of the drug at the site of infection.
- Two drugs may be prescribed at once to treat mixed infections, or to minimise the risk of resistance.
- Prophylaxis is the administration of an antimicrobial drug before there is any evidence of infection, under conditions where the risks of an infection developing are considered very high.

DEVELOPMENT OF RESISTANCE TO ANTIMICROBIAL DRUGS

- Bacteria may exhibit resistance by the production of enzymes which destroy or inactivate the drug, by a change in membrane permeability, by an alteration in the binding sites for the drug, or by synthesis of the required compounds via an alternate pathway.
- The high usage of antimicrobial drugs in hospitals provides an environment in which resistant organisms can flourish.
- Strategies to control the spread of antimicrobial resistance include hospital policies for prescribing antimicrobials, use of narrow spectrum antimicrobials, improved surveillance to determine prevalence, infection control procedures to prevent hospital-acquired infections, and a continuing search for vaccines against bacterial infections.

IMPLICATIONS FOR NURSING PRACTICE

- The nurse is responsible for the collection of an appropriate specimen in a sterile, labelled container, using aseptic technique, for arranging transport to the laboratory as soon as possible and for receiving the reports.
- The nurse should be aware of the correct methods of administration of the drugs and any special precautions that apply.
- Patients should be closely monitored for adverse reactions, such as hypersensitivity, which can occur in patients who are allergic to penicillin and may cause anaphylaxis.
- The patient must be observed for signs of improvement and for side effects such as an overgrowth of other microrganisms, causing thrush (*Candida albicans*) or diarrhoea (*C. difficile*).

STUDY QUESTIONS

1. What is meant by the term 'selective toxicity'?
2. Give three examples of ways in which antibacterial drugs can be selectively toxic.
3. Define the terms 'broad spectrum' and 'narrow spectrum' when applied to antimicrobial drugs.
4. Discuss the different ways in which antibacterial drugs can inhibit or damage the bacterial cell.
5. What are some of the major side effects associated with the use of aminoglycosides?
6. Why should tetracyclines not be given to children or pregnant women?
7. Why is chloramphenicol used mainly in topical applications?
8. Discuss the way in which sulfa drugs exhibit selective toxicity.
9. What is the main point of attack of most antifungal drugs?
10. Why is it difficult to design effective antiviral drugs?
11. What are interferons?
12. How is an antimicrobial sensitivity test carried out?
13. Why do doctors prescribe medication before the laboratory results are available?
14. Should specimens for diagnosis of infection be collected before or after the implementation of antimicrobial therapy?
15. What is meant by the half-life of a drug?
16. What is the therapeutic index of a drug?
17. List four ways in which bacteria can resist the action of antibacterial drugs.
18. Why are hospital-acquired infections more likely to be resistant to antibacterial drugs than community-acquired infections?
19. In what situations is the prophylactic use of antimicrobials considered necessary?
20. What are the responsibilities of the nurse in administering and monitoring antimicrobial therapy?

TEST YOUR UNDERSTANDING

1. Why is it preferable to prescribe bactericidal drugs under some conditions, rather than bacteriostatic drugs?
2. Why may bacteria that produce beta-lactamase enzymes exhibit resistance to both penicillins and cephalosporins?
3. What are the advantages of using chemically modified (semi-synthetic) antibiotics?
4. Name two major disadvantages of the indiscriminate use of antimicrobial drugs.
5. Explain why it is more difficult to treat systemic fungal infections than cutaneous infections.
6. Why should travellers to malarious areas seek advice from the Health Department?
7. Explain why analogues of nucleic acid precursors are effective as antiviral agents.
8. Why is it necessary to perform antimicrobial sensitivity tests?
9. What are the advantages/disadvantages of prescribing two drugs simultaneously?
10. Explain how bacteria can become resistant to antimicrobial drugs.

Reference

Therapeutic Guidelines – Antibiotic, 2003, Version 12. Melbourne: Therapeutic Guidelines Ltd.

Haygarth S 1998, 'Howard Florey: a maker of miracles', *Microbiology Australia*, 19(3): 7–9.

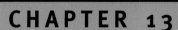

Infection Control in Health-care Facilities

[CHAPTER FOCUS]

- ■ *Why are health-care-associated infections (HCAI) important?*

- ■ *What factors contribute to the incidence of infections in health-care facilities?*

- ■ *How are infections transmitted in hospitals?*

- ■ *What are Standard Precautions and Additional Precautions?*

- ■ *What methods are used to control the spread of infection in hospitals?*

- ■ *Which groups of patients are most susceptible to infection by hospital pathogens?*

The very first requirement in a hospital is that it should do the sick no harm.

Florence Nightingale

Introduction

Pathogenic microorganisms are present everywhere in the environment but are particularly prevalent in health-care facilities. An important aspect of the provision of quality health care is the prevention of transmission of infection to susceptible patients, health care workers or any other people who come in contact with infectious patients in these settings. Health-care facilities include hospitals, doctors' consulting rooms, day-surgery centres, residential aged care, home nursing services and ancillary health services such as dental practices and podiatrists. In these settings infected patients are a major reservoir of infection, but contaminated equipment and instruments, as well as the environment, can also be the source of pathogenic microorganisms. The level of risk of transmission of infection to a susceptible person depends on such factors as the type of facility, the medical procedures being carried out and the health status of the patient (or health-care worker).

In recent years there has been an increasing realisation of the importance of health-care-associated infections (HCAI) – previously referred to as **nosocomial infections**. They are infections contracted as a result of health care and include iatrogenic infections (resulting from a medical procedure) and infections which result from a patient's presence in a health-care facility. They are important not only in terms of patient morbidity and mortality but also because of the wider socioeconomic implications for patient well-being and the overall cost of health care to the community. Government agencies and health facilities have developed infection control guidelines and practices aimed at limiting the spread of infection. However, it was not always this way.

Specialised buildings for the care of the sick have existed for over 2000 years. The word 'nosocomial' is derived from the ancient Greek words *nosos* meaning 'disease' and *komeion* meaning 'to take care of'. In early times these buildings were carefully designed to allow for plenty of fresh air, and bathing and hygiene were considered very important. After the fall of the Roman Empire and the emergence of Christianity there was a decline in hygiene. Ignorance and superstition blamed evil spirits and miasmas ('toxic emanations from the earth') for the occurrence of infectious diseases. Hospitals associated with the Christian church during the Middle Ages were overcrowded, insanitary buildings with several patients in each bed and poor ventilation. More than 50% of hospitalised patients died. During the early 19th century some physicians tried to draw attention to the appalling rate of infection and to devise ways of reducing mortality. However, there were many who did not believe that diseases were contagious and blamed high mortality rates on 'intrinsic defects' in the patients, such as poverty or ignorance.

A major problem during the first half of the 19th century was puerperal fever (childbed fever), a septicaemia that occurred in women following childbirth and had a high mortality rate. OLIVER WENDELL HOLMES published an essay in 1843 claiming that puerperal fever was contagious. This was at a time when most people believed that bad air was responsible for such diseases.

At about the same time, the Hungarian physician, IGNAZ PHILIPP SEMMELWEIS, noticed the smell of cadavers on the hands of doctors and medical students who were in the habit of going directly from a post-mortem examination to a delivery without washing their hands. He suggested that the cause of puerperal fever was being spread from the corpses in the autopsy room to the labour rooms and demonstrated that, when the doctors washed their hands in a chlorinated solution before entering the obstetric ward, there was a dramatic decrease in the incidence of puerperal fever and mortality (see Figure 13.1). We now know that these infections were caused mainly by the bacterium, *Streptococcus pyogenes*. Unfortunately, his classic paper was not published until 1860 and even then was not accepted by his profession. He was later confined to a mental institution where, ironically, he is alleged to have died from a streptococcal infection.

The Scottish surgeon JAMES SIMPSON made a study of the epidemiology and prevention of 'surgical fever' which he believed was similar to puerperal fever. In 1869 he reported that over 40% of amputees in large metropolitan hospitals died after surgery, a rate that was four times higher than for amputations performed by country physicians. He noted that death rates increased with the size of the hospital and reported that in large hospitals pyaemia (infection) accounted for 60% of all deaths. He commented that the bringing together of so many sick people in a confined area was 'perilous' and made a number of recommendations to reduce the incidence of infection, one of which was that dressings should not be reused!

The British surgeon, JOSEPH LISTER, is regarded as the first person to introduce the use of antiseptics in surgery. In the 1860s he began to use a fine spray of carbolic acid to disinfect operating rooms and as an antiseptic in wound dressings, and reported a decrease in mortality after amputation from 46% to 15%.

FLORENCE NIGHTINGALE was also aware of the high mortality rates in hospital wards. She is noted for many achievements in nursing, not least for her efforts in English field hospitals in Turkey during the Crimean War. She was sent there in 1854 as Superintendent of Nursing because of a public outcry over the death rate of British

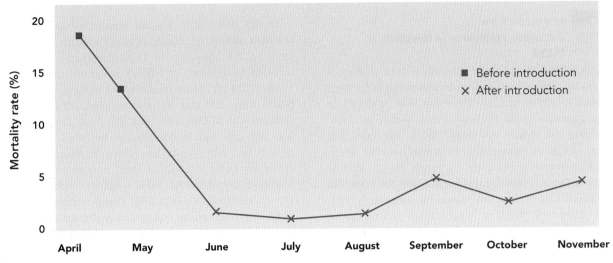

Figure 13.1

Effect of hygienic hand disinfection as introduced by Semmelweis in May 1847 on maternal mortality at the Vienna Lying-in Hospital

Adapted from R.P. Wenzel (ed.), *Prevention and Control of Nosocomial Infections*, Williams & Wilkins, Baltimore, 1987, p. 4.

soldiers in these hospitals. The conditions in these so-called 'medical facilities' were appalling, and the death rate of over 50% was due mainly to infection. Within six months of her arrival the mortality rate had dropped to under 3%, due to the much improved sanitary measures that she introduced. Ten years later, still concerned with infection rates in hospitals, Florence Nightingale wrote that 'in all probability a poor sufferer would have much better chance of recovery if treated at home'. However, Nightingale did not believe that disease could be communicated from person to person or that quarantine was an effective method of control. Instead, she advocated sanitary measures to control the spread of disease.

Towards the end of the 19th century the work of Koch and Pasteur (see Chapter 1) identified microorganisms as the cause of infectious diseases and the 20th century saw moves for hospital reform and the development of methods of infection control. To reduce the spread of infection, specialised disease hospitals such as smallpox hospitals, fever hospitals and tuberculosis sanitoriums were established.

In the 1950s the introduction of antimicrobial drugs led to a significant reduction in mortality from infectious diseases (see Chapter 12). However, this was not matched by a reduction in the number of infections. Despite the many advances in hospital infection control, in Australia in the 21st century 5–10% of patients in hospitals will still develop an infection.

This chapter examines the causes of health-care-associated infections, the risks associated with various medical and hospital procedures and the measures being taken to reduce the incidence of infection in health-care facilities. It is not possible to describe foolproof procedures to prevent the spread of infection. Rather, it is the responsibility of each health-care worker to be able to identify the factors that put patients or themselves at risk, understand the principles of infection control, be aware of national and local guidelines and be able to apply this knowledge in the clinical setting. In this chapter we focus on the hospital scene but the principles described are applicable to any health setting.

The importance of health-care-associated infections

The generally accepted definition of a health-care-associated infection (HCAI) is one that was not apparent or incubating at the time of admission, but appears at least 48 hours after admission or within a specified time (depending on the type of infection and/or facility) after discharge. Apart from an increase in morbidity and mortality, the most obvious outcome of a health-care-associated infection is an increase in the length of hospital stay (or 'hospital days'), but sometimes there are long-term effects on quality of life and even loss of personal income by the patient. In addition, there are other health-related expenses such as the cost of antimicrobial therapy, the costs to the community of replacing workers, reduced productivity and claims on medical insurance. Another important consequence is that, once a patient is infected, they become an additional reservoir of infection in the hospital.

In an Australian national survey of hospital infection rates McLaws et al.[1] found an overall prevalence of 6.3%, which rose to 8.6% in hospitals with more than 500 beds. This compares with a worldwide prevalence rate of 3–21% (average 8.7%) reported by the World Health Organization in 1988.[2] A recent survey by the Public Health Laboratory Service (PHLS) in England[3] found a rate of 7.8% in hospital inpatients and identified a post-discharge rate of 19.1% in patients who had not reported an infection while in hospital.

Prevalence surveys measure the proportion of patients who have an infection *at a given time*. **Incidence** rates

The development and use of penicillin to treat soldiers in World War II was an enormous breakthrough in the fight against infectious disease. Penicillin was produced in large quantities in the 1940s and many lives were saved. However, the success was short-lived. It was found that some strains of *Staphylococcus aureus* quickly developed resistance to penicillin by producing an enzyme (beta-lactamase) which could break down the penicillin molecule. One of these strains was the particularly virulent phage type 80/81, or 'golden staph', which spread around the world between 1955 and 1965.

Golden staph (so named because of the yellow-gold pigment it produces) made headlines in Australia when an epidemic occurred in the neonatal ward of a Sydney hospital in 1953. It then spread rapidly throughout other States, causing major outbreaks of hospital-acquired infections. It was only contained when a number of synthetic derivatives of penicillin, resistant to the beta-lactamase enzyme, were developed. Of these, methicillin became the standard treatment for *Staphylococcus aureus*.

In 1961 the first methicillin-resistant strains of *Staphylococcus aureus* (MRSA) were isolated in Europe. They appeared in Australia in 1966 in the eastern States, and in the United States in 1968. As well, other strains were identified that had a broad pattern of resistance, not only to methicillin but also to the aminoglycosides and cephalosporins.

In the 1970s only a small number of methicillin-resistant strains of *Staphylococcus aureus* were isolated (<2%). However, in 1979, a survey in Victoria reported an increase in MRSA infections and during 1980–82 the incidence reached 50% in some large hospitals. One 700-bed hospital reported 254 patients infected with MRSA, of whom 30% died. The outbreak was not confined to Melbourne, but also spread to Sydney and other Australian States. In Australia there continues to be a constant level of endemic MRSA infections reported from most hospitals, with sporadic serious outbreaks of infection. Using techniques such as DNA typing, phage typing and antibiotic sensitivity patterns, it is possible to identify and track the spread of different strains.

There are three main types of MRSA circulating in Australia. Methicillin-resistant *S. aureus* (also called Eastern Australian MRSA (EAMRSA)) is resistant to all antibiotics except vancomycin. Community MRSA, also called Western Australian MRSA, is sensitive to gentamycin and there are other community strains in Australia and New Zealand which have variable resistance to antibiotics. Strains of MRSA have now emerged with decreased sensitivity to vancomycin. For this reason, careful consideration must be given before prescribing the drug since the search for effective alternatives has so far been unsuccessful. This leaves very few options for treatment of patients infected with MRSA.

Patients and staff are frequently colonised by MRSA without showing any evidence of infection. MRSA does

give the proportion of patients who develop an infection *within a given period of time* and thus more closely reflect the true risk of infection, even though they are much more difficult to measure. Because prevalence rates are biased towards patients who are more seriously ill, they are usually higher than incidence rates.

Mortality data due solely to health-care-associated infections is difficult to interpret, but one estimate in the United States places the death rate at 1–2%.[4] More recently, it has been estimated that there may be as many as 150 000 HCAIs in Australia per year, contributing to 7000 deaths. The cost to the health system is estimated to be of the order of $268 million per year for surgical-site infections and as high as $686 million for bloodstream infections.[5]

A study in the United States estimated that, on average, an infection acquired in hospital extends the length of hospital stay for the patient by 3–4.5 days.[6] However, the PHLS study found that patients stayed an average of 11 days longer with an annual cost to the British National Health Service of 2.5 billion dollars. These figures are influenced by hospital policies regarding discharge but it is obvious that there is a significant increase in patient

bed-days which not only increases costs but also limits the availability of health resources for other patients.

In order to devise strategies to control the spread of infection in hospitals, it is necessary to have information about the extent of the problem, the causative organisms and the major kinds of infection. This requires the establishment of surveillance programs to assess and monitor hospital infections. The SCENIC study in the United States[7] highlighted the value of surveillance programs in reducing hospital infections. However, surveillance data are difficult to compare unless uniform criteria are used (see page 172).

Organisms that cause health-care-associated infections

Bacterial and viral diseases that occur in the community can also occur in the hospital environment. Patients admitted to hospital with an infectious disease or incubating the disease will be a source of infection for other patients and for health-care workers. It is important that the patient is diagnosed as quickly as possible and effective infection control procedures are put in place to protect other patients

not seem to be particularly invasive in healthy individuals. The patients who are most at risk are those who are debilitated or have diminished resistance to infection: infants in neonatal high dependency units; cancer and leukaemia patients; patients who are immunodeficient; patients in whom invasive foreign bodies have been inserted, such as heart valves, joint prostheses, IV lines or catheters; and patients who have undergone extensive surgery.

What can be done to contain MRSA?

There have been numerous reports of MRSA outbreaks and of the many different measures taken to contain the organism. Some common factors emerge. Staff who are colonised with MRSA in the nose do not appear to present a significant risk of transmission. Even so, opinions vary about the need to treat them with an antiseptic nasal cream such as mupirocin. On the other hand, staff who are colonised in skin lesions do present a significant risk of transmission and should not be assigned to high-risk areas until the MRSA is cleared. Infected patients who are shedding MRSA should be isolated and Additional Precautions used. There are varying opinions about the risks posed by patients who are colonised but not infected.

It has been suggested that outbreaks of MRSA infection are indicative of a general breakdown in infection control procedures, due to such factors as overcrowding, pressure of work, or even complacency on the part of health workers that all infections can be dealt with by the use of antibiotics. Countries with a low rate of antibiotic usage, strict infection control measures and a better ratio of nurses to patients seem to have a lower incidence of resistant microorganisms.

MRSA has been shown to be transported on the hands and is readily removed by effective handwashing between patients. Some hospitals advocate surveillance (i.e. routine swabbing of staff and patients), but the results of this have to be measured against the cost and the work created for medical, nursing and laboratory staff.

Nurses should be aware of the risk they pose if they have been working in the environment of a MRSA patient and are then assigned to a high-risk area where patients are particularly susceptible. This applies especially to agency staff who may move from one hospital to another.

Although most strains of MRSA seen in Australia are not nearly as virulent as the golden staph phage type 80/81 of the 1950s, it is still a major cause for concern because of its resistance to all antibiotics except vancomycin. The use of antibiotics in hospitals must be monitored carefully at all times as the appearance of resistant strains of other bacteria is one outcome of the indiscriminate use of antibiotics. In recent years a number of other multi-resistant hospital organisms have appeared. Some strains of *Pseudomonas aeruginosa*, *Acinetobacter* and enterococci are almost untreatable.

It is not possible to rely on antibiotic therapy to cure infections. Rather, it is essential to maintain good infection control practices to prevent the spread of pathogenic microorganisms, of which MRSA is an important example.

and staff. These diseases include viral infections such as colds, influenza, respiratory syncytial virus (RSV), chickenpox and measles as well as more serious bacterial diseases such as tuberculosis. The 2003 epidemic of SARS, severe acute respiratory syndrome, occurred because it was a new viral disease and was spread to patients and health workers before it could be diagnosed; see Spotlight box, page 162.

In addition to these known diseases, patients are at risk of being infected with a pathogen they may be exposed to in the hospital environment as the result of a medical procedure they have undergone or treatment they have received.

The most common site of HCAIs is the urinary tract, followed by surgical wounds and infections of the lower respiratory tract, skin and blood. The relative frequency of each type of infection is influenced by a number of factors including the age of the patient, the type of operation in surgical cases, the degree of immunosuppression and the length of time a catheter or intravenous cannula is in place. Many infections of the urinary tract are associated with indwelling urinary catheters. Although inconvenient, urinary tract infections do not usually lead to a prolonged stay in hospital. On the other hand, wound infections, pneumonia and septicaemia are more serious – they cause significant morbidity and are occasionally fatal. Infections may occur as single cases (sporadic) or in outbreaks or clusters (epidemic).

Bacteria are responsible for most HCAIs, followed by fungi and viruses. The pattern of microorganisms responsible for wound infections has changed over the last 80 years. In the 1920s streptococci, especially *Streptococcus pyogenes,* were the most feared microbes in hospitals. With the introduction of sulfonamide drugs in the 1930s, their importance waned. Within ten years *Staphylococcus aureus* ('golden staph') had virtually replaced streptococci as the dominant cause of hospital infections. Penicillin, the 'wonder drug' introduced in the 1940s, was initially highly effective against staphylococci and streptococci. By the 1950s, however, strains of *Staphylococcus aureus* had appeared that were resistant to this drug (see Spotlight box, above).

Although methicillin (a derivative of penicillin) was introduced in the early 1960s, strains of **methicillin-resistant *Staphylococcus aureus* (MRSA)** soon appeared. Subsequently, strains of *Staphylococcus aureus* emerged that were resistant to methicillin and a number of other drugs and they also became known as **multi-resistant *Staphylococcus aureus*** (**MRSA**). Since then MRSA has been responsible for numerous epidemics in hospitals and is still a major problem. MRSA is considered to be endemic in many hospitals throughout the world, including major teaching hospitals in Australia. In the last few years, strains of MRSA with decreased sensitivity to vancomycin (the only drug available to treat them) have been isolated. They are known as VISA (vancomycin intermediate *Staphylococcus aureus*) or GISA (glycopeptide intermediate *Staphylococcus aureus*) and are the cause of serious infections that usually occur in patients who are already very ill.

Staphylococcus epidermidis and other coagulase-negative staphylococci (organisms commonly found on human skin as normal flora and formerly considered non-pathogenic) are now recognised as being responsible for many cases of infection associated with indwelling intravenous lines, cerebrospinal fluid shunts, prosthetic heart valves and other prostheses. Resistant strains are now common.

In recent years there has also been a re-emergence of virulent strains of the group A streptococcus (GAS), *Streptococcus pyogenes*, as a cause of HCAI. They are often carried in the nose or pharynx. They are a common cause of wound infections and cellulitis and some strains carry virulence factors that cause invasive infections such as necrotising fasciitis. Most strains are still sensitive to penicillin.

Gram-negative rods, especially *Escherichia coli* and *Pseudomonas* spp., and, to a lesser extent, species of *Klebsiella, Proteus, Enterobacter* and other enteric bacteria, have always played a prominent role in HCAIs. Some strains now exhibit resistance to two or more antibiotics (see Chapter 12). Some of these bacteria, in particular the Gram-negative bacilli *Klebsiella* and *E. coli* produce ESBLs (extended spectrum β-lactamases) – enzymes that destroy β-lactam antibiotics such as the cephalosporins.

The 1980s and 1990s saw the emergence of a number of other microorganisms that cause health-care-associated infections. *Acinetobacter baumannii* occurs in some high-dependency or critically ill patients and easily acquires resistance to antibiotics. *Serratia marcescens* is often a problem in high-dependency units.

Enterococci are part of the normal flora but the emergence of vancomycin-resistant strains (VRE) poses another serious infection risk for susceptible patients (see Spotlight box, at right). In immunocompromised patients, such as AIDS patients or those receiving immunosuppressive drugs or chemotherapy for cancer, infections caused by enterococci and mycobacteria have become more common. *Clostridium difficile* usually occurs as an opportunistic infection in patients receiving extensive antimicrobial therapy. It can also be transmitted to other susceptible patients as it readily contaminates the environment and is difficult to remove.

The number of systemic infections caused by fungi is also increasing. These opportunistic infections are occurring

---

SPOTLIGHT ON
Emerging infections – VRE

Vancomycin is a glycopeptide antibiotic which for many years has been used as a last resort in the treatment of serious hospital infections such as MRSA. The emergence around the world of numerous isolates of enterococci resistant to vancomycin (VRE) has therefore been a cause for alarm.

Enterococcus faecium and *Enterococcus faecalis* are normal inhabitants of the human intestine and are sometimes responsible for hospital-acquired infections such as surgical wound infections, urinary tract infections, septicaemia and endocarditis. They are naturally resistant to a number of antibiotics including the cephalosporins and sometimes the aminoglycosides, tetracycline and erythromycin, but serious infections used to be effectively treated with penicillin/amoxycillin and vancomycin.

The first vancomycin-resistant enterococci appeared in Australia in 1994 and a strain resistant to both vancomycin and amoxycillin has been isolated in Brisbane.[8]

Patients in high-dependency areas are most at risk of infection with VRE. Vulnerability to infection is largely determined by the presence of an indwelling device such as a peripheral vascular line, central line, urinary catheter or surgical drainage. Immunological impairment plays a part, although it is not the major factor. Exposure to broad spectrum antibiotics predisposes a patient to colonisation and infection with resistant organisms.

Because VRE is shed in the faeces, transmission of VRE in hospitals is usually due to dissemination by health personnel or contact with fomites. Enterococci can survive for long periods on surfaces so strict attention to infection control practices and **handwashing** are essential. Patients need to be isolated and Additional (contact) Precautions implemented.

Genes for antibiotic resistance can be transferred between related species on plasmids, and already strains of MRSA with reduced sensitivity to vancomycin (VISA) have been isolated overseas. So far, infections with VRE are uncommon in Australia; however, measures such as restricting the use of vancomycin need to be implemented to prevent the organism becoming endemic in hospitals and to reduce the risk of vancomycin resistance occurring in Australian strains of MRSA.

---

because of the increasing use of procedures and medications that lower the resistance of the patient. Not only are immunocompromised patients more susceptible to these previously rare causes of infection but, once infected, they serve as important reservoirs of these pathogens in hospitals. The main fungi are species of *Candida*, of which *Candida albicans* is most common. *Aspergillus fumigatus* is the most common mould, but other moulds such as *Scedosporium* spp. are seen with increasing frequency.

Latent viruses like cytomegalovirus and herpes simplex, which may be reactivated in patients whose immune system is compromised, can be a source of infection for other patients. In specific units or hospitals, other organisms may be important. For example, rotavirus and respiratory syncytial virus (RSV), are important pathogens in paediatric hospitals.

Gastrointestinal infections are common in the community and can also occur in health facilities. Often the source is an infected patient but sometimes contaminated food or poor food handling is responsible. Pathogens include *Campylobacter, Salmonella, Staphylococcus aureus, Clostridium perfringens, Bacillus cereus* and noroviruses.

The common causes and risk factors of hospital-acquired infections are summarised in Table 13.1.

Sources of hospital infections

Infections may be caused by microorganisms that are found either inside or outside the hospital. Those that originate outside and are brought into the hospital by patients, staff and visitors are regarded as **community strains**. They include the normal flora of these people as well as any pathogens they may be infected with or are carrying asymptomatically. If these pathogens are shed they can be transmitted to patients or staff. The patient's own normal flora may also be the source of an infection – for example, gastrointestinal flora that move to the urinary tract, or *Staphylococcus epidermidis* from the skin that infects an IV cannula-insertion site. In general, community strains are likely to be sensitive to antimicrobial drugs.

Many infections are caused by **hospital strains**. As the name implies, these are strains of microorganisms that are found mainly in hospitals or associated with people (patients and staff) who have been in hospitals. Hospital strains differ from community strains in that they usually have a greater resistance to antimicrobial drugs and some disinfectants. Multi-resistant strains of bacteria like *Staphylococcus aureus* (MRSA), *Staphylococcus epidermidis, Pseudomonas, E. coli, Klebsiella, Enterobacter* and *Enterococcus* cause infections that are difficult to treat and

Table 13.1

Common causes and risk factors of hospital-acquired infections

INFECTION	COMMON CAUSES	RISK FACTORS
Urinary tract	*E.coli, Klebsiella* spp., *Enterococcus* spp., *Pseudomonas aeruginosa, Proteus* spp.	Urinary catheter; structural or functional abnormality
Surgical wound	*Staphylococcus aureus, Klebsiella* spp., *Streptococcus* spp., *E. coli, Pseudomonas aeruginosa, Enterococcus* spp., *Enterobacter* spp.	Debility, prosthesis, prolonged surgery, surgery on heavily colonised sites
Pneumonia	*Staphylococcus aureus, Klebsiella* spp., *Pseudomonas aeruginosa, Candida* spp., *Enterobacter* spp., *Streptococcus pneumoniae* viruses	Underlying disorder, surgery, ventilation
Septicaemia	*Staphylococcus aureus, Klebsiella* spp., *E. coli, Staphylococcus epidermidis, Enterococcus* spp.	Indwelling IV catheter, infection
Skin	*Staphylococcus aureus, Candida* spp.	Newborn
Immunocompromised patient	Viruses, *Aspergillus* spp. *Candida* spp.	Transfusion, immunosuppression, immunodeficiency, AIDS

may even be life-threatening. The major sources of hospital strains are the hospital environment, patients with infections and colonised patients and staff.

COLONISATION

Colonisation refers to the presence and growth of a microorganism on the skin or mucous membrane without any evidence of infection. The organisms that make up a person's own normal flora are the usual colonisers. However, hospital strains can colonise patients within days or even hours of admission. The major sites of colonisation by drug-resistant hospital organisms are the nose, the skin, the oropharynx, the lower intestine and the urinary tract. The organisms tend to prefer certain sites, as shown in Table 13.2.

Colonisation may result in the short-term presence of unusual organisms in a particular site – for example, Gram-negative bacteria on the skin or in the oropharynx. Having taken up residence with (or displaced) the normal

flora, these hospital strains may then remain there for weeks or months, even after discharge from hospital. Colonisation with hospital microorganisms becomes increasingly common the longer a person is in hospital, and is favoured if the patient is exposed to antimicrobial drugs. The presence of an antibiotic in the tissues of a patient means that, if colonisation occurs, it will probably be by a drug-resistant strain.

Both patients and hospital staff can be colonised by hospital organisms and thus become carriers of these potential pathogens. For example, approximately 30% of the general community carry *Staphylococcus aureus* in the nose, while as many as 70% of hospital staff may carry it. Some of them may be carrying a multi-resistant hospital strain and are therefore an important reservoir of these pathogens. These organisms do not usually pose a threat to a healthy carrier but are often the cause of infection in an individual whose resistance is lowered.

Burns wounds and surgical wounds are ideal sites for microbial growth and are frequently colonised by hospital organisms that can cause serious infections. These wounds act as important sources of pathogens in the spread of hospital acquired infections.

EXOGENOUS AND ENDOGENOUS INFECTIONS

Identification of the source of the causative agent of an infection is important in the epidemiological investigation of outbreaks, and for the selection of appropriate methods of infection control to prevent further transmission. HCAIs can be divided into two general categories based on the source of the causative organism – *exogenous* and *endogenous*. See Figure 13.2. The distinction between exogenous and endogenous sources can be useful for infection control, but in practice is often difficult to make.

Exogenous infections are infections caused by microorganisms from a source external to the patient, such as the hospital environment, staff, other patients or visitors.

Table 13.2
Sites of colonisation with hospital strains in patients and staff

ORGANISM	COLONISATION SITES
MRSA	Nose
	Skin: hands, perineum, groin, axillae
E. coli, Klebsiella,	Bowel
Enterobacter	Oropharynx
	Urinary tract
Pseudomonas	Bowel
	Oropharynx
Staph. epidermidis	Skin
	Urinary tract
Enterococci	Bowel
Candida	Bowel
	Urinary tract

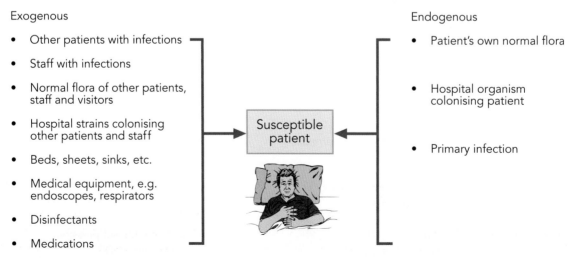

Exogenous

- Other patients with infections
- Staff with infections
- Normal flora of other patients, staff and visitors
- Hospital strains colonising other patients and staff
- Beds, sheets, sinks, etc.
- Medical equipment, e.g. endoscopes, respirators
- Disinfectants
- Medications

Susceptible patient

Endogenous

- Patient's own normal flora
- Hospital organism colonising patient
- Primary infection

Figure 13.2
Sources of infections in health facilities

There are many exogenous sources of potential pathogens. Patients with infections will serve as sources of infection for other patients. For example, in a surgical ward, the patient with an infected wound is a potential source of pathogens for any other patient who has just had surgery. Staff may be colonised with hospital pathogens or be carrying them on their hands. Those who have close patient contact are a particularly important source, especially if they have skin lesions on their hands. Infected patients and staff are not the only human source, since all people carry organisms that can cause infection in a susceptible patient.

Inanimate objects (called *fomites*) in the hospital environment also carry microorganisms capable of causing infection but they are rarely the primary source of pathogenic microorganisms. Mostly they have been contaminated with organisms from human sources. The contribution of the environment to hospital infections is often overestimated. While there is plenty of opportunity for the environment to become contaminated, most microorganisms are unable to multiply and do not survive well on clean, dry surfaces such as floors, walls and furniture. Gram-negative rods such as *E. coli*, *Klebsiella* and *Pseudomonas* are susceptible to desiccation and survive for only a few hours on dry surfaces. However, the endospores of some bacteria (e.g. *Clostridium*) can survive for long periods. *Staphylococcus aureus* is resistant to desiccation and Group A *Streptococcus pyogenes* can survive for several days on surfaces. Standardised cleaning and disinfection procedures are important to minimise the risk of infection from these sources (see Chapter 11).

Environmental organisms such as *Pseudomonas* and *Aspergillus* often cause infections. *Pseudomonas* is found in soil and on flowers and is a common cause of infection in burns patients and patients with cystic fibrosis. The spores of the fungus *Aspergillus* are carried on air currents and cause lung infections, especially in immunocompromised patients. Outbreaks of atypical pneumonia caused by *Legionella* are usually traced to water-cooling towers of air-conditioning units.

Bacteria multiply readily in warm moist environments and items such as sinks, mops, sponges, respiratory equipment, suction apparatus and humidifiers have all been implicated as potential sources of infection (see Figure 13.3). IV fluids, especially TPN (total parenteral nutrition), can also be a source if not handled correctly. Even disinfectant and antiseptic solutions can sometimes become contaminated, especially if not freshly prepared. *Pseudomonas aeruginosa*, for example, will grow in povidone-iodine solutions.

In summary, the most important exogenous sources are places where microbial multiplication can take place. These include infected patients, human carriers, infected wounds and moist areas of the hospital environment. Dry objects and surfaces in the hospital environment are less important, but should not be ignored as potential sources of infection, particularly if they have been *recently* contaminated.

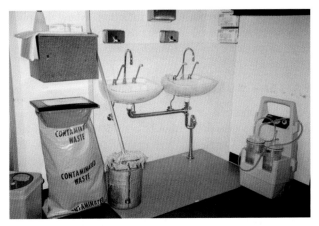

Figure 13.3
Reservoirs of infection in hospitals

Endogenous infections are caused by microorganisms that are part of the patient's own normal flora, or are organisms (including hospital strains) that have colonised the patient after admission to hospital. Often patients who already have an infection transfer the pathogen to another site in the body – the primary infection acts as the source of microorganisms for the second site. The transmission may occur by mechanical transfer on the hands of the patient or staff, or it may be systemic if the organism is carried in the blood or lymphatic system. Latent infections which are reactivated when the patient's immune system is compromised are also considered to be endogenous.

Factors contributing to the incidence of hospital-acquired infections

MICROBIAL FACTORS

The capacity of a microorganism to cause disease (i.e. its virulence) is *not* directly related to its sensitivity or resistance to antimicrobial drugs. A particular strain of an organism can be resistant to a number of drugs but is not necessarily more virulent than a sensitive strain of the same organism. However the use of large amounts of antimicrobial drugs in hospitals favours the selection and persistence of resistant strains (see Chapter 12). A resistant strain is therefore more likely to be responsible for an infection in the hospital environment, and the infection will be serious mainly because of the limited availability of drugs to treat it. Some bacteria have also developed resistance to the disinfectants and antiseptic solutions normally used to control their spread (see Chapter 11).

As explained in Chapters 9 and 10, the outcome of exposure to a microorganism depends on the balance between the virulence of the microbe and the resistance of the host. Generally, the virulence of a microorganism is the major factor in determining whether infection occurs, but an equally important factor is the patient's overall state of health and general resistance to infection. While some hospital pathogens have demonstrated exceptional virulence, such as the outbreaks of 80/81 phage type of *Staphylococcus aureus* ('golden staph') in the early 1950s, this is not a prerequisite for infection. Many hospital infections are caused by organisms of low virulence (e.g. *Staphylococcus epidermidis*) in patients with compromised body defences.

PATIENT SUSCEPTIBILITY

A high proportion of hospitalised patients have lowered immune defences and can thus be considered to be at risk of infection (see Chapter 9). Age is an important factor. The newborn are highly susceptible to infection because of the immaturity of their immune system. Elderly people also have a greater risk of infection because of the deterioration of their immune system, or because of impairment to other body functions such as the blood supply to tissues. Immobility in the aged may lead to stasis of body fluids and hence to infection in organs such as the lungs or bladder.

Lowered resistance may be associated with an underlying disease. For example, patients with leukaemia are more susceptible to infection because they have inadequate numbers of functional white cells. People with diabetes or with liver or renal impairment may have lowered resistance because of vascular changes leading to poor peripheral circulation, causing tissue hypoxia and necrosis. Co-infection may lower a person's resistance. Thus, patients with an influenza virus infection are more susceptible to bacterial pneumonia. A more extreme example is that of HIV infection, which increases patient susceptibility to opportunistic infections because of the effect of the virus on the immune system.

Some medical treatments lower the patient's resistance to infection. Cytotoxic drugs and radiotherapy used for the treatment of cancer both affect the immune system. The drugs given to transplant patients to prevent rejection are designed to suppress the immune system, as are anti-inflammatory drugs, especially the corticosteroids.

Damage to the protective skin barrier such as occurs with skin lesions or pressure sores provides a portal of entry for microorganisms. Patients with burns are also highly susceptible because of loss of skin and fluid imbalance (see Chapter 16). Accident victims or trauma patients with extensive skin damage or crushing injuries to tissues often suffer serious infections because microorganisms may be carried deep into the tissues.

MEDICAL PROCEDURES

As long as the skin and mucous membranes remain intact they provide very effective barriers against infection (see Chapter 9). However, many diagnostic and therapeutic procedures involve the penetration of these barriers by the introduction of a device into a sterile body area, thus providing microorganisms with easy access to susceptible tissues. Infections resulting from medical procedures or treatment are termed **iatrogenic infections**.

Surgery is an obvious example of a procedure that breaches a patient's intact skin. Surgical wound infections are the second most common type of infection in hospitals. Other procedures that carry a risk of infection include the insertion of intravascular cannulae and urinary catheters

and endotracheal and drainage tubes, all of which allow microorganisms to circumvent the body's external barriers.

Urinary catheters allow microorganisms to enter the bladder by travelling either up the outside of the catheter tube or through the tube itself. They are able to colonise the urethra (outside the tube) because the normal flow of urine is not there to wash away the organisms from the tissue surface. If the drainage reservoir is contaminated, organisms can gain entry to the inside of the tube and then spread to the bladder. The use of closed drainage systems reduces the risk of spread of organisms to the bladder via the inside of a catheter tube (see Figure 13.4). The longer a catheter is in place, the greater the risk of infection.

Indwelling intravenous cannulae are frequently used to administer fluids, medication or nutrients to patients. These devices also provide easy access for microorganisms. The cannula and skin around the insertion site can become colonised and subsequently infected, leading to bacteraemia and sometimes septicaemia. *Staphylococcus epidermidis*, a normal skin inhabitant, is frequently

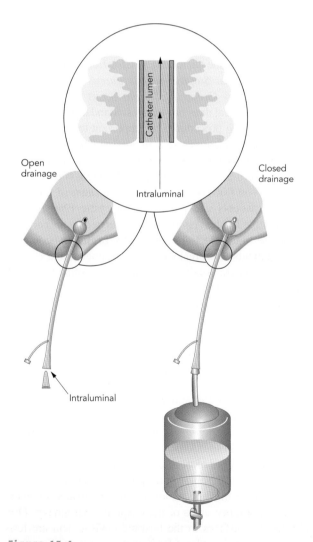

Figure 13.4

Potential sites of infection associated with a urinary catheter. The difference between open and closed drainage systems

the cause of such infections. Again, the longer the device is in place, the greater the risk of infection. Very occasionally, the fluid being administered may be contaminated, or the equipment may become contaminated and microorganisms are passed directly into the bloodstream.

Lower respiratory tract (lung) infections may result from tracheostomy (an opening made into the trachea through the neck) and insertion of a tube into the trachea. Intubation increases the risk of infection because it gives microorganisms direct access to lower airways, and because the procedure often causes injury and irritation to the tracheal lining. The use of respiratory equipment to administer oxygen or medication deep into the lungs can predispose a patient to infection. Nebulisers, humidifiers and other respiratory equipment provide a moist environment for bacteria to multiply, and are difficult to sterilise.

The use of endoscopes to examine mucosal passageways and associated organs increases the risk of infection, since endoscopes are difficult to sterilise. They can irritate or break the delicate mucosal linings of the passageways through which they are passed and thereby increase the risk of infection.

Implantation of prostheses such as heart valves or artificial joints has a high risk of infection, since the site of the operation is exposed to the air for several hours and organisms may be introduced at the time of implantation. The prosthesis may act as a site of colonisation for microorganisms that later enter the bloodstream. Under normal circumstances, small numbers of organisms entering the bloodstream are quickly removed by the body's defences, but inert objects (which do not have a blood supply) provide a site for colonisation that is inaccessible to these defences.

Even the common practice of giving injections using a hypodermic needle brings with it the chance of infection. For such a simple device and common procedure, there are several potential hazards – the needle or syringe may be contaminated, the solution to be injected may be contaminated, or the skin may not have been properly disinfected.

The more severely ill a patient is, the more likely they are to acquire an infection, either as a direct result of their clinical condition or because of the medical or surgical procedures to which they are subjected. The combination of invasive procedures and extensive use of immunosuppressive or antimicrobial therapy that is necessary for some patients leaves them very susceptible to infection. High-dependency units, with severely ill patients, frequently have the highest incidences of infection. As medical science develops, more complex and invasive (lifesaving) procedures are used, with an ever-increasing risk of infection for those subjected to them.

The host factors and medical procedures that predispose patients to hospital infection are summarised in Table 13.3.

MOVEMENT OF PATIENTS

Patients are frequently transferred from ward to ward or from one health-care facility to another. This has the potential to introduce a new pathogen into the environment. For example, a patient transferred from a high-dependency unit to a renal unit may be colonised with MRSA and this would create a new reservoir of infection in the renal ward. Patients transferred from a hospital to a nursing home or *vice versa* might be colonised with a pathogen which is not present in the other facility. Some authorities require the patient to have negative swabs for resistant organisms such as MRSA before they can be moved. However, in practice, when there is a shortage of beds in a hospital or wards are closed, patients have to be transferred. It is important that there is proper communication between the transferring facility and the receiving institution about the requirement for additional precautions. This should also include notification of the ambulance service or other patient transport service.

Trauma patients or patients evacuated from other countries may also introduce new strains of pathogens (see Spotlight box, page 286).

Table 13.3

Factors that predispose patients to hospital infection

FACTOR	SPECIFIC EXAMPLES
Age	The newborn have an immature immune system; the elderly have an immune system that is deteriorating
Underlying disease	Leukaemia, diabetes, cancer, neutropenia
Existing infection	Viral influenza can lead to bacterial pneumonia; HIV infection; herpes virus lesions can be infected by bacteria (e.g. *Staphylococcus aureus*)
Medicines and treatments	Cancer therapy (cytotoxic drugs, radiotherapy); immunosuppression for transplant patients; anti-inflammatory drugs; antibiotics that alter the normal flora; chloramphenicol (suppresses the bone marrow)
Medical procedures	Surgery; indwelling IV catheters; indwelling urinary catheters; intubation of the trachea; tracheostomy; use of respiratory equipment (which is difficult to sterilise); endoscopes; injections; implantation of prosthesis (e.g. heart valves); dialysis
Accidental wounds	Burns, traffic accident, bed sores

Spread of infection in health-care facilities

In every health-care facility there is a risk that infections will be transmitted from an infected patient to another susceptible patient. The number of HCAIs that occur vary from one facility to another, influenced by such factors as:

- the size (number of beds) of the hospital
- the location of the hospital (e.g. inner city or country)
- the type of hospital or unit.

The Australian survey carried out by McLaws and co-workers[1] showed a higher prevalence of HCAIs in large teaching hospitals. To some extent, the figures are a reflection of the hospital facilities as well as the type of patient. Large hospitals usually have high-dependency units,

---

SPOTLIGHT ON
Imported infections

There were many casualties from the bombing of the Sari nightclub in Bali in 2002. Patients were first treated in Bali and some of the more serious cases were flown to Australian hospitals for specialised medical treatment. The patients carried microorganisms derived from Indonesia, the environment and some of the hospital strains circulating in Bali, as well as their own normal flora.

A strain of *Acinetobacter baumannii*, resistant to multiple antibiotics (MDR-AB), including gentamicin, was among the bacteria introduced into one Adelaide hospital on one of these patients. The organism has since been implicated in several outbreaks in the high-dependency unit and other wards of the hospital and has necessitated a surveillance program to monitor its spread. A collaborative infection control effort, including extra cleaning and hand hygiene, had to be instituted to contain the spread of this pathogen.

Comment

Although *Acinetobacter baumannii* is common in the environment, in this case it was introduced on a patient and then persisted in the hospital. Multi-drug-resistant strains pose a serious risk to patients who are immuno-compromised or critically ill. The ability of the organisms to persist in a range of environments and to resist desiccation means they are particularly difficult to eradicate. This case highlights the potential for drug-resistant pathogens to be introduced into a hospital and to spread to susceptible patients.

Regulations differ in other countries and antibiotics are freely available without a prescription in many Asian countries. As a result, there are many multi-resistant strains of bacteria circulating in these communities and they can be carried into Australia by tourists or, in this case, by patients brought for specialist treatment.

Source: H. Brettig et al., Proceedings of AICA Conference 2004.

---

specialised burns units and facilities for transplant operations, all of which act as reservoirs of infection. Patients in these units are particularly susceptible to infection, because of the weakened status of their immune system. Patients admitted to a busy accident/emergency unit are likely to be severely traumatised and therefore at greater risk of infection. In contrast, aged-care facilities do not usually have a population of severely ill patients or patients who are actually infected. There is thus a smaller reservoir of microorganisms present.

A feature of hospitals is the large amount of physical contact that occurs between staff and patients. Depending on the size and nature of the unit, a nurse might be required to perform routine procedures such as temperature, pulse and blood pressure readings, change dressings or administer medication for each patient on several occasions during the day. Other health workers may attend to these patients as well as to patients in other units throughout the hospital. Thus, not only will a staff member have physical contact with many patients, but the patient will have contact with a number of different staff. The contact between patients and staff is thus frequent and varied, allowing easy transmission of microorganisms. Isolation procedures are sometimes instituted to prevent this type of transmission.

Chapter 8 gives a general description of the ways in which diseases can be spread. In the specialised hospital environment, microorganisms can be spread in a number of different ways (Figure 13.5, Table 13.4).

Guidelines for infection control

The actual procedures that are followed to prevent the occurrence of infection may vary from one health-care facility to another, but should all be based on sound microbiological principles and the infection control guidelines published by Commonwealth and State health departments. The CDNA publication, *Infection Control Guidelines for the prevention of transmission of infectious diseases in the health care setting* 2004, is a comprehensive document which presents the strategies that should be used to implement effective infection control. Some of the key points in this document are included in this chapter, but the reader is referred to the guidelines for a complete description. In addition, the national guidelines are interpreted and modified by State health departments and interpreted at a local level for each health facility.

Before the outbreak of HIV/AIDS, hospitals used a number of different procedures to prevent the transmission of various types of organisms. They were based on guidelines proposed by the American Centers for Disease Control (CDC) in 1983 and recommended the use of **category-specific isolation precautions**, which placed specific diseases, together with the secretions, excretions, body fluids and tissues that are infective for each disease, in defined categories; and **disease-specific isolation precautions**, which gave a more specific set of instructions to be implemented for each disease.

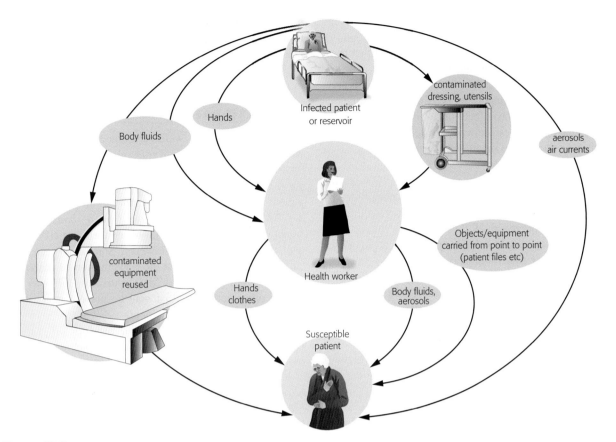

Figure 13.5
Spread of microorganisms in hospital

Table 13.4
Transmission in the health-care environment

SOURCE	METHOD OF TRANSMISSION	PORTAL OF ENTRY
Endogenous (patient)	Patient (hands or systemic)	Wound, IV, or other body site
Environment Contaminated fomites (e.g. patient records, keys, computer terminals)	Hands of health-care workers: doctors, nurses, other personnel	Wounds, IV or injection site, or other break in skin
Environment Air currents and aerosols e.g. bacteria (Legionella, TB), viruses, (influenza, RSV), fungal spores	Air conditioning, inhalation	Upper respiratory tract
Contaminated (non-sterile) equipment or materials, e.g. endoscopes, IV solutions	Iatrogenic	Various, depending on procedure
Contaminated food	Hands Food and food utensils	Oral ingestion
Contaminated material (dressings, used equipment)	Hands Incorrect disposal	Break in skin, IV line, wound
Body substances, faeces	Hands, poor hygiene	Oral ingestion, break in skin, wound, IV line
Body substances, blood (HBV, HCV, HIV), urine (CMV)	Sharps injury	Needlestick (sharps) injury, mucocutaneous splashes

The discovery of the human immunodeficiency virus (HIV), a hitherto unknown deadly virus that is found in blood and body fluids, drew attention to the fact that there may be many other viruses and microorganisms with the potential to cause disease, which have not yet been described. Even more important, there are many situations where patients may be infectious even though they are asymptomatic (i.e. they show no evidence of infection). This is true during the incubation period of a disease or when a person is a carrier.

In Australia, hepatitis B, hepatitis C and HIV are the most important viruses that are known to be transmitted by contact with blood or other body substances from infected carriers. The emergence of these blood-borne diseases changed the way in which health professionals approach the prevention of transmission of infectious agents. It is important to prevent transmission not only from patient to patient, but also from patient to health-care worker and from health-care worker to patient.

UNIVERSAL PRECAUTIONS

In 1987 the CDC issued a document, *Recommendations for the Prevention of Transmission of HIV in Health Care Settings*, which was updated in 1988. This document recommended that Blood and Body Fluid Precautions be used for all patients *regardless of their infection status*. The extension of these precautions to *all* patients was referred to as **Universal Blood and Body Fluid Precautions**.

In 1993 the National Health and Medical Research Council (NHMRC) and the Australian National Council on AIDS (ANCA) issued a joint document on infection control which extended the Universal Precautions recommended by CDC to include 'all blood, body fluids and body substances'. However, in Australia it was perceived that the term 'Universal Precautions' was ambiguous, causing confusion and a false sense of security in its application. Some health-care workers appeared to consider the use of gloves to be a substitute for handwashing, and there was concern that this mistaken perception could increase the risk of transmission of infection.

As an alternative to the term 'Universal Precautions', in 1996 the NHMRC and ANCA recommended adoption of the terms '**Standard Precautions**' (applied as the first-line approach to infection control) and '**Additional Precautions**' where Standard Precautions may be insufficient to prevent transmission of infection, particularly via the airborne route. This change in terminology, reflecting a two-tiered approach based on modes of disease transmission, is in line with changes in terminology adopted by the US Centers for Disease Control and Prevention (CDC).

Because of the changing patterns of health care, professional responsibilities and perceived risks of infection, the guidelines are constantly reviewed. A working party of the Communicable Diseases Network Australia (CDNA) published new guidelines in 2004. This document provides current technical information on best practice for infection control, and aims to establish a nationally accepted minimum standard for infection control. The implementation of the guidelines is the responsibility of individual health-care establishments.

An extract from the current recommendations is set out in the Spotlight box on page 289.

STANDARD PRECAUTIONS

Standard Precautions were developed to protect health workers from the risk of transmission of blood-borne pathogens from patients. The current Australian guidelines cover transmission from health worker to patient as well as patient to health worker. They apply to all pathogens that are likely to be present in *any type of body fluid or substance*. The pathogens of most concern are HIV, hepatitis B and hepatitis C. However, Standard Precautions should also protect against the transmission of pathogens such as cytomegalovirus (CMV) in urine or saliva as well as any other pathogens that may be present in the body fluids of an asymptomatic patient.

Standard Precautions should be used for all patients, whether symptomatic or asymptomatic and regardless of their infective status.

There is a slight, but real, risk of transmission of blood-borne pathogens (such as hepatitis B or C) from an infected health worker to a patient (see Case History on hepatitis C transmission in Chapter 18). CDC has published guidelines dealing with this situation and Australian health departments, both Commonwealth and State, have also issued statements (see below). Dental patients are considered to be at greatest risk because of the invasive nature of dental treatment and the risk of injury to the dentist as well as patient. The Dental Registration Board in each State has regulations for registration of dentists and recommends vaccination for hepatitis B and the use of a steam steriliser for the sterilisation of all instruments.

There have been few documented cases of HIV transmission from health worker to patient worldwide, but a case of transmission of HIV from one patient to another due to a breakdown in surgical aseptic technique was recorded in Australia in 1993. In many cases, it is very difficult to establish definitely the source of an infection and it may be that unrecorded cases of transmission of HIV infection do occur.

Health departments require all health practitioners (including health-care students) to know their own status with regard to the blood-borne pathogens, HIV, HBV and HCV, to follow infection control guidelines, to exercise the duty of care and, if they are carriers of HIV, HBV or HCV, to refrain from carrying out exposure-prone procedures.

Exposure-prone procedures

An exposure-prone procedure is considered to be any situation where there is a potentially high risk of transmission of blood-borne disease from the health-care worker (HCW) to the patient, or vice versa, during invasive medical or dental procedures. Invasive procedures include any surgical entry into tissue, body cavities or organs or repair of traumatic injury. Exposure-prone

Standard and Additional Precautions

Standard Precautions are work practices required for the basic level of infection control. They are designed to cover situations where:

- infectious patients may not show any signs or symptoms of infection
- laboratory tests cannot be completed in time for emergency treatment
- patients may be in the 'window' period of the disease
- people may be placed at risk of infection from other people who are asymptomatic but infectious.

Standard Precautions are recommended for the treatment and care of *all* patients, regardless of their perceived or confirmed infectious status, and in the handling of:

- blood (including dried blood)
- all other body fluids, secretions and excretions (excluding sweat), regardless of whether they contain visible blood
- non-intact skin
- mucous membranes.

Standard Precautions should be implemented for all patient contact and in particular for patients undergoing invasive procedures including catheterisation, cannulation and intubation. They include:

- the use of aseptic techniques, including use of skin disinfectants
- personal hygiene practices, particularly washing and drying hands before and after patient contact
- the use of personal protective equipment which may include gloves, gowns, plastic aprons, masks, eye shields or goggles
- appropriate handling and disposal of sharps and other contaminated or infectious waste
- environmental controls including design and maintenance of premises, cleaning and spills management

- appropriate provision of support services such as laundry and food services.

Additional Precautions are used for patients known or suspected to be infected or colonised with infectious agents that cannot be contained by using Standard Precautions alone and that can cause infection by the following means:

- in respiratory secretions
  - by airborne transmission (e.g. *Mycobacterium tuberculosis*, measles virus, chickenpox virus)
  - by droplet transmission (e.g. mumps, rubella, pertussis, influenza)
- by contact with patients who may be disseminating infectious agents:
  - colonisation with MRSA
  - faecal contamination from carriers of VRE
- other disease-specific means of transmission where Standard Precautions are not sufficient – (e.g. Creutzfeldt-Jakob disease (CJD)).

Additional Precautions should be tailored to the mode of transmission of the particular infectious agent involved and may include:

- allocation of single room with ensuite facilities
- a dedicated toilet (to prevent faecal transmission)
- cohorting (room sharing by people with the same infection)
- special ventilation requirements (negative air pressure)
- additional use of personal protective equipment (e.g. a 0.3 μm particulate filter mask for TB)
- special rostering of duties for health workers
- dedicated patient equipment
- restriction of movement of patients and health workers.

Source: CDNA, *Infection Control Guidelines for the prevention of transmission of infectious diseases in the health care setting*, 2004.

---

procedures are defined by the potential for direct contact between the skin (usually finger or thumb) of the HCW and sharp surgical instruments, needles or sharp tissue (spicules of bone or teeth) in body cavities or poorly visualised or confined body sites (including the mouth).

ADDITIONAL PRECAUTIONS

The implementation of Standard Precautions is the primary strategy for the successful control of health-care-associated infections (HCAIs). However, Additional Precautions may be required for a patient with a suspected or confirmed infection which is carried by the airborne, droplet or contact route (see Table 13.5). The recent outbreak of SARS illustrated the importance of Additional

Precautions to prevent transmission via the airborne route – approximately 21% of all cases occurred in health-care workers exposed to respiratory secretions in the hospital environment, before the causative agent or method of transmission was identified (see Spotlight box, page 162). Respiratory infections such as SARS and tuberculosis are difficult to contain unless the patient is isolated. A single room with negative pressure ventilation and the wearing of suitable masks is necessary.

Additional Precautions should also be used where patients are colonised by pathogens such as MRSA which may be released by excessive shedding of skin cells. Patients infected with vancomycin-resistant enterococci (VRE) or suffering from diarrhoea or viral gastroenteritis, transmitted by the faecal-oral route, may require a single room with dedicated toilet facilities. Additional Precautions are particularly important when nurses are caring for patients with an altered mental state or poor hygiene practices.

See Table 13.5 for an outline of the use of Additional Precautions. Students should refer to the CDNA Guidelines for information on Additional Precautions required for specific diseases.

Prevention of transmission

Strategies to prevent transmission are more likely to succeed if they are based on an understanding of the factors that put patients and health workers at risk.

RISK ASSESSMENT

Although the Infection Control Guidelines provide a framework for the management of infections in the health-care environment, it is important that the health-care worker is able to assess the risk of transmission and susceptibility to infection for each individual patient and situation. Health workers need to be able to identify a potential hazard and implement strategies to prevent transmission.

To evaluate the infection risks involved in any situation, health workers should consider the following questions:

1. *Is there a source (reservoir) of pathogenic micro-organisms?*
   Potential sources should be identified and the nature of pathogen and its method of transmission assessed.

Table 13.5
Outline of Additional Precautions

REQUIREMENT	TYPE OF ADDITIONAL PRECAUTION NEEDED		
	AIRBORNE TRANSMISSION	DROPLET TRANSMISSION	CONTACT TRANSMISSION
Gloves	None	None	For all manual contact with patient, associated devices and immediate environmental surfaces
Impermeable apron/gown	None	None	Use when HCWs' clothing is in substantial contact with the patient (includes items in contact with the patient and their immediate environment)
Respirator or mask	Particulate filter personal respiratory device for tuberculosis only All others, surgical mask*	Surgical mask*	Protect face if splash likely
Goggles/ face-shields	Protect face if splash likely	Protect face if splash likely	Protect face if splash likely
Special handling of equipment	None	None	Single use or reprocess before reuse on next patient (includes all equipment in contact with patient)
Single room	Yes (or cohort patients with same infection) Door closed	Yes (or cohort patients with same infection) Door closed	If possible, or cohort with patient with the same infection (e.g. methicillin-resistant *Staphylococcus aureus*)
Negative pressure	Essential for pulmonary tuberculosis	None	None
Transport of patients	Surgical mask* for patient Notify area receiving patient	Surgical mask* for patient Notify area receiving patient	Notify area receiving patient
Other	Encourage patients to cover nose and mouth when coughing or sneezing and to wash their hands after blowing nose. Provide one metre of separation between patients in ward accommodation	Provide one metre of separation between patients in ward accommodation	Remove gloves and gown, and wash hands before leaving patient's room

*Surgical mask refers to a fluid-repellent, paper filter mask used in surgical procedures (see AS 4381).

Source: CDNA, *Infection Control Guidelines for the prevention of transmission of infectious diseases in the health care setting*, 2004.

2. *What is the risk of the patient acquiring an infection?*

It is necessary to assess factors relating to patient susceptibility, such as the patient's immune status, underlying or contributing illnesses, the presence of wounds or pressure sores, the presence of a urinary catheter or IV line, etc.

3. *What are the risks of transmitting the infection to or from the patient?*

The actual procedures to be carried out when caring for the patient should be examined to assess their potential to spread microorganisms into the environment, to another patient or to a health-care worker.

4. *What protocols and work practices exist to prevent transmission?*

The protocols developed for the prevention of transmission are very similar in all hospitals. They should be ascertained, monitored and modified according to experience.

BREAKING THE 'CHAIN OF TRANSMISSION'

Effective implementation of infection control is based on a sound understanding of the nature and properties of the infectious agent(s) involved, their method of transmission and the strategies that can be used to 'break the chain of transmission'. There are several routes by which a pathogen can reach a susceptible host. The reservoir may be an infected patient or health-care worker, or the pathogen may be present in the environment. The source may be the air conditioning, fomites, or the clothing or hands of a health-care worker (see Figure 13.6).

Ways of 'breaking the chain' are indicated by the corresponding numbers in Figure 13.6.

Handwashing

The oldest, simplest and single most effective method of preventing cross-infection is proper handwashing between each patient contact (see Table 13.6). Handwashing should be carried out immediately *before* and immediately *after* each significant patient contact, even if hands are not visibly soiled. The first washing is to remove microorganisms that may have been picked up from the environment and thus prevent their transfer to the patient. Handwashing after patient contact removes organisms picked up from the patient and prevents their transfer to equipment or to other patients or staff.

Opinion varies considerably among hospitals and various parts of the world regarding the most efficient chemical agent to use for handwashing. Thorough washing with neutral pH soap and water is satisfactory for routine situations. It has been shown to remove transient microorganisms from the hands as well as some of the normal flora. Some hospitals favour the use of antiseptic handwashes, especially those such as chlorhexidine that have a residual action (i.e. they continue to act for a significant time after washing). These are especially useful for surgery, but continual use may sometimes cause skin problems. Damaged skin can then become colonised with

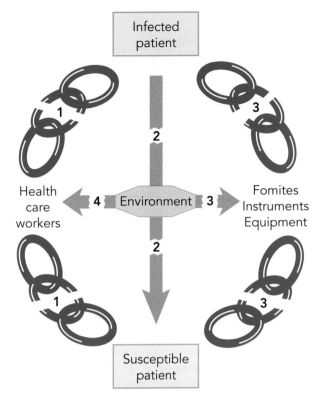

Figure 13.6

Breaking the chain of transmission
Ways of 'breaking the chain' are indicated by the corresponding numbers.
1. HANDWASHING, Standard and Additional Precautions, aseptic technique, protective clothing.
2. Additional Precautions (airborne, contact) use of negative pressure, masks.
3. Cleaning, disinfection, use of sterile equipment.
4. HANDWASHING (personal hygiene, gloves and protective clothing).

potential pathogens and act as a dangerous source of infection. The use of hand lotion is recommended to minimise skin damage.

It is important that staff comply with the handwashing guidelines recommended by their hospital or health-care facility. Unfortunately, studies have shown that compliance does not always occur, but it is generally agreed that even an abbreviated handwash is preferable to not washing at all. The use of alcoholic handrubs between patients is useful when access to hand basins is not available. Posters are often used to remind staff about the importance of handwashing (see Figure 13.7).

Patients should also be instructed about the importance of handwashing. Many hospital-acquired infections are caused by the patient's normal flora and may actually be transmitted to a wound site (portal of entry) by the patient's own hands.

Gloves are an important means of reducing cross-infection but their use *does not remove the need for handwashing*. Handwashing should still be performed, preferably before and after using the gloves. *Gloves should also be changed between patients* and when moving from a 'contaminated' area (e.g. a surgical wound site) to a 'clean'

Table 13.6

Handwashing techniques

TYPE	TECHNIQUE (HOW)	DURATION	DRYING	EXAMPLE (WHEN)
Routine handwash	Remove jewellery Wet hands thoroughly and lather vigorously using neutral pH liquid handwash Rinse under running water Do not touch taps with clean hands If elbow or foot controls are not available, use paper towel to turn taps off	10–15 seconds	Pat dry using paper towel	Before eating or smoking After going to the toilet Before significant contact with patients, e.g. physical examination, emptying a drainage reservoir (catheter bag) Before injection or venepuncture Before and after routine use of gloves After handling any instruments or equipment soiled with blood or body substances
Aseptic procedures	Remove jewellery Wash hands thoroughly using an antimicrobial skin cleanser Rinse carefully Do not touch taps with clean hands. If elbow or foot controls are not available, use paper towel to turn taps off	1 minute	Pat dry using paper towel	Before any procedures that require aseptic techniques (such as inserting intravenous catheter)
Surgical wash	Remove jewellery Wash hands, nails and forearms thoroughly and apply an antimicrobial skin cleanser (containing 4% w/v chlorhexidine) or detergent-based povidone-iodine (containing 0.7% available iodine) Rinse carefully, keeping hands above the elbows No-touch techniques apply	First wash for the day, 5 minutes; subsequent washes, 3 minutes	Dry with sterile towels	Before any invasive surgical procedure

Source: CDNA, Infection Control Guidelines for the prevention of transmission of infectious diseases in the health care setting, 2004, Table 12.1.

site (e.g. an IV line) on the same patient. The aim is always to protect both the patient and the health-care worker.

Aseptic technique

Asepsis refers to the absence of all disease-producing organisms. It is a relative term as, in practice, the complete absence of all microorganisms is difficult to sustain for long periods.

Aseptic technique describes the practices and procedures used by health-care workers to *limit* the spread of microorganisms. Aseptic technique may be described as 'clean' or 'sterile'.

Clean technique includes practices designed to confine microorganisms in a specific area and the use of procedures to prevent the transfer of infectious agents from one site or person to another. It covers personal hygiene practices, especially handwashing, which reduce or limit the number of organisms that may be present on skin. It also involves the correct cleaning and processing of equipment between each patient use and the cleaning and disinfection of all surfaces and equipment that come into contact with the patient in a non-invasive manner. Clean technique should be used to protect both patients and health workers from infection.

Sterile technique is intended to render and maintain objects and areas free from *all* microorganisms. It applies to operating rooms and to any other situation that involves invasive procedures such as the insertion of intravenous (IV) cannulas. It requires that all instruments, gloves, surgical drapes, sutures, dressings and other items that come within a defined

CLINICAL "HANDWASHING" PROCEDURE

"The objective is to remove soil and any transient microorganisms which may have been acquired through patient contact or normal duties."

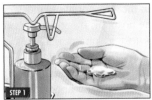

STEP 1
- Remove all rings, watches & jewellery.
- Wet hands with warm water.
- Apply recommended hand cleanser as per directions.

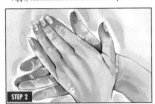

STEP 2
- Wash hands thoroughly beginning with palm to palm.

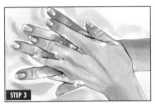

STEP 3
- Pay special attention to backs of hands and wrists...

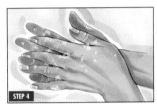

STEP 4
- ...Interdigital spaces...

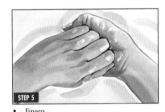

STEP 5
- ...Fingers...

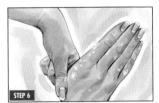

STEP 6
- ...and thumbs...

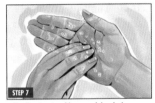

STEP 7
- Finally using tips of fingers and thumb cleanse palms using rotational motion.

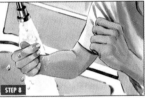

STEP 8
- Rinse hands thoroughly with warm water.
- Dry with a clean disposable towel.

Johnson & Johnson MEDICAL PTY. LTD.

*Trademark

Figure 13.7
Procedure for medical handwash

radius of the patient must be *sterile* (i.e. completely free of all microorganisms and their spores) – see Chapter 11.

Sterilisation and disinfection of equipment
The risk of transmission of infection on instruments or equipment is determined by the number of microorganisms present on the instrument, the area of the body where it is to be used and the procedure to be undertaken. Instruments used in areas of the body classified as critical must be sterile, those used in semi-critical areas must be sterile or subjected to high-level disinfection and those in non-critical areas must be clean. See Table 13.7.

Procedures for disinfection and sterilisation of instruments are described fully in Chapter 11.

Table 13.7
Spaulding classification system for possible contact sites of instruments

APPLICATION	CLASSIFICATION	DESCRIPTION	EXAMPLES
Entry or penetration into sterile tissue cavity or bloodstream	Critical	Sterile	Surgical procedure with entry into sterile tissue; intravascular cannulation
Contact with intact non-sterile mucosa (or non-intact skin)	Semi-critical	Sterile or high-level disinfection	Respiratory therapy; gastrointestinal endoscopy
Contact with intact skin	Non-critical	Clean	Non-invasive procedures (e.g. palpation, abdominal ultrasound)

Source: CDNA, *Infection Control Guidelines for the prevention of transmission of infectious diseases in the health care setting*, 2004, Table 4.2.

Isolation

Patients are placed in single rooms (isolation) to prevent the transmission of infectious agents either to or from the patient or health worker. Standard and Additional Precautions are used to prevent transmission from infectious patients to other patients or health-care personnel. Patients with an infection transmissible by the airborne route (e.g. TB) are ideally placed in a room with negative pressure ventilation.

Patients whose immune system is compromised, either from illness or treatment, pose a particular problem in the hospital setting. They are extremely susceptible to infection by the many microorganisms to which they may be exposed, including opportunistic pathogens (i.e. microorganisms that cause infections mainly in immunodeficient hosts). These patients should be accommodated in a room with positive pressure to prevent the entry of pathogens.

However, these patients may sometimes already have an infection (e.g. tuberculosis) that would be hazardous if transmitted to hospital personnel and/or other patients. Thus, measures must also be taken to prevent the spread of this infection by containing it within the patient's environment. The isolation procedures therefore must involve the prevention of the passage of microorganisms *in either direction* across a 'barrier'.

It should be noted that these procedures cannot protect patients from endogenous infections (i.e. microorganisms derived from their own body) nor from recurrence of a latent infection.

Personal protective equipment

Protective clothing is used in the hospital to:

- protect health-care workers from having their hands, eyes or clothing contaminated by microorganisms from an infected patient
- prevent microorganisms on health-care workers' hands, clothing or body (e.g in the respiratory tract) being transferred to a susceptible patient.

The selection of appropriate protection (disposable or reusable gowns, plastic aprons, gloves, masks, goggles or eye protection, face shields and overshoes) is determined by the *risk* of exposure and the *amount* of body fluids likely to be encountered.

Microorganisms are transported around the hospital on the clothing of the health-care worker. Clean, freshly laundered clothing carries very few microorganisms. However, current practice is for hospital staff to 'live out' and to wear their uniform outside the hospital environment – on public transport, for example. The responsibility therefore lies with health professionals for the cleanliness of their clothing and person.

Gowns can also be used to limit the transfer of organisms from an infectious patient to the clothing of the health worker, and their subsequent spread around the hospital. Plastic aprons or impermeable gowns should be used when there is a risk of splashes of blood or body substances. However, it is important that the gowns are used correctly,

that they are put on and removed so that other clothing is not contaminated. Also, if they have been used while caring for an infectious patient, they must be left in the infectious area or put in the appropriate laundry container and not worn around the hospital. If a gown becomes wet, the protective effect is lost as microorganisms can pass through wet material. Staff are responsible for the correct disposal of soiled or contaminated clothing.

There is considerable discussion about the usefulness of masks in the prevention of infection. Surgical masks are used routinely in surgery and for other procedures where there is thought to be a risk of microorganisms from the nose/throat of the health worker being transmitted to the patient. The use of masks can also guard against microorganisms in airborne droplets from an infectious patient entering the respiratory tract of the health worker. Many of the cases of SARS in health workers occurred before the cause of the disease was identified as an airborne virus and staff realised the importance of wearing masks. Special particulate filter masks should be worn to protect staff from exposure to cases of SARS or TB.

In practice, most paper masks have been shown to be somewhat ineffective as bacterial filters, especially when moist. The universal habit of continually adjusting masks may in fact transfer microorganisms to the hands of the health worker, where they are potentially more hazardous.

Protective eyewear and face shields should be worn when there is a risk of splashing, splattering or spraying of blood or body substances such as might occur during surgery, dental procedures or cleaning.

Gloves are used to prevent transmission of infection on the hands of health-care workers and to protect the health worker from infection. They are not an alternative to handwashing. Hands should be washed before and after using gloves. Gloves must be changed regularly otherwise they may become a source of infection. The correct gloves should be used, sterile gloves for sterile procedures and clean gloves for clean technique. Latex hypersensitivity and irritant contact dermatitis associated with powdered gloves are two problems that have emerged with the increasing use of gloves.

The use of protective clothing by staff is sometimes seen as creating a psychological problem for patients, who are already feeling isolated in a strange environment. For this reason, health workers should ensure they use only the appropriate clothing and explain its use to the patient.

Providing a safe environment

The prevention of transmission of infection and the protection of staff and patients are paramount in the design and implementation of a safe working environment in health-care facilities. The provision of a safe environment requires the development of policies and procedures and the cooperation of all staff to ensure that these policies are put in place.

INFECTION CONTROL TEAMS

In recent years there has been an increasing awareness of the importance of infection control in Australian hospitals. The first infection control nurse was appointed in 1965. Since then infection control programs have evolved to deal with the ongoing problem of health-care-associated infections. There is now a strong Infection Control Association throughout Australia (AICA) with a network of members in every State.

In most large city hospitals the policies and procedures for infection control are the responsibility of the Infection Control Committee. This committee usually comprises representatives of the Medical Board, Nursing Administration, Microbiology, Pharmacy, Theatre Staff, Clinical Nurse Consultants and other hospital departments. In practice, the responsibilities and composition of this body will vary considerably depending on the size of the hospital, the resources available and financial considerations. In large city hospitals an infection control team, consisting of one or two Clinical Nurse Consultants and the Microbiologist and Infectious Diseases specialist, is responsible for the daily implementation of infection control policies. In smaller country hospitals the responsibility may rest with one part-time Clinical Nurse Consultant.

Infection control personnel are usually responsible for the production of a hospital infection control manual containing details of procedures for infection control, including cleaning, disinfection and sterilisation, that should be followed by all medical and ancillary staff. Procedures should comply with Australian and New Zealand Standards. Increasingly, infection control programs are included in the quality assurance audits for accreditation of health-care facilities. An ongoing responsibility of the infection control team (usually the Clinical Nurse Consultant) is to conduct information sessions for all hospital staff, to make them aware of the importance of preventing transmission and of their own responsibility to observe correct practices. See Figures 13.8 and 13.9.

Infection control practitioners have a range of information services at their disposal. In Australia, the Communicable Diseases Network Australia (CDNA) published new guidelines for use by health facilities in 2004. These guidelines are interpreted and administered at a State or Territory level by the State health departments, who also issue guidelines for hospitals and health practitioners. Individual hospitals and health facilities use these guidelines to develop their own procedures and policies. Advisers within the health departments and hospitals provide advice to practitioners about dealing with particular disease problems.

The New South Wales *Nurses Act 1991 Regulation*, relating to infection control standards in New South Wales, was amended in 1995 to include penalties for improper practice. The Australian Government Department of Health and Ageing publishes the quarterly *Communicable Diseases Intelligence (CDI)* which reports on current outbreaks of infections <www.cda.gov.au/index.htm>.

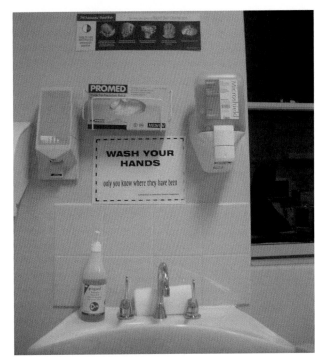

Figure 13.8

The importance of handwashing
Hand basins should be available close to all work areas. Posters are placed above the basins to remind staff of the importance of handwashing.

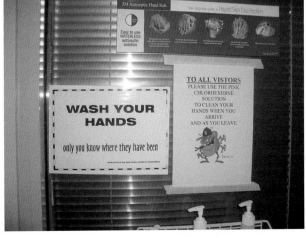

Figure 13.9

Notices such as this are often placed at the entrance to rooms containing seriously ill patients as a reminder to staff and visitors of the importance of handwashing

On a worldwide basis, the US Centers for Disease Control (CDC) in Atlanta, Georgia <www.cdc.gov> publishes the *Morbidity and Mortality Weekly Report (MMWR)*, which reports disease outbreaks and the results of surveillance studies, mainly in the United States. They also issue guidelines for infection control policies and warnings about the emergence and distribution of new strains of pathogenic microorganisms (e.g. multi-resistant *Mycobacterium tuberculosis*, which is now a major problem in the United States). *Eurosurveillance Weekly* <www.eurosurveillance.org> covers infection control issues in Great Britain and Europe. With the increase in worldwide travel, the sharing of this type of information is vitally important in containing the spread of disease.

Sometimes, the ideal infection control situation is not achievable because of space, staffing or financial constraints. Alternative procedures may need to be instituted by the infection control practitioner. Under these circumstances a sound understanding of microorganisms, disease transmission and methods of control can lead to a practical and successful solution. All these factors must be taken into account when developing policies and procedures to prevent cross-infection in a hospital. The purpose of infection control programs is to provide high-quality patient care and a safe working environment for staff and patients.

Surveillance

An important function of the infection control team is to monitor the incidence of infections within the hospital. Infection control staff are in a position to collect epidemiological data on the type of hospital infections and patterns of antibiotic resistance of isolated organisms. This constant surveillance helps to detect an increase in infection rates or an outbreak or cluster of similar infections in the hospital, so that measures can be taken to determine the source and means of transmission and prevent further cross-infection. Surveillance is essential for quality assurance and to monitor the effect of interventions designed to reduce infection.

Effective surveillance requires the collection of good quality-controlled data using accepted case definitions and calculations of infection rates. The Australia Infection Control Association (AICA) has developed standardised definitions for surgical-site infections (SSI) and bloodstream infections (BSI) <www.aica.org.au>. This type of data can be used as a measure of the quality of health-care outcomes in a particular facility. If data from different facilities are to be compared, they must be appropriately standardised and adjusted for risk factors. They can then be compared and used to provide information about the incidence of HCAIs, possible causal associations and various prevention strategies.

ACCOMMODATION

Health-care facilities, especially new buildings, need to be designed to comply with infection control requirements. These include the provision of single rooms, correct ventilation and access to handwashing facilities. The provision of safe, clean accommodation is an essential part of health care.

Ideally, it is preferable to care for a patient with an infectious disease in a single room. However, for a variety of reasons, this may not always be possible or desirable. With a thoughtful approach to infection control it is often possible to create an effective 'barrier' between the source of the infection and the environment. The implementation of the barrier will depend on the type of infection and the way it is transmitted as well as an analysis of perceived risk factors.

The current approach to infection control requires that the procedures to be implemented are assessed individually for each patient. The need to contain an infection means that patients may be cared for differently, depending on such factors as their dependence on staff, whether they are losing excessive blood or other fluids, their ability to comply with personal hygiene, whether they are mobile and other relevant factors. During a seasonal outbreak of an infection, it may be possible to nurse 'in cohort'; that is, patients with the same infection can be accommodated in the same room.

Patients with a highly communicable disease, such as SARS or active tuberculosis, should ideally be accommodated in a respiratory isolation room until they are deemed not to pose a significant risk to other patients or personnel. Patients with communicable diseases such as MRSA or GI infections should also be isolated – if possible in a single room with private toilet facilities. For identifiable bacterial diseases that can be treated with antibiotics, the patient is not considered infectious once therapy is established and symptoms are alleviated. For viral infections there is usually no effective therapy, so patients are considered to be infectious until asymptomatic. Patients who are carriers of the blood-borne viruses, HIV and hepatitis B and C, do not require special accommodation unless they have other infections. Obviously, a patient suffering from an unknown infection should be isolated until a diagnosis is made or symptoms disappear.

It should be remembered, however, that in some diseases (e.g. typhoid fever) carriage or shedding of the organisms can occur well after clinical recovery. In such cases, patients continue to be a source of infection even though they may be asymptomatic.

HOSPITAL CLEANING

Regular cleaning is essential for the establishment of a safe working environment. Procedures for routine hospital cleaning are established by the hospital infection control committee. Cleaning procedures should not disperse dust which may contain infectious particles. Most hospital cleaning is carried out using a neutral detergent and water and it is important to avoid the generation of aerosols. The use of disinfectants is usually only necessary when significant contamination (e.g. with blood or body substances) has occurred. Sodium hypochlorite (bleach) is recommended for this purpose. The chlorine in household bleach is effective against HIV, hepatitis B and other viruses. Areas contaminated with blood or body substances should first be washed with soap and water. If there is a possibility that the area could come in contact with bare skin, it should be treated with a suitable disinfectant (e.g. a fresh solution of 0.1% sodium hypochlorite). Household bleach contains 5% available chlorine; a 1:50 dilution gives a 0.1% solution. The use of Standard Precautions (gloves and protective clothing) is recommended for all cleaning procedures.

Hospital disinfection and sterilisation

The use of disinfectants, antiseptics and different methods of sterilisation are all important in maintaining good aseptic technique (see Chapter 11). Bacteria do not multiply on clean, dry surfaces. They need a warm, moist environment in which to reproduce. If surfaces and equipment are kept clean, dry and well ventilated, their contribution as a source of infection is greatly reduced. Many hospitals have a central sterilising department (CSD) where equipment and supplies are cleaned and sterilised. The effectiveness of this department is monitored regularly by the microbiology laboratory. Most hospitals now use disposable presterilised instruments, needles, syringes, dressing packs and other items.

Spills management

It is inevitable that spills of blood and other body substances will occur in any health facility. Standard Precautions should be used to contain and clean up the spill. The management of the spill will depend on the size, location and type of infectious material involved. In general, the spill should be cleaned up with paper towels and the area cleaned with neutral detergent and water (avoiding aerosols). The use of disinfectants is not usually necessary unless there is the possibility of the area coming into contact with bare skin. Protective clothing should be worn.

Waste management

Health facilities generate various categories of waste material which must be disposed of correctly in specially marked containers to avoid the spread of infection and reduce hazards for health personnel. The procedures are established by the infection control committee and should conform with Australian standards (AS/NZS 3816). Personnel should use protective clothing and observe Standard Precautions. See Figure 13.10. Sharps should be

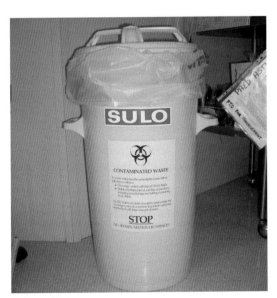

Figure 13.10

Waste management
Separate containers are used for different types of waste. This yellow bin is for contaminated waste, which has to be disposed of safely.

CASE HISTORY 13.1
Food poisoning due to *Clostridium perfringens*

An outbreak of gastroenteritis occurred at a Melbourne nursing home. One elderly woman died and 25 of the 80 residents became ill with stomach cramps, nausea and diarrhoea. The outbreak prompted investigations to determine the cause and source of the illness. Food and faecal samples were tested, environmental swabs taken and food-handling procedures were reviewed.

At the nursing home, the cause of the infection was shown to be *Clostridium perfringens* which had contaminated the pureed food prepared for the residents. The temperature of the cool-room at the nursing home was found to be 8–12°C, well above the maximum recommended temperature of 5°C. The prepared food was usually pureed and then kept warm until eaten. It was not reheated thoroughly before serving.

Comment
Clostridium perfringens is an endospore-forming Gram-positive bacterium which occurs widely in the environment. It is a common cause of gastroenteritis, especially in institutions or at large gatherings. Bacterial endospores survive the cooking process and germinate in warm food, multiplying rapidly at temperatures up to 45°C. Unless the food is reheated to over 70°C to kill the bacteria, after ingestion they continue to multiply in the intestine, producing enterotoxins which cause the typical disease symptoms. In this outbreak the prepared food was held for several hours at ambient temperatures, allowing the bacteria to multiply and cause illness when the food was eaten. Although the illness is usually of short duration, this case highlights the widespread occurrence of this organism and the risk to elderly or susceptible patients. In the investigation at the nursing home the contract caterer was held to have contributed to the death of the patient by failing to reheat the food properly. These outbreaks illustrate the importance of hygiene and correct temperature controls for the preparation of food.

Source: Aust NZ J Public Health 1999; 23(4): 421–423. Table 8.3.

---

placed in special containers and health workers should be particularly aware of the risk of infection from sharps injury.

FOOD STORAGE AND HANDLING

Gastrointestinal (GI) infections occur as a result of the ingestion of contaminated food or water. This can occur in health-care facilities as well as in the community and has the potential for a serious outcome.

Patients in health facilities are in close proximity to one another and have regular contact with staff. GI infections are transmitted by the faecal-oral route so strict hygiene is required to prevent transmission of an infection to other patients or health workers. The effect of a GI infection may be more serious in patients who are debilitated or frail, and the disease itself or the associated dehydration can result in serious morbidity or even death.

The main pathogens are *Clostridium perfringens* (which has heat-stable endospores), *Salmonella* and *Campylobacter*. *Bacillus cereus* and *Staphylococcus aureus* can produce heat-stable toxins in food left at room temperature for any length of time. Noroviruses (Norwalk-like viruses) can also cause infections.

Handling of food requires correct transport, storage and preparation. Many raw ingredients are contaminated with bacteria and it is essential that the food preparation process either removes or destroys these organisms. Microorganisms will multiply rapidly in food kept between 20°C and 40°C, so food should be chilled to below 5° or heated above 63°. It is important that kitchen hygiene is maintained and that food handlers are careful with their personal hygiene, especially handwashing.

All food preparation and hygiene should comply with Australian standards. The Hazard Analysis Critical Control Point (HACCP)-based food safety program identifies specific hazards and describes measures for their control. In many health facilities the food is precooked, then chilled and reheated. Health workers should follow the correct procedures for the storage and reheating of food delivered to their ward. Pureed food can be easily contaminated if cooked, pureed and served without thorough reheating. There should be policies for the correct use of microwave ovens and ice machines. Refrigerators should be inspected regularly to ensure they comply with standards for temperature control.

Enteral feeding presents a particular hazard as it is generally used for seriously ill patients who are unable to feed themselves. Most feeds are prepared commercially in sterile packs and must be administered using aseptic technique. Unused portions should be discarded.

ROLE OF THE MICROBIOLOGY LABORATORY

The hospital microbiology laboratory works closely with infectious disease physicians and the Clinical Nurse Consultant to monitor the occurrence of infections, particularly those caused by resistant hospital strains such as MRSA. Specimens from patients with a suspected infection are sent to the laboratory for analysis. Appropriate types of specimen and collection methods are described in Chapter 15. For correct identification and subsequent diagnosis it is important that specimens sent to the microbiology laboratory are collected properly, in an aseptic manner, labelled correctly and despatched to the laboratory as soon as possible.

The staff of the microbiology department are responsible for identifying the pathogen causing the infection and, if necessary, alerting the infection control team so that appropriate infection control measures can be taken. Often they are the first to recognise an outbreak of an infection when the number of isolates of a particular pathogen is higher than normal. See Figure 13.11.

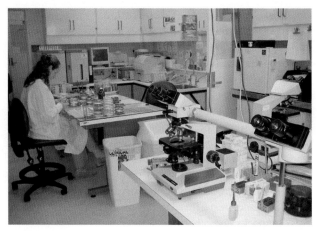

Figure 13.11

The microbiology laboratory
The identification of bacteria and viruses responsible for infections in the hospital is carried out by microbiologists in a laboratory such as this. A microbiologist is examining plates of bacterial cultures that have been grown overnight.

Microbiologists work closely with infectious diseases physicians, advising on treatment for infections caused by antibiotic-resistant organisms and carrying out molecular typing for epidemiological investigations.

DEALING WITH AN OUTBREAK

Often, an outbreak is detected first by the microbiologists, who alert infection control staff. It may be confined to one ward or spread throughout the hospital. To contain the outbreak, it is necessary to analyse the situation and implement measures to limit the spread of the infection. These measures may involve:

- examination of all work practices
- a focus on staff handwashing
- identification of shared equipment and disinfection of contaminated equipment
- monitoring of patient movements
- identification of a procedure that may have created a risk
- identification of staff or patients who are shedding the pathogens
- appropriate isolation measures.

The infection control team is responsible for devising, implementing, and monitoring the outcome of an outbreak management plan.

Specific problems in infection control

Although the general principles of transmission and cross-infection (described above) apply to all areas of the hospital, there are various situations where the risk of infection is very high and Additional Precautions need to be taken. In these situations, patients and staff are more susceptible to infections because of the nature of the treatment, the state of their immune system or the type of microorganisms to which they are exposed. Some units of the hospital are more likely than others to harbour a population of resistant organisms. These tend to be units where there are seriously ill or compromised patients and thus an associated high level of antibiotic usage. Staff working in these units are much more likely to be nasal carriers of resistant organisms and have the potential to spread them around the hospital. Continual surveillance of hospital staff would help to prevent this kind of cross-infection, but is not always cost-effective.

Some specific examples are described below.

DEALING WITH THE UNKNOWN: ACCIDENT AND EMERGENCY

Health-care workers have no way of knowing the infective status of patients who present to the accident and emergency department of a hospital so it is important that appropriate infection control precautions are in place. Standard Precautions should always be used and Additional Precautions when necessary. For example, the outbreak of severe acute respiratory syndrome (SARS), a new disease that originated in China in November 2002 and spread rapidly via Hong Kong in March 2003 to about 30 other countries, resulted in more than 8000 cases of atypical pneumonia and 774 deaths worldwide. Approximately twenty-one per cent of the cases occurred in health-care workers.

This event highlighted the need for health-care workers to be continually aware of the possibility of the emergence of new diseases and the need to protect themselves as well as patients. SARS is caused by a previously unknown corona virus, now called SARS-CoV. It is highly infectious to close contacts, especially the health workers providing clinical care and support. Because the patients presented with ordinary respiratory symptoms, many of the health workers were infected before a diagnosis was made. This might have been avoided if additional respiratory precautions to prevent contact and droplet transmission had been used. The use of ventilation equipment, suctioning devices, endotracheal intubation and medicinal sprays created aerosols that contributed to the ease of transmission of viral particles.

Handwashing, protective clothing and particulate filter masks are necessary to prevent transmission of SARS by contact or aerosol droplets.

It is important to take a complete patient history, including details of overseas travel, from anyone presenting with unusual symptoms (see also SARS Spotlight box, page 162).

The emergence of avian influenza H5N1 as well as SARS has prompted CDNA to release a set of guidelines to help health practitioners assess patients who present with fever and respiratory symptoms. They are available on the website: <http://www.health.gov.au/avian_influenza/>

OPERATING THEATRES AND SURGICAL PATIENTS

Surgical procedures carry a high risk of infection because the patient's external defences are breached during

---

SPOTLIGHT ON
Accident and Emergency

Scenario 1 A patient comes to the emergency department complaining of headache, high temperature for the last two days, some congestion and difficulty in breathing and generally feeling unwell.

Scenario 2 Trauma patients from a road accident are brought by ambulance to A&E. One has head injuries, one has a compound fracture of the leg. Both are losing a lot of blood.

Scenario 3 A 68-year-old man is admitted having suffered a heart attack at home but was resuscitated by ambulance officers.

Scenario 4 A 21-year-old man is brought in with a suspected drug overdose.

Comment

Any of these scenarios could occur in the A&E department of a hospital. The staff and any other people in the waiting room are at risk from any infections carried by these patients. The infection risks are immediate – before any laboratory diagnoses can be made.

What if . . .?

Scenario 1	The patient has SARS
Scenario 2	One patient is a hepatitis B carrier
Scenario 3	The man has (reactivated) TB
Scenario 4	The man is hepatitis C positive

How should Standard and Additional Precautions be implemented in these scenarios? Would they prevent transmission of infection?

---

surgery. Patients may develop postsurgical infections at the site of the wound or in the organs or spaces accessed during the operation. In many cases the source of these infections is the patient's own normal flora (endogenous infections). These may be skin flora such as aerobic Gram-positive cocci or enteric organisms such as *E. coli* when the incision is near the perineum or groin. Seeding of the operative site from a distant focus of infection can occur, particularly in patients having a prosthesis implanted.

Exogenous infections are caused by bacteria from the environment, from the air or from personnel in the operating theatre and are mainly skin flora such as staphylococci and streptococci. As many as 50% of hospital personnel carry *Staphylococcus aureus* in the nose or on broken skin. Group A streptococcal infections have been traced to colonised operating room personnel and *Clostridium perfringens* (the most important cause of gas gangrene) is commonly carried in the human intestine.

Occasionally, wounds can become contaminated by exposure to non-sterile surfaces or equipment.

In general, there are different levels of risk associated with different types of surgery. Reliable predictors of the risk of infection include:

- pre-existing microbial contamination at the surgical site
- the duration of the operation – the length of time that tissues are exposed to the air in the operating theatre
- host susceptibility, including infections at other body sites and underlying health factors.

The level of microbial contamination at the surgical site can be placed in one of four categories and is used to predict the likelihood of the occurrence of a surgical-site infection (SSI).

1. *Clean/clean*: an uninfected wound in which no inflammation is encountered and no body organs are entered. The wound is closed or closed drainage is used.
2. *Clean/contaminated*: a wound in which the alimentary, respiratory, urinary or genital tract is entered under controlled conditions and no evidence of infection is encountered.
3. *Contaminated/open*: fresh accidental wounds, or operations where a break in surgical technique occurs or inflammation is encountered.
4. *Dirty/infected*: traumatic wounds with retained or devitalised tissue and those involving pre-existing infection or perforated viscera. The organisms causing the infection were present in the operating field before surgery.

STRATEGIES TO REDUCE WOUND INFECTION RATES

The risk of surgically acquired infections can be reduced by various methods, including operating room procedures, reduced hospital stays and prophylactic antibiotics.

Operating rooms

These are cleaned after each operation or as indicated by the nature of the medical risk involved. Most hospitals use a filtered air-flow system into the operating suites, and overnight disinfection with UV light to minimise the number of microorganisms in the air space. Air contains dust particles and bacteria, so traffic is limited to prevent the spread of microorganisms.

All personnel wear sterile gowns, masks and gloves. See Figure 13.12. Medical and nursing staff scrub hands and arms with antiseptic wash before gloving. All equipment, drapes, sutures and dressings that come into contact with the patient are sterilised. Patients are no longer shaved preoperatively as this has been shown to cause irritation to the skin and allow microorganisms to enter. The surgical site is disinfected (usually with povidone-iodine or chlorhexidine) before the incision is made.

Additional Precautions such as single-use equipment are taken when the patient is harbouring an infection such as MRSA or TB, and the order of surgical cases (or 'list') is arranged to minimise the risk of transmission. Special Precautions have been introduced to prevent transmission of the infective agent responsible for Creutzfeldt-Jakob disease (CJD) (see Spotlight box, page 240).

Patients should be carefully monitored after surgery for any sign of wound infection. Inflammation, drainage from the suture line, purulent discharge and fever are all indicators of infection. If the wound is infected, a swab is taken and sent to the microbiology laboratory for identification of the causative organism and determination of antibiotic sensitivities.

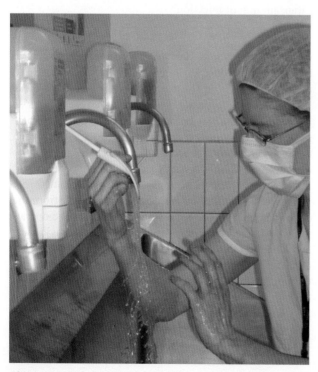
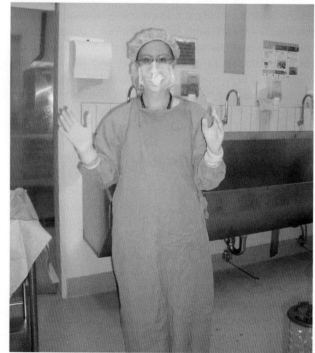

Figure 13.12

Staff working in operating theatres 'scrub' and put on special protective clothing in order to minimise the risk of transmission of infection.

Reduced hospital stays

Wound infections are potentially more serious, even life-threatening, when the infection is due to a resistant hospital organism. One way in which this problem has been addressed is by minimising the patient's stay in hospital, especially preoperatively. Patients undergoing major operations (e.g. open heart surgery) used to be admitted two to three days before the operation in order to carry out tests and stabilise the patient. However, it was found that this allowed time for patients to become colonised with resistant hospital organisms, replacing their own normal flora. If wound contamination occurred, the outcome was often quite serious. Patients for major surgery are now admitted as close as possible to the time of surgery, to minimise exposure to hospital strains. Many operations are now done in day-surgery facilities which not only reduces costs but also the risk of infection.

Although these measures may lead to an apparent reduction in infection rates, it is difficult to obtain accurate data on the incidence of SSIs which may not present until after the patient has left the health facility.

Prophylactic antibiotics

The use of prophylactic antibiotics in all surgical cases has been widely discussed. Their use for surgery of previously contaminated sites is obviously indicated. They are also useful for surgery on the bowel or genital tract where there is already a large population of resident normal flora that may be released into the body cavity. However, widespread use of antibiotics for all types of surgery creates a dilemma as it has the potential to lead to an increase in resistant bacterial strains that pose a threat, not only to the individual patient, but also to the hospital environment. On the other hand, the medical profession is increasingly aware of the risks of litigation if preventive treatment is not given (see Chapter 12).

THE BURNS UNIT

The survival rate of patients with extensive burns has improved in recent years, partly because of improved infection control practices, as well as new treatments. Burns vary in their degree of severity, depending on the cause of the burn and the area of the body affected. A large percentage of children admitted to Accident and Emergency are suffering from burns caused by boiling water, which can cause extensive damage to children's delicate skin. Inhalation burns from smoke or fire damage the epithelial lining of the lungs and may predispose to pneumonia.

Patients suffering from burns to a large part of their body are at increased risk of infection since one of the primary body defences (an intact skin) has been destroyed (see Chapter 9). Shock and fluid loss mean that the patient may also be receiving IV fluids, which creates another possible point of entry for microorganisms. The burn site itself provides a moist area, full of nutrients, ideal for the growth of organisms. In addition, the nature of the tissue damage means that phagocytic cells and antibodies are unable to reach the damaged area and prevent bacterial multiplication from taking place.

When burns become infected, it is difficult to treat them with systemic antibiotics because damage to the vascular tissue around the burn site prevents the antibiotics from reaching the infection. Similarly, topical application of antibiotics is not always successful because of large quantities of dead tissue. The two most common organisms found in infected burns are *Pseudomonas aeruginosa* and *Staphylococcus aureus*. Both pathogens have strains that are resistant to many antibiotics and some disinfectants. It is therefore very important to maintain asepsis in a burns unit.

As the burns unit can be such a significant source of antibiotic-resistant microorganisms, staff should exercise appropriate infection control precautions when moving from burns units to areas of the hospital that have particularly susceptible patients (e.g. transplant units, oncology and HDUs).

HIGH-DEPENDENCY (INTENSIVE CARE) UNITS

Patients in high-dependency units (HDUs) are usually seriously ill and so their body defences are highly compromised. The invasive nature of their treatment, which may involve procedures such as intubation and the use of ventilators and monitoring equipment, renders patients in HDUs very susceptible to hospital-acquired infections.

Usually, patients in HDUs are receiving a number of different medications, administered for convenience via a central line. Studies have shown that these lines are associated with a high level of sepsis, which has been correlated with high rates of morbidity and mortality. Central vein lines carry a much higher risk of causing infection than peripheral vein cannulae.

Sepsis associated with peripheral vein cannulae can be reduced by adhering to strict infection control protocols. Control of sepsis in central lines is more difficult because the patient is usually seriously ill and the cannula may need to be in place for a longer period. The length of time the cannula is in place affects the likelihood of infection and opinions vary about the optimum time for replacement of cannulae.

The most common organisms associated with infections are *Staphylococcus aureus* and coagulase negative staphylococci. Sepsis due to *Candida albicans* is found with central lines, especially when used for total parenteral nutrition (TPN), but is not common with peripheral vein cannulae. Unfortunately, due to the high antibiotic usage in HDUs, many of the infections acquired there are caused by resistant organisms. Staff who work in these units are also often colonised by antibiotic-resistant pathogens. Handwashing, the maintenance of strict aseptic technique and the use of protective clothing (gowns) are essential to minimise the risk of infection. Special care should be taken when handling intravenous cannulas.

TRANSPLANT AND ONCOLOGY WARDS

Patients in transplant and oncology wards, in addition to being critically ill, are usually being treated with immuno-suppressive drugs. These wards are thus important areas of the hospital where opportunistic infections and resistant organisms can flourish, and patients require special care to prevent cross-infection.

MATERNITY WARDS

Patients in a maternity ward are often thought of as 'well' because their hospitalisation is not due to illness. However, there are significant infection risks associated with child-birth. These include infections that may occur at the site of a caesarean section, or in the perineal area where tearing or tissue damage may occur. A significant number of women carry potentially pathogenic microorganisms (e.g. *Streptococci* spp.) in the normal flora of the vagina and these can readily invade damaged tissue. Faecal bacteria can also contaminate the wound. Group B streptococci (GBS) are usually responsible for puerpural, or childbed, fever which, until the 1930s, carried a 10% mortality rate. At risk patients can be screened for GBS during pregnancy and administered antibiotics intra-partem.

Care of the patient involves education about personal hygiene and careful monitoring for any signs of infec-tion (e.g. fever, inflammation, pus). Patients should also be instructed about breast care, as cracked nipples can lead to mastitis (infection of the milk glands). Although these infections are often caused by normal flora there is a real risk that hospital strains can be transported to the mother, either on the nurse's hands or on the baby after being handled in a communal nursery. Standard Precautions should be observed for all blood and body substances.

Neonatal infections

All women carry a population of normal flora in the vagina. Most of these organisms pose no infection risk to either mother or baby. However, sometimes, the mother is carrying opportunistic pathogens in the vagina or has acquired a sexually transmitted disease. Babies born to infected mothers are at risk of being infected either transplacentally or during passage through the birth canal. These infections include organisms such as *Candida albicans* (thrush), herpes simplex virus, Group B strepto-cocci, *Chlamydia*, *Mycoplasma*, *Neisseria gonorrhoeae*, *Treponema pallidum* (syphilis), hepatitis B, hepatitis C and HIV/AIDS.

All these infections are very serious for the neonate whose immune system is immature and who may not have maternal antibodies for protection. Some of these infec-tions are highly contagious and can be transmitted to other babies in the nursery, usually on the hands of hospital staff. Organisms can enter through the eyes, umbilicus or any breaks in the skin. Infections such as herpes are easily transmitted; babies must be isolated if possible and the mothers instructed about the disease and ways to prevent transmission.

Neonates are also at risk of acquiring hospital infec-tions caused by *E. coli*, *Staphylococcus aureus* and many other pathogens. Neonates should be regarded as parti-cularly susceptible because of their immature immune system and the constant handling they receive. Isolation, handwashing and careful hygiene procedures when handling nappies are essential to prevent the spread of infection.

A SPECIAL PROBLEM WITH CHILDREN

Everything that has been said about the prevention of cross-infection applies to paediatric wards, but there are some additional factors to be considered. Children are highly mobile. Adults can usually be expected to stay in one place but children are very active and are therefore more likely to spread an infection around a ward. Spills and injuries often occur when staff have to control strug-gling, frightened children. In particular, needlestick (sharps) injuries and body fluids and substance exposures are likely to be more common, and staff must be encour-aged to report all incidents. It is often more difficult with children to contain faeces, vomitus and other excreta.

Small children tend to put articles such as toys in their mouths and this facilitates the spread of organisms that may be present in the saliva or respiratory secretions. Unless careful infection control procedures are followed, respiratory infections and gastrointestinal infections, such as rotavirus, can easily spread.

During epidemic outbreaks of diseases such as RSV (respiratory syncytial virus) in the winter months, hospi-tals may be besieged with cases. Isolation may not be possible and it may be necessary to nurse 'in cohort' (i.e. place patients with the same infection in the same ward) or with other patients who are immune.

Occasionally, children may develop an infectious disease such as chickenpox after admission for some other procedure. It is then necessary to identify all susceptible patients and staff and take steps to protect them from this highly contagious disease. A vaccine for chickenpox is now available in Australia and is advisable for non-immune staff. Leukaemia patients are particularly suscept-ible to infection and need to be protected from contact with people who may be infectious. Each situation needs to be assessed carefully by the infection control team.

Occupational exposure for hospital staff

The hospital environment can be hazardous, for patients and staff, so all health workers need to understand the potential risks involved in their work. These will vary depending on the type of health facility. The CDC has issued comprehensive guidelines on infection control for health personnel. In general, hospital staff are healthy and thus have very low susceptibility to the many pathogens found in hospital, unless they have underlying risk factors such as depression of the immune system, a broken or weeping skin condition, or pregnancy. However, staff are

A registered nurse working in an HDU notified the Infection Control Nurse that her daughter had chicken-pox. The daughter's skin lesions had appeared five days prior to the notification. The staff member did not have a history of having had the disease and was in the first trimester of her second pregnancy. Blood tests on the RN for antibody to varicella zoster virus (VZV) were negative. She was rostered off work and given varicella zoster specific immunoglobulin by her obstetrician, although it is only considered effective if given within 96 hours of exposure. She subsequently developed chickenpox.

Comment

This case illustrates a number of infection control issues. Chickenpox is a highly contagious disease which is more serious in adults. The virus also causes shingles. There is a small (1–2%) but significant risk of congenital abnormalities if the disease is contracted during pregnancy. In this case the nurse contracted the disease from her own daughter, but non-immune health workers are always at risk, especially if working in paediatric wards.

The other major risk is to patients and staff the nurse comes into contact with. As with many infectious diseases, the patient is infectious before symptoms appear, so the disease can be passed on during the incubation period. A vaccine is now available and is recommended for non-immune health workers, especially those working in HDUs or in contact with immunosuppressed patients.

The RN delivered a normal baby and, because of the thorough action by the Infection Control Nurse, there were no other cases.

Source: K Doolan, personal communication.

susceptible to many infections that a patient may have – especially respiratory diseases such as TB or SARS.

It is important that all health workers are up to date with the immunisation schedule recommended by the Department of Health for hepatitis B, as well as for the usual childhood diseases (especially for HCWs working with neonates or children). Staff working in institutions, mental health facilities and day-care centres should also be immunised against hepatitis A. Immunisation of staff against influenza also protects elderly and immunosuppressed patients.

Exposure to blood-borne pathogens such as hepatitis B and C and HIV poses a significant risk and all staff should be educated about observing Standard Precautions. This is particularly important for staff responsible for the disposal of contaminated waste.

NEEDLESTICK (SHARPS) INJURIES

A major risk factor is needlestick injuries – that is, when a health worker is accidentally cut or pricked by a sharp object, usually a needle, that has been contaminated by blood or body substance. Hospital guidelines require that needles should *not* be resheathed and that all sharps should be disposed of in a sharps container. Recappable needles have largely been replaced by single-use safety devices in most hospitals.

Nevertheless, many health workers still receive needle-stick injuries and they should always be reported. Each hospital has its own procedures for assessing the situation, and the worker may be offered prophylactic treatment if the injury is known to have been caused by a sharp from a patient with hepatitis B or HIV. It should be noted here that health workers should be immunised against hepatitis B. If injury does occur and the staff member is not immunised, hyperimmune anti-hepatitis B globulin can be administered.

In the case of HIV, antiretroviral therapy is available but to be effective should be initiated within a couple of hours of injury. Data on the protective efficacy of these drugs are still limited, and staff are usually counselled at the time of injury before deciding to undertake the therapy, which has some side effects. At present, there is no treatment for hepatitis C exposure.

TUBERCULOSIS

Another major risk to health workers is exposure to tuberculosis (TB) (see page 408). After its virtual eradication in Australia in the 1950s by a mass X-ray screening and immunisation campaign, there has been a resurgence of the disease. The highest number of cases occurs in indigenous Australians and in immigrants from Asian countries, where it is endemic. Patients who are immunodeficient are particularly susceptible to infection or reactivation of latent TB and thus can act as a significant reservoir of the organism in the hospital environment.

TB is transmitted in aerosol droplets from respiratory secretions of patients with pulmonary disease. Health-care workers can be exposed during procedures such as sputum (cough) induction, bronchoscopy, intubation and autopsy. Undiagnosed TB presents the greatest risk to health personnel so suspected patients should be diagnosed as soon as possible. Additional airborne precautions should be used and particulate filter masks worn.

Staff should be tested for previous exposure to TB and the effect of exposure to TB can be monitored using the Mantoux test. There is some difference of opinion regarding the value of the BCG vaccination for health workers and recommendations vary in different States (see Chapter 14). At present, the multi-resistant strains that are common in the United States have not reached Australia. Only about 2% of notified cases are resistant to more than two drugs.

RISKS ASSOCIATED WITH PREGNANCY

Health-care workers who are pregnant should be aware of the possible congenital effects of some infections. Rubella can cause serious birth defects if contracted in the first trimester. Although a vaccine has been available for many years, there are groups within the community (e.g. some males and immigrants) who may not be immune. They can be a risk to a pregnant health worker, so all health workers (male and female) are advised to be immunised.

Cytomegalovirus (CMV) is a mild infection in children and adults but can cause severe infections in immuno-compromised patients. Women contracting CMV during pregnancy risk serious damage to the foetus (see Chapter 19). CMV infection, which is often asymptomatic, is transmitted in body fluids so staff can minimise risks by following Standard Precautions, especially for urine and saliva.

Chickenpox can be a serious illness in pregnancy and workers who are not immune should avoid contact with children. Staff can discuss the occupational exposure risks associated with pregnancy with the infection control team (see Case History 13.2 on page 303).

Conclusion

The control of infection in health-care facilities is the responsibility of all health workers. Each situation is unique – with different patients, procedures, risks and pathogens.

Health professionals must have a good understanding of the different types of pathogens – their habitat and properties and the way they are transmitted. It is important to be able to assess the risk to individual patients, to identify reservoirs and sources of infection. In this way it is possible to implement the appropriate infection control procedures for each situation.

SUMMARY

- Health-care-associated infections (HCAIs) are infections acquired by patients in a hospital or other health facility.
- Infections that are acquired in non-hospitalised people are called community-acquired infections.

THE IMPORTANCE OF HCAIs

- The prevalence of hospital-acquired infection in Australia ranges from 6.3 to 8.6%.
- Hospital-acquired infections increase patient suffering, prolong the length of hospital stay and increase the cost of medical care.

ORGANISMS THAT CAUSE HEALTH-CARE-ASSOCIATED INFECTIONS

- The most common sites of nosocomial infections are the urinary tract, surgical wounds, lower respiratory tract, skin and blood.
- Bacteria are the most common cause of HCAIs, followed by fungi and viruses.
- Methicillin-resistant *Staphylococcus aureus* (MRSA) emerged in the mid-1970s in Australia and is still a major concern in hospital infection control.
- Antibiotic-resistant Gram-negative organisms cause serious infections in very ill patients.
- In immunocompromised patients, organisms such as enterococci, mycobacteria, fungi and certain viruses frequently cause infections.

SOURCES OF HOSPITAL INFECTIONS

- Community strains are organisms that originate from outside the hospital and are generally sensitive to most antimicrobial drugs.
- Hospital strains originate from within the hospital and can be difficult to treat because they are frequently resistant to antimicrobial drugs and disinfectants.
- Colonisation is the presence and growth of a microorganism on the skin or mucous membrane without infection. Major sites are the nose, skin, oropharynx, lower intestine and urinary tract.

- Colonisation with hospital strains can occur after admission and becomes more likely the longer the stay in hospital. Exposure to antimicrobial drugs also favours colonisation.
- Hospital staff are frequently colonised by hospital organisms and are thus carriers of these potential pathogens.
- Patients with lowered resistance (e.g. surgical or burns patients) may be infected by a multi-resistant hospital strain, and then become important reservoirs of these organisms.
- Hospital infections may be exogenous (derived from outside the patient's body, e.g. from other patients or staff or the hospital environment) or endogenous (derived from the patient's own body).
- Clean, dry surfaces are not a significant source of microorganisms unless freshly contaminated, but the numbers of microorganisms contaminating moist areas or objects may be very high.

FACTORS CONTRIBUTING TO THE INCIDENCE OF HOSPITAL-ACQUIRED INFECTIONS

- Infections acquired in hospital are more serious and difficult to treat because they are frequently caused by drug-resistant strains of microorganisms.
- Many hospital patients have lowered resistance to infection due to age (young or old), immobility, underlying disease or infection, or surgical or traumatic wounds.
- Medical treatments can lower a patient's resistance to infection: these include cancer therapy, immunosuppressive drugs, anti-inflammatory drugs and some antimicrobial drugs.
- Diagnostic and therapeutic procedures (e.g. injections, the use of intravascular and urinary catheters, endotracheal tubes and drainages, and endoscopes) involve the penetration of the protective skin and mucous membrane barriers.
- Infections that are brought about by some medical procedure or treatment are called iatrogenic infections.
- Implanted prostheses are favoured sites of colonisation by microorganisms.

- Transfer of patients from one ward to another can spread infection.

SPREAD OF INFECTION IN HEALTH-CARE FACILITIES

- HCA transmission involves the infection of a susceptible patient by the transfer of organisms from another patient. The risk of transmission varies among hospital facilities.
- Microorganisms can be spread on hands, clothing, equipment and utensils, air currents and contaminated material.
- Standard Precautions are a set of procedures to be followed to prevent patient-to-staff, staff-to-patient and patient-to-patient transmission of pathogens present in blood or any body substances, especially HIV, HBV, HCV and CMV.
- Health workers who are infected with a blood-borne virus should not carry out exposure-prone procedures.
- Additional Precautions may be required for a patient with an infection carried by the contact or airborne route, such as SARS or pulmonary tuberculosis.
- Infection control procedures should be used for all patients until they are deemed to be no longer infectious.

PREVENTION OF TRANSMISSION

- The health worker needs to evaluate the risks of transmission for each patient.
- An understanding of the nature of the infection is essential to 'break the chain of transmission'.
- Handwashing is the most effective method of preventing cross-infection.
- Asepsis refers to the absence of all disease-producing organisms.
- Aseptic technique comprises practices and procedures designed to limit the spread of infections.
- Sterile technique is intended to render and maintain objects and areas free from all microorganisms.
- Equipment should be disinfected or sterilised according to the risk involved for its use.
- Isolation of patients in a single room with correct ventilation is used to prevent transmission.
- Patients whose immune system is compromised need to be protected from infection.
- Various kinds of protective clothing are worn to prevent the spread of microorganisms.
- Gloves are an important means of reducing cross-infection but their use does not remove the need for handwashing.

PROVIDING A SAFE ENVIRONMENT

- In large city hospitals the policies and procedures for infection control are the responsibility of the Infection Control Committee.
- The infection control team monitors the incidence of infections within the hospital and conducts information sessions for hospital staff.
- Methods for cleaning, disinfection and sterilisation are contained in each hospital's infection control manual.
- Strict protocols for hygiene and correct handling and storage of food should be followed to avoid gastrointestinal infections.
- The microbiology department is responsible for identifying the pathogen causing the infection and informing the infection control team, so that appropriate infection control measures can be taken.

SPECIFIC PROBLEMS IN INFECTION CONTROL

- Patients in some units of the hospital are more susceptible to infection than others (e.g. surgical patients, because their defences have been breached).
- Health-care workers in Accident and Emergency are at risk from patients with undiagnosed illnesses.
- Various methods have been introduced to reduce the incidence of postoperative wound infections, such as attention to sterilisation and disinfection, reduced hospital stays and the use of prophylactic antimicrobial drugs.
- Other patients who are particularly susceptible to infection are those with burns, those in high-dependency units, the immunocompromised, and those who are susceptible because of the nature of the treatment they require.
- Infection risks in maternity and neonatal wards include postpartum infections of the mother as well as the baby.
- There are special risk factors associated with paediatric wards, because of the nature of children.

OCCUPATIONAL EXPOSURE FOR HOSPITAL STAFF

- Hospital staff are at risk of becoming infected via needlestick injuries and exposure to respiratory diseases such as TB.
- Staff should be fully immunised.
- Pregnant staff should be aware of the infection risks associated with pregnancy.

STUDY QUESTIONS

1. Differentiate between hospital-acquired infections and community-acquired infections.
2. What was the major contribution of Ignaz Semmelweis to hospital infection control?
3. List the most common sites of hospital-acquired infections.
4. What is MRSA?
5. What is an important difference between hospital strains of bacteria and community strains?
6. What is meant by 'colonisation' in relation to microorganisms and the human body?
7. List the factors that can make a patient immunocompromised.
8. What is a iatrogenic infection? Give three examples.
9. Define the terms 'exogenous infection' and 'endogenous infection'.
10. What are the important sources of organisms that cause exogenous infections in hospitalised people?
11. Dry objects and surfaces do not generally support the growth of microorganisms, but can still act as a source of infection. Explain.

12. List the common ways that microorganisms can be spread in the hospital.
13. What are the major responsibilities of a hospital's infection control committee?
14. Define the terms 'asepsis' and 'aseptic technique'.
15. Handwashing at the appropriate times is an extremely important means of reducing cross-infection in hospitals. When are the appropriate times? Explain your answer.
16. Describe the basic principles of Standard and Additional Precautions, and explain why they are necessary.
17. What procedures are followed in Standard Precautions?
18. Describe the major ways in which the incidence of surgical wound infections can be reduced.
19. List the types of patients that are particularly susceptible to hospital-acquired infections.
20. What procedures are used to reduce the incidence of needle-stick injuries?
21. Which infections are particularly serious if contracted while pregnant?

TEST YOUR UNDERSTANDING

1. Why are hospital-acquired infections often more serious than those acquired in the community?
2. Explain why patients in the burns unit are particularly susceptible to infection.
3. Discuss how the use of Standard and Additional Precautions is important to protect health-care workers.
4. What special precautions should be used when caring for a patient who is immunocompromised?
5. Discuss the merits of the various types of protective clothing that can be worn by health workers.

RESOURCES

Standards and Guidelines

AS/NZS 3816 (1998) *Management of clinical and related wastes.* Standards Australia.

Bolyard EA, Tablan O, Williams W, Pearson M, Shapiro C, Deitchman MD & the Hospital Infection Control Practices Advisory Committee, 1998, 'Guideline for infection control in health care personnel', *American Journal of Infection Control*, 26, pp. 289–354.

CDC 1987, 'Recommendations for the prevention of transmission of HIV in health care settings', *Morbidity and Mortality Weekly Report* 6: Suppl. 25, pp. 1S–18S.

CDC Update 1988, 'Universal precautions for prevention of transmission of human immunodeficiency virus, hepatitis B virus and other blood-borne pathogens in health care settings', *Morbidity and Mortality Weekly Report* 37, pp. 377–88.

Communicable Diseases Network Australia (CDNA) 2004, *Infection Control Guidelines for the prevention of transmission of infectious diseases in the health care setting.* Canberra, Australian Government Publishing Service. This comprehensive document replaces the guidelines from 1996 and introduces new terminology for methods of infection control. It details the types of infections that can be transmitted in health-care establishments, the modes of transmission of infectious diseases, risk assessment and methods for prevention of cross-infection.

Mangram AJ, Horan TC, Pearson M, Silver L & Jarvis WR, 1999, 'Guideline for prevention of surgical site infection', *American Journal of Infection Control*, 27(2), pp. 97–134.

National Health & Medical Research Council/Australian National Council on AIDS, 1993, *Management Guidelines for the Control of Infectious Disease Hazards in Health Care Establishments,* Canberra: Australian Government Publishing Service.

National Health & Medical Research Organisation and Australian National Council on AIDS, 1996. *Infection Control in the Health Care Setting: Guidelines for the Prevention of Transmission of Infectious Diseases*, Canberra: Australian Government Publishing Service.

Further reading

Mallon DFJ, W Shearwood, SA Mallal, MAH French & RL Dawkins 1992, 'Exposure to blood-borne infections in health-care workers', *Medical Journal of Australia* 157, pp. 592–95. (This article reports on the incidence and nature of occupational exposures to blood and body fluids in health-care workers in a large Australian hospital.)

Selwyn S 1991, 'Hospital infection: the first 2500 years', *Journal of Hospital Infection* 18 (suppl. A), pp. 5–64. (This review article examines the history of hospital infection and the development of infection control procedures over time.)

References

1. McLaws M, J Gold, K King, LM Irwig & G Berry, 1988, 'The prevalence of nosocomial and community-acquired infections in Australian hospitals', *Medical Journal of Australia*, 149, pp. 582–90.
2. Mayon-White RT, G Ducel, T Kereselidze & E Tikomirov, 1988, 'An international survey of the prevalence of hospital-acquired infection', *Journal of Hospital Infection*, 11 (suppl. A), pp. 43–48.
3. DoH/PHLS, 1999, *Socio-economic Burden of Hospital Acquired Infection*, Public Health Laboratory Service, London.
4. Wenzel RP (ed.), 1987, *Prevention and Control of Nosocomial Infections*, Baltimore: Williams & Wilkins.
5. Australian Council for Safety and Quality in Health Care. *National Strategy to Address Health Care Associated Infections.* July 2003.
6. Haley RW, DR Schaberg & KB Crossley, 1981, 'Extra charges and prolongation of stay attributable to nosocomial infections: A prospective interhospital comparison, *American Journal of Medicine*, 70, pp. 51–58.
7. Haley RW & RH Schachtman, 1980, 'The SCENIC Project', *Journal of Epidemiology* 111(5), pp. 574–91.
8. McAlister T, George N, Foaogali J & Bell J, 1999, 'Isolation of beta-lactamase positive vancomycin-resistant *Enterococcus faecalis*: First case in Australia', *Communicable Diseases Intelligence*, 23(9), pp. 327–39.

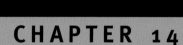

CHAPTER 14

Issues in
Public Health

[CHAPTER FOCUS]

■　*Which infectious diseases are the most important in Australia?*

■　*How is information about the incidence and prevalence of infectious diseases in Australia collected and distributed?*

■　*Which aspects of primary health care are concerned with the prevention of infectious diseases?*

■　*What are the special infection control problems in child-care centres?*

■　*What are the particular challenges facing the provision of health care in rural and remote areas of Australia?*

■　*How do public health issues in New Zealand differ from those in Australia?*

The Australian health scene

The 20th century saw remarkable improvements in the standard of health and health care in the developed world. This was particularly true in countries such as Australia, which has one of the highest standards in the world. However, even in developed societies with a high standard of living, major inequalities in health status and quality of health care may exist between different groups within the population.

One of the most dramatic changes has been in the number of deaths attributable to infectious diseases. At the beginning of the 20th century more than 60% of all deaths were due to infections but, by the close of the century, less than 5% of deaths were directly caused by microorganisms. However, although the mortality rate has fallen, infectious diseases are still the cause of serious morbidity in our everyday lives and make up a significant proportion of the overall cost of the health system.

The decline in mortality due to infectious diseases can be attributed to three main factors.

1. The ability to isolate and identify the microorganisms responsible for causing infections. This has enabled scientists and health professionals to develop and implement procedures to prevent or control the spread of many diseases. Improvements in general standards of hygiene, sanitation facilities, housing and quality of water supply have all contributed to an improved standard of living and a decrease in the incidence of disease.
2. The discovery of antibiotics in the 1940s provided drugs that were able to selectively kill the bacteria responsible for many life-threatening illnesses (see Chapter 12).
3. The use of vaccines has dramatically reduced mortality from the so-called 'childhood diseases', and from 'adult' diseases such as influenza and pneumococcal disease. Vaccines are a valuable preventive measure against viral infections, which are difficult to treat with antibiotics for reasons discussed in Chapters 5 and 12. The use of vaccines and the value of immunisation are discussed more fully later in this chapter.

The responsibility for the delivery of health care in Australia rests with a number of government bodies at Commonwealth, State and Territory level, as well as with the private sector. At the local level, each State or Territory is organised into Area or District Health Services which report to the State Health Department on matters of public health.

The Australian Department of Health and Aged Care has the responsibility of providing guidelines and information in regard to health policies of national importance. The National Health and Medical Research Council (NHMRC) is a statutory authority within the portfolio of the Minister for Health, and its objective is to:

- raise the standard of individual and public health throughout Australia
- foster the development of consistent health standards between States and Territories
- foster medical research and training, and public health research and training, throughout Australia
- foster consideration of ethical issues relating to health.

This involves the publication of recommendations covering areas such as immunisation schedules, child health, communicable diseases, infection control, nutrition, mental health and other health issues. Another function of the NHMRC is to advise the government on the funding of competitive grants for medical and public health research.

An important function of the health authorities is to collect epidemiological data (see Chapter 8) and carry out surveillance of the occurrence of communicable diseases. Information supplied by doctors, laboratories, hospitals and health services is sent to local, State and Commonwealth authorities and used to develop policies to control the spread of disease.

The control of infectious diseases is one area of public health for which there are intervention strategies of proven efficacy. Immunisation is available to prevent previously fatal childhood diseases and to protect against illnesses such as influenza and hepatitis B. Antimicrobial therapy is a valuable tool for treatment and prevention of infection. Hospital infection control programs based on a knowledge of the aetiology (cause) and transmission of disease can reduce the incidence of hospital-acquired infections.

Notifiable diseases

A number of communicable diseases are required by law to be notified to the health authorities when diagnosed in a patient. The National Notifiable Diseases Surveillance System (NNDSS) was established in 1990 under the auspices of the Communicable Diseases Network, Australia (CDNA). The NNDSS coordinates the reporting of notifiable diseases at a Commonwealth level. Sources of surveillance data include doctors, hospitals and laboratory notifications. The diseases or syndromes that are nationally notifiable are listed in Table 14.1. Laboratory-confirmed influenza, invasive pneumococcal disease and cryptosporidiosis became notifiable in all States in 2001. Standard case definitions for all notifiable diseases have been developed and were adopted in 2004.

A number of additional diseases are required to be reported in the different States. These are conditions or diseases that occur in certain regions – for example, melioidosis in the Northern Territory – or that have significant implications for public health in that region. When the diagnosis can be made largely by symptoms, the responsibility for notification rests with the general practitioner. Diagnostic microbiology and serology laboratories are required to notify any cases of communicable diseases that they identify. The chief executive officers of hospitals and general managers of health services have the responsibility of coordinating notifications of diseases in hospitalised patients, although, in practice, this often

Table 14.1
Nationally notifiable diseases in Australia

Acquired immunodeficiency syndrome (AIDS)
Anthrax
Arbovirus infections
    Barmah Forest virus
    dengue virus
    Japanese encephalitis virus
    Kunjin virus
    Murray Valley encephalitis virus
    Ross River virus
    other arbovirus infections
Botulism (food-borne)
Brucellosis
Campylobacteriosis
Chlamydia
Cholera
Cryptosporidiosis
Diphtheria
Donovanosis
Gonococcal infection
Haemolytic uraemic syndrome (HUS)
Haemophilus influenzae type b (invasive)
Hepatitis A
Hepatitis B
Hepatitis C
Hepatitis D
Hepatitis E
Human immunodeficiency (HIV) infection
Influenza (laboratory confirmed)
Legionellosis

Leprosy
Leptospirosis
Listeriosis
Lyssavirus – Australian bat lyssavirus (ABL)
Lyssavirus – rabies
Malaria
Measles
Meningococcal infection (invasive disease)
Mumps
Pertussis (whooping cough)
Plague
Pneumococcal infection (invasive)
Poliomyelitis
Psittacosis (ornithosis)
Q fever
Rubella or congenital rubella syndrome
Salmonellosis
Shiga toxin and verotoxin producing *Escherichia coli*
  (STEC/VTEC)
Shigellosis
Smallpox
Syphilis or congenital syphilis
Tetanus
Tuberculosis
Tularaemia
Typhoid
Viral haemorrhagic fevers
Yellow fever

involves direct notification from a hospital doctor or laboratory to the State or Territory surveillance centre.

The data collected for each notification include an identification number, the State or Territory, sex and age of the patient, date of onset, date of notification, Aboriginality or ethnicity and post code. This information is important for epidemiological studies and for identification of epidemics. The incidence of notifiable diseases is updated regularly on the *Communicable Diseases Intelligence (CDI)* website at <www.cda.gov.au/index.htm.> and a quarterly review with case reports and comments on outbreaks of disease is published online and also in hard copy. The data are analysed on the basis of age, sex, geographical distribution and seasonal variation and provide a valuable resource for health practitioners.

Notification data compiled by the NNDSS should be interpreted with some caution. They are influenced by a number of factors. For example, diagnostic laboratories are not always able to distinguish between incidence and prevalence statistics (see Chapter 8) – they may test the same patient more than once and record the disease each time they carry out the test, even though only one patient is involved. A disease that is rare or severe is more likely to be notified. A proportion of cases of some diseases,

such as rubella or hepatitis C, may be asymptomatic or too mild to seek medical attention and so the number of cases reported may underestimate the true incidence. Reporting procedures vary somewhat from State to State – for example *Campylobacter* is not notifiable in New South Wales.

As well as NNDS, a number of other surveillance schemes are coordinated through *CDI*. Reports are published regularly on the *CDI* website. They include:

- National Influenza Surveillance Scheme
- Australian Gonococcal Surveillance Program
- Sentinel Chicken Surveillance (for early detection of arbovirus outbreaks)
- Virology and Serology Laboratory Reporting Scheme (LABVISE)
- Australian Paediatric Surveillance Unit (APSU), which carries out surveillance of rare childhood diseases
- National Enteric Pathogens Surveillance System
- Australian Tuberculosis Reporting System, conducted by the Australian Mycobacterial Reference Laboratory Network (AMRLN)
- National Neisseria Network, which examines cases of invasive meningococcal disease

- HIV and AIDS surveillance, coordinated by the National Centre for HIV Epidemiology and Clinical Research (NCHECR)
- Oz Food Net. This was established in 2000 as a collaborative project between Federal, State and Territory authorities, academic institutions, CDNA and the National Centre for Epidemiology and Population Health. Its aim is to improve surveillance and carry out research on food-borne diseases. It is estimated that approximately five million people in Australia experience a food-borne illness every year, but most are not reported. Surveillance is a fundamental part of ensuring a safe food supply. Food safety also depends on the implementation of quality assurance and control programs in the food industry, based on Hazard Analysis Critical Control Point (HACCP) principles.

It is important to be able to detect changes in the pattern of infectious diseases and implement control measures. The ability to collect data and disseminate information rapidly via an electronic medium (website) is an indication of the technological advances available for use in public health strategies in the 21st century.

INFECTIOUS DISEASES IN AUSTRALIA

Data in this section are extracted (with permission) from the *CDI* reports. The numbers of notifications for the most common diseases in each State in 2003, together with the national five-year mean for each disease, are listed in Table 14.2. These figures provide a useful overview of the major infectious diseases and their distribution in Australia. Although the numbers vary from year to year, reflecting seasonal outbreaks, the pattern of distribution is fairly constant. The most recent data can be accessed on the *CDI* website.

Usually, the highest *number* of notifications comes from Queensland, which probably reflects a comprehensive reporting network, but the highest *rate* of notifications (i.e. notifications per 100 000 population) comes from the Northern Territory, which highlights the high incidence of communicable diseases in the susceptible Aboriginal population in that part of Australia. This is discussed later in this chapter. Changes from year to year in the number of notifications of certain diseases, such as hepatitis B and C, may reflect a change in reporting procedures.

Australia is free of some of the diseases that present major problems in other parts of the world. This is either because there are no reservoirs of infection for the microorganisms or the appropriate vector is not found in Australia. This situation may change with increasing global travel. For example, the number of cases of dengue fever has varied from year to year (see Figure 14.1), but in each outbreak the index case was identified as an overseas traveller, usually from South-East Asia. In 2000, there were several cases of dengue fever in soldiers returning from peacekeeping duties in East Timor. In February and March of 2003 there were nearly 500 confirmed cases of dengue fever around Cairns. The index case was a woman who had been to Papua New Guinea. There were other outbreaks in the Torres Strait Islands and a mosquito eradication project was initiated to bring the outbreaks under control.

Notifications of malaria usually occur in people who have contracted the disease outside Australia. However, in 2002, an outbreak of malaria affecting ten people in far north Queensland involved local transmission of *Plasmodium vivax*. The index case was identified as an overseas traveller. A few cases of Japanese encephalitis have been reported. These occurrences highlight the need

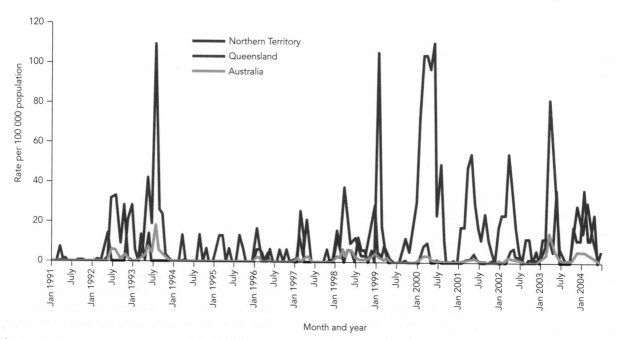

Figure 14.1

Notification rate of Dengue 1991–2003 in Northern Territory, Queensland and Australia
Source: Communicable Diseases Intelligence 2005 29(1), Figure 53, page 48, © Commonwealth of Australia, reproduced by permission

Table 14.2
Incidence of selected notifiable diseases in 2003 by state

DISEASE	ACT	NSW	NT	QLD	SA	TAS	VIC	WA	TOTAL	5 YEAR MEAN
Blood-borne										
Hepatitis B (incident)	0	70	15	40	10	10	147	45	337	373
Hepatitis B (unspecified)	57	2632	NN	805	221	70	1629	419	5833	6971
Hepatitis C (incident)	12	114	NN	NN	74	13	105	142	460	498
Hepatitis C (unspecified)	241	5172	208	2761	574	342	3705	1166	14169	17310
HIV	4	394	5	186	44	0	265	44	882	
Gastrointestinal										
Campylobacteriosis	406	NN	268	3857	2644	624	5596	1977	15372	14440
Cryptosporidiosis	9	202	94	164	80	26	209	437	1219	n/a
Haemolytic uraemic syndrome	0	5	1	1	3	0	4	1	15	14
Hepatitis A	5	124	40	48	13	14	89	85	418	738
Listeriosis	1	28	0	9	1	2	22	6	69	64
Salmonellosis	80	1858	360	2201	445	151	1302	614	7011	7019
Shigellosis	3	59	131	52	32	4	49	110	440	506
SLTEC, VTEC	0	0	0	6	37	0	3	3	49	48
Sexually transmissible										
Chlamydial infection	523	7556	1602	7661	1990	609	6457	3763	30161	21135
Gonococcal infection	30	1194	1399	1042	297	23	1172	1454	6611	6129
Syphilis	12	826	316	375	21	14	356	136	2056	1994
Vaccine-preventable										
Diphtheria	0	0	0	0	0	0	0	0	0	0
Haemophilus influenzae type b	0	6	2	5	2	2	1	1	19	27
Measles	0	18	1	11	24	0	38	0	92	122
Mumps	2	35	0	10	12	-	4	13	76	132
Pertussis	357	2786	5	716	233	132	639	256	5106	6083
Pneumococcal disease (invasive)	40	784	72	466	176	43	443	150	2174	n/a
Rubella	0	24	0	23	1	1	1	3	53	253
Tetanus	0	1	0	2	0	0	1	0	4	4
Vector-borne										
Barmah Forest virus infection	1	451	14	872	2	0	8	22	1370	939
Dengue	7	69	20	727	9	1	18	17	868	327
Malaria	18	120	40	253	28	27	59	56	601	693
Murray Valley encephalitis	0	0	0	0	0	0	0	0	0	†
Ross River virus infection	1	492	120	2517	33	4	13	661	3841	3419
Zoonoses										
Leptospirosis	0	37	4	67	2	0	9	6	125	218
Q fever	1	278	1	224	13	1	13	19	550	624
Other										
Legionellosis	1	60	3	39	65	2	93	65	328	410
Meningococcal infection	13	199	11	104	32	20	125	46	550	627
Tuberculosis	18	378	29	96	42	4	309	68	944	1021

Source: Communicable Diseases Network Australia New Zealand; National Notifiable Diseases Surveillance System. 2005, 29 (1) Table 2.

http://www.health.gov.au/pubhlth/cdi/cdihtml/htm

† 2 cases recorded in 1996, 5 cases in 2001, 2 cases in 2002

for good preventive measures. The appropriate mosquito vector for each of these diseases occurs in Australia so they have the potential to become established here. There have been no reported cases of poliomyelitis, rabies, plague, botulism, yellow fever or other haemorrhagic fevers in Australia in recent years.

The *CDI* data reveal marked differences between the incidence of various diseases in different parts of Australia. Health workers should be aware that, if they choose to work in rural or remote areas, the diseases and health problems they are likely to encounter will be quite different from those in a big city hospital. For example, the Northern Territory has diseases such as melioidosis and donovanosis that are rarely seen in the southern States. Diseases such as hydatids (dog tapeworm) are seen mainly in rural areas where dogs are fed raw offal, and Q fever, a rickettsial disease carried by ticks, occurs mainly in cattle-raising areas. Leptospirosis occurs mainly in rural Victoria, Queensland and the Northern Territory see Figure 14.23.

The distribution of diseases is also influenced by climate and environmental factors. Where a vector such as a tick or mosquito is required for transmission, the disease is confined to areas where the vector is found. In addition, seasonal variations occur, often linked to breeding seasons for vectors such as mosquitoes. For example, Ross River fever occurs in most parts of the country, with the highest rates in north Queensland, and is most common in late summer or after a period of heavy rain and flooding when the mosquito population is high (see Spotlight box, page 336).

ANALYSIS OF NOTIFICATION RATES

The highest number of notifications of infectious diseases in Australia is for the sexually transmissible infections (STIs), chlamydia, gonorrhoea and syphilis. There has been a significant increase in STIs in recent years but this may partly reflect the use of more sensitive detection methods (for chlamydia) and improved reporting procedures. Nationally, the trend in rates of notification for chlamydia shows a steady increase in all age groups: there were more than 30 000 notifications in 2003, up from 24 000 in 2002 (see Figure 14.2).

The highest *rate* of STI notifications is in the Northern Territory and the Kimberley region of Western Australia. In these regions, as in previous years, the recorded incidence of chlamydia is about six times the average for the whole of the Australian population. Gonorrhoea and syphilis are about 25 times the national average.

Gastrointestinal infections notified to authorities represent only a small proportion of those occurring in the community as most infections are mild and self-limiting. Food-borne illnesses due to *Salmonella, Campylobacter,* hepatitis A, *Shigella, Listeria* and toxigenic *E. coli* are notifiable. *Campylobacter* is the predominant food-borne pathogen reported in Australia, but Oz Food Net reports *Salmonella* as responsible for most outbreaks of gastroenteritis. Salmonellosis peaks in the summer months, see Figure 14.3. Most cases of non-pregnancy-associated listeriosis occur in people who are elderly or immunocompromised, and some of these are fatal. Food-borne illnesses are increasing with the growing use of ready prepared or takeaway food. Health departments set standards for food preparation and monitor food outlets to prevent outbreaks of gastroenteritis.

There is also the potential for food-borne diseases to be imported and to spread nationally.

A number of diseases are preventable by vaccination but a significant number of cases still occur, sometimes with serious outcomes. The actual incidence of vaccine-preventable diseases varies from year to year but is unacceptably high in a country like Australia where a free childhood vaccination program is available to all (see page 317). The introduction of meningococcal and

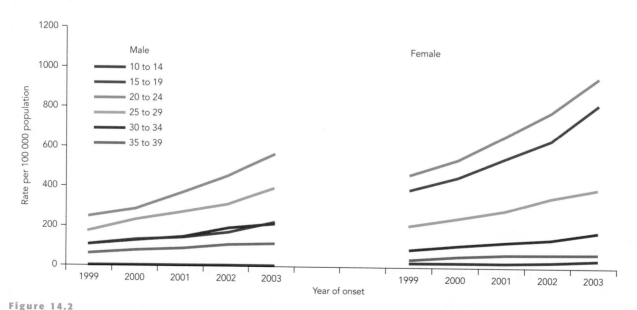

Figure 14.2

Trends in notification rates of chlamydial infection in persons aged 10–39 years in Australia 1999–2003
Source: Communicable Diseases Intelligence 2005 29(1), Figure 27, page 33, © Commonwealth of Australia, reproduced by permission

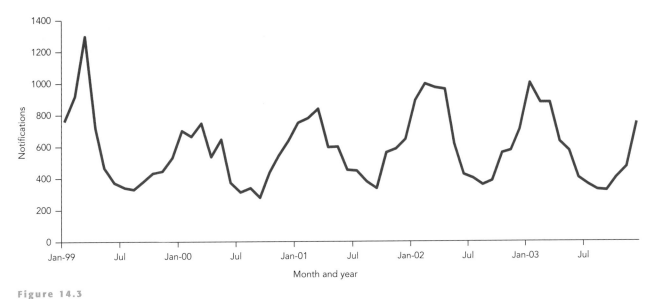

Figure 14.3

Notifications of salmonellosis in Australia 1999–2003
Source: Communicable Diseases Intelligence 2005 29(1), Figure 21, page 28, © Commonwealth of Australia, reproduced by permission

pneumococcal vaccines for children should lead to a lowering of cases of these diseases.

As mentioned above, LABVISE records the incidence of diseases that are diagnosed by serological techniques. These are mainly viral diseases, but other organisms such as *Chlamydia*, which are slow or difficult to grow in the laboratory and for which there is a specific antibody test available, are also diagnosed in this way. Outbreaks of viral diseases tend to occur mainly in the winter months. Among the viruses that affect children, the highest incidence of infections is usually due to respiratory syncytial virus (RSV). Rotavirus, which causes serious gastroenteritis, is the most commonly reported viral infection in the 1–4 years age group.

An important aspect of surveillance data is the information that is obtained about risk factors. Unfortunately, these data are often incomplete, but Figure 14.4 shows the major risk factors associated with the diseases diagnosed by serological methods. As can be seen, injecting drug users are at substantial risk of acquiring serious infections. Patients whose immune system is compromised are also at risk (e.g. HIV-positive people (7.8%) and transplant recip-

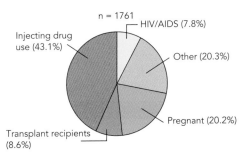

Figure 14.4

Risk factors for acquiring serious infections
Source: Communicable Diseases Intelligence 19/23, 30 October 1995, p. 598, © Commonwealth of Australia, reproduced by permission

ients (8.6%)). More sensitive indicators such as ethnicity (Aboriginality) and poverty are harder to obtain.

INCIDENCE OF HIV/AIDS

The annual number of newly diagnosed HIV infections in Australia declined since testing began in 1985, from about 1700 in 1985 to an annual figure of about 700 (see Table 14.2 and Figure 14.5). However, there has been a recent rise in the number of new HIV diagnoses to over 800 per year. Men with a history of homosexual contact account for the majority of infections see Figure 19.7. The change in numbers occurred only among men; the incidence in females remains constant at 60–80 per year. More than 50% of heterosexual transmissions in Australia occur when the partner or sexual contact is from a high-incidence country, see Figure 14.6. Current data on the incidence of HIV infections and AIDS is accessible on the National Centre for HIV Epidemiology and Research website: <www.med.unsw.edu.au/nchecr>.

The spread of HIV in Australia has been contained, largely because of a massive public education campaign and the introduction of needle exchange programs. The availability of a number of new anti-HIV drugs which have been effective in reducing viral load and illness in people with HIV infection has also contributed to a reduction in AIDS cases. The incidence in surrounding Asian countries is much higher (see Figure 14.7) and heterosexual transmission is common in the sex industry there.

Although HIV is a notifiable disease, people who are infected are often asymptomatic for a long time and testing is voluntary so the true incidence is not known.

Primary health care

Primary health care, in its broadest sense, is a philosophy of promoting equal health care at all levels of the social system. It involves the provision of services on the basis of

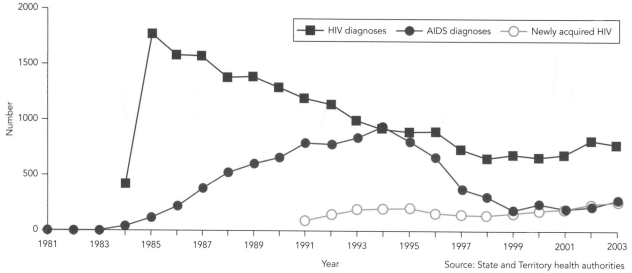

Source: State and Territory health authorities

Figure 14.5

Diagnoses of HIV infection* and AIDS in Australia
*HIV diagnoses adjusted for multiple reporting. AIDS diagnoses adjusted for reporting delays.
Source: NCHECR Annual Report 2004.

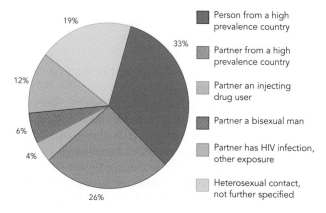

- Person from a high prevalence country
- Partner from a high prevalence country
- Partner an injecting drug user
- Partner a bisexual man
- Partner has HIV infection, other exposure
- Heterosexual contact, not further specified

Source: State and Territory health authorities

Figure 14.6

HIV infection attributed to heterosexual contact, 1999–2003, by exposure category
Source: NCHECR Annual Report 2004.

the needs of the population, the provision of health education and the development of a balanced system of health promotion, disease prevention and treatment of illness.

In Australia there is firm evidence that, despite an overall high standard of health, there are disadvantaged groups of people in the community whose health status is poor. For example, Aborigines and Torres Strait Islanders have a much lower general standard of health than the rest of Australia, due in part to the poor standard of housing and physical environment in which many of them live. The infectious diseases that affect indigenous people are examined later in this chapter.

Some of the most important factors that influence health are socioeconomic. Factors such as marital status, sex, ethnicity, level of education and place of dwelling (urban or rural) can also affect health. Some of the social circumstances that can cause inequalities in health status are:

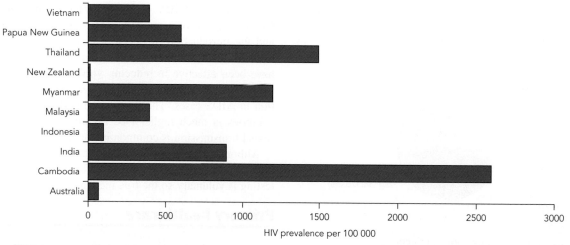

Figure 14.7

HIV prevalence in selected countries in the Asia–Pacific region in 2003
Source: NCHECR Annual Report 2004.

- level of education
- level of economic resources
- living conditions, including quality of housing, clean water supply, air pollution, hazardous environments
- working conditions
- availability of social support.

Numerous studies show that people in the lowest socio-economic groups, with low levels of education, have the poorest health. They tend to delay seeking treatment, so their illnesses have often become more severe by the time they present to the hospital or health service. Other untreated, underlying illnesses often contribute to morbidity. They are also less likely to seek out preventive services such as screening and immunisation.

Two aspects of primary health care that can directly affect the level of infectious diseases in the community are immunisation and preventive screening programs. Other activities of primary health care are beyond the scope of this text, but should be kept in mind as being essential for good health. They include:

- basic education, including health education
- provision of adequate food and nutrition
- provision of a safe water supply and proper sanitation
- control of endemic diseases
- provision of maternal and child care, and family planning information
- provision of appropriate medication and treatment.

The changing lifestyle in Australia, with many women in the workforce, has meant that more children aged 0–5 years are in child-care centres. These pose special problems in infection control and are discussed in a later section of this chapter.

Immunisation

The development of vaccines and the implementation of immunisation programs were among the major reasons for the improvement in health last century. One of the great success stories of vaccination campaigns is the worldwide eradication of the dreaded disease, smallpox; and in many developed countries polio has been virtually eliminated. During the polio epidemics in Australia in the 1940s and 1950s, there were up to 1000 cases of paralytic polio disease and 100 deaths each year. The introduction of the **Salk vaccine** (a killed preparation) and later the **Sabin vaccine** (an attenuated virus) saw a dramatic fall in the occurrence of the disease. The last recorded case of polio in Australia was in 1978 and in 2000 Australia was declared free of polio.

The principles behind the development of immunity to an infectious disease are fully described in Chapter 9. To summarise: when a person is exposed to a foreign organism, the body responds by producing antibodies, activated lymphocytes and long-term memory cells against that organism. If the person is subsequently exposed to the same organism, the preformed antibodies and memory cells (which produce more antibodies and activated T lymphocytes) combine to kill or remove the invading organism before disease can occur. The person is said to be *immune* to that disease. Immunity is specific for each disease and sometimes even for each different strain of a pathogenic organism. Thus, if the organism is slightly different (due to a mutation, such as occurs with the influenza virus) then the person may not be immune to the altered form of the pathogen.

The possibility of producing immunity by artificial means was recognised as far back as 1796 when EDWARD JENNER noticed that milkmaids who had suffered from cowpox, a mild disease with lesions similar to smallpox, appeared to be immune to smallpox. He first used a preparation derived from cowpox (caused by *Vaccinia* virus, hence the word 'vaccine') to immunise people successfully against smallpox. The milder cowpox virus induced immunity to smallpox.

Jenner's work laid the basis for our modern immunisation programs. In practice, the terms 'vaccination' and 'immunisation' are used interchangeably. However, **vaccination** is used by some people in a general sense to denote the administration of any vaccine without regard to whether the recipient is made immune. **Immunisation** is a more specific term, denoting the process of inducing or providing immunity artificially. It may be active or passive.

Active immunisation is the administration of a vaccine in order to stimulate the body's immune system to produce both specific antibodies and cellular immunity to the antigens contained in the vaccine. It takes several days for this process to occur and immunity to be developed.

Passive immunisation is the provision of temporary immunity by the administration of preformed antibodies derived from another person or animal. They may be in the form of pooled, non-specific human immunoglobulin, specific antitoxins (e.g. tetanus) or specific antibody preparations (e.g. hepatitis B immunoglobulin). These products are used mainly when a person has been accidentally exposed to a serious disease and requires immediate protection because they have no immunity. The antibodies circulate only for a short time (weeks to months) before being degraded by normal body processes.

Maternal antibodies that cross the placenta in the late stages of pregnancy are a natural type of passive immunisation which protects the infant from infection during the first months of life. At birth the neonate has a range of maternal antibodies which represent the exposure of the mother to previous infectious diseases. Premature infants (less than 32 weeks) have not yet received maternal antibodies transplacentally and so are at a significantly higher risk of infection. Further passive protection is afforded by the antibodies present in colostrum and breast milk, especially against gastrointestinal infections.

As the immune system develops during the first year of life, the maternal antibodies are destroyed and the infant builds up its own immunity to the various microorganisms to which it is exposed. The development of protective immunological memory in early childhood can be stimulated by the administration of appropriate vaccine preparations, before significant risks of exposure to the infectious agents occur. This is called **artificial active immunity**.

TYPES OF VACCINES

Obviously, it would not be safe to administer live pathogens in order to promote an immune response. It has been necessary to develop suitable preparations which contain the specific immunogenic groups (antigens) of the pathogen but which are unable to cause disease (see Chapter 9). Table 9.4 (page 205) lists the properties of vaccines in common use. Some (e.g. measles, mumps, rubella, Sabin polio, OPV) consist of live, attenuated (weakened) forms of the pathogen. They have the advantage of being able to multiply in the host, producing a high level (titre) of antibody formation from a single dose of vaccine, without producing disease. There is always a very slight risk that these preparations may revert to a virulent (disease-producing) strain, but this is extremely rare.

Toxoids are inactivated forms of bacterial toxins that retain their ability to induce immunity. Toxoids are used when the disease symptoms are due mainly to the formation of a toxin; for example, tetanus toxoid and diphtheria toxoid.

The safest vaccines are preparations that use only part of the pathogenic organism to induce effective immunity. They do not contain any nucleic acid, so replication (and disease) is not possible. For example, the vaccine for hepatitis B consists of the surface antigen HBsAg from the outer layer of the virus. It is produced by placing the viral gene for HBsAg into cells of the yeast, *Saccharomyces cerevisiae*, inducing the synthesis of large quantities of the antigen, which is then extracted and purified for use in the vaccine.

The vaccine against *Haemophilus influenzae* type B (Hib) is a **conjugate vaccine**, consisting of the antigenic polysaccharide from Hib, bound to a protein carrier. The new pneumococcal vaccine suitable for children under two years is a polyvalent conjugated vaccine consisting of

seven of the polysaccharide antigens from *Streptococcus pneumoniae* bound to a protein carrier. A cell-free pertussis (whooping cough) vaccine, which has fewer side effects than the old 'killed whole cell' preparation, is now used in Australia.

Vaccines containing non-replicating antigens require the administration of several doses to build up adequate levels of immunity. Theoretically, live vaccines should require only one dose, but some of the newer attenuated viral vaccines have only been available since the 1970s and are still being evaluated to determine how long the artificially acquired immunity will last. In some cases (e.g. rubella, hepatitis B), antibody titres are known to fall over time. Measurements of antibody titre at various time intervals after immunisation sometimes show wide variations among individuals, and it is not known whether this represents a lowered level of immunity.

At present, it is recommended that women intending to become pregnant should have their rubella antibody level checked; if seronegative they should be vaccinated or, if their antibody titre is low, have a booster dose of vaccine. This should be done at least two months before becoming pregnant. Since it is a live vaccine, its use close to or during pregnancy is not advised, although there are no reports of congenital abnormalities due to vaccine use.

VACCINATION SCHEDULES

Until the widespread introduction of childhood immunisation, many children died from infectious diseases. However, the last 50 years has seen a dramatic decrease in infant mortality due to vaccine-preventable diseases (see Table 14.3).

The Australian Health Department provides free vaccination for most childhood diseases. The current recommended childhood vaccination schedule is shown in Table 14.4. This is now the standard schedule for all Australia.

Highlights of the schedule
Some of the changes in the last few years include the replacement of whole cell pertussis vaccine with an

---

Table 14.3

Deaths from diseases commonly vaccinated against, Australia 1926–2002

PERIOD	DIPHTHERIA	PERTUSSIS	TETANUS	POLIOMYELITIS	MEASLES*	POPULATION
1926–1935	4073	2808	879	430	1102	6 600 000
1936–1945	2791	1693	655	618	822	7 200 000
1946–1955	624	429	625	1013	495	8 600 000
1956–1965	44	58	280	123	210	11 000 000
1966–1975	11	22	82	2	146	13 750 000
1976–1985	2	14	31	2	62	14 900 000
1986–1995	2	9	21	0	32	17 300 000
1996–2002	0	15	6	0	0	18 900 000

Sources: Feery B. One hundred years of vaccination *Public Health Bull* 1997; 8:6–13; Feery B. Impact of immunization on disease patterns in Australia. *Med J Aust* 1981; 2:172–6. Deaths recorded for 1966–1975 and 1996–2002 updated with data provided by AIHW Mortality database.

* Excludes deaths from subacute sclerosing panencephalitis.

▨ Indicates decade in which community vaccination started for the disease.

Table 14.4

National Immunisation Program Routine schedule of vaccines

AGE	VACCINE
Birth	Hepatitis B
2 months	Hepatitis B* Diphtheria, tetanus and acelluar pertussis *Haemophilus influenzae* type b Poliomyelitis vaccine, OPV/IPV Pneumococcal conjugate vaccine
4 months	Hepatitis B* Diphtheria, tetanus and acellular pertussis *Haemophilus influenzae* type b Poliomyelitis vaccine, OPV/IPV Pneumococcal conjugate vaccine
6 months	Hepatitis B* Diphtheria, tetanus and acellular pertussis Poliomyelitis vaccine, OPV/IPV Pneumococcal conjugate vaccine
12 months	Heptatitis B* *Haemophilus influenzae* type b Measles, mumps and rubella Meningococcal C Pneumococcal conjugate vaccine (eligible children only+)
18–24 months	Pneumococcal polysaccharide vaccine (eligible children only+) Chickenpox
4 years	Diphtheria, tetanus and acellular pertussis Poliomyelitis vaccine, OPV/IPV Measles, mumps and rubella Pneumococcal polysaccharide vaccine (eligible children only+)
10–13 years	Hepatitis B* Chickenpox (eligible children only) *Arrangements vary. Contact your State or Territory health department.*
15–17 years	Diphtheria, tetanus and acellular pertussis *Arrangements vary. Contact your State or Territory health department.*
65 years and over	Influenza Pneumococcal polysaccharide vaccine

* Total 3 doses required following birth dose.

The brands of vaccines and age of administration vary slightly among States and Territories. Immunisation providers should contact their health department for further information on the National Immunisation Program specific to their State or Territory. This schedule should be read in conjunction with the National Health and Medical Research Council's *Australian Immunisation Handbook 8th Edition 2003* at <http://www1.health.gov.au/immhandbook>, which provides detailed information on available vaccine choices and the administration of vaccines.

For more general information about the National Immunisation Program, visit Immunise Australia at <http://www.immunise.health. gov.au> or contact the Immunisation Infoline on 1800 671 811.

acellular preparation, the inclusion of hepatitis B for all infants, and the introduction of free meningococcal vaccine in 2003 and free pneumococcal vaccine in 2005.

A vaccine against chickenpox (varicella) for infants aged 18 months and children 10–13 years old, was also added to the free schedule in 2005.

Meningococcal infections are caused by *Neisseria meningitides*. There are 13 known serogroups distinguished by differences in the surface polysaccharides of the outer membrane capsule. Globally, serogroups A, B, C, W135 and Y most commonly cause disease. In Australia, serogroups B and C occur most frequently – approxi-

mately 32% of cases are serogroup C and most of the remainder are group B. The overall notification rate of meningococcal disease of both serogroups B and C to the National Notifiable Diseases Surveillance System has been increasing gradually, during the past 10 years. The new meningococcal vaccine, MenCCVs, is a conjugate vaccine that confers protection against serogroup C only, but it is more effective than previous vaccines and can be administered to children under two years of age. In the period 2003–05, there was a scheduled school-based 'catch-up' immunisation program for children over five years of age.

Pneumococcal vaccine was added to the schedule for all children in 2005. *Streptococcus pneumoniae* is a leading cause of otitis media, pneumonia, bacteraemia and meningitis and is responsible for significant morbidity and mortality, especially in infants, the elderly and people with a predisposing illness. Invasive pneumococcal disease (IPD) occurs when the bacteria infect a normally sterile site. IPD is usually a disease of the very young and very old, see Figure 14.8. The highest rates of invasive disease occur in indigenous people in the Northern Territory, see Table 14.5 and Figure 14.9. Ninety different serotypes are identified by the polysaccharides in the capsule of *S. pneumoniae* and this has made vaccine development difficult. In 2005, the 7-valent pneumococcal conjugate vaccine against *Streptococcus pneumoniae*, which is suitable for young children, was added to the free recommended schedule at 2, 4 and 6 months. (See Figure 14.10.) A free 'catch-up' campaign for children born between 2003 and 2005 was also included. In addition, a free program of immunisation against invasive pneumococcal disease with a 23-valent vaccine is available to all adults over 65.

In the latest schedule (see Table 14.4), the inactivated injectable vaccine IPV (Salk) is recommended instead of

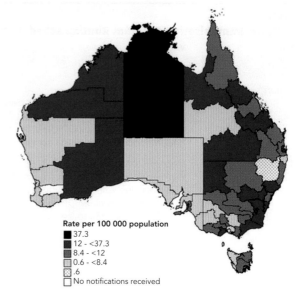

Figure 14.9

Notification rates of invasive pneumococcal disease Australia 2003 by statistical division of residence

Source: Communicable Diseases Intelligence 28(4), Map p 445, © Commonwealth of Australia, reproduced by permission

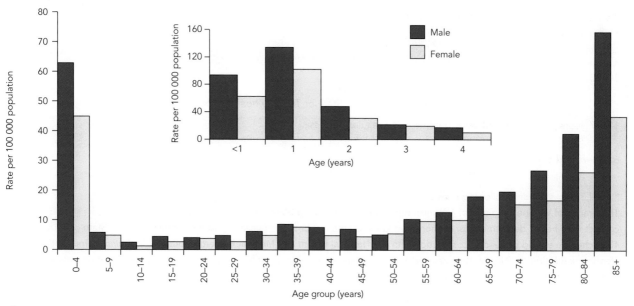

Figure 14.8

Notification rates of invasive pneumococcal disease by age and sex, Australia 2003

Source: Communicable Diseases Intelligence 2004 28(4), Figure 2, p 445, © Commonwealth of Australia, reproduced by permission

Table 14.5

Notifications and notification rate per 100 000 population, invasive pneumococcal disease, Australia, 2003*

	ACT	NSW	NT	QLD	SA	TAS	VIC	WA	AUSTRALIA
Notifications	40	784	72	466	176	43	443	150	2 174
Rate per 100 000 population	12.4	11.7	37.3	12.3	11.5	9.0	9.0	7.7	10.9

* By date of disease onset.

Source: CDI 2004 28(4), Table 5, p 445.

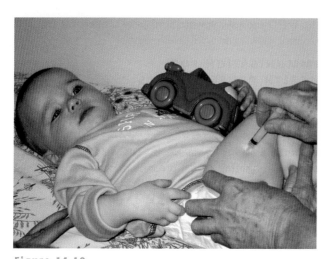

Figure 14.10

Baby receiving 12 month vaccinations

the live oral polio vaccine OPV (Sabin) in order to prevent the very slight risk of vaccine-associated disease. This is now included in the schedule of free vaccines. The fourth dose of DTPa, which was previously given at 18 months of age, is no longer required. Instead, the fourth dose of DTPa is now recommended at 4 years of age with a fifth dose at 15–17 years.

To improve protection against measles, a two-dose vaccination schedule (given in the combined measles-mumps-rubella, MMR, preparation) is now recommended at 12 months and 4 years. In addition, a 'catch-up' campaign of measles vaccination for school-age children was carried out in 1998. A campaign is under way to increase measles vaccine coverage in susceptible young adults born since 1966 who do not have evidence of two doses of the vaccine in the past.

Haemophilus influenzae type b (Hib) is responsible for the invasive diseases meningitis, pneumonia and epiglottitis in young children, with an overall fatality rate of 2–5%.

Sequelae to Hib meningitis, ranging from mild hearing loss to neurological impairment, occur in 20–30% of cases. Hib vaccines suitable for infants of two months were introduced in 1993 in Australia and are now included in the routine immunisation schedules. The result has been a dramatic decrease in the incidence of Hib (see Figure 14.11). In children under five years there has been a marked reduction in the number of notifications to 1.7 per 100 000 population in 2000 (and in 2003 only 3 cases were notified). The impact of herd immunity following the vaccination of young children has led to a reduction in infections across all age groups.

Indigenous Australians have a high risk of acquiring tuberculosis so BCG vaccine, which is most effective in children, is recommended for neonates in regions of high incidence. There are differences in schedules used in Australia and other countries – for example, New Zealand). The schedules are continually modified to include new vaccines and to take into account new knowledge and changes in the prevalence of various diseases.

PROCEDURES FOR VACCINATION

The NHMRC publishes up-to-date comprehensive information on immunisation procedures and recommendations for administration in the *Immunisation Handbook*. Recommendations change from time to time and updates are available on the website <www.immunise.health.gov. au>. Vaccines should be administered by the correct route and at the optimal site (for injections). The age at which vaccines are administered is also important. Maternally derived antibodies (IgG) seem to lower the infant's response to live (attenuated) vaccines, but do not interfere with the response to the non-replicating (killed) vaccines. For this reason, DTP (triple antigen: diphtheria, tetanus, pertussis) can be given as early as two months of age, but the live MMR (measles, mumps, rubella) vaccine is better delayed to 12 months. Since premature infants are lacking

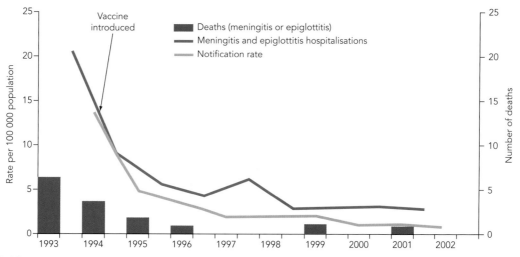

Figure 14.11

Incidence of Hib

Hib notifications, Hib hospitalisations and deaths of children aged 0–4 years, Australia, July 1992 to June 2002.
Source: Communicable Diseases Intelligence 2004 128, Supplement 2, Figure 3, page 512, © Commonwealth of Australia, reproduced by permission

in maternal antibodies, immunisation should begin at the chronological age and not be delayed because of prematurity.

ADULT IMMUNISATION

Although the major emphasis in all vaccination campaigns is on childhood vaccination, there is a large number of adults who, for various reasons, are not fully immunised. This may be because they are recent immigrants from countries where vaccination is not readily available, or it may be because of their age and the previous unavailability of vaccines. There is significant morbidity and mortality among adults from vaccine-preventable diseases and there is a need to develop a national strategy aimed at immunising adults. Currently, influenza vaccine is available to all Australians 65 years and older.

Aboriginal people and Torres Strait Islanders have a high incidence of invasive pneumococcal disease. The Northern Territory has developed an adult immunisation schedule which, in addition to influenza vaccine, includes:

- influenza and pneumococcal vaccines for Aboriginal people 50 years and older; and for those 15 years and older who fall into high-risk groups
- measles-mumps-rubella vaccine for adults 18–40 years
- adult diphtheria tetanus (ADT) every 10 years.

IMMUNISATION AGAINST OTHER DISEASES

As discussed above, it is important that adults as well as children are fully immunised against the vaccine-preventable diseases. There are other, less common diseases that are also preventable by vaccines, but immunisation is usually only recommended for high-risk groups. Vaccines are available to protect against influenza, pneumococcus, Q fever, meningococcal meningitis and tuberculosis.

Other vaccines (e.g for cholera, typhoid, yellow fever) are required only by travellers to countries where the disease is endemic. Travellers should consult their State health department for current recommendations for vaccination or refer to the *Immunisation Handbook* <www.immunise.health.gov.au>. Information about infectious diseases in other countries is available online from the WHO site <www.who.int/ith/> or Centers for Disease Control <www.cdc.gov/travel/index>.

IMMUNISATION FOR HEALTH PROFESSIONALS

Due to the nature of their work, health professionals are at significantly higher risk of encountering infectious diseases. Health workers are advised to ensure they are vaccinated against hepatitis B. The value of the BCG vaccine in offering partial protection against tuberculosis is a controversial area. Some States recommend vaccination for all health workers while others favour regular Mantoux testing, followed by antibiotic prophylaxis if required. In some institutional facilities, vaccination for hepatitis A may be advisable.

All health-care workers, especially those working with children, should ensure they have adequate immunisation against all the 'childhood diseases', especially as some of these diseases – for example, measles and chickenpox – are much more severe in adults. Immunisation is also necessary to protect susceptible children (and adults) such as those suffering from leukaemia, who are particularly vulnerable to infection. A vaccine for chickenpox is available and should be given to all non-immune paediatric staff and those working with immunocompromised patients.

COMPLIANCE WITH IMMUNISATION: HERD IMMUNITY

The success of immunisation programs in developed countries has meant a dramatic reduction in infant morbidity and mortality. However, to maintain this situation it is essential that parents continue to have their children immunised. An important factor in maintaining a community free of disease is the proportion of individuals in the community who are immune to a particular disease. This is described as group or **herd immunity**. As we saw in Chapter 8, to control the spread of disease the reservoirs of infection must be eliminated, in this case by immunisation. If the number of immune individuals is high, then the disease can affect only a few susceptible people and so the likelihood of exposure of unimmunised individuals – and therefore transmission of the disease – is low. *Thus, a high group immunity protects not only the immunised members but also the susceptible ones* (see Figure 14.12).

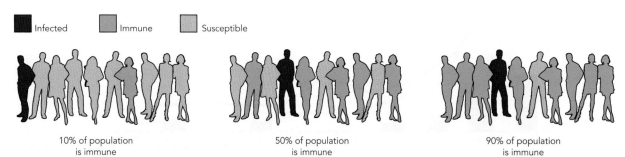

■ Infected   ■ Immune   ■ Susceptible

10% of population is immune   50% of population is immune   90% of population is immune

Figure 14.12

Herd immunity

The greater the percentage of immune persons in a population, the less likely a susceptible individual is to be exposed to the disease.

SPOTLIGHT ON
Measles and herd immunity
Case Report 1: Family, Queensland[1]

In May 2000 five children from the same family in north Queensland were confirmed as having measles. None of the children had been vaccinated because the parents did not believe in vaccination. Two of the children had travelled to the United Kingdom with a stopover in Sri Lanka. The first child became unwell in England and was seen by two different GPs, but continued the tour in Scotland, England and Wales. The family was billeted in private homes during their trip. On their return the second child became ill and visited a medical centre on three occasions. The family also travelled to a nearby town and stayed in a caravan park. Another child became ill and was seen by a GP there and later presented at the local hospital where the diagnosis was confirmed and the disease notified to the authorities.

The family said they were not advised the disease was contagious or of the need for isolation and so continued to travel. In all, they made four visits to GPs, four visits to the local medical centre and one to hospital. Everywhere they travelled they came in contact with people who were possibly susceptible to measles. All the patients and staff at the health facilities and other contacts had to be traced and, if necessary, offered vaccination.

Case Report 2: Young adults, Victoria[2,3]

In February 2001 an outbreak of measles affected 31 people aged 15–34 and one infant aged 10 months. Seventeen of the cases required hospitalisation. The index case was a 19-year-old male who had recently returned to Melbourne from a holiday in India. Eight of the cases (including the infant) were directly linked to the primary case as they had all attended the same restaurant on the same evening.

This was similar to a previous outbreak in Victoria in March 1999, when there were 41 cases of measles in people who had attended a seminar together. They were mainly young adults, with one case in a 10-month-old infant; the index case was a young man recently returned from a holiday in Bali. Forty per cent of the patients had to be hospitalised.

Comment

Measles is a highly contagious, notifiable, vaccine-preventable disease which was responsible for 2223 hospitalisations and seven deaths in Australia between 1993 and 1998. A vaccine was introduced in Australia in 1968 and, since 1989, infants aged 12–15 months have received the combined measles-mumps-rubella vaccine, MMR. The measles epidemic of 1993–94 prompted the introduction of a second dose of this vaccine which is now given at 4 years. A highly successful 'catch-up campaign' for 1.7 million school children was carried out between August and November 1998. However, in Australia there still exists a pool of young adults born between 1966 and 1989 who are susceptible to measles because they were born before the MMR was introduced for infants and missed out on catching the wild-type virus because the incidence of the disease had dropped after the vaccine was introduced. These people make up a susceptible population who are not only at risk of catching the disease themselves but can also transmit it to unimmunised infants, which explains the outbreaks described in Case Report 2.

As discussed in the text, a compliance rate of 90–95% is required to provide 'herd immunity'. Until the coverage in the Australian population reaches this level, outbreaks such as the one in Victoria are likely to continue. In both reports cited here the index case contracted the disease outside Australia, in an area where measles was endemic. In the Victorian outbreak the susceptible population were young adults who, for reasons described above, were not immune. In the Queensland case, the victims were members of a family who had chosen not to be vaccinated. An unknown number of their contacts may have contracted the disease.

The World Health Organization has identified measles as a disease which, theoretically, could be eradicated worldwide because humans are the only reservoir and the disease is transmitted directly from person to person. The side effects of vaccination are much less than the serious effects that can result from having the disease.

These two reports highlight the need for *everyone* to comply with vaccination in order to maintain coverage in the community and protect children too young to be immunised. If the level of protection in the community is not maintained, the disease can easily be reintroduced by a traveller from an endemic area. Currently, Australians travelling to an area where measles is endemic are advised to have a second dose of MMR.

Sources
1. *Comm Dis Intell* 2000; 24: 211–12.
2. *Comm Dis Intell* 2001; 25: 12.
3. *Comm Dis Intell* 1999; 23: 75.

This is particularly important for a disease like pertussis (whooping cough). Older children and adults suffer a severe but usually non-fatal illness. However, for babies under six months pertussis may be fatal. If the older children and adults are immunised, they do not contract the disease and so the susceptible babies are protected because they have less chance of being exposed to an infected person.

It is necessary to understand the concept of herd immunity in order to realise the importance of continuing vaccine programs after the incidence of a disease has declined – for example, polio. If a person with polio (e.g. a traveller from a country where the disease is still prevalent) enters a country which has been declared 'polio free', and has discontinued its vaccination program, there is the potential for an epidemic to occur. This will continue to be the case until the disease is eradicated worldwide (see Spotlight box, page 499).

An individual's response to a vaccine preparation depends on their immune system. Not all vaccines are 100% effective. For example, the measles vaccine produces immunity in only 90–95% of people vaccinated but that is usually high enough to protect everyone because of herd immunity. If there is low compliance with immunisation programs, then the level of protection can fall as low as 50% in the community. Figures from the Australian Bureau of Statistics for the period 1989–90 showed that, overall, only 52.9% of children under six years were *fully* immunised. This lack of full immunisation greatly increases the risk of epidemics, as is shown by the outbreaks of measles in Australia (see Figure 14.13).

The epidemic of measles that began in 1992 continued into 1994 with 4895 cases being reported. Measles can be a serious and sometimes fatal disease; it also has a rare postviral complication – subacute sclerosing panencephalitis (SSPE) – which is usually fatal (see Chapter 5). Immunisation of all school-age children provides herd immunity which also protects susceptible children under 15 months (see Spotlight box, page 321). Catch-up vaccination campaigns targeting measles have greatly improved the coverage (see Figure 14.15).

There are various reasons why people do not comply with immunisation recommendations. These include:

- ignorance or complacency about the serious nature of vaccine-preventable diseases
- fear of complications of vaccination
- lack of correct information about side effects and/or contraindications.

In 1996 the Australian Childhood Immunisation Register was established and in 1997 a seven-point plan was devised to increase immunisation levels to a target coverage of 95%. Various initiatives were introduced and the level of vaccine coverage is now monitored by the National Centre for Immunisation Research and Surveillance of Vaccine Preventable Diseases (NCIRS). The level of coverage has since increased steadily, especially in the Northern Territory (see Figures 14.14 and 14.15). By the end of 2003 vaccine coverage had reached the target of 90% in all states except ACT (88%). The percentage of 6 year olds classified as fully vaccinated remained steady at about 85%.

RISKS AND COMPLICATIONS OF VACCINATION

In the past there have been instances of adverse reactions, even some deaths, following administration of vaccines. The standard of vaccine production and administration is now very high. Health professionals should be familiar with the contraindications for vaccination. Children with immunodeficiencies require special consideration. The *Australian Immunisation Handbook 2003* (8th edition) is

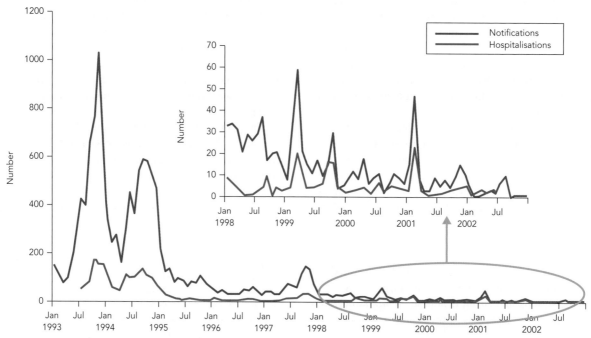

Figure 14.13

Measles notifications and hospitalisations by month of onset or admission, Australia 1993–2002
Notifications where the month of onset was between January 1993 and December 2002; hospitalisations where the month of admission was between 1 July 1993 and 30 June 2002.
Source: Communicable Diseases Intelligence 2004 28, Suppl 2, Figure 12, page 528, © Commonwealth of Australia, reproduced by permission

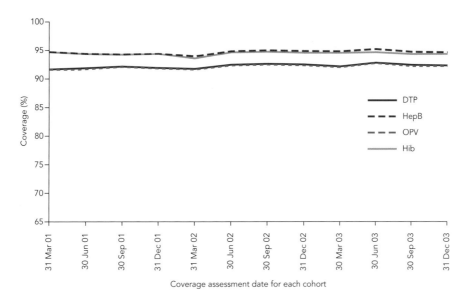

Figure 14.14

Trends in vaccination coverage estimates for individual vaccines: children vaccinated for 3 doses of DTP, OPV, Hib and Hep B at the age of 1 year

Source: Communicable Diseases Intelligence 2004 (28), Supplement 2, Figure 41, page 572, © Commonwealth of Australia, reproduced by permission

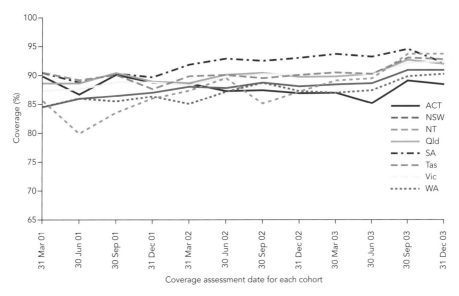

Figure 14.15

Trends in vaccination coverage estimates by jurisdiction: children fully vaccinated for four DTPa and Hib, 3 doses of OPV and 1 dose of MMR at the age of 2 years

By 3-month birth cohorts born between January 1999 and 31 December 2001.
Source: Communicable Diseases Intelligence 2004 (28), Supplement 2, Figure 43, page 573, © Commonwealth of Australia, reproduced by permission

available online at <www.immunise.health.gov.au/hand-book.htm> and contains complete information about the use of the recommended vaccines together with a description of any adverse reactions that might be expected and contraindications for use (see Table 14.6).

An adverse reaction is defined as "a serious uncommon or unexpected event following administration of a vaccine. Such an event *may or may not* be caused by the vaccine or it may be caused by chance after the vaccination. Any vaccine may cause an adverse event. Adverse events following immunisation fall into three categories that are

not mutually exclusive: local, systemic or allergic". (*Immunisation Handbook*, 8th edn, p. 30)

Reports of suspected adverse events following immunisation are collated in a central database by the Adverse Drug Reactions Advisory Committee. NCIRS carries out an analysis of the reports which is published regularly in the *CDI* bulletins. The most commonly reported adverse reactions are local swelling and pain at the site of the injection. Fever may occur less commonly. There is a very low reporting rate of serious events, which demonstrates a high level of safety in Australian vaccines.

Table 14.6

Comparison of effects of vaccines and diseases

DISEASE	EFFECTS OF DISEASE	SIDE EFFECTS OF VACCINATION
Diphtheria: contagious bacteria spread by droplets; causes severe throat and breathing difficulties.	About 1 in 15 patients die. The bacteria release a toxin which can produce nerve paralysis and heart failure.	DTPa vaccine: about 1 in 10 have local inflammation or fever. Serious adverse events are very rare and much less common than DTPw.
Hepatitis B: contagious virus spread mainly by blood, sexual contact or from mother to newborn baby; causes acute hepatitis or chronic carriage.	About 1 in 3 chronic carriers will develop cirrhosis or liver cancer.	About 1 in 15 to 1 in 100 have pain and fever. Anaphylaxis occurs in about 1 in 600 000.
Hib: contagious bacteria spread by droplets; causes meningitis, epiglottitis (respiratory obstruction), septicaemia, osteomyelitis.	About 1 in 20 meningitis patients die and 1 in 4 survivors have permanent brain or nerve damage. About 1 in 100 epiglottitis patients die.	About 1 in 20 have discomfort or local inflammation. About 1 in 50 have fever.
Influenza: contagious virus spread by droplets; causes fever, muscle and joint pains, pneumonia.	Causes increased hospitalisation in the elderly. High-risk groups include the elderly, diabetics, alcoholics, etc.	About 1 in 10 have local reactions, Guillain-Barré syndrome occurs in about 1 in 1 million.
Measles: highly infectious virus spread by droplets; causes fever, cough, rash.	1 in 25 children with measles develop pneumonia and 1 in 2000 develop encephalitis (brain inflammation). For every 10 children who develop measles encephalitis, 1 dies and up to 4 have permanent brain damage. About 1 in 25 000 develop SSPE (brain degeneration), which is always fatal.	About 1 in 10 have discomfort, local inflammation or fever. About 1 in 100 develop a rash, which is non-infectious. 1 in 1 million recipients may develop encephalitis (inflammation of the brain).
Meningococcal infections: bacteria spread by respiratory droplets. Cause sepsis (infection of the blood stream) and meningitis (infection of the tissues surrounding the brain).	About 1 in 10 patients dies. Of those that survive, 1 in 30 has severe skin scarring or loss of limbs, and 1 in 30 has severe brain damage.	Polysaccharide vaccine: Local reactions common. Mild fever, headache, malaise in 1 in 30. Conjugate vaccine: About 1 in 10 has local inflammation, fever, irritability, anorexia or headaches.
Mumps: contagious virus spread by saliva; causes swollen neck glands, fever.	1 in 200 children develop encephalitis (brain inflammation). 1 in 5 males past puberty develop inflammation of the testicles. Occasionally mumps causes infertility or deafness.	1 in 100 recipients may develop swelling of the salivary glands. 1 in 3 million recipients develop mild encephalitis (inflammation of the brain).
Pertussis: contagious bacteria spread by droplets; causes whooping cough and vomiting, lasting up to 3 months.	About 1 in 200 whooping cough patients under the age of 6 months die from pneumonia or brain damage.	As for DTPa vaccine (see diphtheria).
Pneumococcus: bacteria spread by droplets; causes fever, pneumonia, septicaemia, meningitis.	About 1 in 10 meningitis patients die.	Fewer than 1 in 20 have pain or local reactions.
Polio: contagious virus spread by faeces and saliva; causes fever, headache, vomiting and may progress to paralysis.	About 1 in 20 hospitalised patients die and 1 in 2 patients who survive are permanently paralysed.	Fewer than 1 in 100 recipients develop diarrhoea, headache, and/or muscle pains. 1 in 2.5 million recipients or close contacts develop paralysis.
Rubella: contagious virus spread by droplets; causes rash, fever, swollen glands, but causes severe malformations to babies of infected pregnant women.	About 5 in 10 patients develop a rash and painful swollen glands; 5 in 10 adolescents and adults have painful joints; 1 in 3000 develop thrombocytopenia (bruising or bleeding); 1 in 6000 develop inflammation of the brain; 9 in 10 babies infected during the first 10 weeks after conception will have a major congenital abnormality (such as deafness, blindness, brain damage or heart defects).	About 1 in 10 have discomfort, local inflammation or fever. About 1 in 20 have swollen glands, stiff neck or joint pains. About 1 in 100 have a rash, which is non-infectious. Thrombocytopenia (bruising or bleeding) occurs after a first dose of MMR at a rate of 1 in 30500.
Tetanus: caused by toxin of bacteria in soil; causes painful muscle spasms, convulsions, lockjaw.	About 1 in 10 patients die. The risk is greatest for the very young or old.	As for DTPa vaccine (see diphtheria).
Varicella (chickenpox): caused by highly contagious virus; causes low-grade fever and vesicular rash. Reactivation of the virus later in life causes herpes zoster (shingles).	1 in 5000 patients develop encephalitis (brain inflammation). About 3 in 100 000 patients die. Infection during pregnancy can result in congenital malformations in the baby. Onset of infection in the mother from 5 days before to 2 days after delivery results in severe infection in the newborn baby in up to one-third of cases.	About 1 in 5 has a local reaction or fever. A mild varicella-like rash may develop in 3–5 per hundred recipients.

Source: The Australian Immunisation Handbook 8th edn 2003.

Reactions to the combined 'triple antigen' DTaP have decreased since the introduction of acellular pertussis vaccine. Much publicity was focused on the side effects of the old whole cell pertussis vaccine. It was common for infants to be feverish and crying after the DTP vaccination. These effects have been greatly reduced with the use of the new vaccine. Although the old whole cell DTP vaccine was blamed for serious brain damage, several large controlled case studies failed to show any permanent neurological damage that was directly attributable to the pertussis vaccine.

On the other hand, pertussis (whooping cough) is a serious, sometimes fatal, respiratory infection that is particularly serious in infants under six months of age. Encephalopathy occurs in 1.1% of all infants under six months of age who contract pertussis. Acute neurological complications from an attack of whooping cough occur in 2–7% of unimmunised individuals. Worldwide, about 250 000 babies are infected with pertussis each year and many of them suffer brain damage. The vaccine has been very effective in reducing the incidence of the disease in Australia (see Table 14.3).

Lack of compliance with vaccination by some parents puts babies who are too young to be immunised at risk. In the five years between 1993 and 1998 nearly 35 000 cases of pertussis were notified in Australia, and nine babies died in the 1996–97 outbreak. Figure 14.16 shows pertussis admissions and hospitalisations between 1993 and 2002 and illustrates the importance of maintaining herd immunity to prevent epidemics.

Vaccination with the combined measles-mumps-rubella (MMR) vaccine is recommended at 12 months and again at 4 years. The first of these, measles, is a serious, highly infectious viral illness. Acute encephalitis occurs in 2–10 people per 10 000 reported cases of measles, with a mortality rate of 10–15%. About 15–40% of survivors have permanent brain damage. Mumps is an unpleasant but less serious infection and permanent adverse sequelae are rare. Orchitis may occur in up to 20% of postpubertal males, but subsequent sterility is rare. Rubella is a mild, often subclinical infection. However, when contracted during the first 8–10 weeks of pregnancy it results in foetal damage in up to 90% of pregnancies. Malaise, fever and a rash may occur 7–10 days after MMR vaccination. Febrile convulsions occur in about 0.1% of children. Symptoms can be alleviated with paracetamol. Reports of the vaccine being linked to autism are unfounded (see Spotlight box, page 326).

It is obvious that the risks associated with immunisation are much less than the risks from having the disease. More importantly, as explained before, a high level of immunisation in the community protects not only immunised individuals, but also the infants who are not old enough to be immunised. Thus, the process of immunisation has wider implications for the community than merely protecting the health of the individual.

The NHMRC has issued recommendations regarding the attendance at school and day-care centres of children who are not adequately immunised. Victoria, the ACT and New South Wales have enacted legislation requiring the provision of immunisation certificates prior to school entry. Children who are not vaccinated against particular diseases are excluded from school when an outbreak of one of the diseases occurs.

HOMOEOPATHIC IMMUNISATION

Some natural health practitioners advocate homoeopathic immunisation as a safe alternative to the recommended schedule. However, the NHMRC childhood immunisation schedule has been shown to prevent tetanus, diphtheria and poliomyelitis and give a high level of protection against whooping cough, measles, mumps and rubella. 'Homoeopathic "immunisation" has *not* been shown to give protection against infectious diseases; only conventional

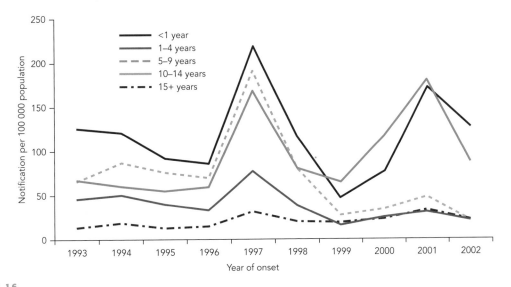

Figure 14.16

Pertussis notifications rates, Australia 1993–2002 by age group

Source: Communicable Diseases Intelligence 2004 (28), Supplement 2, Figure 22, page 543, © Commonwealth of Australia, reproduced by permission

In 1998 a group of British researchers reported the occurrence of an apparently new syndrome of an unusual type of inflammatory bowel disorder (IBD) in a small group of children, in association with developmental disorders such as autism.

The researchers suggested that the MMR vaccine caused IBD, which then resulted in decreased absorption of essential vitamins and nutrients through the intestinal tract. They proposed that this could result in developmental disorders such as autism. However, MMR vaccination and the onset of autism may coincidentally appear associated in time, because the average age at which parents report concerns about child development is 18–19 months, and over 90% of children receive the MMR vaccine before their second birthday in the UK.

More thorough, large epidemiological studies by the World Health Organization have found no evidence of an association. The Global Advisory Committee on Vaccine Safety (GACVS) concluded that:

*no evidence exists of a causal association between measles, mumps, and rubella (MMR) vaccine and autism or autistic disorders.**

However, many parents in Britain decided not to vaccinate their children with MMR and the overall coverage rate has fallen to less than 50%. This creates a potential risk for outbreaks of measles and mumps and the possibility of more cases of congenital rubella. Some parents in Australia have also opted not to vaccinate their children, thus decreasing the protective effect of herd immunity for other susceptible people.

* WHO, Global Advisory Committee on Vaccine Safety, 16–17 December 2002. *Wkly Epidemiol* Rec 2003; 78: 17–18. <http://www.who.int/wer/pdf/2003/wer7804.pdf>

immunisation procedures produce measurable immune response' (*Immunisation Handbook*, 8th edn, p. 315).

Screening procedures

Another important aspect of primary health care is the implementation of screening programs for the detection of infectious diseases. Early detection often allows intervention which can reduce or prevent morbidity and mortality.

ANTENATAL SCREENING TESTS

Among the most useful screening programs are antenatal screening tests. Some infections that are transmitted from mother to baby are not apparent in the mother and can affect the outcome of the pregnancy. If infection can be detected before or during pregnancy, appropriate treatment can be given.

Serological screening before pregnancy to detect the presence or absence of rubella antibody is used to determine the woman's susceptibility to infection so that vaccination can be offered. If exposure occurs during pregnancy, the measurement of IgG and IgM antibodies can assist in counselling. In some cases the presence of antigen or antibody indicates chronic infection (e.g. hepatitis B (HBV), syphilis, human immunodeficiency virus (HIV). For most diseases, the presence of specific IgG antibodies alone indicates past infection and the absence of IgG antibodies indicates susceptibility. The presence of specific IgM antibody suggests recent infection.

Routine screening is only recommended if there is a suitable sensitive test available and there is significant risk of damage to the foetus or infant *that is preventable*.

One of the most important screening procedures is the investigation of pregnant women to determine their status with respect to immunity to rubella. Rubella is a mild disease in adults, but is known to cause serious congenital defects if contracted during the first trimester of pregnancy. Antenatal screening identifies women who are not immune and who should therefore be advised to avoid exposure to people who have the disease. Measurement of the woman's immune status also enables the risk to the foetus from exposure to rubella during pregnancy to be determined. Vaccination of pregnant women is not advised but postnatal immunisation is offered to women who are not immune. Mass immunisation of the whole population with MMR vaccine at 12 months and again at four years is recommended, as well as screening.

Screening for hepatitis B is particularly useful. Mothers who are chronic hepatitis B carriers have a high risk of their baby being infected at term or during delivery. Babies who are likely to be exposed to the virus can be identified by maternal screening during pregnancy, allowing prophylactic treatment to be given. The baby is given anti-hepatitis B immunoglobulin at birth, followed by a course of vaccination. This treatment breaks the chain of vertical transmission.

If syphilis infection is detected early during pregnancy, treatment with antibiotics (penicillin) can be given to the mother to prevent birth defects, which do not usually occur until after 20 weeks' gestation.

Babies are also at risk of infection during passage through the birth canal from organisms present in the vagina. Of these, Group B streptococci (GBS) are the commonest cause of neonatal sepsis (about 1–2 cases per 1000 live births). Detection of GBS in the vagina by screening at 26–28 weeks allows for intra-partum antibacterial prophylaxis for high-risk women (administration of antibacterials just before and during labour).

TUBERCULOSIS

The **Tuberculin skin test (TT)**, or **Mantoux test (Mx)**, consists of a simple skin test to determine whether a person has been exposed to and infected by the tubercle bacillus. It does not always reveal the state of the infection but allows follow-up investigations to be carried out. The test looks for a delayed hypersensitivity reaction to the intradermal injection of a small dose of purified protein from *Mycobacterium tuberculosis*. The injection site is examined after 48–72 hours and the diameter (in mm) of the resulting **induration** is measured as an estimate of the strength of the reaction.

A Mantoux test may be positive if the person has a latent infection or active disease, has recovered from active disease, or has been vaccinated against tuberculosis with the BCG (Bacille Calmette Guerin) vaccine. It may also give a positive result if the person has been infected with a non-tuberculous mycobacterium (e.g. leprosy). Most Mantoux-positive people have a latent infection and do *not* have active disease when investigated further.

Preventive treatment may be offered to those with a latent infection. Individuals who are infected with the human immunodeficiency virus have a high risk of reactivation of a latent TB infection.

SCREENING OF BLOOD PRODUCTS

In Australia all blood and blood products supplied by the blood bank are screened for the presence of infectious agents. These include the human immunodeficiency virus (HIV), hepatitis B virus (HBV) and hepatitis C virus (HCV), cytomegalovirus (CMV), *Treponema pallidum* (syphilis) and human T cell leukaemia virus I (HTLVI). Blood is not accepted from donors who are classified as 'high-risk' on the basis of their medical history or sexual preference, who are intravenous drug users or who have had previous blood transfusions. A ban has been placed on blood or organ donation by people who have lived for a cumulative period of more than six months in Britain between 1980 and 1996, because of fears of transmission of variant Creutzfeldt-Jakob disease (see Spotlight box, page 240).

Although there is always the possibility of as yet undiscovered viruses or infectious agents being present, current screening procedures ensure that the supply of blood and blood products is as safe as possible.

CERVICAL CANCER DETECTION

Sexually mature women are advised to have regular cervical smear tests (Pap smears) to detect any changes in the cells of the cervix which may lead to invasive carcinoma. Although this is not strictly an infection, many cases of cervical cancer have been associated with prior infection by the human papilloma virus (HPV). Regular screening can detect early cellular changes so that treatment can be given to minimise the risk of progression to cancer (see Spotlight box, page 98).

Infectious diseases in child-care centres

More than half a million children in Australia attend preschool or long-day-care centres.

This is a reflection of changing lifestyles, with many more mothers in the workforce than in previous years. The centres cater for children from a few weeks of age up to five years. Babies, whose immune system is not mature, and toddlers who have not been fully immunised are therefore exposed to a community of people who may be carrying a range of infectious diseases. There is considerable evidence that children attending these centres suffer from more infectious diseases than children cared for at home. Some of these diseases are minor but some can be life-threatening, especially in unimmunised babies. Staff employed in child-care centres are also at risk of contracting some of these infections.

It is important that child-care workers have a thorough knowledge of the important diseases of childhood and understand the principles of transmission of microorganisms and control of infection. These principles are similar to those applied in any health facility. Many trained nurses and health workers are employed in child-care centres and can contribute to the general standard of health and hygiene.

The child-care centre is a unique environment, populated by a large number of people (and microorganisms) from a range of diverse backgrounds. It is different from the child's own home where the population of microorganisms is similar in all members of the family. At home, infants do not come into contact with a large number of people and those they meet are usually immune to childhood diseases and so cannot transmit them.

A feature of this type of facility is the close personal contact between babies, infants and carers, allowing for easy transmission of microorganisms. It is not possible to prevent the spread of all infections, but certain measures can be taken to minimise outbreaks of serious illness. The ways in which pathogens are transmitted are described in Chapter 8.

Special precautions therefore need to be used in these settings to minimise the risk of infection. The NHMRC 2001 publication, *Staying Healthy in Child Care: Preventing Infectious Diseases in Child Care*, deals with all aspects of infection control in child-care centres. It is available online at <www.health.gov.au/nhmrc/publications/pdf/ch40.pdf>. Here, we look briefly at some of the most important points.

MODES OF TRANSMISSION

Aerosol droplets

One of the most common methods of transmission is via aerosol droplets. Pathogens may be shed in secretions from the nose and mouth and transmitted to other children by direct inhalation or by contamination of an object which is handled or placed in the mouth. The diseases transmitted in this way include colds and influenza, diphtheria, whooping cough, measles, meningitis, rubella, respiratory syncytical virus (RSV), viral gastroenteritis and chickenpox, as well as bacterial infections such as *Streptococcus pneumoniae* and *Haemophilus influenzae* (Hib). It is difficult to prevent airborne transmission in confined areas. Secretions from the nose and mouth can be contained by using tissues for nose-blowing, by careful handwashing and by regular washing and disinfection of utensils and toys.

Faecal-oral transmission

A significant part of the daily activities of child care involve toileting. Babies and infants require nappies to be changed; older children need to be toilet trained and are prone to accidents. The potential exists for the microorganisms present in the faeces to be liberally spread around. Viruses, bacteria and parasites may be present not only in the faeces of ill children with obvious signs of diarrhoea but also in the faeces of infected but asymptomatic children. It is very easy for the microorganisms to be transferred from one child to the next, via hands contaminated in the toilet area being put in the mouth. They may also be present on other objects or equipment such as toys, cups, toilets, tap handles, toilet flush buttons, or in nappy-changing areas, on the floor or table tops.

The types of infection transmitted in this way include those responsible for viral or bacterial gastroenteritis: *Shigella*, *Campylobacter*, *Salmonella* and rotavirus, as well as hepatitis A, hand, foot and mouth disease (coxsackie virus) and the protozoan *Giardia.*

Suspected outbreaks of gastroenteritis should be notified to the relevant health authorities so that investigations and control measures can be implemented. Children with diarrhoea should be excluded.

Children need to be taught how to wash their hands after going to the toilet. Staff also need to be thoughtful about handwashing. The spread of organisms around the centre can be minimised by following correct procedures for nappy-changing areas and use of the toilet. Contaminated areas should be cleaned and disinfected promptly, but care must be taken that infants do not come into contact with harsh disinfectant solutions. The use of protective nappy covers, and the wearing of pants and other clothing can also reduce the spread of faecal microorganisms.

Skin infections

Children are very prone to skin infections, associated usually with minor scratches, abrasions or mosquito bites. The infections are often caused by staphylococci or streptococci; they can easily develop into impetigo and, in severe cases, cause systemic infections. It is important that infected skin sores are treated with antibiotics and the sore is covered to prevent shedding of the bacteria onto floors, carpets or bedding where they can be transmitted to other children. Children sitting on the floor when they have uncovered infected sores on their legs is a common way of spreading these skin infections. In serious cases of impetigo, the child may be excluded from the centre unless the sores can be adequately covered.

Pathogens in blood and body fluids

Hepatitis B, hepatitis C and human immunodeficiency virus (HIV) are transmitted by direct contact with blood or body secretions. Contact with urine and saliva can be responsible for the transmission of mumps and cytomegalovirus. Staff should be aware of the use of Standard Precautions.

PREVENTION OF CROSS-INFECTION

Various strategies can be employed to prevent cross-infection. Many of these are derived from similar practices in hospitals and health facilities. They are based on a knowledge of the different types of microorganisms responsible for infectious diseases and an understanding of the method of transmission of each pathogen.

Handwashing

Regular handwashing before and after each task and contact with children (especially with respiratory secretions) is the most effective method of infection control. Gloves should be worn when handling body substances and hands should be washed after removing the gloves. Good hygiene, thorough cleaning and disinfection procedures all play an important part in preventing the transmission of infections. Children should also be encouraged to wash their hands when they arrive and before they leave the centre, after toileting or nappy changing, before eating and after playing outside (see Figure 14.17).

Separation of tasks

It is important that child-care workers are aware of the importance of separate areas for different tasks. For example, staff who are involved with food preparation should not also change nappies. There is always the possibility of contamination of their clothing as well as their hands so it is preferable that these duties are performed by different personnel. If this is not possible, staff should use protective clothing and be aware of the importance of thorough handwashing between tasks. If any of the surfaces, taps or door handles in the kitchen are contaminated, there is the potential for the organism to contaminate the food or eating utensils and thus be spread to all the children.

Food preparation is an important area where infection can easily be spread (see Spotlight box on the next page). Staff should be aware of regulations regarding the handling of food. Hands should be washed before preparing food and all surfaces and utensils involved in food preparation kept scrupulously clean. Children's hands should be washed before eating and they should not share food or utensils or anything else they may put in their mouths (e.g. dummies, toothbrushes). The food should be well heated and served at once or else covered and refrigerated. It should not be allowed to stand at room temperature for any length of time before eating (see Figure 14.18).

Sharing of toys is a common way for pathogens to be transmitted from one child to another. Toys should be washable and cleaned or disinfected at least once a week to minimise the transfer of microorganisms. Children should have their own personal items such as toothbrushes.

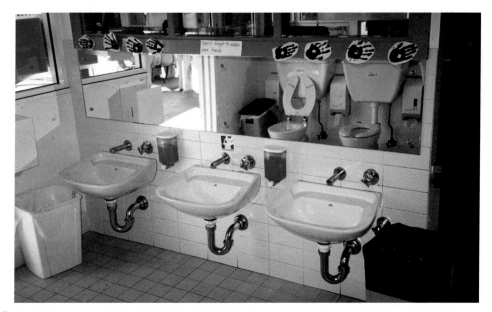

Figure 14.17

Well designed toilet and handwashing facilities encourage good hygiene

SPOTLIGHT ON

Gastroenteritis

Case Report: Outbreak of gastroenteritis due to *Salmonella typhimurium* in a child-care centre

In December 2002, 17 people (12 children, 4 staff and one parent) associated with a large child-care centre in Brisbane reported symptoms of gastroenteritis. Investigations by health authorities included surveillance, and inspection of food-preparation facilities and procedures. It was concluded that the cause of the outbreak was most likely the presence of *Salmonella* on the shells of unwashed eggs purchased from a local supplier who did not comply with health regulations for cleaning eggs.

Comment

Children are particularly vulnerable to the consequences of *Salmonella* infection. The organism is frequently associated with poultry and poultry products. Legislation and standards are in place for food handling in child-care centres. All food should have been produced under a quality assurance program that guarantees the produce. Eggs should be cleaned and checked for cracks. Food handlers should be aware of this when purchasing and preparing eggs, and of the importance of handwashing after handling eggs.

Adapted from BJ McCall et al. 2002, *CDI Bulletin*, 26: 257–9.

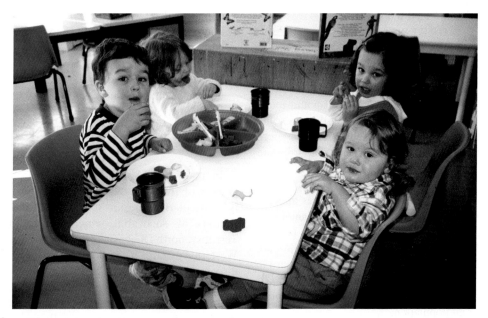

Figure 14.18

The use of separate plates and utensils can minimise transmission of infection

Sometimes the most effective way of preventing the spread of disease is to place children in separate groups or play areas depending on their level of susceptibility (i.e. age and immune status).

Protection against disease

Immunisation was discussed earlier in this chapter. It is the most effective method of protection against many childhood diseases. Legislation allows schools and child-care centres to exclude unimmunised children when there is an outbreak of an infectious disease for which a vaccine is available. The recommended schedule for childhood immunisations is given in Table 14.4.

Immunisation not only protects the person who has been immunised, but also children who are too young to be immunised or those who have been vaccinated but did not respond. As discussed earlier in this chapter, it is essential to establish a high level of **herd immunity** in these susceptible communities. Parents who refuse to have their children immunised are placing at risk all children who are too young to be fully immunised. This is very important in the child-care setting where close contact allows for easy transmission of pathogens, especially by the respiratory route. The serious, vaccine-preventable diseases, diphtheria and whooping cough, can be fatal in small infants.

Exclusion of sick children

To prevent the spread of disease in a centre, it is sometimes necessary to exclude sick children and their contacts from the centre until they are no longer infectious to others. Exclusion of infectious children is an important way of breaking the chain of infection in a centre. The NHMRC has published guidelines for the recommended minimum periods of exclusion of infected children *and their contacts* from school, preschool and child-care centres.

OCCUPATIONAL RISKS FOR CHILD-CARE WORKERS

Staff in child-care centres are also exposed to the infectious diseases that affect the children. Scrupulous attention to handwashing can prevent the transmission of some of these infections to staff. All staff should make sure they are fully immunised, especially as some childhood diseases, such as chickenpox, can be more serious in adults. Additional vaccines that are appropriate for child-care workers are hepatitis A, hepatitis B and chickenpox.

Children who are born overseas are sometimes infected with tuberculosis (as indicated by a positive Mantoux or Tuberculin test) and their dormant infection may become active after their migration to Australia. Child-care workers should be aware of the increased risk of disease in children from countries with a high prevalence of TB. Regular Mantoux testing of staff may be advised in centres with a high migrant population.

Pregnancy

Child-care workers should be aware that some infectious diseases can have serious consequences if contracted during pregnancy. It is especially important for women to be protected against rubella, for which a vaccine is available. If the mother suffers from **rubella** during the first trimester, the baby may be born deaf or blind, or with heart or lung damage. Women intending to become pregnant can have a blood test to determine their rubella antibody titre from previous disease or vaccination, and a booster vaccination may be advisable before becoming pregnant.

Cytomegalovirus (CMV) is a mild disease that is very common in young children. Infection in early pregnancy can have serious effects on the unborn child. Staff can be tested before becoming pregnant to ascertain their level of previous exposure. No vaccine is available. If there is a suspected case in the child-care centre, pregnant women should avoid contact with urine and saliva and have a blood test to determine their immune status and thus assess the risks involved.

Chickenpox infection during pregnancy has been shown to lead to a slightly increased risk of congenital damage. Infections with **human parvovirus**, *Erythema infectiosum* (fifth disease), causes miscarriage in a small percentage of women.

Health care in rural and remote areas

The challenges of the provision of health care in remote areas of Australia are often quite different from those encountered in large city hospitals. Various factors influence the type and severity of the infectious diseases encountered. They include:

- climate and environmental conditions that favour some microorganisms that are not commonly found in other parts of Australia
- socioeconomic factors such as education, unemployment and lifestyle, as well as availability of good housing, sanitation and clean water supplies
- availability and access to health services, and the level of compliance with public health measures such as immunisation.

In many areas of rural Australia, certain diseases occur with a frequency above the national average. This is particularly true in the unique tropical northern regions of Australia, which include the Northern Territory, north Queensland and the Kimberley region of Western Australia. The range and incidence of infectious diseases vary between regions and are significantly different from the rest of Australia. These areas have a wide range of vegetation and a tropical climate, and are the habitat for organisms not usually found in other parts of Australia. When humans disturb the natural ecology of these regions they may be exposed to new micro-organisms.

The special health problems faced by the people in the northern parts of Australia are the subject of a number of ongoing projects at the Menzies School of Health Research in Darwin. As well, the Northern Territory Department of Health and Community Services collects and coordinates the publication of reports of infectious diseases in the quarterly *Northern Territory Disease Control Bulletin*, which is also available online at <http://www.nt.gov.au/health/cdc/bulletin/index.shtml>.

ABORIGINAL HEALTH

The northern tropical areas of Australia have a larger proportion of Aborigines and Torres Strait Islanders than other regions. There have been numerous studies and reports dealing with the health status of indigenous people. They highlight the disparity in general health and incidence of infectious diseases that exists between indigenous and non-indigenous people.

Aboriginal and Torres Strait Islander people are disadvantaged in terms of most socioeconomic indicators (income, education, employment, housing). They experience a greater burden of both communicable and non-communicable disease and have a lower life expectancy (up to 20 years less) than other Australians. This is notice-able in the high mortality rate among young adults (20–40 years). The mortality rate for Aborigines is between two and four times the rate for the Australian population as a whole. Although many deaths are due to circulatory diseases, hypertension, chronic heart disease, diabetes, alcohol abuse and trauma, there are also significant differences in the morbidity and mortality rates for infectious diseases. Underlying diseases contribute to the severity and morbidity of infectious diseases (see Figure 14.19).

Approximately 25% of Aborigines and Torres Strait Islanders live in remote areas, mainly the Northern Territory, including the Top End and Central Australia. While many Aborigines living in urban environments experience poorer health and lower socioeconomic conditions than other Australians, Aborigines in the north are also exposed to a number of unique tropical diseases. The overall notification rate for communicable diseases from the Northern Territory is six times the national average, and mortality rates are three to four times greater than the rate for non-Aboriginal people in the Territory.

There are significant differences in the incidence of infectious diseases between Central Australia and the Top End, and between Aboriginal and non-Aboriginal people in each region (Table 14.7). The rate for Central Australian Aborigines is 20 times the national average, and for the

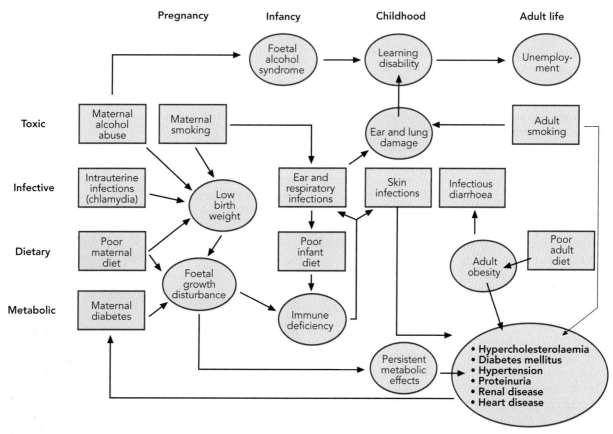

Figure 14.19

Diagram of Aboriginal health

Source: Mathews J. et al. Aboriginal Health, Menzies School of Health Research, Darwin. Reproduced with permission from *Today's Life Science*, 1995; 7(8): 24.

Table 14.7

Rate ratios of Northern Territory nationally notifiable diseases; Australian rates as reference

LOCATION AND ETHNIC ORIGIN	RATE RATIO AUSTRALIA = 1
Top End Aboriginal	11.1*
Top End non-Aboriginal	0.8*
Top End total	6.9
Central Aboriginal	20.6
Central non-Aboriginal	2.9
Central total	8.3
Total Northern Territory Aboriginal	14.3*
Total Northern Territory non-Aboriginal	1.9*
Total Northern Territory	6.0

* 46.7% of the data from the Top End is missing and therefore these are the minimum rate ratios.

Source: A. Ruben, Master of Applied Epidemiology thesis, ANU, 1994.

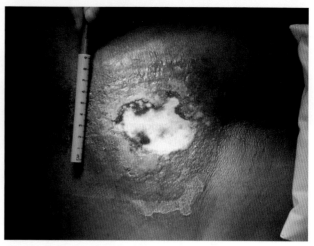

Figure 14.20

Severe staphylococcal abscess resulting from a delay in seeking medical treatment

Top End 11 times the national average. The variations between the Top End and Central Australia are explained, in part, by the differences in climate and socioeconomic conditions. Notification data are often incomplete, so the figures are probably an underestimate of the true incidence of infections.

At all stages of their lives, Aboriginal people in remote areas experience poorer health than non-Aboriginals. Despite improvements in recent years, the infant mortality rate (in the first year of life) is still two to three times higher than the rest of Australia. Disorders of growth and nutrition are prevalent among Aboriginal people. Infants are often malnourished and vulnerable to a range of infections and other diseases such as pneumococcal meningitis. In all age groups, there are serious diseases that occur more commonly in Aboriginal than in non-Aboriginal people. They include diabetes, circulatory disorders, eye and ear infections, and other communicable diseases. Many of these are directly related to deficiencies in nutrition, lifestyle and housing. Many Aboriginal people living in remote areas delay seeking medical treatment – often resulting in a more serious outcome (see Figure 14.20).

Among the communicable diseases, Aborigines have a much higher incidence of sexually transmitted infections and tuberculosis than the rest of Australia. The risk of death from cervical cancer for Aboriginal women is much higher than in non-Aboriginals, especially in rural and remote areas. Compliance with vaccination used to be below the national average but has improved in recent years (see Figure 14.15).

To improve Aboriginal health, there is general agreement on the need to coordinate services at the community level, with community-controlled health services and Aboriginal health workers taking a prominent role in the delivery of primary health care and the implementation of specific programs. It is also essential that health professionals have a good understanding of the culture of the people for whom care is being provided.

INFECTIOUS DISEASES IN THE ABORIGINAL POPULATION

Overcrowded living conditions and poor hygiene in many Aboriginal communities lead to a high rate of bacterial colonisation. The carriage of bacteria by infants and young children provides a reservoir of infection and allows cross-infection and reinfection to occur. Bacterial infections are responsible for chronic morbidity (illness) and mortality in many Aboriginal children. Complications (sequelae) of bacterial infections include chronic bronchitis, blindness, infertility, deafness, rheumatic heart disease and renal failure in adult life.

Group A Streptococcus pyogenes (GAS)

Streptococcal impetigo is frequently seen in Aboriginal children. A number of factors contribute to the existence and persistence of skin sores. Skin lesions due to minor trauma, mosquito bites and scabies infestations (see Figure 14.21)

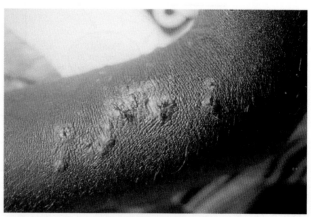

Figure 14.21

Streptococcal skin infection associated with scabies infestation

can become infected with bacteria. Scabies is endemic in most Aboriginal communities and transmission occurs via close body contact, bed linen, etc. Continuous itching and scratching of scabies allow secondary bacterial infections with GAS to occur.

Various sequelae (outcomes) are attributed to infection with GAS, including **rheumatic fever** and **acute post-streptococcal glomerulonephritis** (APSGN). These diseases are commonly seen in Aboriginal communities, attributed largely to overcrowded living conditions. Such diseases are rarely seen in developed countries if streptococcal infections are well managed.

Rheumatic fever may cause damage to the aortic and mitral valves of the heart due to immunogenic reactions to streptococcal antigens. The weakened heart valves are susceptible to further infection and disease later in life (see Chapter 20).

Epidemics of **acute post-streptococcal glomerulonephritis** occur at regular intervals in Aboriginal communities in the Northern Territory and far north Queensland. However, **glomerular haematuria** and/or **proteinuria** (blood and protein in the urine) are also common in non-epidemic circumstances (the incidence is 20% in school-age children) and patients with infected skin sores are more likely to have evidence of renal impairment. The lack of access to renal dialysis machines is another problem as many Aborigines are unwilling or unable to travel long distances to large centres where facilities are available. The incidence of end-stage renal failure is about 100 times greater for Bathurst and Melville Islanders than for other Australians, and rates for other Northern Territory Aborigines are about ten times the national average. The contribution that persistent childhood infections with GAS makes to chronic renal disease is uncertain as other factors, including diabetes, obesity and hypertension, also play a role.

Meningococcal disease

Overall, the incidence of meningococcal disease in indigenous Australians is nearly six times that in non-indigenous people. Serogroup C causes 15% of disease in indigenous people, compared with about 30% in non-indigenous people.

Otitis media

Chronic otitis media (OM) (middle ear disease) and associated hearing loss are prevalent among Australian Aborigines. About 50–80% of school-age children have been shown to be affected, as well as a significant proportion of adults. Perforated eardrums are present in up to 40% of infants aged less than 12 months. Recent studies in the Northern Territory have shown that otitis media develops in Aboriginal infants below the age of three months with a high prevalence of non-inflamed but immobile eardrums, **otitis media with effusion (OME)**. This can progress to **acute otitis media** and develop into **chronic suppurative otitis media (CSOM)** with associated loss of hearing.

The rapid and early onset of otitis media in Aboriginal children is associated with early nasal colonisation by a number of bacteria, in particular *Streptococcus pneumoniae*, *Haemophilus influenzae* and *Moraxella (Branhamella) catarrhalis*, which are able to spread to the middle ear.

Ear infections leading to hearing impairment have serious educational outcomes for the affected individuals. Students with fluctuating hearing loss are likely to exhibit poor behaviour patterns and to experience learning difficulties. Lack of hearing and subsequent poor communication skills may cause children to perform poorly or to stop attending school altogether.

Trachoma

Trachoma is a chronic conjunctivitis caused by repeated episodes of infection with *Chlamydia trachomatis*. If left untreated trachoma can lead to blindness. It begins as conjunctivitis, called 'follicular' or inflammatory trachoma, seen mainly in young children. This can lead to cicatricial trachoma. Scarring of the eyelids causes the eyelashes to turn inwards (trichiasis), the cornea becomes opaque and blindness results. The disease is spread person to person and within the family unit.

Because the prevalence has decreased over the last 20 years, some health workers no longer regard the disease as serious, but the prevalence of follicular trachoma in children in some remote areas in Western Australia is still high, ranging from 15% in the Kimberleys to 55% in the Pilbara. The occurrence of trichiasis increases with age.

A new treatment for trachoma is now available. Azithromycin is a macrolide antibiotic which is effective when used as a single dose. It replaces prolonged courses of tetracycline ointments or drops. In areas where it has been used, a 95% success rate has been recorded.

Haemophilus influenzae type b (Hib) infections

As well as giving rise to otitis media, infections due to invasive *Haemophilus influenzae* type b (Hib) cause meningitis, pneumonia, epiglottitis, septicaemia, osteomyelitis, septic arthritis and cellulitis. Children under five years are particularly susceptible and children in the Northern Territory and far north Queensland, especially Aboriginal children, used to have among the highest rates of Hib infection in the world. The introduction of Hib vaccine has seen a 98% fall in the incidence of Hib disease in the age groups targeted by vaccination programs in the Northern Territory as well as the rest of Australia (see Figure 14.11).

Streptococcus pneumoniae

As well as causing otitis media in children, this organism is a significant cause of pneumonia and meningitis in children and adults. In the Northern Territory, invasive pneumococcal disease is responsible for 40% of community-acquired bacterial pneumonia in adult Aborigines admitted to hospital, with a mortality rate of 21%. The invasive disease is 14 times higher in Aboriginal than non-Aboriginal people in the Northern Territory (see

Figure 14.9). A pneumococcal vaccine is recommended for adult use and a new polyvalent conjugated vaccine is now available for use in children under two years.

Respiratory syncytial virus

Respiratory syncytial virus (RSV) is a major cause of lower respiratory tract infection in young children, causing bronchiolitis, pneumonia and tracheobronchitis that often require hospitalisation. Data from Western Australia and north Queensland show that the rate of hospital admissions for bronchiolitis was at least three times higher for indigenous children than for non-indigenous children.

Gastrointestinal infections

The rates in the Northern Territory for enteric diseases caused by *Shigella*, *Salmonella*, *Campylobacter* and hepatitis A are all significantly higher than in other parts of Australia. The highest incidence occurs in children under five years of age, and the ratio of Aboriginal to non-Aboriginal infections is as high as 30:1. Outbreaks of rotavirus are common. Shigellosis is the most infectious of the bacterial enteric diseases. Seasonal outbreaks of gastroenteritis due to the protozoan *Cryptosporidium parvum* have been reported from Alice Springs.

Hepatitis

A seroprevalence study of Aboriginal children in the Top End has shown a high burden of exposure to hepatitis A by the age of five years. Similar data are not available for non-Aboriginal children in the Northern Territory. The high incidence of hepatitis B carriers in the Aboriginal population has been recognised for some time and the Northern Territory was the first to introduce hepatitis B vaccination into the recommended childhood schedule.

Tuberculosis

The Northern Territory has the highest incidence of notifications of new cases of tuberculosis in Australia about six times the national average. Although there is a high level of TB in the Aboriginal population, two-thirds of all notifications in Australia are for foreign-born individuals.

Leprosy

A few cases of leprosy are notified each year, spread among all States. Early diagnosis and use of the WHO-recommended multi-drug therapy can help to prevent serious neurological damage.

Sexually transmitted infections

Sexually transmitted infections (STIs) account for over 50% of all notifications of communicable diseases from the Northern Territory. They occur mainly in the 15–50 age group, with a higher frequency in Central Australia than in the Top End, which may reflect the higher proportion of Aboriginal people in Central Australia. Syphilis, gonorrhoea and chlamydia are the most commonly notified STIs, followed by genital herpes, non-specific urethritis (NSU) and donovanosis. Donovanosis is now much less common due to programs of treatment with azithromycin. It is rarely seen in the southern parts of Australia.

The high level of STIs in the Northern Territory is of concern because of the possibility of the spread of AIDS. STIs that have ulcerative lesions, such as syphilis and donovanosis, provide an increased risk factor for transmission of the AIDS virus.

UNUSUAL DISEASES OF RURAL AND REMOTE AREAS

As discussed above, the remote areas of Australia provide a unique environment for the occurrence of diseases that are not commonly seen in more settled areas.

Melioidosis

Melioidosis is the most common cause of fatal, community-acquired bacterial pneumonia in the Northern Territory. It is caused by a soil organism, *Burkholderia pseudomallei* (formerly *Pseudomonas pseudomallei*), which is endemic in northern Australia. It usually gains entry to the body through breaks in the skin during exposure to soil or water, especially during the wet season. Percutaneous exposure may be followed by the bacterium spreading to the lungs and causing pneumonia. Melioidosis can cause abscesses in the skin or in deep tissue and body organs (Figure 14.22).

There is a spectrum of presentations from fulminant sepsis with a 25% fatality rate to subclinical infections which may reactivate years later. Risk factors include diabetes, alcohol-related problems and renal disease. Prompt diagnosis and treatment is required to prevent fatal outcomes. Environmental factors such as rainfall contribute to variations in incidence.

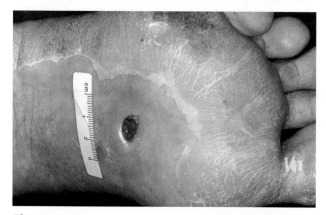

Figure 14.22
Lesion of melioidosis

Leptospirosis

Leptospirosis is a zoonosis with worldwide distribution and is now recognised as an re-emerging disease. The disease is likely to be underdiagnosed in visitors or people returning to Australia and may need to be considered among the many causes of travel-associated febrile illness.

In Australia leptospirosis occurs mainly in rural Victoria, Queensland and the Northern Territory. It is caused by a spirochaete, *Leptospira interrogans*, serovar *australis* being the one most commonly associated with serious infections in Australia. Symptoms include headache, chills, myalgia, rash and, sometimes, meningitis and jaundice; in severe cases there may be pulmonary haemorrhage and liver and kidney failure. The disease is usually a result of occupational exposure to animals and animal urine. See Figures 14.23 and 14.24.

Transmission to humans occurs by skin contact (especially if broken) with the tissues or urine of infected animals or with contaminated water, soil or vegetation. It can also be contracted by recreational exposure to contaminated water (e.g. in national parks). Reservoirs include domestic and native rodents, bandicoots, rabbits, cattle and feral pigs. The incidence is highest in north Queensland, especially among workers in the banana industry.

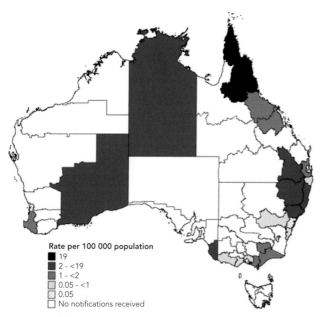

Figure 14.23

Notification rates of leptospirosis Australia 2003, by statistical division of residence

Source: Communicable Diseases Intelligence 2005, 29(1), Map 9, page 51, © Commonwealth of Australia, reproduced by permission

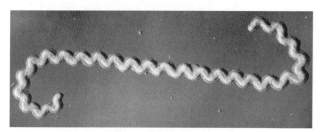

Figure 14.24

Scanning electron micrograph of *Leptospira interrogans*

Scrub typhus

Scrub typhus is caused by the rickettsia *Orientia tsutsugamushi* and is transmitted to humans by the bite of a mite that lives on rodents. It occurs wherever the host mite is found and is widely distributed throughout areas of South-East Asia, the north-west of Western Australia, far north Queensland, the Torres Strait Islands and also in Litchfield Park in the Northern Territory.

It is difficult to diagnose as symptoms are non-specific headache, fever, myalgia and a maculopapular rash affecting the trunk. An eschar may be visible at the site of the bite (see Figure 14.25). Scrub typhus can be successfully treated with doxycycline or azithromycin but has a 50–60% mortality without antibiotic treatment.

Q fever

Q fever is caused by the rickettsia *Coxiella burnetii* and occurs mainly in cattle-raising areas, although it is not seen in the Northern Territory. Transmission is by the airborne dissemination of the organism in dust particles, or by contact with contaminated animals. Abattoir workers, meat packers and stockyard workers are most at risk. A vaccine is available.

Arboviruses

Arboviruses, including Ross River virus, Barmah Forest virus, Kunjin virus and Murray Valley encephalitis virus, are carried by mosquitoes and tend to occur mainly in rural areas where mosquitoes breed in the wet season (see Spotlight box, page 336). The tropical climate of northern Queensland favours the mosquito *Aedes aegypti*, which can act as a vector for **dengue fever**. Although the dengue virus is not endemic in Australia, cases of the disease imported by travellers from overseas can cause an epidemic if the mosquitoes are not controlled (see below).

IMPLICATIONS FOR HEALTH CARE

The range and severity of infectious diseases seen in remote areas, together with the socio-economic conditions that prevail, pose special challenges to health workers. Because of the distances involved, many people living in these areas often do not seek medical care until the disease is well advanced (see Figure 14.20). In addition, underlying illnesses may contribute to the severity of the disease and make diagnosis more difficult. Health workers also need to be aware of the customs and taboos of indigenous people.

Protocols have been developed specifically for these areas and health workers should be aware of their

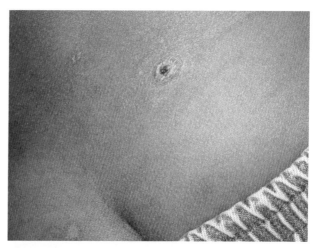

Figure 14.25

Typical eschar of scrub typhus due to infection by the rickettsia *Orientia tsutsugamushi*

SPOTLIGHT ON
Arboviruses

The wet season in Australia usually begins in November with heavy rains and flooding in Central and northern Australia and continues throughout the summer, providing extensive breeding grounds for mosquitoes. Health departments in Western Australia, South Australia and the Northern Territory issue warnings to residents and tourists, especially campers, about the risks of being bitten by mosquitoes that might be carrying Ross River virus, or other mosquito-borne diseases. Outbreaks of disease caused by arboviruses (**ar**thropod-**bo**rne virus) have been increasing in recent years, causing significant morbidity.

Ross River virus (RRV) is the most common of a number of arboviruses that are endemic in Australia. Other endemic viruses that cause significant morbidity and occasional mortality are Barmah Forest virus, Murray Valley encephalitis virus and Kunjin virus. Japanese encephalitis and dengue fever occur in Australia but the index case is usually imported.

Ross River virus infection occurs in cycles dependent on environmental conditions such as tides and rainfall (see Figure 19.13). The virus is carried by a number of mosquitoes, the most common being *Aedes vigilax* or 'salt marsh' mosquito which bites during the day and night, and the common banded mosquito, *Culex annulirostris,* which is found throughout Australia and feeds mainly in the evening and at night. Mosquitoes spread the virus after feeding on an infected animal or person then biting another human. See Figure 14.26.

The highest incidence of the disease is usually in north Queensland with the peak season extending from February until May but in recent years large outbreaks have occurred throughout the summer in other parts of Australia, including the north coast of New South Wales, Western Australia, throughout the Northern Territory and as far as Kangaroo Island in South Australia.

The main preventive measure is to avoid being bitten by mosquitoes. People should wear long-sleeved shirts, loose-fitting protective clothing, use insect repellents, ensure that insect screening is adequate in homes and avoid known mosquito areas and wetlands, especially at dusk and dawn. Residents should control mosquito breeding around homes by emptying water from containers, pools and guttering. Macropods, especially kangaroos, are the main vertebrate hosts for RRV.

Symptoms of Ross River fever and Barmah Forest viral infection are flu-like chills, fever, pain in joints and muscles, chronic fatigue and headaches. The joints may be swollen and stiff and a rash may occur that lasts for 7–10 days. Most people recover in a few weeks but in some the symptoms of polyarthritis persist for months and even up to a year. The disease causes significant morbidity and loss of earning capacity in rural areas. Tourists returning from endemic areas can spread the disease to the city if the appropriate mosquito vector is present.

In the Perth metropolitan area in 2004 a large number of cases were reported, confirming the theory that Ross River virus disease has become more urbanised and that domestic mosquitoes are spreading the virus.

The mosquito-borne disease, Murray Valley encephalitis (MVE) is a potentially fatal illness. The symptoms are severe headache, high fever and drowsiness, which in serious cases can lead to coma and death. Mild cases make a full recovery but serious non-fatal cases can display long-term neurological sequelae, such as paraplegia. The last serious outbreak of MVE was in 1974. It originated along the Murray River and spread to other parts of Australia. There have been sporadic cases since then, located mainly in the northern regions of Australia. Three cases of Murray Valley encephalitis were reported in 2001, two in Alice Springs and one in Mt Isa, and there was one case in Central Australia in 2004. February to May is the peak risk period for the virus in the Northern Territory. People living, visiting or camping overnight within 5 kilometres of swamp, creek and river systems are at greatest risk.

Kunjin virus is closely related to MVE and West Nile virus. It causes encephalitis, but the disease is usually milder. MVE and Kunjin are transmitted by the common banded mosquito which bites only after sundown. The major vertebrate hosts for both viruses are waterbirds.

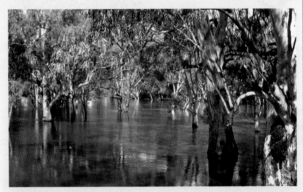

Figure 14.26(a)

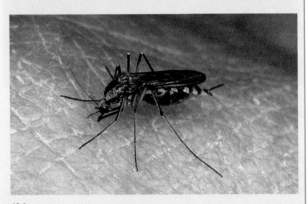

(b)

Flooded river systems (a) provide breeding grounds for mosquitoes (b) which are the vectors for a number of arboviral infections

existence and use them to optimise the treatment and control of infectious diseases. They include:

- specific immunisation schedules
- additions to the list of notifiable diseases
- treatment protocols for use by health workers
- input into the national Antibiotic Guidelines.

Infectious diseases from outside Australia

Australia is fortunate in that, being an island, it is free from some of the infectious diseases that occur in other parts of the world. However, there is always the risk that some of these diseases may be imported into Australia, carried by travellers, tourists, students or immigrants. As more people undertake overseas travel and more tourists and students visit Australia, the potential for the spread of microorganisms and/or their vectors is increased. The entry of illegal immigrants who have not undergone health screening prior to their arrival poses an additional health risk. In this section we look briefly at some of the diseases that pose potential health problems.

Occasionally, a person suffering from one of these diseases may enter Australia but the disease does not spread because of the lack of an appropriate vector, or does not become established because an intermediate host or animal reservoir is lacking. Diseases such as tuberculosis already occur in Australia, but the incidence is much lower than in other parts of the world and the multi-drug-resistant strains of *Mycobacterium tuberculosis* that are found in other countries have not yet reached Australia. Australian residents returning from overseas sometimes present to their doctors with unusual symptoms. Unless a full history, including overseas travel, is obtained, the correct diagnosis may be missed. A number of cases of unusual diseases are diagnosed each year in Australian travellers returning from overseas.

TUBERCULOSIS

Tuberculosis (TB) is a global disease which, according to the World Health Organization (WHO), affects one-third of the world's population and 50% of all refugees. It is estimated that there are eight million new cases worldwide and over two million deaths each year attributable to TB. Infection with HIV increases susceptibility to TB and it is estimated that, HIV will account for an extra 1.5 million cases of TB per year. TB thrives in areas of poverty, malnutrition, natural disasters and political instability. Nearly two-thirds of all notifications of TB come from South-East Asia and the western Pacific region.

Poorly supervised and partially treated TB infections are responsible for the emergence of multi-drug-resistant strains of TB (MDR-TB) in many countries.

Prior to 1945 the incidence of active tuberculosis in Australia was more than 45 per 100 000 population. A national TB campaign of mass chest X-rays, BCG vaccinations and treatment resulted in a large decline in the rate of notifications. Despite the regional threat of disease, the notification rate for the whole country now averages about 1000 cases per year, or 5.5 per 100 000 population. Although this rate compares favourably with other countries, it is still a cause for concern. The rate varies from over 18 per 100 000 in the Northern Territory to 2 per 100 000 in Tasmania.

Almost 80% of all notifications are in foreign-born people, mainly from Indo-China. Notifications in Australia are monitored by the National Mycobacterium Surveillance System (NMSS) which reports in *CDI*.

Tuberculosis is a highly infectious disease that is readily transmitted from person to person on aerosol droplets. The bacterium lodges in the body, usually in the lungs. It may remain latent for many years or it may develop into active TB (see Chapter 17). Although immigrants are screened prior to entry to Australia, it is possible they may develop TB by reactivation of a earlier infection. They also have a high rate of lymphatic TB.

People infected with HIV are particularly susceptible to reactivation of latent TB infection as well as to new infections. At present, MDR-TB strains are rare in Australia but it is possible they can be transported to Australia by returning travellers. There is concern that all these factors may combine to cause a serious epidemic in a population that is largely non-immune.

The NHMRC working party has identified a number of issues that affect the incidence and management of TB in Australia. These include:

- the pattern of immigration and travel
- the increased worldwide incidence of TB
- the emergence of multi-drug-resistant strains
- the interaction of TB and HIV infection.

The BCG vaccine offers some protection against infection by *Mycobacterium tuberculosis*, but does not guarantee immunity. It is currently recommended for health-care workers in some States, for children in high-risk groups (e.g. Northern Territory Aborigines) and for young travellers to high-risk areas. A disadvantage of BCG vaccination is that it interferes with the interpretation of the Mantoux or Tuberculin test which is used to identify whether exposure to TB has occurred and whether preventive treatment is necessary.

MALARIA

Malaria is the most important of the diseases carried by insect vectors (see Chapter 20). It is endemic in the tropical regions north of Australia, especially South-East Asia, Papua New Guinea (PNG) and the Pacific Islands (see Figure 14.27). The cause of malaria, the protozoan *Plasmodium*, is carried by the Anopheles mosquito which is found in many parts of Australia, especially in the north.

The Torres Strait Islands to the north of Queensland are close to Papua New Guniea and there were four locally acquired cases of *P. falciparum* in the 1990s and two more cases in 2001 which were thought to have been introduced by visitors from PNG. For the disease to spread there has

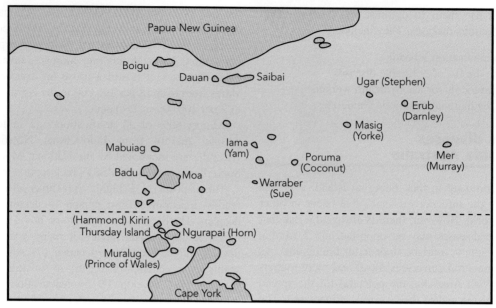

Figure 14.27

Map of Northern Australia and Torres Strait Islands showing proximity to Papua New Guinea and S.E. Asia

to be a reservoir, or pool, of infected people and conditions suitable for the appropriate vector to breed and transmit the disease.

There is a real possibility of the reintroduction of malaria, especially in parts of northern Australia where there is a large number of mosquitoes, many of the dwellings are open and there is an influx of immigrants, tourists and students from high-risk endemic areas. Control of the mosquito vector is the most effective way to prevent reintroduction of the disease.

Australian travellers to endemic areas are at risk of contracting malaria. Between 700 and 1000 cases of malaria contracted outside Australia are notified each year. This is a huge increase in the number of cases compared with 20 years ago and reflects an increase in travel by Australians to endemic areas as well as an increase in immigration. Strains of *Plasmodium* resistant to the antimalarial drug, chloroquine, have appeared in many areas. Although several trials are in progress, there is currently no vaccine against malaria and travellers should consult their health department for up-to-date information on appropriate medication for the areas they intend to visit.

It is important to use preventive strategies to avoid mosquito bites: antimicrobial prophylaxis, insect repellent, long-sleeved clothing, mosquito nets and screens. Travellers should be aware that they may contract malaria, despite taking medication, if the particular strain of the organism is drug-resistant, or if the medication is not appropriate or not taken for long enough.

Malaria should be suspected in any person who has recently returned from a malarious area and is suffering intermittent bouts of fever, headaches and nausea. Microscopic examination of blood films can give a correct diagnosis. Most cases of malaria can be treated successfully if diagnosed early in the course of the disease, but delay can have fatal consequences.

JAPANESE ENCEPHALITIS

Japanese encephalitis is a mosquito borne viral zoonosis, which is widespread in S.E. Asia and Papua New Guinea. Cases have occurred on Badu Island in the Torres Strait during the wet season and there is evidence of activity on the far north tip of Cape York peninsula. A vaccine is recommended for residents in the Torres Strait Islands.

DENGUE FEVER

Dengue fever is a mosquito-borne viral disease occurring mainly in northern parts of Australia. It is carried by the vector *Aedes aegypti*, which is found in some areas of Queensland. Outbreaks of dengue occur from time to time, usually associated with good mosquito-breeding conditions (see Figure 14.1). There are four known serotypes of the virus, all of which have now been isolated in Australia.

The symptoms of dengue fever include acute headache, joint pain, rash and fever, but occasionally haemorrhagic fever and dengue shock syndrome may occur, especially in young children. Haemorrhagic dengue fever appears to occur in people who have a prior history of dengue disease and a second infection with a different serotype of the virus. Dengue fever has been known for many years but has only become a major health problem with extensive global travel, which has allowed circulation of the four serotypes.

Most cases of dengue are acquired outside Australia but returning travellers can pose a threat. This occurred in 2000 when troops returning from East Timor to Townsville imported seven cases of dengue of two different serotypes. None of the cases was haemorrhagic and mosquito control measures ensured the disease did not spread. However, all four serotypes are circulating in Indonesia and there are thousands of cases and hundreds of deaths there each year. Control of the vector *Aedes aegypti* is important in preventing outbreaks of dengue (see Spotlight box, page 468). If different serotypes are involved in separate outbreaks, the risk of haemorrhagic disease is increased.

YELLOW FEVER

Yellow fever is an acute viral disease, transmitted by mosquitoes. It is found in Africa and parts of South America, but does not occur in Australia. A vaccine is available and travellers entering Australia from endemic areas are required to have been vaccinated or to undergo quarantine.

SCHISTOSOMIASIS

Schistosomiasis is a chronic parasitic infection caused by trematodes, or flukes. Their complex life cycle involves a larval form, the free-swimming **cercariae**, which are released from the intermediate host, a freshwater snail. Infection of humans occurs when the cercariae penetrate the skin, usually when the person is working, swimming or wading in contaminated water. A number of cases of schistosomiasis have been recorded in travellers returning to Australia; for example, in a rugby team that had visited Zimbabwe and been white-water rafting on the Zambezi river. Other travellers had been swimming in Lake Malawi.

When correctly diagnosed, schistosome infections can be treated with praziquantel. Travellers should be aware of areas where schistosomiasis is endemic. As long as the species of freshwater snail that is needed as the intermediate host is not imported into Australia, people who are infected will not pose a health risk to other Australians.

Public health issues in New Zealand

Many infectious diseases occur throughout the world, while others are restricted to certain regions. Each country produces its own statistics for the incidence of diseases, and develops policies and regulations appropriate for their control that may differ from their neighbours. Although New Zealand is geographically close to Australia, its climate and population are different. In this section, we examine some of the public health issues that are unique to New Zealand.

The population of New Zealand is about 3.5 million of whom 13% are Maori, 5% are from the Pacific Islands and the remaining 82% are of mainly European origin with an increasing number of people from Asia. The Pacific Islands population living in New Zealand is heterogeneous, consisting of people of the Samoan, Tongan, Cook Islands, Tokelauan, Niuean, Fijian and Tuvaluan ethnic groups, as well as people from Papua New Guinea, Vanuatu and the Solomon Islands. The lifestyles and health problems of the three major groups are different and contribute to the variations in incidence statistics for the various diseases.

SURVEILLANCE

The *New Zealand Public Health Surveillance Report (NZPSHR)* is prepared by the Institute of Environmental Science and Research (ESR) and published jointly by the Ministry of Health and the ESR; it is available online at <www.surv.esr.cri.nz>. The list of about 50 notifiable diseases includes those required by the World Health Organization, as well as other infections for which a public health intervention is required or for which the incidence needs to be monitored. A revised schedule of notifiable diseases came into effect in June 1996, one of the main changes being the addition of vaccine-preventable diseases.

Most sexually transmitted infections (STIs) are not notifiable in New Zealand, and their surveillance has traditionally been based on data from specialist sexual health clinics. STI cases reported through the clinic-based surveillance system underestimate the true burden of disease because a substantial percentage of STIs are diagnosed by other health providers, particularly general practitioners.

Surveillance reports are available for notifiable diseases, influenza, sexually transmitted infections and chemical injuries. The Antibiotic Reference Laboratory at ESR is responsible for the national surveillance of antimicrobial resistance among human pathogens. The ESR public health virology laboratory collates, analyses and reports all-year-round laboratory-based virological surveillance, and the Enteric Reference Laboratory is responsible for the confirmation of isolates of notifiable diseases *Salmonellae*, *Shigellae*, *Vibrio cholera* and VTEC.

Comparison of notification rates of infectious diseases in Australia and New Zealand

Several diseases in New Zealand have a higher rate of notification than in Australia. They include tuberculosis, meningococcal meningitis and rheumatic fever.

The higher incidence of **tuberculosis** in New Zealand is seen mainly in the Maori and Pacific Islander population.

Meningococcal disease is a serious illness caused by *Neisseria meningitidis*. There are three major serogroups – A, B and C – and two minor groups – Y and W-135. A tetravalent vaccine is available for serogroups A, C, W-135 and Y and is used when outbreaks occur. There have been several epidemics of meningococcal disease in New Zealand. When the cases are due to a vaccine-preventable serogroup, a vaccination program for children is instigated. Meningococcal disease presents as meningitis, septicaemia and other diseases. Children under five years are most at risk, especially Maori and Pacific Island children. During an outbreak in 1994, there were 208 cases with 11 deaths, an overall 6.3% mortality rate.

Compared with other developed countries, New Zealand has high rates of post-streptococcal disease such as **rheumatic fever**. The disease presents as arthritis and carditis, affecting the aortic and mitral valves of the heart, and sometimes causing residual damage to the valves of the heart. The person is susceptible to further streptococcal infections and damage to the heart valves. Rheumatic fever is a notifiable disease in New Zealand and a register of patients was set up in 1986. The incidence is highest among Maori and Pacific Island children. In Australia the incidence of rheumatic heart disease is highest among Aborigines.

HEALTH STATUS OF NEW ZEALAND'S ETHNIC GROUPS

The health status of different groups within the community is affected by socioeconomic conditions as well as ethnicity. Various measurements are used to determine the relative health status of the ethnic groups that make up the New Zealand population. These include general health, prevalence of disease or disability, the infant mortality rate, incidence of infectious diseases, and death rates.

At the beginning of the 20th century, a series of epidemics of infectious diseases (influenza, whooping cough, measles), a high mortality rate and land wars drastically reduced the Maori population. The situation was addressed by public health measures such as improvements in hygiene, sanitation, water supplies and vaccination. However, the 1994 report by the Public Health Commission of New Zealand on the health of the Pacific Islands people in New Zealand found that differences still existed in health, incidence of infections and outcome of diseases for the major ethnic groups in New Zealand.

Despite an overall decline in infant mortality in New Zealand in the last 20 years, the rate for Maoris is still almost twice that for Europeans. The rate for Pacific Islanders is similar to that for Europeans. Of the Maori infant mortality rate, 50% is attributed to sudden infant death syndrome (SIDS).

The rate of notification of some infectious diseases varies for people of different ethnic origin. Of the gastrointestinal infections, Pacific Island peoples had higher rates of **hepatitis A** while **campylobacteriosis** was higher among Europeans. Of concern is the high incidence of meningococcal disease in Maoris and Pacific Islanders,

compared with Europeans. The incidence of hepatitis B in New Zealand is quite high, mainly in young adults and injecting drug users. Maoris have a high rate of infection and a greater chance of subsequent **hepatitis B** carriage, leading to chronic hepatic disease.

The incidence of **rheumatic fever** in Pacific Islanders is 20 times that for Europeans and higher than the incidence for Maoris. Hearing loss resulting from **otitis media** affects 6–10% of New Zealand school children. It is more likely to occur in children under seven and is more common among males and Maori children (15%). Pacific Island children have a similar rate to Maori children.

Tuberculosis has declined in most developed countries but there is concern that the incidence will increase as the number of immunosuppressed people rises and there is spread of multi-resistant strains. In New Zealand there is a marked difference in the incidence of TB among ethnic groups. For Europeans the rate in 2004 was 1.5 per 100 000, Maoris 13.9 per 100 000, Pacific Islanders 30.5 per 100 000 and, for other ethnic origins, 78 per 100 000. Of all reported cases, 66% had been born overseas.

IMMUNISATION

The New Zealand Department of Health recommended vaccination schedule (Table 14.8) is contained in the Immunisation Handbook and is available online at <www.immune.org.nz>. This is revised continually and health professionals should ensure they are aware of the most recent schedule. Currently between 80 and 90% of one year olds are fully immunised but this falls to only 60% for 2 year olds. A higher percentage of Maori and Pacific Island people are not immunised compared with children of European origin. Various strategies are being introduced to improve coverage and reach families who do not participate in vaccination programs. A higher coverage is needed to prevent outbreaks of measles and whooping cough.

Table 14.8

New Zealand immunisation schedule – from 1 July 2004

PATIENTS AGE	DTaP-IPV (IM)	Hib-Hep B (IM)	DTaP/Hib (IM)	Hep B (IM)	MMR (SC)	Td (IM)	Influenza (IM)
6 weeks	DTaP-IPV	Hib-Hep B					
3 months	DTaP-IPV	Hib-Hep B					
5 months	DTaP-IPV			Hep B			
15 months			DTaP/Hib		MMR		
4 years	DTaP-IPV				MMR		
11 years						ADT	
45 years						ADT	
65 years						ADT	Influenza

Key: DTaP – diptheria, tetanus, acellular pertussis
      IPV – inactivated polio vaccine (Salk)
      Hib – *Hemophilus influenzae* type b
      Hep B – hepatitis B
      ADT – adult diphtheria/tetanus
Refer to website <www.immune.org.nz> for latest vaccination schedules

SUMMARY

- The decline in mortality from infectious diseases in the 20th century was due to an improved standard of hygiene, the discovery of antibiotics and the development of vaccines.
- Responsibility for the delivery of health care in Australia rests with various State, Territory and Federal authorities.

NOTIFIABLE DISEASES

- A core group of communicable diseases is required by law to be notified to the health authorities when diagnosed in a patient.
- The NNDSS coordinates the adoption of the NHMRC list of diseases for notification and the reporting of notifiable diseases at a Commonwealth level.
- The annual report of the NNDSS is published in the *CDI* bulletin.

PRIMARY HEALTH CARE

- Primary health care involves the provision of services such as health education, health promotion, disease prevention and treatment of illness.
- In Australia the major factors that influence health status are socioeconomic conditions.
- The Aborigines and Torres Strait Islanders have a much lower general standard of health than other Australians.

IMMUNISATION

- Major reasons for improvement in health in the 20th century were the development of vaccines and the implementation of immunisation programs.
- Active immunisation is the administration of a vaccine to stimulate the body's immune system to produce both specific antibodies and cellular immunity.
- The Australian Health Department provides free vaccination for most childhood diseases.
- The NHMRC publishes information on immunisation procedures and recommendations for administration.
- The most effective type of vaccine consists of live, attenuated (weakened) forms of the pathogen. Some vaccines consist of toxoids, some contain killed, whole cells of the pathogen, others consist of fragments of the pathogen.
- The principle of herd immunity means that, for a population to be protected from a disease, a certain percentage must be immunised against that disease.
- In Australia, compliance with immunisation schedules is not complete and there have been epidemics of measles and pertussis.
- The risks from immunisation are much less than the risks from having the disease.
- Children who are not vaccinated against a particular disease will be excluded from school when an outbreak of the disease occurs.
- Vaccines are available for travellers and health workers.
- The NHMRC warns that homoeopathic 'immunisation' has not been shown to give protection against infectious diseases.

SCREENING PROCEDURES

- Screening of women during pregnancy is useful to detect the presence of, or susceptibility to, pathogens that may cause congenital defects.
- The Tuberculin skin test (TT), or Mantoux test (Mx), is a skin test that can determine whether a person has been exposed to and infected by the tubercle bacillus.
- In Australia all blood and blood products supplied by the blood bank are screened for the presence of infectious agents such as the human immunodeficiency virus (HIV), hepatitis B virus (HBV) and hepatitis C virus (HCV), *Treponema pallidum* (syphilis) and human T cell leukaemia virus I (HTLVI).
- Pap smears can detect changes in the cells of the cervix that may lead to invasive carcinoma.

INFECTIOUS DISEASES IN CHILD-CARE CENTRES

- Australian children aged 0–5 years attending child-care centres have a high risk of acquiring infections.
- Infections are transmitted in aerosol droplets, by exposure to faecal material and by handling contaminated toys.
- Skin infections are easily transmitted and can develop into impetigo.
- Cross-infection can be prevented by good hygiene, practising regular handwashing, teaching children to wash hands and by separation of tasks.
- Staff should be immunised and children should be up to date with the immunisation schedule.
- Occupational risks include exposure to childhood infections and pregnant workers should be aware of the risk of congenital infections.

HEALTH CARE IN RURAL AND REMOTE AREAS

- Factors such as climate, socioeconomic conditions and access to health services affect the incidence of infectious diseases in remote areas.
- The Northern Territory Department of Health and Community Services collects and coordinates the publication of reports of infectious diseases in the monthly *Northern Territory Communicable Diseases Bulletin*.

Aboriginal health

- There is a disparity in general health and incidence of infectious diseases between Aboriginal and non-Aboriginal people.
- The overall notification rate for communicable diseases in the Northern Territory is six times the national average.
- The infant mortality rate is 2–3 times higher than the rest of Australia.
- Aborigines have a much higher incidence of sexually transmitted infections and tuberculosis than other Australians.
- Overcrowded living conditions and poor hygiene in Aboriginal communities lead to a high rate of disease and cross-infection.

- Complications (sequelae) of bacterial infections include chronic bronchitis, blindness, infertility, deafness, rheumatic heart disease, and renal failure in adult life.
- Skin infections with Group A *Streptococcus pyogenes* (GAS) may have outcomes such as post-streptococcal glomerulonephritis and rheumatic fever.
- Chronic otitis media (OM) and associated hearing loss are prevalent among Australian Aborigines.
- Trachoma is still a serious disease in some remote areas. It can be treated with azithromycin.
- *Haemophilus influenzae* type b (Hib) infections can cause meningitis, epiglottitis, septicaemia, osteomyelitis, septic arthritis and cellulitis.
- The introduction of the Hib vaccine has reduced the incidence of Hib disease in the Northern Territory as well as in the rest of Australia.
- The incidence of gastrointestinal infections is significantly higher in the Northern Territory than in other parts of Australia.

Unusual diseases of rural and remote areas
- Melioidosis is the most common cause of fatal, community-acquired bacterial pneumonia in the Northern Territory.
- *Leptospira interrogans* is the cause of an acute renal failure with a 5–10% fatality rate. Other unusual diseases include Q fever and dengue fever.
- Arboviral infections occur during the wet season.

Implications for health care
- There are special health-care procedures to be implemented in remote areas – specific immunisation schedules, additional notifiable diseases, antibiotic guidelines for Central and north Australia, and special treatment protocols.

INFECTIOUS DISEASES FROM OUTSIDE AUSTRALIA
- Diseases that are not endemic in Australia may be imported by travellers.

- Eighty per cent of all notifications of active tuberculosis in Australia are in foreign-born people, mainly from Indo-China.
- Multi-drug-resistant strains of *Mycobacterium tuberculosis* (MDR-TB) occur in many countries. At present these strains are not common in Australia.
- Australian travellers to endemic areas are at risk of contracting malaria.
- Dengue fever is an imported viral disease, occurring usually in northern parts of Australia where the vector *Aedes aegypti* is found.
- Yellow fever is an acute viral disease, transmitted by mosquitoes. It is found in Africa and parts of South America, but does not occur in Australia. A vaccine is available.
- Cases of schistosomiasis have been recorded in travellers returning to Australia from Africa.

PUBLIC HEALTH ISSUES IN NEW ZEALAND
- Some public health issues are unique to New Zealand, because of its different climate and population.
- The *New Zealand Public Health Surveillance Report* (*NZPHSR*) is prepared by the Institute of Environmental Science and Research (ESR) and published jointly by the Ministry of Health and the ESR.
- The health status of the different ethnic groups within the community is affected by socioeconomic conditions as well as ethnicity.
- The infant mortality rate for Maoris is almost twice that for Europeans; 50% of it is attributed to sudden infant death syndrome (SIDS). The infant mortality rate for Pacific Islanders is similar to that for Europeans.
- The incidence of several infectious diseases varies among the different ethic groups.
- Vaccine-preventable diseases are now notifiable in New Zealand.

STUDY QUESTIONS

1. What is meant by a 'notifiable' disease?
2. Who is responsible for the notification of infectious diseases?
3. Where can you find information about the incidence of infectious diseases in Australia?
4. What are the functions of the NHMRC?
5. What are some of the public health strategies for the prevention and control of infectious diseases?
6. How does immunisation protect a person from a particular disease?
7. What are the current recommended schedules for childhood vaccination?
8. Why do some vaccines require more than one dose?
9. Why is vaccination for rubella particularly important for pregnant women?
10. What is homoeopathic immunisation? Does it work?
11. Why are antenatal screening tests carried out for some infectious diseases?
12. What information can be gained from a Mantoux test?
13. What is a Pap smear?
14. Which infectious diseases occur most frequently in child-care centres?
15. How are these infections transmitted?
16. Name three ways to minimise the spread of infection in child-care centres.
17. What are some of the major differences between the health of Aboriginal Australians and other Australians?
18. What are some of the infectious diseases that particularly affect Aboriginal people in the Northern Territory?
19. Describe some of the unusual infectious diseases that are seen mainly in remote or rural areas.

20. Name two diseases that are not presently endemic in Australia and describe how they could become established.
21. How does the incidence of infectious diseases in New Zealand differ from that in Australia?

TEST YOUR UNDERSTANDING

1. Why is it important to have comprehensive data on the incidence and prevalence of infectious diseases?
2. What is meant by herd immunity?
3. What are the dangers of non-compliance with vaccination schedules?
4. What are some of the advantages of screening programs?
5. Why should all sexually mature women have regular Pap smears?
6. Why do children in child care have more infections than children cared for at home?
7. What are some of the challenges for the provision of health care in remote areas?
8. Why is Australia free of some serious diseases? How could this change?

Further reading

Currie B 1993, 'Medicine in tropical Australia', *Medical Journal of Australia*, 158: 609.

Currie B 2003, Intensity of rainfall and severity of melioidosis, *Australia. Emerging Infectious Diseases* 9(12): 1538–1542.

'Enough to make you sick': How Income and Environment Affect Health 1992, National Health Strategy Research Paper No. 1, Canberra.

Mathews J, T Weeramanthri & P DíAbbas 1995, 'Aboriginal health', *Today's Life Science*, 7 (8).

Menzies School of Health Research, Darwin, Annual Reports 1991–1999.

NHMRC 2001, *Staying Healthy in Child Care: Preventing Infectious Diseases in Children*, Canberra, Australian Government Publishing Service.

NHMRC, *The Australian Immunisation Procedures Handbook* 2003, 8th edn, Canberra, Australian Government Publishing Service.

New Zealand Ministry of Health, *New Zealand Public Health Surveillance Report (NZPSHR)* <www.surv.esr.cri.nz>.

Ruben A 1994, *Thesis, Masters of Applied Epidemiology*, National Centre for Epidemiology and Population Health, ANU, Canberra.

Taylor HR 1997, *Eye Health in Aboriginal and Torres Strait Islander Communities*, Canberra, Commonwealth Department of Health and Family Services.

Wass A (ed.) 1994, *Promoting Health: The Primary Health Care Approach*, Sydney, Harcourt Brace & Co.

World Health Organization 2000, *Global Tuberculosis Control: WHO Report 2000*. Geneva, World Health Organization.

Websites

Government reports and guidelines and most of the information regarding the incidence of notifiable diseases are available from Internet sites.

- Australian Department of Health and Aged Care: this is the starting point for all information relating to health in Australia.
  http://www.health.gov.au
- This is the introduction to the public health site.
  http://www.health.gov.au/pubhlth
- This is the *Communicable Diseases Intelligence (CDI)* website with links to reports of notifiable diseases, immunisation schedules, etc.
  http://www.health.gov.au.pubhlth/cdi/
- This site provides access to State and Territory government department sites; other university departments and health laboratories; World Health Organization; international government organisations; New Zealand Ministry of Health; US Centers for Disease Control (CDC); International travel information.
  http://health.gov.au/pubhlth/cdi/cdilinks.htm
- National Centre in HIV Epidemiology and Clinical Research.
  http://www.unsw.edu.au/nchecr
- New Zealand public health reports and notifiable diseases data.
  http://www.moh.govt.nz/nzphr.html
- This site provides access to the CDC publication *Emerging Infectious Diseases*, a series of current review articles on world infectious diseases.
  http://wwwcdc.gov.ncidod/EID/index.htm
- A monthly review of notifications of outbreaks of infectious diseases in the European community.
  http://www.eurosurv.org

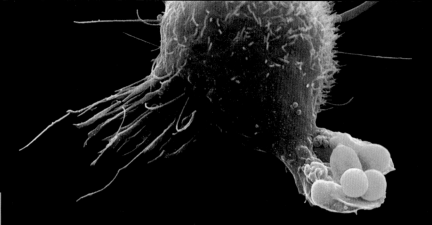

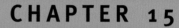

CHAPTER 15

Microbial Techniques for Diagnosis of Infection

Introduction

The main function of the clinical microbiology laboratory is to assist in the diagnosis of infectious diseases. Relatively few infectious diseases can be accurately diagnosed solely on clinical grounds. For an accurate laboratory diagnosis it is essential that an appropriate specimen is properly collected. To achieve this, one must have a good understanding of the pathogenesis and possible cause of infection. If it is suspected that a patient has an infectious disease, certain laboratory tests are requested based on the nature of the symptoms and the likely causative agent. One or more specimens may have to be collected and the doctor, nurse or other qualified health-care worker must perform the collection procedure correctly. The specimen must then be transported promptly to the laboratory for processing. Laboratory findings are made available to the clinical team as soon as possible to facilitate the prompt diagnosis and appropriate treatment of the disease.

A number of different methods are used in the laboratory for the diagnosis of infections. The appropriate method in a given situation is determined by the possible causative agents. Generally, laboratory tests are designed to detect either (1) the microorganism itself or a component of it in a specimen from the patient or (2) evidence of an immune response to the causative organism in the blood of the patient. Five main methods are employed.

1. *Direct microscopic examination of a specimen.* Microscopy is a fundamental technique in microbiology laboratories. A direct microscopic examination of a specimen can provide a very rapid presumptive diagnosis in certain situations. It may also provide information about the host cells present in the specimen, which can indicate the probable type of infection (e.g. viral versus bacterial) as well as the quality of the specimen (e.g. a mucoid versus a purulent sputum).
2. *Culture and isolation of microorganisms from patient material.* A specimen from the patient is used to inoculate appropriate microbiological media (see Figure 15.1) and, after incubation, the cultures are examined for the presence of pathogens. In some cases (e.g. urinary tract infections), the number of microorganisms in the specimen can be estimated. When the causative agent is bacterial, the organism's sensitivity to antibiotics can also be determined. Unfortunately, not all pathogens can be cultured (especially some viruses and protozoa). Another major disadvantage is that culture results may not be available for 18 hours or more for many bacteria, and much longer for viruses. Thus, faster diagnostic methods are continually being sought.
3. *Identification of infection using serologic (or immunologic) reactions.* This involves the detection of specific antibodies to a microorganism in the serum or other body fluid of a patient. A serologic method is generally used when culture of the pathogen is not possible or too difficult, or when culture takes too long (e.g. viruses, protozoa, some bacteria).

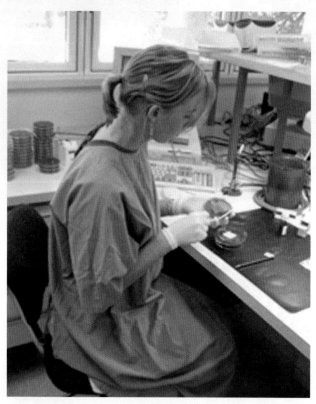

Figure 15.1

Culture of specimens in the microbiology laboratory

4. *Identification of antigens of the microorganism in patient material.* This involves the detection of a particular microorganism or a component (antigen) of it in a specimen from the patient. Antigen detection methods are also useful when culture of the pathogen is not possible, too difficult or too time-consuming. In some diseases, antigens of the microorganism can be detected before the patient produces specific antibodies.
5. *Identification of microbial nucleic acids in a specimen from the patient.* A gene sequence that is specific for a particular microorganism can be detected in patient material by the use of a DNA probe. This method is usually used in conjunction with DNA amplification techniques such as the polymerase chain reaction (PCR). There is immense interest in these DNA techniques, mainly because of their potential speed in identifying microorganisms that are difficult or impossible to isolate by cultural methods.

Time and accuracy are the two key factors in the laboratory diagnosis of infectious diseases. The earlier results become available, the sooner specific steps can be taken for appropriate management of the patient. Not all the methods outlined above are suitable or available for all infections; and the fastest methods are not always the most accurate. The time frames for microscopic and cultural methods, currently the most commonly used, are summarised in Figure 15.2. It should be noted that the times given are for typical organisms and that there are many exceptions to those shown in the figure. There are also many specific methods for some organisms that are not shown in the figure.

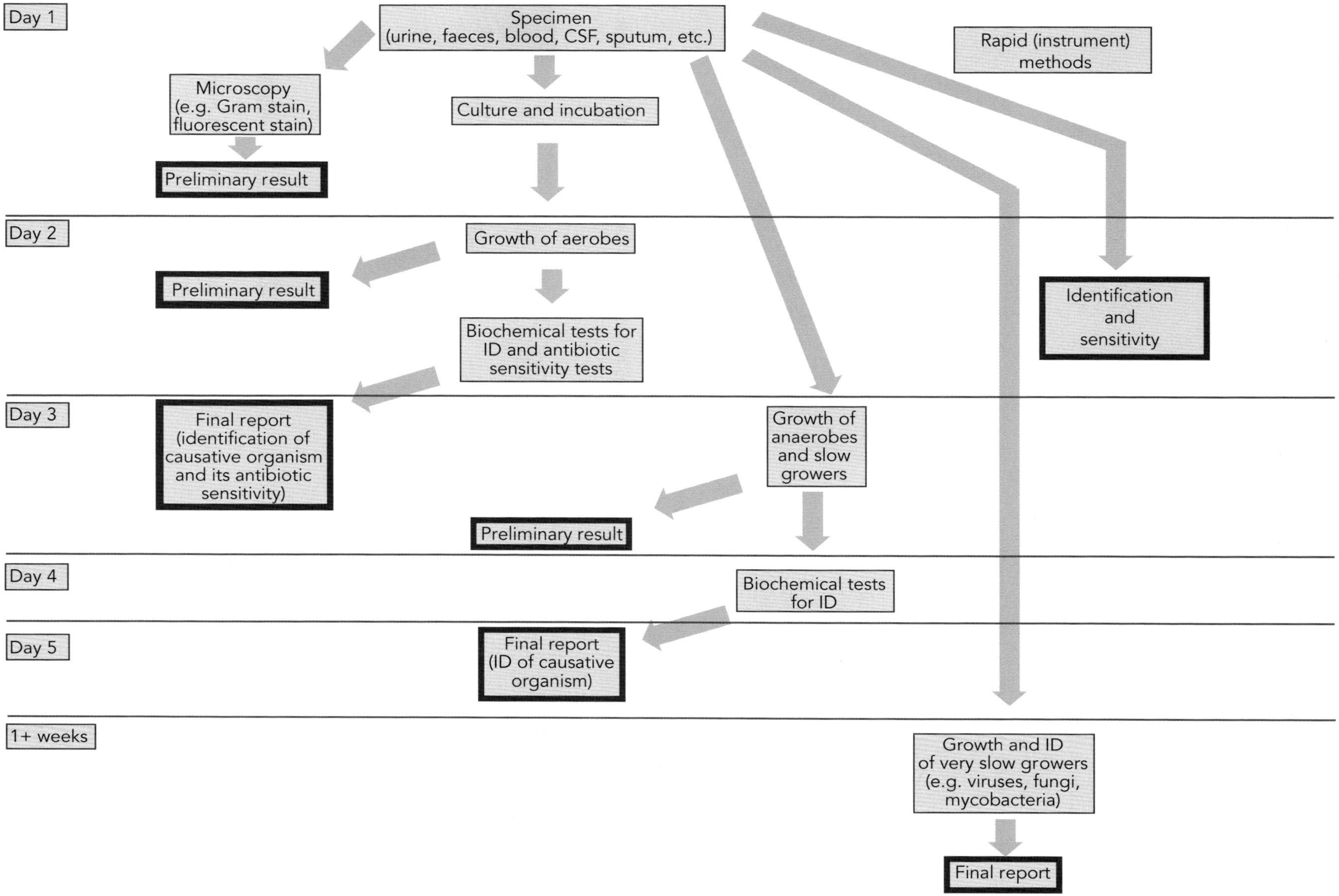

Figure 15.2

Laboratory diagnosis of infectious diseases by culture methods

In relation to the accuracy of a test or method, two terms that are often used are *sensitivity* and *specificity*. The *sensitivity* of a test refers to the proportion (or percentage) of people with a particular disease that can be identified as having the disease by the test. The more people with the disease that are not identified by the test, the less sensitive is the test. A test is also said to lack sensitivity if it can only identify people who are infected with large numbers of the microorganism, and misses people infected with low numbers.

Specificity refers to the proportion (or percentage) of people without the disease who yield a negative test result. The more people without the disease who are indicated by the test as having the disease, the less specific is the test. A positive test result in a person who doesn't have the disease is called a **false positive**. A **false negative** is a negative test result in a person who does have the disease.

Microscopic techniques

Direct microscopic examination of certain specimens can sometimes provide a presumptive diagnosis within an hour, although several hours may be required for more complex staining and microscopic methods. Generally, direct microscopy using a simple light microscope is most useful in the following circumstances.

- When the site of infection is a normally sterile part of the body. For example, in a case of meningitis, a Gram stain of cerebrospinal fluid (CSF) can provide rapid and vital information about the likely cause. The more common causes of acute bacterial meningitis are *Neisseria meningitidis* (a Gram-negative coccus and *Streptococcus pneumoniae* (a Gram-positive coccus), which can be distinguished in a Gram stain (see Figure 15.3).
- When the pathogen is readily distinguishable by its morphology (size, shape and other physical attributes) under the microscope. Certain intestinal parasites can be readily identified in a wet mount of faeces or other specimen – for example, *Giardia* (a protozoan) and *Ascaris lumbricoides* (a roundworm), as shown in Figure 15.4. Malaria is diagnosed by microscopic examination of a blood smear. In the case of parasites such as these, microscopy can be crucial since culture of these organisms is not possible.
- When the pathogen can be differentially stained so that it can be specifically identified under the microscope. For example, mycobacteria (causing tuberculosis) can be distinguished from other microorganisms in a Ziehl-Neelsen stained (acid-fast stain) smear of sputum. *Cryptococcus neoformans* can be identified in CSF using an India ink stain. Another particularly useful staining technique involves the use of fluorescent dyes attached to antibody molecules specific for a particular microorganism. The organisms are identified if they fluoresce under a microscope using an ultraviolet light source. This technique can be used in many situations,

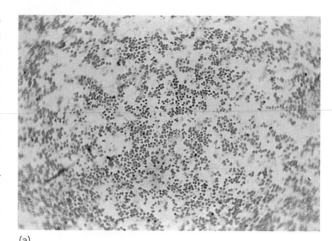

(a)

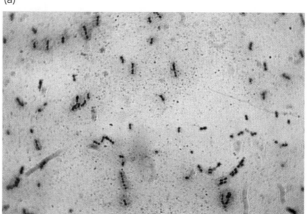

(b)

Figure 15.3

Gram stains of the common causes of bacterial meningitis
(a) *Neisseria meningitidis* and (b) *Streptococcus pneumoniae*.

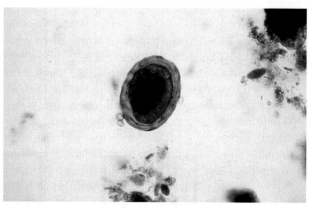

Figure 15.4

Egg of *Ascaris lumbricoides* as seen in a light microscope

such as for the identification of *Legionella*, *Pneumocystis jiroveci*, and for *Treponema pallidum* in fluid from a genital lesion (see Figure 15.5). It is also useful as a rapid diagnostic tool for acute viral infections when large numbers of viruses are present.

A further important advantage of direct microscopic examination of a specimen is that the host cells present in the specimen can be identified. This can provide infor-

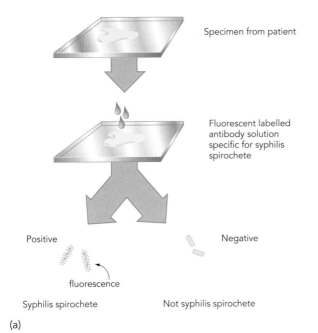

Specimen from patient

Fluorescent labelled antibody solution specific for syphilis spirochete

Positive

Negative

fluorescence

Syphilis spirochete

Not syphilis spirochete

(a)

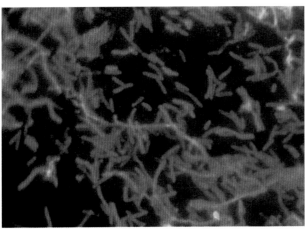

(b)

Figure 15.5

The fluorescent antibody technique
(a) Fluorescent antibody stain results of *Treponema* and an unrelated microorganism in a specimen; (b) photomicrograph of treponemes fluorescing.

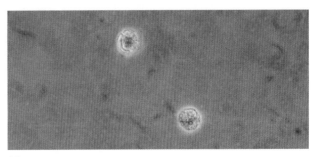

(a)

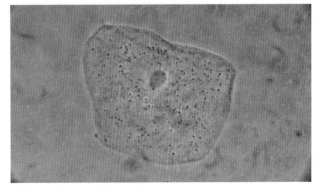

(b)

Figure 15.6

Direct microscopic examination of urine
(a) Pus cells (polymorphonuclear leukocytes) in urine are indicative of infection; (b) epithelial cells suggest poor specimen collection.

electron microscopy is that the microscope is a highly specialised piece of equipment, usually affordable only by specialist virology laboratories or research establishments.

Specimen collection for culture

An infectious disease is most accurately diagnosed when the causative agent is isolated and identified from patient material. The specimen is cultured on appropriate microbiological media and then an identification of the causative organism is made. Identification is usually based on colony morphology, and/or biochemical properties, and/or antigenic properties (see page 193) of the microorganism. The microbiological analysis in the laboratory is only as reliable as the quality of the specimen allows. Thus, the correct selection, timing, collection and transport of patient specimens are of the utmost importance.

When specimens are not properly collected and handled:

- the causative organisms may not be present in the specimen at all, or
- the organisms may die if subjected to adverse conditions, or
- the causative organisms may be overgrown by indigenous microbial flora also present in the specimen.

As stated earlier, a major disadvantage of cultural methods is the length of time required for a result. It should

mation about whether or not infection exists, the type of infection and the quality of the specimen. For example, the presence of pus cells (polymorphonuclear leukocytes) in a sample of urine is suggestive of infection (see Figure 15.6), whereas large numbers of epithelial cells in urine suggest that the specimen was improperly collected (i.e. not a mid-stream sample). The presence of pus cells in CSF suggests an acute bacterial infection, whereas lymphocytes suggest that a non-bacterial cause (e.g. virus, fungus) or a tuberculous meningitis is more likely.

Electron microscopy is a complex procedure that generally takes much longer than light microscopy, mainly because of the more complicated specimen preparation that is required. However, it can be a valuable tool for the identification of very small microbes, such as viruses. Virus culture takes days or even weeks and some viruses can't be cultured at all. The major limitation of

be recognised that results of culture can take up to 18 hours or even much longer (e.g. as long as 1–2 weeks for some organisms in blood cultures). Then another 5–24 hours may be required for antibiotic sensitivity results.

SPECIMEN SELECTION

Many different types of specimens are sent to the laboratory for culture, including blood, urine, faeces, sputum, pus and swabs from sites of infection. These specimens are generally readily obtained. However, for some infections, tissues or body fluids from less accessible sites may have to be collected, such as fluid from a deep abscess, bone marrow, cerebrospinal fluid or peritoneal exudate. The selection of the most appropriate specimen type(s) to be collected should be based on the nature of the infection and the suspected sites of organism persistence. That is, the specimen should be collected from a site where the organism is most likely to be found. For example, a patient with urinary frequency and pain during urination should have a specimen of urine collected for microscopy and culture. Similarly, a patient with respiratory symptoms and a productive cough should have sputum collected for examination.

However, it is not always so straightforward. For instance, *Salmonella typhi*, the cause of typhoid fever, is most likely to be isolated from blood in the first two weeks of infection, but then from faeces or urine in the next two weeks. A good knowledge of the course of the infection is obviously necessary.

TIMING OF SPECIMEN COLLECTION

It is important that, wherever possible, specimens for laboratory culture are collected before antibiotic therapy is initiated. Once antibiotic therapy has begun the likelihood of culturing the causative organism from the specimen is lessened. Antibiotics may not only quickly reduce the numbers of pathogenic microorganisms in the tissues, but they may also interfere with the growth of the organisms in culture. In certain situations, however, it may not be possible to delay antibiotic therapy until a specimen is collected. For example, in a case of meningitis, which can be life-threatening, antibiotic therapy may have to be initiated before a lumbar puncture for cerebrospinal fluid (CSF) collection can be performed.

A knowledge of the usual clinical course of a given infection, combined with a careful observation of the patient's signs and symptoms, should indicate the appropriate time for specimen collection. For most infections, the collection of the specimen should simply be done as soon as possible but, for some, more precise timing is required. For example, early morning sputum specimens should be collected for the diagnosis of tuberculosis to maximise the chance of finding organisms.

Correct timing of the collection of blood samples for culture is critical because organisms may only be intermittently released from the infection source. In septicaemia, chills followed by fever represent the showering of microorganisms into the bloodstream. Cultures are most likely to be positive when they are collected during such episodes.

PROPER COLLECTION OF SPECIMENS

The proper collection of specimens is vital for three main reasons: (1) to obtain an appropriate and useful specimen; (2) to prevent contamination of the specimen during collection; and (3) to prevent harming the patient during specimen collection. The following general procedures should be observed.

- Hospital Standard Precautions guidelines should be followed at all times. All specimens should be treated as potentially hazardous.
- Sterile, leak-proof containers of an adequate size to hold the specimen should generally be used. Care should be taken not to contaminate the external surface of the collection container and its accompanying paperwork. If contamination does occur, appropriate steps for their disinfection or disposal must be taken.
- Specimen collection should be performed with care and tact to avoid harming the patient, or causing discomfort or undue embarrassment. If the specimen is to be collected by the patient (e.g. sputum or urine) he/she should be given clear and detailed instructions.
- All specimens should be collected in a manner that will keep contamination by commensal microflora and external microorganisms to a minimum.
- A sufficient quantity of the specimen should be obtained to enable all necessary tests to be performed. The volume of specimen may be critical. For instance, cerebrospinal fluid needs to be concentrated by centrifugation before it is cultured because the number of organisms is often low.
- The specimen container must be properly labelled and accompanied by the appropriate laboratory requests. The label and request form should identify the patient and the source of the specimen, and the date and time of collection. Any information that will aid the laboratory in performing the appropriate analyses should be included in the clinical history.
- Specimen containers should always be sterile. Faecal specimen containers are an exception since faeces has a very high microbial load and is cultured on highly selective media.
- Certain specimen types, especially swabs, may require special transport systems to protect the pathogens from drying or being overgrown by commensals.

Swabs are frequently used to collect specimens for microbiological analysis. There is a tendency to take a swab of an infected site, rather than some other type of specimen (e.g. a volume of pus or a tissue biopsy) because the former is easier to collect. In some situations (e.g. pharyngitis) a swab may be the only possible type of specimen, but in other situations it is less than ideal. The main problems with swab specimens are that only a limited amount of material can be collected and specimens are highly susceptible to desiccation, leading to reduced viability of microorganisms. After collection, swabs should usually be placed into a transport medium for transport to the laboratory.

SPECIMEN TRANSPORT

Specimens should be delivered promptly to the laboratory so that microbiological examination can begin as soon as possible. Also, it is important that the results of the analysis accurately represent the microbiological population present in the specimen at the time of collection. If delivery is delayed, some fragile pathogens may die; and if the specimen is from a site in the body with an indigenous microflora, the more hardy or faster growing members of the flora may overgrow the pathogens.

While it is most desirable to submit specimens to the laboratory quickly and in an unaltered state, this is not always possible. Therefore, certain specimens should be sent to the laboratory in a transport device, containing a **transport medium**. This is a liquid or semi-liquid, designed to prevent the specimen from drying and to maintain microorganism viability, while retarding their growth prior to culture. It is designed to maintain the microbial population in the specimen as close as possible to its composition at the time of collection.

Not all specimens need to be transported in transport medium, but it is strongly recommended for specimens that could easily dry out, such as swabs and small amounts of fluid, tissue or biopsy material. For some specimens (e.g. a small amount of biopsy material) the medium may simply be 0.85% NaCl. There is a variety of specialised devices, such as swab transport systems, anaerobe transport systems and viral transport media.

It should always be remembered that clinical specimens for culture are collected and sent to the laboratory because they may contain pathogenic microorganisms. Careless handling of the specimen during collection or transport could result in contamination of the outside of the container and the accompanying paperwork. Anyone who handles these (e.g. nurse, orderly, laboratory technologist) may then be exposed to any pathogens present.

Common specimen types for culture

BLOOD CULTURES

A blood culture is usually performed in the investigation of a patient with fever or other manifestations of systemic infection. The blood is inoculated into one or two bottles of culture medium, depending on the type(s) of organisms expected. One bottle is for growth of aerobes and is routinely used, and a second bottle is inoculated if anaerobes are suspected. Less than one bacterial cell may be present in a millilitre of blood, even in serious illness. Thus, the volume of blood collected for culture is critical. The recommended volume of blood for the blood culture system in use should be followed.

Because the number of microorganisms is often low, and because they may be shed into the bloodstream only intermittently, it is recommended that three sets of separately collected blood cultures are obtained over a 24–48 hour period. A single blood culture may miss

intermittently occurring bacteraemia. Also, a differentiation between pathogens and contaminants is possible if more than one sample is collected. Timing of the collections is important because intermittent bacteraemia usually coincides with the onset of fever or chills, although these symptoms may occur as much as an hour after the organisms are shed into the bloodstream.

It is essential that blood for culture is collected aseptically. This is done by first disinfecting the venipuncture site with an alcohol pad (70% isopropyl or ethyl alcohol). The intended venipuncture site should not then be touched except with similarly disinfected gloved fingers. After the venipuncture, any residual antiseptic should be removed with an alcohol pad. The stoppers of the culture bottles or collection tubes should be disinfected with alcohol prior to their inoculation.

Optimally, the blood should be inoculated directly into the culture bottles with the same syringe and needle at the bedside of the patient. Figure 15.7 shows blood culture bottles inoculated with blood.

In the laboratory, cultures are incubated for up to seven days in an automated blood culture system (see Figure 15.8). Automated systems regularly monitor the blood cultures for microbial growth as they incubate. Such systems are designed to provide as early a detection of positive cultures as possible. Once a culture becomes positive it is then subcultured onto agar plates for ultimate identification and sensitivity testing of the organism, if necessary. Manual blood culture methods, in which cultures are visually examined for evidence of growth by laboratory staff, are virtually obsolete in modern laboratories.

INTRAVASCULAR CATHETERS

Intravascular catheters may become colonised and serve as a source of microorganisms in septicaemia. Culturing of a catheter tip may help to determine if there is a relationship between the catheter and infection. A distal segment of the catheter (approximately 5 cm) should be obtained by aseptically clipping off the end of the catheter directly into a

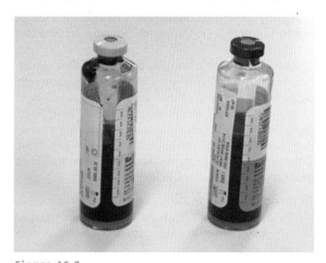

Figure 15.7

Blood culture bottles inoculated with blood from a patient

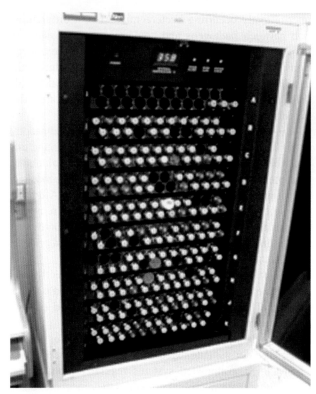

Figure 15.8

Automated blood culture system
The incubator and detection unit are connected to a computer that signals when a culture becomes positive.

screw-cap sterile container at the time the catheter is removed. This specimen should be sent immediately to the laboratory before excessive drying occurs. The number and type of viable bacteria in the catheter specimen may then be determined.

SPECIMENS FOR URINARY TRACT INFECTIONS

Bladder urine is normally sterile. However, it is usually contaminated during urination by the normal microflora of the urethra. Contamination can be reduced by collecting a 'clean-catch' or mid-stream urine specimen. If this method is properly performed, the urethra is flushed out with the first portion of urine and the middle portion is collected for urinalysis.

Proper instruction of patients on how to collect a mid-stream specimen of urine (MSU) is critical to ensure the collection of a good specimen and hence the accuracy of laboratory results. An understanding by health-care personnel of the proper methods for obtaining urine specimens from bedridden patients is also very important. If the patient is collecting the specimen, he/she should be given detailed instructions, including diagrams.

To collect an MSU specimen from a female

1. The urethral opening and vaginal vestibule are cleansed with soapy water or clean gauze pads soaked with liquid soap.
2. The area is rinsed well with sterile water or wet gauze wipes.

3. The labia are held apart during voiding.
4. A few millilitres of urine are allowed to pass. The flow of urine should not be stopped.
5. The mid-stream portion of urine is collected into a sterile container.

To collect an MSU specimen from a male

1. The foreskin is retracted (if not circumcised) and the penis is washed with soapy water.
2. The area is then well rinsed with sterile water.
3. With the foreskin still retracted, a few millilitres of urine are allowed to pass. The flow of urine should not be stopped.
4. The mid-stream portion of urine is collected into a sterile container.

Soap rather than disinfectants should be used for cleaning the urethral area, because disinfectants introduced into the urine during collection may inhibit the growth of microorganisms.

Urine is an excellent growth medium for microorganisms. If a urine sample is left standing at room temperature, contaminating bacteria may increase from low to high numbers. In large numbers they may inhibit the growth of the pathogen or be mistaken for the pathogen. Specimens should be sent to the laboratory within one hour of collection. If this is not possible, they should be refrigerated.

Urine is cultured quantitatively for bacteria, since the number of viable bacteria or colony-forming units (CFU) per litre is critical in the interpretation of urine cultures. A urinary tract infection is indicated if the number of bacteria in a clean-catch MSU exceeds 10^8 organisms per litre and if increased numbers of white cells are present. Lower numbers of organisms may be considered significant in certain situations (e.g. if antibiotic therapy has been commenced, or in a patient with high urine output). Chapter 21 gives a more detailed description of how urinalysis is interpreted.

Contamination of the urine by urethral or vaginal bacterial flora may be avoided by suprapubic aspiration. This involves the collection of urine directly from the bladder by needle aspiration. It may be used for patients with clinical evidence of urinary tract infection but in whom bacterial counts in MSU specimens are low and indeterminate. It is also useful for neonates and young infants, and for other patients who can't produce an MSU and in whom catheterisation is contraindicated.

In patients with indwelling urethral catheters attached to a closed drainage system, urine is collected by disinfecting the wall of the catheter at its juncture with the drainage tube and puncturing it with a needle attached to a syringe (see Figure 15.9). The connection between the catheter and the drainage tube should not be broken for specimen collection and the material in the drainage bag, which may have been standing for several hours, must not be used. Urine may also be collected for culture during the course of cystoscopy or retrograde pyelography.

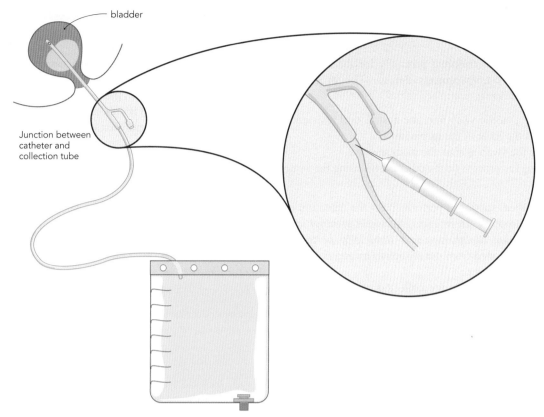

bladder

Junction between
catheter and
collection tube

Figure 15.9

Collection of a catheter specimen of urine
A needle is inserted just below the junction between the catheter and collection tube.

SPECIMENS FOR CENTRAL NERVOUS SYSTEM INFECTIONS

In a case of suspected meningitis, cerebrospinal fluid (CSF), obtained by lumbar puncture, is investigated. A lumbar puncture must be performed under conditions of strict asepsis to protect the patient. Also, if contamination of the specimen occurs, the isolation and identification of the true causative agent may be impaired.

The skin at the puncture site should be disinfected with an antiseptic such as povidone-iodine. Specimens should be collected in sterile containers that are sealed with a screw cap to prevent leakage and loss or contamination of the contents. Usually, three portions of 2–5mL each are placed in separate containers for microbiology, cytology and biochemistry testing. The most turbid (cloudy) tube should be sent to microbiology. If only one tube of CSF is obtained, it should be submitted to the microbiology laboratory first so that it can be opened aseptically.

Meningitis is a life-threatening infection, warranting rapid transport of the CSF specimen to the laboratory, rapid diagnosis and treatment. Blood cultures should also be collected from patients suspected of having meningitis.

SPECIMENS OF OTHER BODY FLUIDS

Apart from blood, urine and CSF, other normally sterile body fluids that may be collected include pleural, peritoneal and synovial fluids. These are usually collected by percutaneous needle aspiration using strict aseptic technique.

The number of microorganisms in these specimens may be low, primarily because of their dilution by fluid accumulation at the site. It is therefore necessary to collect as large a specimen sample as possible.

SPECIMENS FOR UPPER RESPIRATORY TRACT INFECTIONS

A number of different types of specimens may be collected from the upper respiratory tract, including throat, nasal and nasopharyngeal swabs, nasopharyngeal fluid and nasal washings. The type of specimen is determined by the type of organism suspected.

Throat swabs (pharyngeal specimens) are collected primarily for the detection of infection by Group A streptococci (*Streptococcus pyogenes*), *Neisseria gonorrhoeae* (in pharyngeal gonorrhoea), *Candida albicans* (thrush) and *Haemophilus influenzae*. The procedure involves:

1. depressing the tongue gently with a tongue depressor
2. extending a sterile swab between the tonsillar pillars and behind the uvula (avoiding contact with the cheeks, tongue, uvula and lips)
3. sweeping the swab back and forth across the posterior pharynx, tonsillar areas and any inflamed or ulcerated areas to obtain the sample.

A throat sample should not be collected if the epiglottis is inflamed, as sampling may cause serious respiratory obstruction.

Nasal swabs are collected primarily for the detection of carriers of *Staphylococcus aureus*. The procedure involves:

1. inserting a sterile swab into one nostril until resistance is met at the level of the turbinates
2. rotating the swab against the nasal mucosa
3. repeating the process on the other nostril using the same swab.

Nasopharyngeal suction is performed for the detection of carriers of Group A streptococci, *Neisseria meningitidis*, *Corynebacterium diphtheriae* and *Bordetella pertussis*. Material is suctioned from the nasopharynx and collected into a sterile container.

Nasopharyngeal swabs are collected primarily for the detection of carriers of *Neisseria meningitidis* and to diagnose *Bordetella pertussis* infections. In this procedure a flexible wire swab is carefully inserted through the nose into the posterior nasopharynx. The swab is rotated, keeping it near the septum and floor of the nose.

Nasal washings are collected primarily for culture of viruses. The patient should be instructed not to swallow during the procedure. With the patient's head hyper-extended (about 70° angle), approximately 5 mL of sterile isotonic saline is instilled into each nostril. To collect the material, the head is tilted forward and the fluid allowed to run out of the nares into a sterile container; or the fluid is aspirated using a rubber bulb syringe. The nasal washings are placed in an equal volume of viral transport medium, or transported in a sterile container.

SPECIMENS FOR LOWER RESPIRATORY TRACT INFECTIONS

The specimen most often collected in the investigation of lower respiratory infection is sputum (purulent mucus). Specimen quality is of utmost importance. Health-care personnel should be aware of the need for a fresh, clean specimen of purulent material produced from a deep cough. In some patients sputum may need to be induced by having them inhale a warmed saline aerosol. A poor quality specimen (predominantly saliva) is more likely to be contaminated with oropharyngeal flora, some of which may be incorrectly assumed to be the cause of infection. This can make it difficult to determine which of the organisms isolated is responsible for the infection. Thus, culture of sputum does not always yield clear-cut results.

Specimen quality may be assessed in the laboratory by performing a Gram stain. Sputum specimens with excessive squamous epithelial cells are judged to be unsatisfactory because such specimens are likely to contain a large amount of saliva and to be significantly contaminated with oropharyngeal flora.

A better specimen may be obtained by bronchial aspiration through a bronchoscope, or by inserting a needle into the trachea below the glottis (trans-tracheal aspiration).

Needle biopsy of the lungs may be necessary for the diagnosis of infections in which there is no productive cough (e.g. fungal and viral infections).

If tuberculosis is suspected, extreme care should be exercised in handling the sputum specimen because the organism can be transmitted from the specimen to the health-care worker. Specimens for TB culture may be refrigerated for several hours without significant loss of viability.

SPECIMENS FOR GASTROINTESTINAL TRACT INFECTIONS

Faeces (stools) may be collected for the culture of bacteria causing gastroenteritis or for the detection of protozoa, helminths or viruses. The proper collection and preservation of faeces are frequently neglected, but are important requirements for the isolation of microorganisms responsible for intestinal infections.

A stool specimen can be effectively obtained by:

- passing the stool directly into a wide-mouth, leak-proof container with a tight-fitting lid; or
- passing the stool into a clean, dry bedpan and then transferring the stool into a sterile leak-proof container with a tight-fitting lid.

Toilet paper should not be used to collect the stool because it may contain chemicals that are inhibitory for some faecal pathogens. The specimen should be transported to the laboratory promptly, or refrigerated if a delay is unavoidable. If a stool specimen cannot be processed within several hours of collection, it may be mixed with a suitable transport medium. Deterioration of parasites (protozoa and helminths) in stool samples may be prevented by the use of appropriate fixatives, which preserve the morphology of the protozoa and helminths.

In selected circumstances, such as in the detection of rectal gonorrhoea, a rectal swab may be necessary. The swab should be passed beyond the anal sphincter, carefully rotated and withdrawn. The swab should be placed in a screw-cap tube containing a preservative such as Cary-Blair medium and transported to the laboratory.

Other specimens that may be required include gastric aspirates for certain parasites (e.g. *Giardia*, *Cryptosporidium*) and gastric biopsies (for detection of *Helicobacter pylori*).

A single negative stool culture or examination for eggs and parasites cannot be regarded as sufficient for ruling out a particular gastrointestinal pathogen. For many infectious diarrhoeas, up to three stool specimens may need to be collected and examined.

SPECIMENS FOR GENITAL TRACT INFECTIONS

Genital tract specimens are submitted mainly for the detection of such pathogens as *Neisseria gonorrhoeae*, *Chlamydia trachomatis*, herpes simplex virus, genital wart virus, *Trichomonas*, *Haemophilus ducreyi*, Group B streptococci, *Candida albicans* and certain anaerobic bacteria.

In females, a number of specimens may be collected depending on the site of infection. For example:

- cervical swab
- vaginal swab
- urethral swab
- amniotic fluid
- rectal swab
- vesicle fluid (e.g. on vulva).

In males, typical specimens include:

- urethral swab
- fluid or swab from penile lesion
- rectal swab.

SPECIMENS FROM INFECTED WOUNDS AND TISSUE

A number of different specimens may be collected from infected wounds and tissues. As for other specimen types, specimen quality is of utmost importance. A sample of tissue, pus or fluid is generally superior to a swab specimen.

Tissue and biopsy specimens should be placed into a sterile, screw-cap container and transported immediately to the laboratory. If the specimen is small, it should be immersed in sterile isotonic saline to prevent it from drying out. From an infected wound a volume of pus should be collected if possible. There are circumstances, however, when only a swab specimen can be obtained. In such cases, the swab should be used to sample as much of the lesion as possible. Swabs should be transported to the laboratory in transport medium.

SPECIMENS FOR ANAEROBIC BACTERIA

Anaerobic bacteria can cause a variety of infections in humans, including appendicitis, cholecystitis, periodontal infections, endocarditis, endometritis, brain abscess, osteomyelitis, peritonitis, empyema, salpingitis, sinusitis, and wound infections following bowel surgery or trauma. These bacteria may be overlooked or missed if the specimen is not properly collected and transported to the laboratory and then subjected to appropriate laboratory procedures.

Anaerobes vary in their sensitivity to oxygen, but a brief exposure of less than 10 minutes to atmospheric oxygen is enough to kill the more sensitive organisms. If anaerobes are suspected, the laboratory request form should indicate it, and the specimen should be exposed to air for as brief a time as possible.

One of the best specimens for anaerobic culture is pus, obtained by using a needle and syringe. In a volume of pus the bacteria are somewhat protected from oxygen and drying. The material, however, should *not* be transported in the needle and syringe. Needle transport is very unsafe because there is the potential risk of a needlestick injury, and syringe transport poses a risk because the specimen may be expelled during transport, creating a threat to people and the environment. So, aspirated material should

be transferred to an anaerobic transport vial. Large volumes of purulent material may be transported in a sterile, screw-cap container. The needle and syringe should be disposed of in the appropriate way (see Chapter 13).

Tissue and biopsy samples are also very good specimens for anaerobic culture. After collection they should be placed into an anaerobic transport device, or a sterile tube or petri dish, which is then placed into a sealable plastic bag that generates an anaerobic atmosphere. Large pieces of tissue can be transported in a sterile jar. When a swab must be used to collect a specimen a commercial anaerobe swab system should be used.

Extremes of heat or cold should be avoided. If delays are unavoidable, the specimens should be held at room temperature until processing.

SPECIMENS FOR FUNGAL CULTURE

A variety of specimens may be collected for the culture of fungi, depending on the site of infection. For superficial infections, skin scrapings, hair or nail clippings from the site of infection are most appropriate. For subcutaneous infections, possible specimens include sputum, blood and pus. Specimens for the culture of fungi should be collected aseptically, placed in sterile containers and delivered to the laboratory within several hours. Swabs are the least suitable, but specimens from certain body sites, such as the ear canal, nasopharynx, throat, vagina and cervix, are not readily collected by other means.

Specimens should be transported in sterile, humidified, leak-proof containers. Only dermatological specimens should be transported in a dry container. Transport medium should not be used unless the specimen can be easily and completely retrieved from the medium.

SPECIMENS FOR VIRAL CULTURE

Typical specimens for viral culture are listed in Table 15.1. In addition to a specimen from the clinical site of infection, blood, throat washings and faeces are also often collected. The chance of virus recovery is best if the specimen is collected within three days of the onset of symptoms; for many viruses it is greatly reduced beyond five days. Specimens other than fluids should be placed in a sterile, leak-proof container with viral transport medium.

Culturing bacteria and fungi

CULTURE MEDIA

A nutrient composition prepared for the growth of microorganisms is called a **culture medium**. Culture media are sterilised when they are made so that they have no microorganisms in them before they are used. When microbes are grown on a culture medium the growth is called a **culture**. It is possible to grow the majority of bacteria and fungi in artificial (chemically prepared) culture media, but there is no single medium in which all types of bacteria and fungi are able to grow.

Table 15.1

Specimens required for viral culture

CLINICAL DISEASE	SPECIMENS REQUIRED
Measles (rubeola)	Blood, urine, nasopharyngeal secretions
German measles	Throat and nasal swabs, blood, urine
Chickenpox	Vesicle fluid
Respiratory syncytial virus	Nasal washings
Herpes simplex – skin lesions	Vesicle fluid
Herpes simplex – encephalitis	Cerebrospinal fluid, brain biopsy
Diarrhoea (e.g. rotavirus infection)	Faeces, rectal swab

Some bacteria have very special nutrient requirements. For example, *Streptococcus pyogenes* can grow only if red blood cells are supplied in the medium, and *Neisseria gonorrhoeae* can grow only if the blood is heated (to release the nutrients) before being added to the medium. Microorganisms that require special growth factors, such as these, are said to be **fastidious**, requiring **enriched media**. There are some bacteria that are so fastidious they can't be grown in culture media at all; for example, *Treponema pallidum* and *Mycobacterium leprae*, and others such as the chlamydia and rickettsia, can't be grown in artificial media but can be grown in cell cultures (cultures of living animal cells).

Some culture media are designed to allow the growth of certain microorganisms, while inhibiting the growth of others. For example, Sabouraud dextrose medium has a low pH and high sugar content, which inhibits bacteria but allows fungi to grow. MacConkey medium contains bile salts which inhibit non-enteric bacteria. These are called **selective media**. MacConkey medium is also an example of what are termed **differential media**, because certain bacteria can be differentiated from others by the particular nature of their growth on the medium (see Figure 15.10). Chromogenic media are recently developed types of differential media on which different organisms can be distinguished by their different coloured colonies (see Figure 15.11).

PURE CULTURES

Culture media may be liquid, but most of the time they are made solid by the addition of a gelling agent, called *agar*. A solid medium contained in a petri dish (a circular plastic dish) is called an **agar plate**. Solid media are often used because bacteria and fungi can grow on the surface of the media, forming colonies composed of millions of cells. All the cells in a colony are identical because they are the progeny of a single cell that was initially implanted onto the surface of the agar. If a single colony is transferred to a fresh agar plate and spread over the surface, numerous colonies will grow on the plate and all the colonies will comprise the same species of organism. This is called a **pure culture**. In order to perform tests on a microorganism it is essential to have a pure culture, so that the test results reflect the attributes of that organism alone.

The way in which pure cultures are usually prepared is

called the **streak plate method**. Bacteria are picked up by a sterile wire loop and, as the loop is moved lightly over the surface of the agar in lines (or streaks), they are deposited on the surface of the plate on the lines. The loop is sterilised by flaming between different areas of streak-

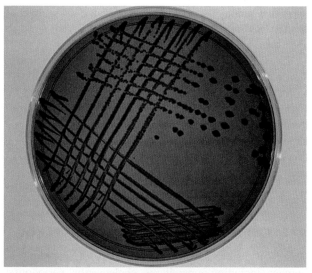

(a)

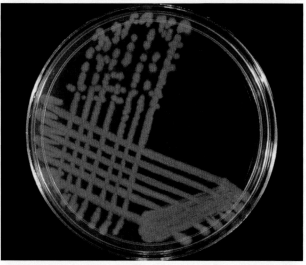

(b)

Figure 15.10

Differential growth medium

Differentiation of (a) *E. coli* and (b) *Pseudomonas aeruginosa* on MacConkey agar.

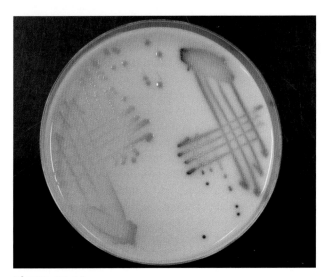

Figure 15.11
Chromogenic medium
A newer type of differential medium.

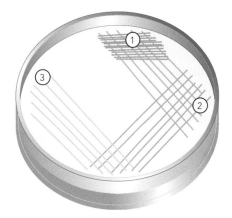

(a)

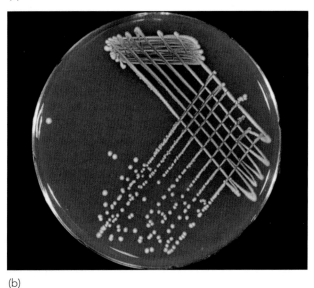

(b)

Figure 15.12

The streak plate method for obtaining pure cultures
(a) Organisms are picked up on a sterile wire inoculating loop and lightly streaked across the agar in region 1; the loop is sterilised by flaming and more streak lines are made in region 2; the loop is sterilised again and the streaking is repeated in region 3; after incubation, well-separated colonies of bacteria appear on streak lines, especially in region 3; (b) a streak plate after incubation.

ing, resulting in fewer and fewer bacteria being deposited. This has a diluting effect and results in single bacterial cells being deposited in the areas that are streaked last. When the plate is incubated, a separated, single colony will grow where each cell is deposited (see Figure 15.12).

Streak plating to obtain pure cultures is necessary because the majority of clinical specimens contain mixtures of microorganisms, particularly if the specimen has been taken from a body site which has a normal microbial flora. Streak plating allows the separation of different organisms and their subsequent purification.

Sometimes, liquid media are used first to increase the numbers of organisms, followed by culture on solid media. Liquid media are used for culturing blood, because the numbers of bacteria in a sample of blood may be very small. Liquid media are also used for culturing of swabs if the presence of anaerobic bacteria is suspected. These are often liquid media containing particles of meat (called a cooked meat medium – see Figure 15.13), within which anaerobes can grow. A liquid medium has the added advantage of diluting any interfering substances in the specimen, such as antibiotics.

INCUBATION

The majority of bacteria and some fungi (yeasts) grow from single cells to macroscopic colonies on an agar plate in 18–24 hours, although anaerobes often require 48 hours or longer. Some bacteria (e.g. Mycobacteria) and moulds grow much more slowly and can take several days or sometimes weeks to form visible colonies. Cultures for anaerobic incubation are placed in an airtight container together with a satchel that chemically removes the air.

IDENTIFICATION OF CULTURED ORGANISMS

Once a culture of a pathogenic bacterium is obtained, various criteria and tests are used to establish the identity of the organism. Different criteria are needed to identify

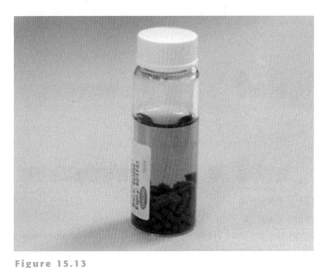

Figure 15.13
Cooked meat medium for the growth of anaerobic bacteria

different organisms, but a presumptive identification is usually based on:

- Gram reaction (see Chapter 4)
- cell morphology (i.e. the shape and arrangement of the cells)
- colony morphology (i.e. the characteristics of the colonies on solid culture media)
- ability to grow aerobically (in the presence of oxygen) or anaerobically, or both
- specialised growth requirements.

To confirm the identity of an organism other properties usually need to be examined, such as:

- the production of special enzymes (e.g. coagulase by *Staphylococcus aureus*)
- biochemical activities (e.g. the ability to metabolise different sugars)
- its motility (ability to swim through liquid).

The biochemical profile is usually performed using commercially available multi-test systems, such as that shown in Figure 15.14. These require incubation for 4–24 hours, depending on the type of kit used. In recent years a number of automated bacterial identification systems have been developed, aimed at achieving a more rapid identification. In such systems an identification and antibiotic sensitivity profile can be obtained for many bacteria in 4–8 hours.

Fungi are usually identified on the basis of their colony appearance (e.g. colour) and the microscopic morphology of their cells and reproductive structures (see Chapter 6). A biochemical analysis is used for some yeasts.

Overall, for most bacteria and yeasts, culture and identification results are usually available 24–48 hours from the time of arrival at the laboratory. However, slow-growing bacteria and moulds can take up to several weeks to culture.

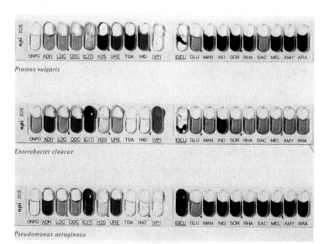

Figure 15.14

Multi-test systems are used to perform multiple biochemical tests on a microorganism simultaneously

Shown here is the commercially prepared API 20E system being used to distinguish between three different bacteria.

ANTIBIOTIC SENSITIVITY TESTS

Bacteria isolated in pure culture may also have their sensitivity to different antibiotics determined. This is required for organisms whose antibiotic sensitivity pattern cannot be predicted. Many of the bacteria that cause hospital-acquired infections certainly fall into this category. Antibiotic sensitivity testing is generally performed on agar plates.

One method, using filter paper discs impregnated with antibiotics, is described in Chapter 12. Briefly, colonies from a culture of the test bacterium are used to seed the whole surface of a plate, and antibiotic discs are then placed on the plate. During incubation, growth of the bacterium is inhibited around the discs containing the antibiotics to which it is sensitive. Thus, antibiotic sensitivity testing requires a further overnight incubation period, although a number of automated sensitivity testing instruments can now give results for some bacteria in 3–8 hours. To obtain a quantitative antibiotic sensitivity result, called a *minimal inhibitory concentration* (MIC) (see Chapter 12), a culture method with an overnight incubation may be required. Automated methods, if available, can provide an MIC in 4–8 hours.

Culture of other microorganisms

Viruses and the bacteria belonging to the genera *Chlamydia* and *Rickettsia* are obligate intracellular parasites and must therefore be grown in cell or tissue cultures, as described in Chapter 5. Growth in cell cultures usually requires a minimum of several days.

Cultured viruses are identified by the cytopathic effect the virus has on the cells it has been grown in and/or by electron microscopic examination of the cultured viruses. Although virus isolation gives the most accurate diagnosis of infection, in most clinical settings it is not practical. The culture of viruses (as well as *Chlamydia* and *Rickettsia*) is time-consuming and involves highly specialised techniques, so alternative diagnostic methods, especially PCR (polymerase chain reaction) and serology, are generally used by clinical microbiology laboratories. Culture is done mainly by specialist virology or research laboratories.

Very few protozoa and helminths can be cultured *in vitro*. Thus, laboratory diagnosis of parasitic infections is usually done by non-cultural methods. Many parasites can, in fact, be quickly identified on morphological grounds by microscopic examination of the specimen. Infections caused by other parasites are usually diagnosed by immunological methods, antigen detection or PCR (see following sections).

Serology (immunologic diagnosis)

The study of antigen-antibody reactions in the laboratory is called **serology**. A serologic diagnosis of infectious disease is based on the principle that when a person has an infection they ultimately produce antibodies that are specific for the microorganism causing the infection (see

Chapter 9). These antibodies are detectable in serum (or blood) and other body fluids. Thus, a serologic diagnosis is performed by testing a person's serum (or sometimes other body fluid) for antibodies against antigens of the microorganism thought to be causing the infection. The antigens may be whole microorganisms, or parts of them, such as viral coats, or bacterial walls, flagella or toxins. Serological tests are useful:

- if the microorganism is impossible or difficult to grow (e.g. *Treponema pallidum*, viruses and parasites); or
- if the microorganism grows slowly (e.g. *Cryptococcus*, *Legionella* and viruses).

The detection of antibodies can also be used to assess a person's immune status to a particular microorganism. For instance, immunity to rubella in pregnant women is determined by measurement of antibodies to the virus in serum. Serological techniques are also used in non-microbiological tests, such as in blood banks for typing blood, for typing tissue before transplant operations and for typing of immunoglobulins in certain immunological disorders.

Most serologic diagnoses are based on measurements of antibody concentration (titre) in serum. These have the disadvantage that usually one to several weeks or more must elapse from the time of infection before a clearly detectable antibody response is produced. Another drawback is that a positive test only represents exposure to the organisms at some time and not necessarily active disease (see Chapter 9).

For a positive diagnosis it is most desirable to demonstrate **seroconversion** in a patient – that is, no (or low) antibodies to the microorganism in the early stage of an illness, and then demonstration of a significant amount (or increase) of antibodies to it a week to several weeks later. An alternative criterion for a positive serological diagnosis is demonstration of a fourfold increase in antibody content in sera collected two weeks apart (usually termed *acute* and *convalescent sera* – see clinical stages of disease, page 144ff).

The principle of antibody titration is shown in Figure 15.15. The patient's serum antibody titre is determined by adding the microbial antigens to serial dilutions of the patient's serum; for example, tube 1 = 1/20, tube 2 = 1/40, tube 3 = 1/80, tube 4 = 1/160, tube 5 = 1/320, etc. The greatest dilution that shows a positive reaction is the antibody titre of the patient's serum. Nowadays, these titrations and reactions are performed in microtitre plates (see Figure 15.16), which can be automated, or in a variety of other automated systems. An antibody titration can also be performed on other body fluids (e.g. urine, CSF).

Several methods are available to determine the amount of antibody in an individual's serum. The method used depends mostly on whether the antigen is a whole cell, a toxin, a cell component or a virus. Because all antibodies have two or more antigen-binding sites (see Chapter 9), a reaction between antibody and antigen forms a latticework (or aggregate) of many antigen-antibody molecules that

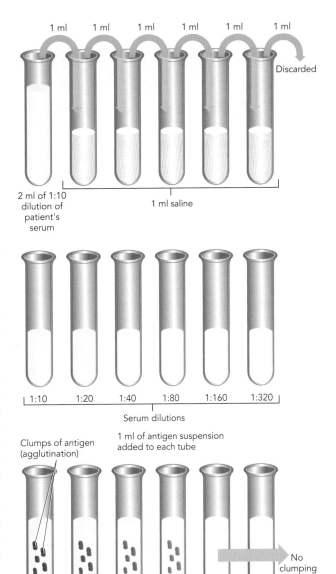

Figure 15.15

The principle of serial dilution for antibody titration
The titre is the last tube that shows a positive reaction (clumping), which in this example is 160.

becomes quite large in appropriate conditions. If the antigen is on or fixed to particulate material, such as a bacterial cell or latex particles, the end result is a clumping of the particles, or **agglutination**. If the antigens are fixed to red cells the positive reaction is called a **haemagglutination**.

Other methods measure the gain or loss of a certain property of the antigen. An example of this is a reaction between antibodies and a bacterial toxin, resulting in neutralisation of the toxin; such antibodies are given the general name **antitoxin**. A similar principle is used in tests that use antibodies to neutralise viruses, thus preventing the viruses from infecting cells.

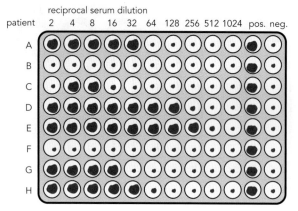

Figure 15.16

Serological assay performed in a microtitre plate
Serial dilutions of patients' serum are made in horizontal rows; in this haemagglutination test, a diffuse layer of cells in the bottom of the well represents a positive reaction, whereas a small button of cells is a negative reaction.

Other commonly used assays are the complement fixation test, the fluorescent antibody test and the enzyme-linked immunosorbent assay (ELISA).

IgM TESTING

A major drawback of serological diagnosis of infection is the need to demonstrate an increase in antibody titre in paired sera (acute and convalescent). For this reason a serological diagnosis is usually retrospective. This can be overcome if specific IgM antibodies can be detected. As we saw in Chapter 9, IgM is present early in infection and usually disappears after several weeks. It is therefore indicative of active, rather than past infection, permitting a diagnosis to be made from a single specimen. The technology to test for specific IgM antibodies has been developed for only some diseases.

Antigen detection

Detection of antigens of a microorganism in an appropriate specimen is a method used for diagnosis of some infections. Like serological methods, antigen detection methods are most commonly used for diseases caused by organisms for which culture is not possible, too difficult or too time-consuming. Antigen detection methods are also useful in providing a rapid, presumptive diagnosis in emergency situations, such as bacterial meningitis. Commercial antigen detection kits are available for a range of viruses (e.g. norovirus, respiratory syncytial virus, herpes simplex viruses, cytomegalovirus), a number of parasites (e.g. *Cryptococcus*, *Giardia*) and some bacteria (e.g. *Legionella*, *Clostridium difficile* toxin, *Neisseria meningitidis*, pneumococcus).

In some diseases, antigens of the microorganism can be detected before the patient produces specific antibodies. For example, cryptococcal antigen can be detected in the CSF of patients with cryptococcal meningitis early in the infection. Antigens of the human immunodeficiency virus

(HIV) can be detected in blood during the antibody negative (window) period, which can exceed three months in some people (see Chapter 19).

Antigen detection methods utilise specific antibodies to identify antigens of the organism in patient material. The methods used include a variety of enzyme immunoassays and latex agglutination tests.

Detection of microorganisms using molecular techniques

Molecular-based techniques have been proclaimed by many people to be the most significant development in diagnostic microbiology in decades. These methods identify the cause of an infection by detecting fragments of nucleic acids of the microorganism in a specimen from the patient or from a culture of the isolated organism. A variety of molecular-based techniques have so far been developed (see Table 15.2), allowing a faster and more sensitive detection of microorganisms than conventional methods.

Molecular techniques are particularly useful for:

- diagnosis of infections caused by organisms that are difficult or impossible to diagnose by other methods (e.g. herpes simplex encephalitis)
- diagnosis of infections for which speed of diagnosis is vital (e.g. gonorrhoea or *Chlamydia* genital infection)
- quantifying the amount of nucleic acid, and hence the numbers of microbes, in a clinical specimen (e.g. to monitor the course of human immunodeficiency virus or hepatitis C infection)
- the detection of specific virulence or antibiotic resistance genes in bacteria
- the subtyping of viruses (e.g. hepatitis C subtypes)
- epidemiological studies.

Only a limited number of commercial molecular kits are currently available for diagnostic laboratory use. However, with technological improvements, the development and introduction of these methods is proceeding rapidly and they will, undoubtedly, become common procedures in the clinical microbiology laboratory in the

---

Table 15.2

Molecular techniques used in clinical microbiology laboratories

- Hybridisation with nucleic acid probes
- Polymerase chain reaction (PCR)
- Ligase chain reaction (LCR)
- Nucleic acid sequence-based amplification (NASBA)
- Trans-mediated amplification (TMA)
- Branched chain DNA signal amplification (bDNA)
- Strand displacement amplification (SDA)
- Pulse field gel electrophoresis

future. They also promise to play vital roles in cancer diagnosis, human genetics, forensic science and archaeology.

NUCLEIC ACID PROBES

Virtually all microorganisms contain some unique nucleotide sequence in their genome which, in theory, can be utilised as a fingerprint for rapid identification. A nucleic acid probe is a single-stranded segment of DNA or RNA that is complementary to the nucleic acid that is to be detected. The probe binds to a complementary nucleic acid sequence, if present, to form a novel duplex molecule (see Figure 15.17). The binding of the labelled probe with the target nucleic acid is called *hybridisation*. Probes are labelled with radioisotopes (such as ^{32}P), enzymes or substances that give colour or fluorescent reactions, so that the formation of duplex molecules can be readily detected. Probes can be made that are specific to the genus, species or even strain, by varying the nucleotide sequence that is used.

A probe can be used to identify unknown organisms growing in culture. For example, gene probes for *Mycobacterium tuberculosis* and *M. avium intracellulare* have reduced the time required to identify cultures of these organisms from weeks to hours. To date, a limited number of commercially available probes have been produced for culture confirmation.

Gene probes can be used to detect genetic sequences that code for antibiotic resistance. One of the best characterised genes that can be detected with gene probes is the *mecA* gene of *Staphylococcus aureus* which codes for methicillin resistance.

Another use for probes is in the detection of pathogens in a specimen. The direct detection of microbial nucleic acid in a clinical sample is the most exciting potential for probes because it has the advantage of speed and specificity. Probes for enterotoxins of *Escherichia coli* or cholera toxin have been applied directly to faeces. A commercially available ^{125}I-labelled DNA probe directed against sequences specific for *Mycoplasma pneumoniae* has been used successfully to detect the organism in sputum specimens.

A major limitation of this technology is that gene probes are generally unable to detect low numbers of organisms (few copies of the gene) in clinical specimens. Gene amplification methods (e.g. the polymerase chain reaction) are a possible solution to this problem.

POLYMERASE CHAIN REACTION

The main drawback of probe technology is its inability to detect very small amounts of nucleic acid (i.e. low sensitivity). The **polymerase chain reaction (PCR)** is a technique that can increase the quantity of a specific nucleotide sequence contained within a sample by a process of directed DNA synthesis. The PCR is a powerful amplification and detection technique that can theoretically generate billions of copies of DNA from a single molecule of the nucleic acid in a few hours.

PCR is a relatively new technology, first described in 1985. In this process, DNA is first extracted from the clinical specimen and then passed through a temperature-controlled cycle that amplifies a specific segment of the target DNA (see Figure 15.18). The target DNA is mixed with sequence-specific primers (that are complementary to, and select, the segment of DNA of interest), free nucleotides and the enzyme DNA polymerase.

The mixture is first heated to 90–95°C to separate the two strands of the target DNA. Each strand of the DNA acts as a template for DNA synthesis. The mixture is then cooled to 45–60°C to allow annealing (joining) of the primers to a specific part of the target DNA. The primers are extended by DNA polymerase by the addition of nucleotides complementary to the target DNA, ultimately yielding two identical replicas of the original target DNA. The cycle of heating and cooling is repeated (by an automated thermocycler) to exponentially increase the number of copies of the target DNA.

PCR has been used to great effect in the diagnosis and management of some diseases and offers enormous potential in diagnostic microbiology in general. For example, it is now commonly used for the diagnosis of some infections caused by organisms that are slow-growing or difficult to grow, such as viruses, *Mycobacterium tuberculosis* and *Chlamydia trachomatis*. These microbes typically take two or more weeks to grow, making culture of limited clinical usefulness.

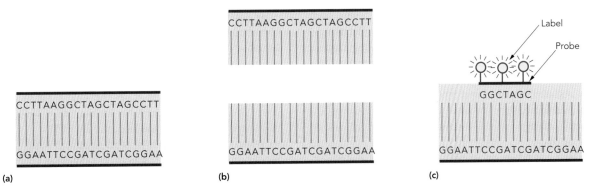

Figure 15.17

Use of a DNA probe to identify a particular DNA sequence
(a) A sample of double-stranded DNA for testing; (b) separation of the DNA segment; (c) binding of the labelled probe DNA to the sample DNA, thereby identifying it.

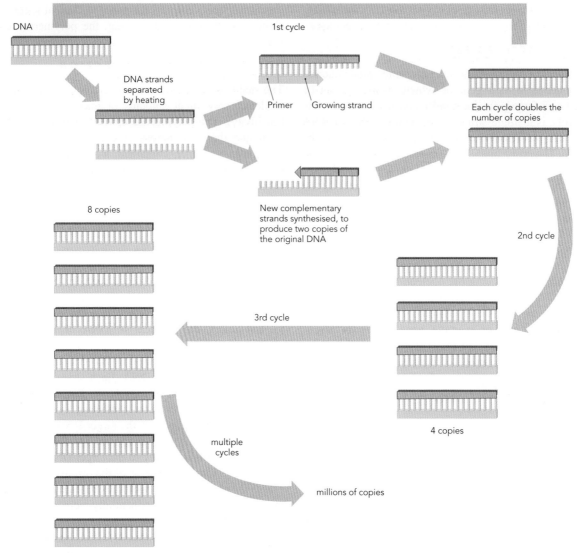

DNA

1st cycle

DNA strands
separated
by heating

Primer   Growing strand

Each cycle doubles the
number of copies

New complementary
strands synthesised, to
produce two copies of
the original DNA

8 copies

3rd cycle

2nd cycle

4 copies

multiple
cycles

millions of copies

Figure 15.18

Mechanism of the polymerase chain reaction
The polymerase chain reaction is a nucleic acid amplification technique allowing a small number of molecules of DNA to be copied many times over.

CASE HISTORY 15.1

Herpes simplex encephalitis

A 10-year-old girl, who was previously well, presented with a nine-day illness, characterised by fevers and headache. On the day before her admission her temperature was noted to be 'very high'. She had rigors, seemed delirious with abnormal speech and was becoming increasingly drowsy. By the day of admission, she was agitated, abusive and incomprehensible. She was admitted to a base hospital where investigations were all normal, except for a CT scan that showed left uncal haemorrhage.

The CSF taken on the day of admission contained 100×10^6/L red blood cells, 400×10^6/L lymphocytes, 100×10^6/L polymorphs, 3.7 mmol/L glucose, 0.88g/L protein, intracranial pressure 13–15 cm.

Polymerase chain reaction (PCR) for herpes simplex

virus (HSV) DNA was positive. Serum taken on Day 2 of admission was negative for HSV IgM and low positive for IgG.

A second CSF was taken on Day 3 of admission, containing 420×10^6/L red blood cells, 550×10^6/L lymphocytes, 24×10^6/L polymorphs, 2.8 mmol/L glucose, 0.8 g/L protein. The CSF was sterile for both bacteria and viruses, negative for HSV IgM and IgG, and again positive by PCR. A third CSF taken eight days after admission had borderline HSV IgM and positive HSV IgG, but was negative by PCR.

When the PCR results were known, ceftriaxone therapy was ceased and aciclovir treatment was continued for a total of 14 days.

Adapted from J. Montanaro, 'Early detection of herpes simplex encephalitis by polymerase chain reaction', *Communicable Diseases Intelligence* 16/4, 24 February 1992, pp. 76–77.

PCR also plays a vital role in assessing disease progression, patient infectivity and prognosis, and the effectiveness of therapy in some very important viral infections (e.g. human immunodeficiency virus (HIV), hepatitis B and hepatitis C). A further application of PCR is in the subtyping of viral infections (e.g. herpes simplex viruses 1 and 2 and subtypes of hepatitis C).

PCR shows great promise in other medical areas such as the amplification of genes associated with genetic diseases like cystic fibrosis and haemophilia and is expected to be useful in the examination of museum and archaeological specimens.

The basic process of PCR has been modified in a variety of ways to expand its versatility and applications:

- Multiplex PCR is a modification in which multiple sets of primers are used to detect several target DNA sequences simultaneously.
- RNA can be detected by converting RNA into complementary DNA and then amplifying it in a process called reverse transcriptase PCR (RT-PCR). This modification is useful for the identification of RNA viruses and for distinguishing between active (viable) and inactive (latent) infection.
- If broad-based primers are used (called broad-range PCR), DNA in clinical specimens can be randomly amplified and unknown microbes can be detected and possibly characterised. This methodology was responsible for the relatively rapid identification of the cause of SARS (severe acute respiratory syndrome) as a coronavirus within weeks of the start of the outbreak in late 2002. This was a major factor that led to the early control of the outbreak.

- A significant development of the PCR technology is real-time PCR. In this method, amplification and detection of amplified products occur in the same reaction vessel. This is a major breakthrough because it enables quantitation of the product to occur simultaneously with the amplification process. By comparison with controls, the amount of starting DNA in the sample can be quantified. This has become an important means of monitoring viral load and the effectiveness of therapy in some viral infections (e.g. hepatitis C).

PCR has some important limitations. It requires scrupulous technique and considerable technical skill to perform. Even then, false positive and false negative results are a constant concern. Also, if antibiotic sensitivity is required, culture of the causative agent must still be performed. Other limitations are that most methods (except RT-PCR) do not distinguish between viable and non-viable organisms, and they are less effective in identifying an infection caused by multiple organisms (except multiplex PCR).

The cost and availability are also limiting factors. Perhaps the greatest limitation of PCR is that it requires a fairly accurate preliminary diagnosis to be effective. PCR cannot detect an organism for which primers have not been provided in the reaction, although multiplex and broad-range methods have reduced this problem to some extent. Despite these limitations, PCR technology has great potential in the diagnosis of infectious disease.

SUMMARY

- The main function of the clinical microbiology laboratory is to assist in the diagnosis of infectious diseases.
- For an accurate laboratory diagnosis it is essential that an appropriate specimen is properly collected and transported promptly to the laboratory for processing.
- Laboratory tests are designed to detect either (1) the microorganism itself or a component of it in a specimen from the patient, or (2) evidence of an immune response to the causative organism in the blood of the patient.
- Direct microscopic examination of certain specimens can sometimes provide a presumptive diagnosis within an hour.
- An infectious disease is most accurately diagnosed when the causative agent is isolated and identified from patient material.
- A major disadvantage of cultural methods is the length of time required for a result; this may be up to 18 hours and, for some specimens, as long as several weeks.
- Many different types of specimens can be sent to the laboratory for culture: blood, urine, faeces, sputum, pus and swabs from sites of infection.
- Wherever possible, specimens for laboratory culture are collected before antibiotic therapy is initiated.

COMMON SPECIMEN TYPES FOR CULTURE

- A blood culture is usually performed when investigating a patient with fever or other manifestations of systemic infection.
- Intravascular catheters may become colonised and serve as a source of microorganisms in septicaemia. Culturing of a catheter tip may help to determine whether there is a relationship between the catheter and infection.
- Bladder urine is normally sterile, but urine usually becomes contaminated with the normal microflora of the urethra during urination. Contamination of urine can be reduced by collecting a 'clean-catch' or mid-stream specimen of urine (MSU).
- In a case of suspected meningitis, cerebrospinal fluid (CSF), obtained by lumbar puncture, is investigated.
- Other normally sterile body fluids that may be collected include pleural, peritoneal and synovial fluids; they are usually collected by percutaneous needle aspiration.
- Several types of specimens may be collected from the upper respiratory tract – throat, nasal and nasopharyngeal swabs; nasopharyngeal fluid; nasal washings.
- The specimen most often collected in the investigation of

lower respiratory infection is sputum. Other specimens include bronchial aspiration through a bronchoscope, transtracheal aspiration and needle biopsy of the lungs.

- Faeces (stools) may be collected for the culture of bacteria causing gastroenteritis, for the detection of specific toxins or for the detection of protozoa, helminths or viruses. Other specimens that may be required for certain infections include rectal swabs, gastric aspirates and gastric biopsies.
- In females, specimens that may be collected for the diagnosis of genital tract infections include a cervical swab, vaginal swab, urethral swab, amniotic fluid, rectal swab and vesicle fluid. In males, typical specimens include a urethral swab, fluid or a swab from penile lesions, and a rectal swab.
- When collecting a specimen from an infected wound or sample of tissue, pus or fluid is always superior to a swab specimen.
- From an infected wound a volume of pus should be collected if possible. When only a swab specimen can be obtained, the swab should be used to sample as much of the lesion as possible and transported to the laboratory in transport medium.
- If anaerobes are suspected, the specimen should be exposed to air for as brief a time as possible.
- One of the best specimens for anaerobic culture is pus, obtained by using a needle and syringe, and transferred to an anaerobic transport vial.
- Tissue samples and biopsy samples are very good specimens for anaerobic culture.
- For superficial fungal infections, skin scrapings, hair or nail clippings from the site of infection are most appropriate.
- For culture of viruses, a specimen from the clinical site of infection plus blood, throat washings and faeces are often collected.

CULTURING BACTERIA AND FUNGI

- A nutrient composition prepared for the growth of microorganisms is called a culture medium.
- When microbes are grown on a culture medium, the growth is called a culture.
- Culture media may be liquid, but most are made solid by the addition of a gelling agent called agar.
- A solid medium contained in a petri dish is called an agar plate.
- Solid media are used because bacteria and fungi can grow on the surface of the media, forming colonies.
- A pure culture is one in which all the colonies comprise the same species of organism.
- Most bacteria and some fungi (yeasts) grow from single cells to macroscopic colonies on an agar plate in 18–24 hours.

- Bacteria isolated in pure culture may have their identification and sensitivity to different antibiotics determined.
- Viruses, and bacteria of the genera *Chlamydia* and *Rickettsia*, are obligate intracellular parasites and must therefore be grown in cell or tissue cultures.

SEROLOGY (IMMUNOLOGIC DIAGNOSIS)

- A serologic diagnosis of infectious disease may be carried out by examination of body fluids and detection of antibodies against certain antigens of an infectious agent.
- Serological tests are useful if the microorganism is impossible or difficult to grow, or if it grows slowly.
- The detection of antibodies is also used to assess a person's immune status to a particular microorganism.
- For a positive diagnosis of infection it is most desirable to demonstrate seroconversion in a patient.
- IgM specific antibody is present early in infection and is indicative of active infection.

ANTIGEN DETECTION

- Detection of antigens of a microorganism in an appropriate specimen is used to diagnosise some infections.

DETECTION OF MICROORGANISMS USING MOLECULAR TECHNIQUES

- Molecular techniques identify the cause of an infection by detecting fragments of nucleic acids of the microorganism in a specimen or from culture of a specimen.
- Molecular techniques allow a faster and more sensitive detection of microorganisms and are particularly useful for infections that are difficult/impossible to diagnose by other methods.
- A nucleic acid probe is a single-stranded segment of DNA or RNA that is complementary to the microbial nucleic acid that is to be detected.
- The direct detection of microbial nucleic acid in a clinical sample is the most exciting potential for probes because it has the advantage of speed and specificity.
- The polymerase chain reaction (PCR) is an amplification and detection technique that can produce billions of copies of DNA from a single molecule of nucleic acid in a sample.
- PCR is used in the diagnosis and management of some diseases caused by organisms that are slow-growing or difficult to grow.
- PCR plays a vital role in assessing disease progression, patient infectivity and prognosis, and effectiveness of therapy in some important viral infections (HIV infection, hepatitis B and hepatitis C).

STUDY QUESTIONS

1. What are the major advantages of a direct microscopic examination of patient material where possible?
2. How does one determine what type of specimen should be collected for the diagnosis of a particular infection?

3. Why should specimens be collected before starting antibiotic therapy where possible?
4. List the important procedures that should be followed when collecting a specimen for microbiological examination.

5. Although swabs are commonly collected for microbiological analysis, they are not always the most appropriate specimen to collect. Explain.

6. What is a 'transport medium' and why is it used?

7. Why are three samples of blood often collected over a 24–48 hour period from a patient suspected of having a septicaemia?

8. What is a 'mid-stream specimen of urine' and why is this the preferred specimen for the diagnosis of urinary tract infections?

9. What is the main problem associated with the delayed transport (several hours) of urine to the microbiology laboratory?

10. What is the main problem associated with the delayed transport (several hours) of sputum to the microbiology laboratory?

11. What important principles should be considered when collecting a specimen from an infected wound?

12. In general, what are the best specimens to collect for the diagnosis of anaerobic infections?

13. What, in microbiological terms, is a 'culture'?

14. Explain the purpose of the streak plate method in microbiology.

15. What type of organisms cannot be grown on agar plates?

16. What is serology?

17. What are detected in serological tests?

18. What is meant by the term 'seroconversion'?

19. Define the terms 'agglutination' and 'haemagglutination'.

20. What are nucleic acid probes? What are their potential uses in microbiology?

21. What is PCR, and what are its potential clinical applications?

TEST YOUR UNDERSTANDING

Case History 15.1 Herpes simplex encephalitis

1. What is the advantage of PCR in this case?

2. Why were antibody tests initially negative?

3. How is PCR able to detect infection so early?

Further reading

Brooks GF, JS Butel & SA Morse 2004, *Jawetz, Melnick & Adelberg's Medical Microbiology*, 23rd edn, New York: McGraw-Hill. (A general text of medical microbiology that covers specimen collection handling and diagnostic methods in a brief but comprehensive fashion.)

Gilbert GL, GS James & V Sintchenko 1999, 'Molecular methods for diagnosis of infectious diseases', *Medical Journal of Australia* 171: 536. (This brief review article outlines the major advantages and disadvantages in the use of molecular biology techniques in diagnostic laboratories.)

Shanson DC 1999, *Microbiology in Clinical Practice*, 3rd edn, Oxford: Butterworth-Heinemann. (A comprehensive text that focuses on the diagnostic aspects of infectious disease.)

Yang S & RE Rothman 2004, 'PCR-based diagnostics for infectious diseases: Uses, limitations, and future applications in acute care settings', *Lancet Infectious Diseases* 4: 337. (A review article that details the method, applications and limitations of the polymerase chain reaction in the clinical microbiology setting.)

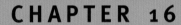

CHAPTER 16

Skin, Wound and Eye Infections

[CHAPTER FOCUS]

- ■ *What microorganisms cause infections of the skin?*

- ■ *What are the clinical features and important infection control considerations of skin infections?*

- ■ *What are the common causes and clinical features of surgical wound infections and burns wound infections?*

- ■ *What infection control procedures prevent infections of surgical and burns wounds?*

- ■ *What are the common causes and clinical features of eye infections?*

Introduction

The skin accounts for approximately 15% of body weight. Except when damaged, the skin provides an effective barrier against invasion by most microorganisms. It acts as a structural barrier and has various chemical attributes that inhibit microorganisms, such as a low pH, high salt concentration, lysozyme and fatty acids (see Chapter 9). Although the skin is a relatively inhospitable place for microorganisms, it does have a normal flora that helps to defend against potential pathogens. The flora includes a variety of aerobic and anaerobic organisms such as staphylococci, micrococci, diphtheroids and propionibacteria. Many other organisms, such as streptococci and Gram-negative enteric bacteria (e.g. *Escherichia coli*, *Proteus* spp.), may transiently colonise the skin. The moister areas of skin such as the axilla (armpit) and groin support relatively large numbers of organisms.

The eye is also exposed to the outside world and is therefore vulnerable to microorganisms and other foreign particles. It too has a number of highly effective defences which generally keep it free of infection. The exposed surface of the eye and the interior surface of the eyelid are covered by the conjunctiva, a thin, mucus-secreting epithelial membrane. As described in Chapter 9, mucous membranes are armed with both non-specific and specific defences. In addition, tears mechanically flush the eye and contain the inhibitory substance, lysozyme. The eye has a normal flora, similar in composition to the skin, but in smaller numbers.

Infections of the skin

Tissue damage is the most common factor leading to infection of the skin, although in some situations apparently normal skin is infected. Minor trauma, such as abrasions, small cuts or cracks, can lead to infection of the skin. More severe trauma, such as that due to surgery, puncture wounds or burns, can lead to serious skin infection, often with involvement of underlying soft tissue. In addition, there are some systemic infections in which organisms are carried in the bloodstream and localise in skin tissue. A skin rash may be the major manifestation of these infections, such as occurs in measles, rubella and chickenpox. The terms used in dermatology to describe different types of lesions on skin are listed and explained in Table 16.1.

BACTERIAL SKIN INFECTIONS

Folliculitis, boils and carbuncles

Staphylococcus aureus is a common cause of skin infections because it is often present on the skin and mucous membranes, particularly the nasal mucosa. Thus, the staphylococci that cause skin infection often come from a person's own flora, or from another person's skin flora. Infection can occur when the organism invades a hair follicle, causing **folliculitis**, also referred to as a **pustule**. These occur mostly on the scalp, face or limbs and are

---

Table 16.1

Dermatological terms for skin lesions

• Erythema	Area of redness due to vasodilation
• Macule	A circumscribed, flat area of altered skin colour
• Papule	A circumscribed, elevated area of skin, less than 1 cm in diameter
• Nodule	A circumscribed, elevated area of skin, larger than 1 cm in diameter
• Vesicle	A small blister containing clear fluid, less than 0.5 cm in diameter
• Bulla	A large blister containing clear fluid, more than 0.5 cm in diameter
• Pustule	A vesicle or bulla containing cloudy fluid
• Wheal/Urticaria	A raised, often itchy erythematous lesion
• Erosion	A superficial, circumscribed loss of epidermis, which heals without scarring
• Ulcer	An area of tissue loss, varying in depth; an ulcer may involve skin only, or may extend more deeply
• Excoriation	An area of skin denuded of epidermis by scratching
• Scale	An abnormal accumulation of keratin; scaling may occur on normal skin, but more often forms on abnormal skin
• Crust ('scab')	The dried exudate from an erosion or ulcer
• Petechia	A small flat haemorrhage
• Purpura	Numerous petechiae

---

often precipitated by some irritation (e.g. following shaving, use of a loofah sponge or dermatitis). *Pseudomonas aeruginosa* may also cause folliculitis, often associated with use of a spa or hot tub. When the deeper areas of a hair follicle are affected, a larger, deeper, pus-filled nodule develops, called a **furuncle** or **boil**. Usually, a boil continues to expand slowly, eventually coming to a head on the surface of the skin. Nasal carriers of virulent *Staphylococcus aureus* may suffer recurrent boils anywhere on the skin.

Boils may discharge to adjacent areas of skin, resulting in multiple abscesses, called a **carbuncle**. (See Figure 16.1.) Carbuncles tend to develop at particular sites, such as on the neck, upper back and buttocks. In addition to the abscesses, there are often systemic symptoms such as fever, malaise and lymphadenopathy. Septicaemia may complicate even simple lesions, especially in the immunocompromised. Boils and carbuncles are encapsulated

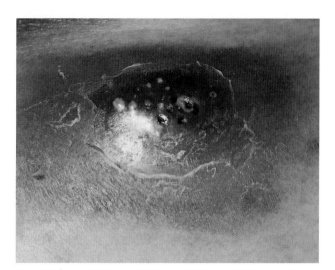

Figure 16.1
Carbuncle

abscesses, representing the body's attempt to localise the infection (see Chapter 9).

Diagnosis is usually made on clinical grounds, but a laboratory confirmation of the causative organism is readily achieved by culture of pus. In general, antibiotics enter abscesses poorly and, when they do, they are inactivated by neutrophil enzymes in pus. For this reason, treatment of these infections usually requires surgical drainage of the lesions.

Impetigo

Impetigo is a highly infectious, pyogenic (pus-forming) infection caused by staphylococci, streptococci, or both (Figure 16.2). It occurs predominantly in young children, where minor skin damage due to insect bites, eczema and scabies is the usual predisposing factor. Lesions often start on the face around the nose and may then spread to other sites of the body. Scratching and other abrasions can result in new lesions, as well as transmission of the organism to others in close contact. It is readily spread on hands, toys and furniture, and can be spread through schools and day-care centres.

There are two main forms of impetigo – the bullous form, caused mainly by *Staphylococcus aureus*, and the non-bullous form caused by staphylococci and/or Group A streptococci (especially *Streptococcus pyogenes*). The non-bullous form is characterised by small vesicles which rupture easily, resulting in weeping, honey-coloured crusts that dry and self-resolve. Bullous lesions are larger, with clear fluid that later becomes cloudy and yellow. After rupture, brownish crusts form. There is generally no systemic illness unless deeper tissues are involved.

Laboratory diagnosis is based on culture of a swab of the lesions under the crusts.

Scalded skin syndrome is caused by strains of *Staphylococcus aureus* that produce a toxin called **exfoliatin** (or **epidermolysin**). It can occur as a complication of minor skin lesions or impetigo. Exfoliatin causes layers of cells in the epidermis to separate, and the outer sheets of skin are shed, exposing layers of inner skin that have the appearance of being scalded. A septicaemia may develop, often with a fatal outcome. The neonatal form is sometimes referred to as *Ritter's disease*.

Erysipelas

Erysipelas is an infection that begins as a small, raised, rubbery lesion, often on the face, and spreads rapidly. Typically, it develops into a bright red, swollen lesion with a sharply demarcated edge (Figure 16.3), followed by

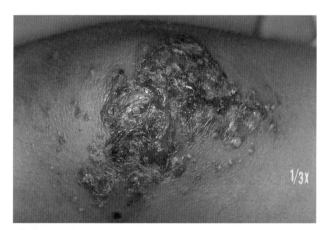

Figure 16.2
Impetigo
A highly contagious disease characterised by vesicles on the skin which break down to a crust form.

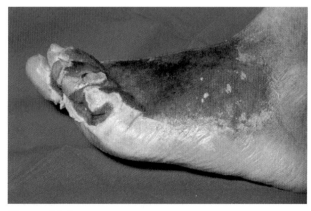

Figure 16.3
A severe case of erysipelas

bullae that rupture and weep. Systemic symptoms of fever, headache and vomiting often precede the cutaneous signs. Erysipelas is usually caused by Group A streptococci, although other bacteria such as *Staphylococcus aureus* or *Haemophilus influenzae* are occasionally responsible. It occurs most often in young children and the elderly. The streptococci usually enter through a break in the skin, but sometimes there is no apparent predisposing lesion. Without appropriate antibiotic treatment the organisms may spread through the lymphatics and cause nephritis, septicaemia, pneumonia and even gangrene.

The diagnosis is usually based on clinical appearance, but the causative agent can be confirmed by culture of fluid from the edge of the lesion.

Cellulitis

Cellulitis is an acute bacterial infection of the skin that spreads to subcutaneous tissues. The infected tissue becomes hot, painful, red and swollen. Fever, chills, bacteraemia and local lymph node enlargement may be present. It may occur following a superficial skin infection or after skin trauma. Following trauma, streptococci (especially *Streptococcus pyogenes*) are usually responsible, but other organisms such as *Staphylococcus aureus*, *Pseudomonas aeruginosa* and *Streptococcus pneumoniae* may be involved. *Clostridium perfringens* and other anaerobes can cause cellulitis in poorly oxygenated tissue, especially after deep wounds and fractures.

Culture of aspirates of the leading edge of the lesion, or skin biopsy, are the usual means of laboratory diagnosis. Blood cultures should also be taken.

Bairnsdale ulcer

Bairnsdale ulcer is a chronic, relatively painless cutaneous ulcer caused by *Mycobacterium ulcerans* (see Figure 16.4). This infection was first reported in 1948 in a group of six patients in Australia, five of whom came from the Bairnsdale district of Victoria. Outbreaks have occurred in Victoria, and it has been made notifiable in that state. It is also endemic in far north Queensland, but rare elsewhere in Australia. It occurs in many other parts of the world including South America, Papua New Guinea and Africa, although it has an unusually uneven and unexplained distribution. It is also referred to as *Buruli*

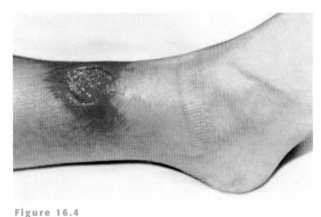

Figure 16.4
Bairnsdale ulcer

ulcer because it has been seen so frequently in the Buruli region of Uganda. In the media it is often called the 'flesh-eating bug'.

Infection is often associated with exposure to water (e.g. swamps, slow-flowing rivers) but the exact mode of acquisition is not currently known. Infection leads to a slowly progressive ulcer which does not respond to the antibiotics normally used for skin infections. The ulcer often leads to scarring and permanent skin deformity and disfigurement. The disease is usually diagnosed by PCR or culture, because of doctors' unfamiliarity with it.

Treatment/prevention of bacterial skin infections

For small, minor skin infections, local measures, particularly wound drainage and gentle debridement of crusted lesions, are often all that is necessary. Sometimes, treatment with topical antibiotics and bathing with antiseptics are required as an adjunct to drainage. In general, systemic antibiotic therapy is given when there are systemic symptoms such as fever, or when the infection is severe or widespread, or involves deeper tissue. Underlying skin disease, scabies infection or eczema should also be treated.

Impetigo and other streptococcal infections are highly contagious and are usually treated with an oral antibiotic such as penicillin, flucloxacillin or erythromycin, or intravenous flucloxacillin or cephalothin in severe infections. Patients with severe infections (especially children) should be isolated until the infection is under control.

Eradication of nasal and skin carriage of *Staphylococcus aureus* in patients with recurrent staphylococcal skin infections may be attempted with a nasal spray of the antibiotic, mupirocin, and a skin antiseptic such as triclosan.

Treatment of Bairnsdale ulcer can be effected with combination therapy such as rifampicin plus streptomycin, plus surgical debridement if tissue damage is extensive.

Acne

Acne is a skin disorder that affects around 80% of teenagers and many adults. *Propionibacterium acnes*, an anaerobic Gram-positive rod that is a normal inhabitant of skin, has been strongly implicated in the pathogenesis of acne. The organism colonises the pilosebaceous follicles (hair follicle and associated sebaceous gland) and appears to be present in both normal and acne-affected follicles in the same individual. Its presence on the skin of some individuals appears to be totally innocuous. Because of this there is some uncertainty about the organism's role in the disorder, but there is other evidence that supports its role. The responsiveness of some cases to antibiotics is part of this evidence.

The lesions of acne have classically been divided into closed lesions (whiteheads), open lesions (blackheads) and inflammatory lesions (papules, pustules or nodules). Whiteheads and blackheads are non-inflammatory lesions that are usually referred to collectively as comedones. These lesions develop when hair follicles and sebaceous glands become blocked with sebum. The inflammatory lesions are postulated to develop when *P. acnes* grows in the blocked follicles and activates the inflammatory response.

Acne is treatable in some people, but some cases do not respond. The mainstay of treatment is frequent cleansing of the skin, antiseptics and topical keratolytics (benzoyl peroxide or tretinoin). Topical or oral antibiotics (e.g. tetracycline or clindamycin) may be prescribed for persistent cases, but some antibiotic resistance in *P. acnes* has been demonstrated.

VIRAL SKIN INFECTIONS

Some viruses cause skin lesions by localising in and infecting cutaneous tissue. The wart viruses and most poxviruses are the major groups of this type. Other viruses cause skin lesions as well as infecting other body sites. The common systemic viral diseases that produce skin lesions as the major manifestation are herpes simplex infections, chickenpox, measles and rubella.

Rubella

Rubella, or **German measles**, is one of several systemic human viral diseases that cause a skin rash. It is caused by a togavirus that is spread mainly by the airborne route from infected individuals. It is highly contagious for about a week before and a week after the rash appears. Despite the availability of an effective vaccine (see below), the National Notifiable Diseases Surveillance System reported an epidemic level of rubella activity in 1992 to 1995, but since then the incidence has decreased, and was under 300 cases in 2002.

Except for the congenital form (described below), rubella is generally a mild, often subclinical, disease. The incubation period is 2–3 weeks. In adults, a short period of mild fever, malaise and upper respiratory symptoms may occur first. The rash is the main symptom of rubella; it appears first on the face or trunk but quickly spreads to the rest of the body. The lesions are macular with a light rose-pink colour (Figure 16.5). Lymph nodes are usually enlarged and in severe cases conjunctival infection may be marked. The rash usually disappears after three days.

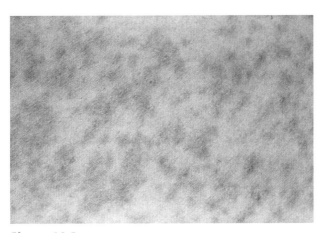

Figure 16.5

Rubella
The patient shows the macular rose-pink spots typical of this disease.

Many infected individuals do not have a rash but are still able to transmit the virus to others.

Congenital rubella syndrome results from infection of a developing foetus when the virus crosses the placenta from the mother's circulation. The effect on the foetus varies with the gestational age at the time of maternal infection. The virus slows cell replication and differentiation, so the most severe damage occurs if the woman is infected in the first trimester, when foetal organ systems are developing. The most severe effects of congenital rubella include stillbirth, mental handicap, deafness, eye defects, cardiac abnormalities, hepatomegaly, splenomegaly, pneumonitis and low birth weight. Major abnormalities are rare if infection occurs after the 16th week of pregnancy.

The link between rubella infection in early pregnancy and congenital defects in infants was first suggested in 1941 by NORMAN GREGG, an ophthalmologist working at the Royal Alexandra Hospital for Children in Sydney.

Rubella cannot be reliably diagnosed by clinical means, so when the diagnosis must be confirmed (e.g. in a pregnant woman or someone in contact with a pregnant woman, or in an affected neonate) serological tests are required. Serology is also used to assess the immunity of pregnant women in prenatal screening tests.

A live attenuated rubella vaccine was licensed in Australia in 1970 and a mass vaccination program commenced in 1971. The principal aim of rubella vaccination is to prevent congenital rubella syndrome. To achieve this, not only must females be immunised prior to child-bearing age, but the circulation of rubella virus in the whole community should ideally be stopped. Hence, both males and females need to be immunised. Rubella vaccine is now a component of the MMR (measles-mumps-rubella) vaccine recommended for all children at 12 months of age, with a

---

CASE HISTORY 16.2
Congenital rubella

A 32-year-old shop owner was pregnant for the first time. She could not recall having received rubella vaccination at school, but remembered that her mother always said that vaccinations were a waste of time. At her first visit to the obstetrician (about six weeks after becoming pregnant), blood was taken for rubella serology and she was found to have no detectable antibodies. Three weeks later she became ill with what she thought was a cold and conjunctivitis. She did not recall having any rash.

Her son was born at full term, but his birth weight was only 2450 g; his Apgar scores were 9 at 1 minute and 10 at 5 minutes (i.e. normal). The paediatrician made a diagnosis of congenital rubella syndrome based on clinical findings, including microphthalmia, a cataract in the right eye and profound deafness, and on the mother's history.

second dose at 4 years of age. Vaccination is also recommended for non-pregnant, seronegative women of childbearing age. Since it is a live vaccine, it is not recommended for women in early pregnancy, and vaccinated women should be advised to avoid becoming pregnant for 28 days after vaccination. Vaccination has been extremely successful, resulting in a significant reduction in congenital rubella.

Measles

Measles, or **rubeola**, is a highly infectious, acute illness caused by a paramyxovirus. In Australia, the incidence of measles has declined over the last decade, especially since 1998 when the Measles Control Campaign (which involved the mass vaccination of primary school children) took place. In 2002 there were 31 confirmed cases, representing a national rate of 0.2 cases per 100 000 population. The highest rate of notification tends to be in the 0–4 years age group although outbreaks can also occur in non-vaccinated young adults, who can then act as a reservoir of disease for the younger age group (see Spotlight box, page 321).

The measles virus is mainly spread from infected people by the airborne route via respiratory secretions. An acute case of measles is infectious 3–5 days before the onset of symptoms and for as long as fever is present. After an incubation period of 9–14 days symptoms of fever, runny nose, dry cough and watery eyes typically develop. **Koplik's spots**, which are areas of white necrosis

on a reddened mucosa, may appear in the mouth 3–4 days later. They may also appear on other mucosa such as the conjunctiva. Usually, within another two days, a dusky red, maculopapular rash develops, often starting behind the ears, then spreading to the face and down the body, eventually reaching the lower extremities (Figure 16.6). The Koplik's spots disappear shortly after the rash appears. The rash fades in several days, starting from the top of the body and progressing in a way similar to its appearance. There is usually a generalised, but minor, lymph node enlargement. The virus may invade the lungs, kidneys or brain, especially in the immunocompromised, and then is often fatal.

Even in immunocompetent people, measles is potentially a very serious disease. **Measles encephalitis** is a severe complication, occurring in approximately one patient per 1000. Many of these patients recover without problems, but 15–40% suffer permanent neurological injury and 10–15% become comatose and die. Malnutrition increases the risk of mortality. In approximately one in 25 000 cases, the virus is not completely cleared from the body but persists in the brain. Six to eight years later, **subacute sclerosing panencephalitis (SSPE)** develops and is always fatal, due to viral destruction of nerve cells with progressive mental deterioration, muscle rigidity and coma. In some areas of the world, such as Africa, mortality rates due to measles or its complications can be as high as 10–20%. Other less serious complications of measles are secondary bacterial bronchopneumonia and middle ear infections.

Measles is usually diagnosed clinically by the initial catarrhal symptoms and dry cough, fever and a rash. It can also be diagnosed serologically by detection of specific IgM antibodies in serum. Treatment is limited to alleviating symptoms and dealing with complications. Secondary, bacterial infections can be effectively treated with antibiotics.

The availability of measles vaccine now prevents major epidemics in developed countries. It is usually used in the form of the MMR vaccine (containing attenuated viruses

---

CASE HISTORY 16.3

Measles

The Victorian Department of Human Services was advised on 1 February 2001 of a suspected case of measles in a 19-year-old female who had been admitted to Royal Melbourne Hospital. The following day, two more cases (a 22-year-old female and a 28-year-old male) were reported, and by 16 February a total of 31 laboratory-confirmed cases had been identified. All the cases except one (a 10-month-old female) were aged between 15 and 34 years. Seventeen cases were hospitalised.

It was subsequently determined that the primary case was a 19-year-old male who returned to Sydney on 4 January 2001 after holidaying in India. He had then visited Melbourne from 17–20 January during his infectious period. The onset of his rash was 20 January, and the onset of rash of all the other cases was between 28 January and 13 February. Eight of the other cases, including the baby girl, were directly linked to the primary case because all had attended the same restaurant on the same night as the primary case. Secondary spread to at least two other cases appeared to have occurred at a nightclub.

Adapted from A. Andrews, 2001, 'Measles outbreak among young adults in Victoria', *Communicable Diseases Intelligence* 25(1): 12.

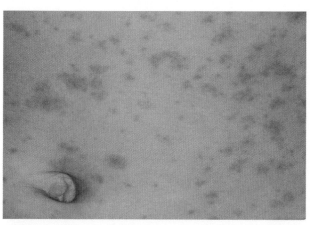

Figure 16.6

Measles

The disease is characterised by small, raised maculopapular lesions.

of measles, mumps and rubella). Measles vaccination should occur at around 12 months of age, followed by a second dose at 4 years of age. Malaise, a moderate to high fever or a rash may occur 7–10 days after vaccination, and last 2–3 days. Encephalitis is a very rare complication of measles vaccination (one in two million doses), much rarer than in natural infection. Anaphylaxis following the administration of MMR is also very rare (less than one in one million doses).

It has been suggested that measles-mumps-rubella (MMR) vaccination might be linked with inflammatory bowel disease and autism, but there has been no scientific evidence to support this claim.

Since measles vaccine comprises living viruses, it should not be used in immunocompromised people or pregnant women. Normal immunoglobulin is used for people who are non-immune and exposed to a confirmed case, or exposed to others who are non-immune and who have been exposed to a confirmed case.

Chickenpox and shingles

The varicella zoster virus (VZV), a member of the herpes family, causes both chickenpox (varicella) and shingles (zoster). Chickenpox is a common, highly contagious disease, transmitted by the airborne route from the respiratory secretions or saliva of infected people, or by direct contact with skin lesions. Over 90% of people have had chickenpox by the age of 15 years. Like other herpes viruses, VZV enters sensory nerve endings during primary infection and becomes latent in sensory ganglia. After remaining latent there for decades, it can be reactivated to cause shingles.

Chickenpox is usually a mild disease, but it is more severe in adults. After an incubation period of around two weeks there may be a short period of fever, malaise, runny nose and a skin rash (see Figure 16.7). The rash comprises different types of lesions at different stages of development, from macules to papules to vesicles and pustules. The lesions dry and crust over in a few days. They start on the scalp and trunk and spread to the face and limbs, sometimes to the mouth, throat and vagina. More severe infection and complications can occur, particularly in adults. Complications include interstitial pneumonia, secondary bacterial pneumonia and meningitis. Infection can be severe in women who are pregnant and in neonates infected after birth. People are infectious 1–2 days before the rash appears and up to the time when the lesions form crusts.

In **shingles**, clusters of painful, vesicular lesions like those of chickenpox develop. The lesions are usually confined to one side of the body, following the unilateral location of affected sensory nerves (Figure 16.8). This infection is most common in the elderly, in whom the immune system is becoming less effective. It is also common in immunocompromised patients who can suffer widespread infections, sometimes involving internal organs, which can be fatal. Some people experience recurrent attacks, often marked by pain but with no skin lesions. Chronic infections can occur in patients with HIV infection.

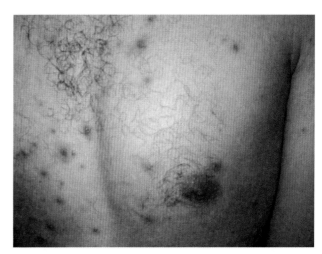

Figure 16.7
Chickenpox skin rash

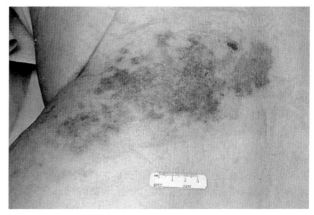

Figure 16.8
Shingles rash

When reactivated, the virus spreads from a ganglion along the pathway of its associated nerve or nerves. The rash may be preceded by a burning sensation or severe pain in the area of the nerves. The lesions are localised in certain areas and may be minor to severe. The rash can be accompanied by headache, fever and malaise. Most patients experience background pain with intermittent sharp stabs, although some are pain-free. Lesions often appear on the trunk but may also occur on the face and eye. These symptoms usually last 2–5 weeks. The pain can persist for up to a year (post-herpetic neuralgia). As in chickenpox, the lesions are rich in virus particles and therefore highly infectious.

Diagnosis of chickenpox and shingles is generally based on clinical signs and symptoms. Laboratory confirmation is rarely required but, in uncertain cases, serology or culture, antigen detection or PCR on a scraping from lesions can provide a definitive diagnosis. Therapy consists of supportive care, such as calamine lotion and soothing baths to relieve itchiness and scratching in chickenpox, and analgesics to relieve the pain in shingles. Aciclovir, famciclovir or valaciclovir may be used for shingles, especially in immunocompromised patients, to prevent spread of infection and complications and to reduce post-herpetic neuralgia. These drugs are very effective if given within a few days of diagnosis and may prevent recurrent attacks. Zoster immune globulin should be given within 96 hours to those in whom varicella may be life-threatening and who have been exposed to the virus – for example, immunosuppressed people, pregnant women, neonates and premature babies.

Vaccination for varicella-zoster is now part of the Australian standard vaccination schedule. It is recommended for children at age 18 months, with a second dose at 10–13 years unless they have had a clinical history of chickenpox. Varicella vaccine is recommended for non-immune adolescents and adults, especially those in high-risk groups such as health-care workers, teachers, child-care-centre staff and household contacts. The vaccine is protective for non-immune individuals exposed to an infected person if given within 3–5 days of exposure. It is also recommended for non-immune women prior to pregnancy. Since the vaccine contains live attenuated viruses, it is not recommended for pregnant women or immunocompromised people.

Warts

Warts are caused by human papillomaviruses (HPV), of which there are over 50 different types. HPV specifically attack skin and mucous membranes, but different types tend to infect different body sites. For example, HPV 2, 3 and 10 typically cause the common warts seen on fingers and knees, whereas HPV 6, 11, 16, 18, 31, 33 and 35 cause genital warts. It is thought that infection lasts a lifetime and, when warts disappear or are removed, the virus still remains dormant in the cells of surrounding tissue.

HPV are transmitted by direct contact, usually between people, or via fomites. Dermal warts occur when the virus enters the skin through abrasions. The virus replicates slowly, stimulating the cells to divide in an uncontrolled way to form a benign mass which protrudes above the skin surface. The incubation period varies from one week to 12 months for dermal warts. Genital warts, which are sexually transmitted, are discussed in Chapter 21.

Warts vary in appearance in different areas of the body. On normal skin, warts develop as small, painless nodules. Often several in number, they occur in areas of friction or minor trauma. Some may be hardly visible. Plantar warts occur in the thick skin on the soles of the feet, level with the skin surface, but with deeper underlying growth. Pressure on them when walking can cause severe discomfort.

Dermal warts usually regress spontaneously, all at the same time, presumably when the immune system gains control, although this may take several years. There appears to be an association of some HPV with cancer, particularly serotypes 16, 18 and 31 with cervical cancer.

Diagnosis of warts is based on clinical observation. Warts can be removed by local freezing of the tissue with liquid nitrogen or by curetting, cautery or laser. Topical treatments include podophyllin and salicylic acid. Recurrences after such treatment are common.

Herpes simplex

Primary infection with herpes simplex virus type 1 (HSV-1) usually involves the skin around the mouth or nose. Occasionally it affects other sites such as the genitalia, cheeks or forehead. Herpes simplex virus type 2 (HSV-2) involves mainly the genitalia but sometimes other sites, including the mouth. Genital herpes infections are dealt with in Chapter 21.

Most primary herpes skin infections are minor or subclinical in immunocompetent people, but may be severe in the immunocompromised. In fact, a severe herpes infection often indicates underlying immune disorder. Primary HSV-1 infection occurs when a susceptible individual comes into close contact with a person with primary or recurrent infection, who may be symptomatic or shedding the virus asymptomatically in saliva. Most primary infections occur in childhood and are asymptomatic.

Herpes skin lesions (cold sores) usually begin as areas of tender erythema, followed by the development of closely grouped vesicles (Figure 16.9) which ultimately progress through pustular and crusting stages. The lesions usually develop on the edge of the lips but may occur elsewhere on the face. They contain large amounts of virus. In patients with impaired cellular immunity (see Chapter 9) due to corticosteroids, cytotoxic drugs or HIV infection, the lesions may be more extensive and spread into the mouth, and resolve more slowly.

Primary infection can sometimes occur at other sites such as the finger (called herpetic whitlow), the conjunctiva (keratoconjunctivitis) or areas of the face subject to frequent rubbing (e.g. 'scrum pox' in rugby footballers).

During primary infection, herpes viruses enter sensory nerve endings and travel along peripheral sensory axons to the sensory ganglion, where they remain latent (see Figure 16.10). The virus remains in the sensory ganglion for life in the form of double-stranded DNA without expressing any viral proteins, which is how it remains hidden from the immune system in periods of latency. The virus can be reactivated by many stimuli, such as sunlight, trauma, viral respiratory infection, menses, stress or immunosuppression, and it then travels back down the same sensory nerves to cause lesions at the same site. The

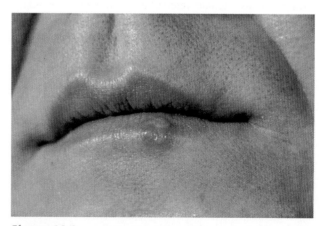

Figure 16.9

Cold sores caused by herpes simplex virus

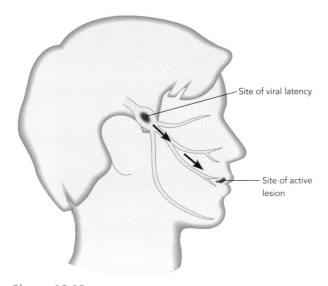

Figure 16.10

Site of latency of herpes virus type 1 in the trigeminal nerve ganglia

interval between recurrences of symptoms can vary from several months to a year, or there may be no recurrence at all. Higher incidences of clinical infection and associated malignancies are seen in immunocompromised people.

The infection is readily recognised clinically, so a laboratory diagnosis is often not necessary. Isolation of the virus from lesion fluid, scraping or biopsy is the definitive diagnostic method, but a diagnosis can also be made by direct antigen detection or PCR on lesion material.

In the immunocompetent, lesions usually resolve spontaneously in 4–5 days. Treatment with saline bathing, peroxide or other astringents may help. In the immuno-compromised, treatment is usually with aciclovir, valaci-clovir or famciclovir, which suppress symptoms and recurrences but do not eliminate latent infection. Secondary infection of herpes lesions by *Staphylococcus aureus* or streptococci may occur.

Molluscum contagiosum

Molluscum contagiosum is a common viral infection, with worldwide distribution, caused by viruses of the pox group. It is most commonly seen in school-age children or young adults. It is transmitted from person to person by direct contact, or indirectly, via clothing, gym equipment or swimming pools, for example. A genital form of the disease, spread by sexual contact, also exists. The infec-tion is characterised by clusters of small (2–5 mm), flesh-coloured papular lesions scattered over the skin. The lesions are disseminated to other areas by scratching. The virus infects epidermal cells, causing epidermal hyper-plasia. The infection is generally mild, but in the immuno-compromised (e.g. people with AIDS) it can result in a severe disfiguring disease.

Diagnosis is usually made by the clinical appearance. PCR or electron microscopic examination of biopsy material may be used to confirm the diagnosis. Spontaneous resolution in the immunocompetent usually occurs within 6–9 months, but therapy is desirable to

prevent spread of infection. Treatment has traditionally been achieved with physical means (e.g. superficial curet-tage or cryotherapy) or with chemical paints (podophyllin or trichloroacetic acid). For serious, chronic disease in the immunocompromised, treatment with antiviral agents (e.g. cidofovir) may be required.

FUNGAL SKIN INFECTIONS

Tinea (ringworm)

The fungi that infect keratinised tissue, causing **tinea** (or **ringworm**), are called **dermatophytes**. Fungal skin infec-tions are called **dermatomycoses**. These diseases can be caused by any one of several organisms from three genera: *Epidermophyton*, *Microsporum* and *Trichophyton*. They cause the disease commonly referred to as athlete's foot, and tinea of the skin, nails, scalp, beard and groin. Different species have a preference for different body sites.

Tinea is spread by contact with arthrospores of the fungi, which may be acquired directly from another person or indirectly from communal bathrooms, dressing sheds or swimming pools. Superficial abrasions or wounds increase the risk of infection. The fungi use keratin as a nutrient and therefore invade skin, nails and hair. The characteristic lesion of tinea is an annular (hence the name 'ringworm', although a worm is not involved), scaling patch of dry skin with a red, raised margin. In hairy parts of the body, the hair might be lost where the lesions develop. The lesions are often itchy. Dermatophytes occasionally penetrate subcutaneous tissues after invading follicles, and may then cause severe pustular lesions.

In **tinea pedis**, or **athlete's foot**, infection usually starts between the toes as a result of maceration from sweating and occlusive footwear. It produces dry, scaly lesions between and under the toes, and subsequently causes the skin to crack and peel (Figure 16.11). The toenails are often infected (**tinea unguium**, tinea of the nails) and may become discoloured, thickened and brittle. Secondary infection by bacteria or *Candida* leads to itchy, soggy, white areas between the toes.

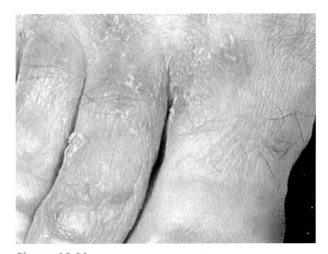

Figure 16.11

***Tinea pedis*, or athlete's foot, caused by fungi called dermatophytes**

Tinea corporis (tinea of non-hair-bearing parts of the body) is characterised by one or more annular, scaly lesions, often on the trunk. **Tinea cruris** (tinea of the groin) occurs in skin folds in the pubic region, and sometimes extends down the thighs. **Tinea capitis** (tinea of the scalp) is most common in children. There are several different forms, depending on the organism involved. At least some hair loss and scaling of the skin are typical.

A clinical diagnosis of tinea is usually adequate. If necessary, a laboratory diagnosis is made by direct microscopic examination of skin scrapings or nail or hair clippings. Sometimes, culture of these specimens is performed but this can take up to two weeks. Some species of dermatophytes fluoresce under ultraviolet light and can be seen when the light is shone onto the infected skin. Treatment generally involves the use of a topical, antifungal cream, powder or ointment and/or a keratolytic agent such as Whitfield's ointment (benzoic acid compound). If lesions are widespread or involve nails or hair, oral griseofulvin or terbinafine is usually used.

Prevention of athlete's foot depends on maintaining healthy, clean, dry skin and avoidance of contact in communal facilities.

Candidiasis

Candida albicans, an oval, budding yeast, is present among the normal flora of the digestive, respiratory and urogenital tracts of humans. It can cause **candidiasis** (or **moniliasis**) in a number of body sites. Superficial infection of mucous membranes causes **thrush**, which appears as milky white patches of inflammation on mucous membranes. *Candida albicans* can also cause **vaginitis**.

Candida skin infections generally occur in areas of warmth, moisture and maceration, such as in skin folds and under tight clothing and in association with nappy rash. *Candida albicans* is an opportunistic pathogen (see Chapter 7), usually requiring some predisposing factor such as diabetes mellitus or antibiotic therapy to cause infection. Obesity also predisposes to *Candida* skin infection, the moist skin folds providing an ideal site for the yeast to grow (see Figure 16.12).

Skin infection is characterised by areas of moist erythema with an irregular, soft, white edge. Satellite areas of infection in the form of red papules or pustules are usually present. If the lesions become generalised, an underlying immune disorder may be present.

In immunocompromised individuals, *Candida* can invade the lungs, kidneys and heart (see Chapter 19). Candidiasis is the most commonly seen fungal infection in hospitalised patients with serious disease such as leukaemia or AIDS.

Diagnosis is usually based on clinical examination. A laboratory diagnosis is made by microscopy and culture of a swab of the lesion. Treatment usually involves the use of topical creams or ointments containing an imidazole. Systemic therapy may be necessary in severe infections.

Tinea versicolor (pityriasis versicolor)

Tinea versicolor is a common, superficial infection caused by the yeast *Malassezia furfur*. The trunk is most often

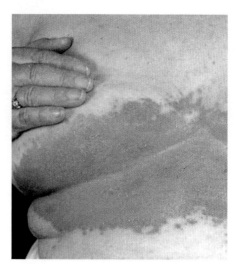

Figure 16.12

***Candida albicans* infection of the skin**
The infection is characterised by areas of moist erythema.

affected, but there may be spread to other areas including the upper arms, neck and abdomen. The lesions are small, sharply demarcated, scaling macules. The organism interferes with pigment production – on white skin the lesions are dark and on dark skin they are lighter, hence the name 'versicolor'. The infection is basically cosmetic, causing little irritation, but it can persist for years if untreated.

The organism has recently been implicated as a cause of or contributor to seborrhoeic dermatitis, or dandruff.

Treatment consists of topical applications of selenium sulphide or the antifungal agent, econazole. Recurrence is common.

ARTHROPOD INFESTATIONS

Scabies

Scabies is caused by the mite *Sarcoptes scabiei* var. *hominis*. The adult female is about 0.4 mm in length, just visible to the naked eye. It burrows in the epidermis of various body sites, laying eggs as it goes (Figure 16.13(a)). The typical scabies lesion is the burrow, but papules, pustules and nodules are also usually seen (Figure 16.13(b)). Itchiness, representing a sensitisation to mites, eggs and faeces in the skin, is severe and is often worse at night. Secondary infection of the lesions by streptococci or staphylococci is a common complication when they are scratched.

Norwegian (crusted) scabies is characterised by formation of thick crusts on the face, scalp, hands, feet and pressure-bearing areas. It is typically found in patients who are either immunologically or neurologically impaired, such as AIDS patients, transplant patients receiving immunosuppressive agents, patients with leukaemia and individuals with trisomy 21. In this form, the host may be harbouring thousands of mites and their epithelial debris may be highly infectious.

The mites are spread by close personal contact. In adults, the usual source is a sexual partner. Because scabies is a highly contagious disease, outbreaks can occur

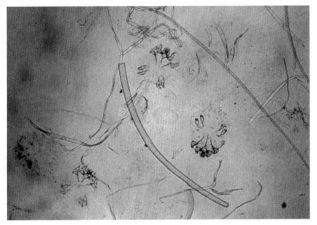

(a)

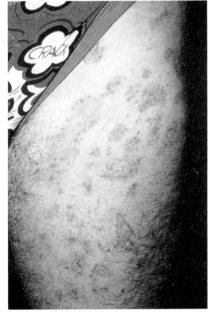

(b)

Figure 16.13

(a) An adult scabies mite; (b) scabies infection

in hospitals and nursing homes. It can be spread directly from patient to patient, or via health-care personnel, visitors and fomites.

The clinical presentation of scabies infestation is variable and often misdiagnosed. Nevertheless, diagnosis is based on clinical examination and microscopic demonstration of mites or eggs in a skin burrow, scraped with a needle point. A number of scabicides, such as permethrin, provide effective treatment. Although scabies rarely seems to be transmitted by clothing, towels or bedding, dry cleaning or machine washing in hot water of these items is recommended. Patient contacts should also be evaluated for infestation.

Pediculosis

Pediculosis, or lice infestation, may involve the scalp, the pubic area or the body. Three species of lice infest these different sites: *Pediculus humanus capitis* (head louse), *Pediculus humanus corporis* (body louse) and *Phthirus pubis* (crab louse). The major symptoms of pediculosis are itching and a maculopapular rash. Scratching can cause crusting and secondary bacterial infection. Enlarged lymph nodes are common.

Head lice infestation affects mainly young school children. The head louse (Figure 16.14) lays its eggs (called nits) at the base of hairs, to which they are firmly attached. After 8–10 days the eggs hatch, leaving translucent shells fixed to the hair. Pink or white dots can be seen near the scalp. Transmission is by hair-to-hair contact, brushes or hair apparel.

Body lice infestation is generally related to poor hygiene, especially when clothes are infrequently laundered. The body louse lives on the clothing, depositing eggs there, and then travels to the body to feed.

Louse infestation of the pubic area (sometimes called 'the crabs') is usually sexually transmitted. Patients with this infestation often have another sexually transmitted disease, such as gonorrhoea. *P. pubis* prefers the pubic area, but can infest other sites such as the perianal area, thighs and trunk.

Lotions or shampoos of permethrin or other insecticides kill lice and nits, which can then be removed with a fine-tooth comb. Family and other close contacts should be examined and treated if necessary. Clothes and linen should be dry cleaned or washed in hot water.

Wound infections

Wound infection results from microbial invasion of a cutaneous lesion. The common types of wound infection and their causative agents are listed in Table 16.2. Some people are hospitalised because of wounds (trauma or burns) and many people in hospital suffer wounds from surgery, intravascular catheters or pressure sores, all of which increase their risk of infection. Most wounds contain a serous exudate which, together with any dead tissue, provides an excellent culture medium for bacteria. Thus, it can be expected that virtually any open skin wound will contain microorganisms. However, this does not necessarily mean that the wound is infected.

If the wound contains non-replicating microorganisms only it is said to be *contaminated*. If there are replicating

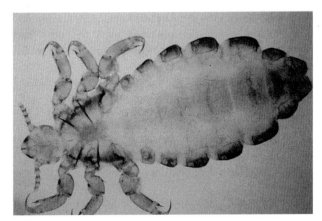

Figure 16.14

The head louse, *Pediculus humanus capitis*

Table 16.2

Types of wound infections and the common causative organisms

TYPE OF WOUND	COMMON CAUSES
• Surgical wounds (clean)	*Staphylococcus aureus* Gram-negative enterobacteria
• Surgical wounds (dirty)	As above, plus anaerobes and enterococci
• Burns	*Pseudomonas aeruginosa* *Staphylococcus aureus* Gram-negative enterobacteria Enterococci
• Intravascular catheters	*Staphylococcus aureus* Coagulase negative staphylococci Gram-negative enterobacteria *Corynebacterium jeikeium*
• Pressure sores	*Staphylococcus aureus* Group A streptococci Gram-negative enterobacteria Enterococci
• Dog/cat bites	*Pasteurella multocida* *Capnocytophaga canimorsus* Oral anaerobes
• Accidental wound (soil or faecal contamination)	Clostridia *Pseudomonas aeruginosa* *Bacteroides fragilis*

microorganisms adhering to the wound surface without causing any tissue damage, the wound is said to be *colonised*. Wound infection can be defined as the invasion of replicating microorganisms into the wound with evidence of tissue injury.

Clinical signs and symptoms of wound infection include increased pain and exudate, excessive inflammation (greater than the normal inflammation of healing), an unhealthy friable appearance of the wound and a failure of the wound to heal. However, it should be recognised that certain factors (e.g. age, poor nutrition, diabetes, immunodeficiency, some medications) can mask the signs and symptoms of infection so that failure to heal may be the only sign.

Whether or not a colonised wound progresses to infection depends on a number of factors, particularly:

• the total number of microorganisms present
• the number of different species present
• the virulence of the organisms present
• the synergistic interactions between the different species
• the immune capacity of the affected person.

There is evidence to suggest that bacteria in infected wounds reside within biofilms (see Chapter 10), in which the bacteria are protected from host defences and also from antibiotics.

SURGICAL WOUND INFECTIONS

Infections of surgical wounds are among the more common types of health-care-associated infections (see Chapter 13) and are a major cause of morbidity in patients following surgery. About 5–6% of all surgical wounds become infected, but the infection rate varies considerably with the type of surgery, the body site involved and patient susceptibility.

The term **postoperative infection** is used for any infection that occurs as a result of surgery. It includes infection involving the operative field, specifically called **surgical site infection** (SSI), and other infections that may follow surgery but occur in a part of the body not involved in the surgical procedure. In this section our focus is on SSI.

Infection of clean, closed wounds is most likely to be due to organisms introduced during surgery, since in most closed wounds the skin edges are sufficiently sealed within several hours to prevent the entry of microorganisms during postoperative care. However, in situations where skin closure is delayed, microorganisms acquired postoperatively become more important. If surgery involves a site that is normally heavily colonised, such as the colon, the number of organisms that can contaminate the wound from surrounding tissue can be very large, and there is a much greater risk of infection. Thus, in bowel surgery, for example, part of the preoperative preparation may involve the reduction of this microbial load with antimicrobial drugs.

The most common causes of postoperative wound infections are bacteria, particularly *Staphylococcus aureus* (including MRSA – multi-resistant *Staphylococcus aureus*), *Escherichia coli* and other Gram-negative enterobacteria, *Pseudomonas aeruginosa*, enterococci and various anaerobes (e.g. *Bacteroides* spp.). However, the common causative agents vary from one hospital setting to another. Most surgical wound infections become apparent within several days of the surgery, and some can be extremely quick, occurring within hours. However, infection of some surgical wounds can appear as much as 30 days after surgery.

Epidemiology of surgical wound infections

Most surgical wound infections are probably acquired at the time of the operation. Possible sources of the organisms include:

- the operating room environment
- the hands of operating personnel
- other body parts of operating room personnel
- the patient's own body.

Strict environmental control and stringent sterilisation and disinfection practices help to reduce infection, as do preoperative scrubbing with an antiseptic with residual action and the use of surgical gloves. Dermatitis on the hands of surgical personnel increases the risk because of the heavy colonisation of these lesions by bacteria. Materials used for gowns and drapes may not be effective barriers for bacteria, especially if they become moist, since microbes on underlying skin may then penetrate the gown and enter the operative field.

The major source of organisms in surgical wound infections is thought to be the patient's own skin and mucosal membranes. These include the patient's normal flora as well as any organisms that the patient may have been colonised with since entering hospital. As explained in Chapter 13, hospital-derived organisms can be resistant to antibiotics, and thus the infections they cause can be difficult to treat.

Factors that increase the risk of surgical wound infection

It has been shown that the duration of the patient's preoperative stay in hospital significantly affects the risk of acquiring a surgical wound infection. Infection rates are approximately doubled if the patient spends a week, as opposed to a day, in hospital prior to surgery, and approximately trebled after two weeks. The longer patients are in hospital, the greater the possibility that they will be colonised by drug-resistant hospital bacteria.

If the patient already has an infection in another part of the body, there is an increased risk of the wound being infected. When organisms have access to the bloodstream, their spread to the surgical wound site is facilitated.

The duration of the operation is a major risk factor for surgical wound infection. Longer procedures are thought to have a higher risk of wound colonisation because of the length of time the tissues are exposed. Longer procedures also usually involve greater amounts of tissue and more extensive damage.

Other factors that increase the risk of infection are:

- age, due to the waning of the immune system
- the presence of underlying debilitating disease (e.g. diabetes or cancer)
- obesity, because a large amount of fat tissue can prolong the operation
- surgery involving a normally colonised site of the body (gastrointestinal, respiratory, genital tracts)
- the implant of a foreign body during surgery (e.g. prosthetic heart valve, vascular graft)
- inappropriate use (or omission) of wound drains.

Classification of surgical wounds

It is common to classify operations into one of four types. A typical scheme is detailed in Table 16.3. This allows the risk of infection for different types of surgery to be estimated. Actual infection rates can then be assessed.

Preventive measures

Given the usual sources of infecting organisms and the factors that increase the risk of infection, the major measures for preventing surgical wound infections are:

- reducing the preoperative hospitalisation of patients
- eradication of other infections prior to surgery, where possible
- appropriate prophylactic use of antimicrobial drugs
- washing of the skin and the application of antiseptics at the incision site
- promoting adequate oxygenation of the wound with exercise and warm water cleansing
- strict aseptic technique when changing dressings, especially for open wounds.

Laboratory diagnosis

The most common specimen collected for the identification of the cause of surgical wound infection is a swab. The swab should be used to collect as much purulent material as possible from the base of the wound, and transported to the laboratory in transport medium. Where large amounts of pus are present, this should be collected into a syringe and then transferred to an anaerobic transport vial. Where anaerobes are suspected, a tissue specimen should be collected and sent in a sterile container. These procedures are described more fully in Chapter 15. Blood cultures should be collected if the patient is febrile.

Cultures of wound specimens are often difficult to interpret. The main reasons are that pathogenic organisms can simply colonise a wound without causing infection, and that common colonisers (e.g. coagulase negative

Table 16.3

Classification of surgical wounds – a typical scheme

CLASSIFICATION	DESCRIPTION
• Clean	No infection encountered Gastrointestinal, respiratory and genital tracts not entered No break in aseptic technique
• Clean–contaminated	Gastrointestinal, respiratory or genital tract entered Minimal spillage of contents
• Contaminated	One of above tracts is entered with significant spillage of contents Or acute inflammation without pus encountered Or surgery involving a minimally contaminated traumatic wound Or a major break in aseptic technique
• Dirty	Pus encountered Or perforated viscus found Or heavily contaminated traumatic wound involved

staphylococci) can sometimes cause infection. Also, mixed infections are common, and pathogens and colonisers may be difficult to differentiate. Poor specimen quality and insufficient clinical information on request forms can add to the problem.

Treatment

Superficial infections often do not require antimicrobial therapy; local measures, including drainage, debridement and irrigation are often adequate. Basic wound cleansing is important because it reduces bacterial numbers and their toxins in the wound and also reduces the nutrients in debris and devitalised tissue that the infecting microbes utilise.

Antimicrobial drugs are generally used when the infection is extensive or involves deeper tissues, or if the patient has impaired immune defences. In these situations, empirical therapy with a broad spectrum agent is usually commenced when the clinical diagnosis is made, and then modified, if necessary, when the sensitivity of the causative agent(s) has been determined. Local measures should accompany this treatment, since pus and necrotic tissue can prevent antimicrobial drugs from reaching the organisms and can also inactivate the drugs.

BURNS WOUND INFECTIONS

Burns wounds are highly susceptible to infection for a number of reasons. First, they are moist and full of nutrients and necrotic tissue, ideal for microbial growth and proliferation. Second, not only has the skin barrier been lost but other defences may be impaired. Extensive and deep wounds lead to depressed immune system function, with both humoral and cellular defences affected. There is evidence that cytotoxic T cell activity can be suppressed, serum immunoglobulin and complement levels may be reduced, and neutrophil activity impaired (see Chapter 9). Even functional defence cells have difficulty in reaching the infection because of the damage to the vascular system. In addition, blood-borne antimicrobial drugs do not readily reach the infection site.

Patients who survive severe burns may suffer fatal infections while in hospital. In patients with burns affecting more than 30% of the body surface infection is very common. The vast majority of burns wounds become infected after the patient is admitted to hospital, and are therefore appropriately regarded as hospital-acquired infections.

The thick crust or scab that forms over a burn is called an **eschar**. Microbes growing in or on the eschar are usually not a problem but, if they invade beneath the eschar, infection of adjacent tissue occurs. If they then enter the blood vessels, septicaemia, with a potentially high mortality, ensues.

Causative organisms, sources and transmission

Like other wounds, burns wounds are generally colonised by bacteria, some of which may subsequently cause infection. *Staphylococcus aureus* and a variety of Gram-negative organisms, particularly *Pseudomonas aeruginosa* and enterobacteria, are the most common causes of burn infections. *Candida albicans* and filamentous fungi such as *Aspergillus* spp. cause about 5% of infections. In a given burns unit, certain organisms tend to predominate, but the predominant types may vary over time.

Burns wounds quickly become colonised and thus constitute a huge reservoir of microbes for cross-contamination to other hospitalised patients. Organisms may be transmitted from patients with old burns to new patients by hands, clothing, other fomites and air. The gastrointestinal tract contains many potential pathogens and may be an important source of infection, especially where faecal contamination is likely (e.g. burns involving the groin, buttocks or upper thigh).

Hospital staff can carry pathogens on their hands and are also an important reservoir of organisms in burns infections. In addition, their hands are important vectors for the transmission of microbes from other sources to the wound. Hands of staff may become contaminated directly from contact with a patient, or indirectly from contaminated environmental surfaces. This emphasises the importance of proper handwashing immediately before and after contact with a patient.

Diagnosis and treatment

A wound biopsy is the preferred specimen for the diagnosis of burns wound infection, because a quantitative culture can be performed and histologic evidence of infection (as opposed to colonisation) can be obtained. However, the invasiveness of the technique and the time taken for collection and processing of this specimen means that swabs or excised necrotic tissue are most often collected. Blood cultures should be collected if systemic symptoms are present.

Antimicrobial therapy has only a supportive role in the treatment of infected burns wounds. Debridement or surgical excision of dead tissue is the most important aspect of treatment, and this will also aid in the delivery of antimicrobial drugs to the infected site. Because infection is usually acquired in hospital, antibiotic sensitivity tests are essential.

Prevention of burns wound infections

Prevention of burn infections is difficult, even when patients are maintained within specialised hospital burns units. Prevention involves prompt excision of dead tissue, skin graft closure of the wound, good wound care, the use of topical antimicrobials to suppress the multiplication of organisms on the wound surface, and strict environmental control. Environmental control includes strictly enforced handwashing, the use of good aseptic techniques, and gowns and gloves, and fastidious sterilisation and disinfection of fomites.

NECROTISING INFECTIONS

Necrotising infections (sometimes called **gangrenous infections**) are infections of the soft tissue below the dermis (the superficial fascia), resulting in extensive tissue necrosis. **Necrotising fasciitis** is the name for the inflammation that develops in this tissue. Necrotising infections usually occur in tissue following trauma, surgery, ischaemia or other causes of tissue damage. These infections progress rapidly and can quickly be fatal without appropriate treatment (see Figure 16.15).

Most necrotising infections are caused by multiple organisms. Since there is often local hypoxia due to the tissue damage, anaerobic bacteria – especially *Bacteroides* spp. or *Peptostreptococcus* spp. – are usually involved, in combination with facultative anaerobes such as β-haemolytic streptococci or Gram-negative enterobacteria (e.g. *E. coli*, *Enterobacter*, *Klebsiella* or *Proteus*). However, there are two major types of necrotising infections caused by a single bacterial species. Streptococcal gangrene is usually caused by Group A streptococci, and gas gangrene (or clostridial myenonecrosis) is most often caused by *Clostridium perfringens* or occasionally by

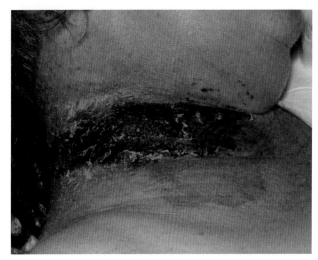

Figure 16.15
Necrotising fasciitis

other clostridial species such as *C. novyi*, *C. septicum* and *C. bifermentans*.

The Group A streptococci that cause necrotising fasciitis have sometimes been referred to as 'flesh-eating bacteria' in the media (see Spotlight box, below). Rather than eating flesh, these bacteria cause disease by releasing toxins and other factors that probably interact with host defence mechanisms to cause a rapidly progressing destruction of subcutaneous tissue. The tissue destruction has been reported to be as rapid as 5 cm per hour!

 SPOTLIGHT ON
Flesh-eating bacteria probe launched
2 November 2000

Unit 5 has uncovered an alarming number of flesh-eating bacteria cases in Illinois, much higher than previously thought. Now a state investigation has been launched.

Toxic bacteria eat away at Bonnie Kowalski's flesh and muscle. 'I went back to surgery four or five times and every time I went in the hole was bigger and bigger and bigger,' she said.

Lisa Carroll feels helpless as necrotising fasciitis, known as flesh-eating bacteria, tunnels through her skin. 'It looked raw, like rancid meat,' she said.

Kowalski and Carroll, within months of each other, had undergone weight-reduction surgery at the same hospital by the same doctor, at Northwest Suburban Community Hospital in Belvidere, near Rockford. They believe that's where the flesh-eating bacteria invaded their bodies, leaving them deformed. Both women have hired attorneys.

Officials at the hospital say they have had no cases of necrotising fasciitis in the past three years, and that it is impossible to determine the source of the women's infections.

Adapted from the NBC 5 News Page

Predisposing factors include penetrating injuries, burns, blunt trauma and childbirth. Early treatment with antimicrobials, supportive care and possibly surgical intervention are essential, but in some cases they may not alter the outcome of the disease. Death may result despite early diagnosis and treatment.

Gas gangrene, caused by clostridia, can occur within hours of tissue damage or surgery. Spores of clostridia are found in soil and in human and animal faeces. They can be introduced into tissues by accidental puncture wounds, or during surgery if improperly sterilised instruments are used, or faecal contamination of the wound occurs. In tissue that is damaged and hypoxic, the spores germinate and the bacteria multiply rapidly, producing toxins that kill more tissue cells, thereby extending the anaerobic environment in which they can grow. The major toxin, alpha toxin, is a lecithinase which hydrolyses lipids in cell membranes, causing cell lysis and death. This allows the organism to invade deeper into the muscle tissue.

As the organisms grow they produce bubbles of gas, which further distort the tissue. This crepitant (rattling) tissue sometimes makes a popping sound when the patient moves, and the bubbles of gas can sometimes be seen in the wound. As the infection progresses, the tissue becomes black and clearly dead. Symptoms also include the sudden onset of pain, high fever and shock.

Diagnosis of gas gangrene is usually based on clinical findings. Because of the infection's rapid progression and potentially fatal outcome, treatment is commenced before laboratory test results are available. Wide debridement of the affected area is mandatory, and benzylpenicillin (or metronidazole) is administered. Amputation of badly infected limbs may sometimes be necessary to prevent the spread of infection.

Gas gangrene can be prevented by adequate cleansing and debridement of wounds to remove dead and damaged tissue and by the use of prophylactic antibiotics for surgery when faecal contamination of tissues is likely to occur.

Infections of the eye

Infections of the eye most often involve the conjunctiva, which is a thin mucous membrane that covers the outer surface of the eye and the inner surface of the eyelids (Figure 16.16). This infection and the resulting inflammation is called **conjunctivitis**. Bacteria and viruses are the most common infectious causes of conjunctivitis, but noninfectious causes are also common, particularly irritation by foreign particulate matter and allergic reactions.

Other infections of the eye may involve the cornea (**keratitis**), the eyelid (**blepharitis**), both the cornea and conjunctiva (**keratoconjunctivitis**) or both the eyelid and conjunctiva (**blepharoconjunctivitis**).

BACTERIAL EYE INFECTIONS

Common causative agents

A wide range of bacteria comprise the normal flora of the eye, including *Staphylococcus epidermidis*, *Propioni-*

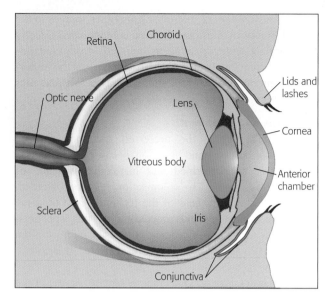

Figure 16.16
Structures of the eye

bacterium, streptococci and corynebacteria. Some of these organisms can cause conjunctivitis, but usually only in the immunocompromised. Bacterial conjunctivitis primarily affects infants and young children. The most common causes are *Streptococcus pneumoniae*, *Staphylococcus aureus*, *Haemophilus influenzae* and *Moraxella catarrhalis*. Contact-lens-related conjunctivitis can be caused by *Pseudomonas* or other Gram-negative bacteria, especially in individuals using extended-wear soft lenses.

Bacterial conjunctivitis (see Figure 16.17) typically develops abruptly, with patients usually experiencing redness, watery eyes, a feeling of grittiness in the eyes, a burning or stinging sensation and photophobia. The watery discharge usually becomes mucopurulent or purulent. On awakening the eyelids can be stuck together by this discharge. The infection usually starts in one eye but

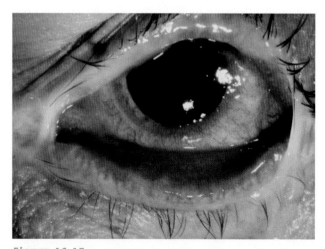

Figure 16.17
Bacterial conjunctivitis

Conjunctivitis

Michael was an active 7-year-old who awoke with the eyelid of his left eye stuck to the lower lid. When he opened this eye he said it felt like he had sand in it, and that it felt a bit 'stingy'. His mother, who was very busy that day, took him to school, intending to take him to the doctor in the afternoon. Apart from his eye problem he felt all right. As soon as she got to work she had a phone call from Michael's teacher, asking her to take him home. The teacher said that he wasn't permitted to stay at school with an eye infection.

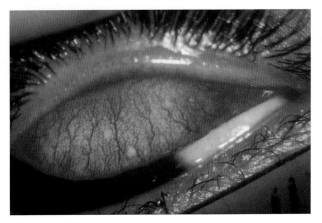

Figure 16.18

Trachoma

A conjunctivitis caused by *Chlamydia trachomatis*. Note the follicles on the conjunctival membrane.

may spread to the other eye in 1–2 days. Even without treatment, many patients will recover completely without permanent sequelae.

Conjunctivitis is extremely contagious, especially among children, and can spread rapidly through schools and day-care centres. Children rub itchy, running eyes and transfer organisms to their playmates.

Neisseria gonorrhoeae infections

In Australia and other developed countries *Neisseria gonorrhoeae* is now an uncommon cause of conjunctivitis, but in underdeveloped countries the disease is still prevalent. It is a potentially serious problem in neonates, who usually acquire the infection from their mother during passage through the birth canal. It is an important cause of **ophthalmia neonatorum**, purulent conjunctivitis in an infant less than 14 days old.

It can also be spread among children, and a number of outbreaks have been recorded in Aboriginal communities in Central and Northern Australia. Early last century, 20–40% of children in European institutions for the blind had suffered from this disease. Sexual transmission is also possible. The infection requires prompt treatment, because it can cause **keratitis** (inflammation of the cornea); this can progress rapidly to ulceration and scarring of the cornea, and even perforation leading to blindness. Perforation can occur within three days of onset of infection.

Chlamydia trachomatis infections

Chlamydia trachomatis serotypes D to K are able to cause conjunctivitis. Transmission is usually by contact, with fingers, towels and flies being important vectors. Some serotypes of *C. trachomatis* can infect the genital tract as well as the conjunctiva and so sexual transmission, autoinoculation from genital infection or infection of the newborn during birth can occur.

Trachoma (Figure 16.18), from the Greek word meaning 'pebbled' or 'rough', is caused by *Chlamydia trachomatis* serotypes A to C. It is the leading cause of preventable blindness worldwide; it is estimated that 500 million people are infected and over 20 million are already blind. The disease is widespread in parts of Asia, Africa and South America, in some areas affecting 90% of the population. It is especially prevalent in arid conditions and in communities with poor hygiene, poor water supply and crowded living conditions. It is still endemic in some remote Aboriginal communities. Flies are important mechanical vectors and close mother–child contact facilitates transfer.

Trachoma is a chronic follicular conjunctivitis, with follicles being more prominent on the upper eyelid. In chronic or repeated infection, fibrosis may occur, which can cause contraction of the eyelid tissue and a turning under of the eyelashes. The lashes abrade the cornea, leading to blindness.

Laboratory diagnosis and treatment

Laboratory tests are usually not necessary for diagnosis of bacterial conjunctivitis, except for severe cases, cases that don't respond to therapy, or when *N. gonorrhoeae* or *C. trachomatis* are suspected. Gonococcal conjunctivitis is confirmed by culture of a conjunctival swab. For suspected chlamydial infections, a swab is rolled firmly several times across the conjunctiva. A diagnosis of chlamydial infection can be confirmed by polymerase chain reaction (PCR) detecting chlamydial antigen in this swab. Sexually active patients with chlamydial conjunctivitis should also be assessed for systemic infection (e.g. urethritis, cervicitis, vaginitis).

As stated above, many cases of acute bacterial conjunctivitis are self-limiting and antimicrobial therapy is not always required. However, appropriate treatment will shorten the course of infection, relieve patient discomfort and limit the spread to other individuals. Topically applied antimicrobials, such as chloramphenicol, are the main form of treatment for bacterial conjunctivitis, except for gonococcal and chlamydial infections. Children should not return to school until their infection has cleared.

Treatment of *N. gonorrhoeae* conjunctivitis involves the use of a topical broad spectrum antibiotic such as a fluoroquinolone (e.g. ciprofloxacin) plus a systemic broad spectrum antibiotic such as ceftriaxone. Preventive measures have almost eradicated the disease in developed countries. Formerly, a 1% solution of silver nitrate in the eyes of neonates was used to prevent infection, but this preventive measure has been replaced by the use of anti-microbial drugs.

Treatment of chlamydial infection is with azithromycin or erythromycin in very young children. When sexual transmission is possible, treatment should also be provided for the patient's sexual partner.

VIRAL EYE INFECTIONS

Viruses are a common cause of infectious conjunctivitis. Adenoviruses cause most of these infections but other viruses, such as the herpes simplex virus, varicella zoster virus, enteroviruses, coxsackie viruses and cytomegalovirus, may also be involved. The typical history is of a recent upper respiratory infection or contact with someone with a red eye. Like bacterial conjunctivitis, viral infection usually begins in one eye but may spread to the other eye within days.

Adenovirus infections

Epidemic keratoconjunctivitis (EKC) is caused by adenovirus serotypes 8, 19 and 37. After an incubation period of about a week, the conjunctiva becomes inflamed and the patient usually complains of a burning irritation and a watery discharge. In contrast to bacterial conjunctivitis, the discharge usually remains watery. Within days the infection may spread to the corneal epithelium and sometimes to deeper corneal tissue.

Direct contact with infected individuals or contaminated fomites is the most common form of transmission.

CASE HISTORY 16.5
Pharyngoconjunctival fever

On 19 October 2000 the principal of north Queensland primary school contacted the Tropical Public Health Unit regarding a high rate of absenteeism. Investigations revealed that 34 students were unwell from 17 to 23 October. The most common symptoms were fever, headache, sore throat, nausea and eye irritation. Between 11 and 13 October some children from the school had been to a school camp at a coastal resort in far north Queensland. The camp had a large saltwater swimming pool. Of the 34 students who were ill, 25 (74%) had attended the camp. The nine affected students who did not attend the camp were assumed to be secondary cases, who acquired the infection from siblings within households or from the school community.

Laboratory investigations confirmed the adenovirus 3 was the cause of this outbreak. Although the virus could not be isolated from the swimming pool, it was strongly implicated as the source of the outbreak. There was evidence that the pool was not appropriately maintained, with an inadequate chlorine level.

Adapted from D. Harley et al. 2001. 'A primary school outbreak of pharyngoconjunctival fever caused by adenovirus type 3,' *Communicable Diseases Intelligence* 25(1): 9–12.

EKC has often been transmitted in epidemic form in eye clinics and ophthalmologists' offices via contaminated equipment or hands. Particular care should be taken in washing hands and disinfecting instruments with alcohol. The virus has been found to be still infectious after two months on unsterilised equipment. Patients should be informed of the extremely contagious nature of this disease, advised to wash their hands frequently and to avoid touching their eyes, sharing towels and having close contact with other people for about two weeks.

Another less common disease, caused by adenovirus serotypes 3 and 7, is pharyngoconjunctival fever. This disease mainly affects children under 10 years of age and is characterised by pharyngitis, fever and conjunctivitis. This is also a highly contagious, person-to-person contact disease. Outbreaks often involve children in summer camps and infection from swimming pools or small lakes.

Viral conjunctivitis is typically self-limiting, normally resolving spontaneously within 2–6 weeks. There is no evidence that topical antiviral drugs improve outcomes. Supportive treatment may be provided, including cold compresses, topical vasoconstrictors and analgesics.

Herpes simplex eye infections

Ocular herpes infections are most often due to herpes simplex type 1 virus. It can produce a number of different clinical manifestations, the most serious being a keratitis, which can result in severe visual impairment. The peak incidence is in children between the ages of 1 and 10 years who have not previously been exposed to the virus and lack protective antibodies. Inoculation of the conjunctiva usually results from direct contact with a person who is shedding the virus from skin or mucous membrane lesions, or by self-inoculation from a primary infection elsewhere in the body.

As with other herpes simplex infections, there is the chance of recurrence due to the latency of the virus in a nerve ganglion, and factors that cause suppression of the immune system (e.g. HIV infection) increase the risk of recurrence. Herpes simplex type 2 virus can also cause conjunctivitis and is most commonly associated with congenital and neonatal disease after acquisition from the mother's genital tract.

Treatment of herpes conjunctivitis or keratitis is with topical antiviral agents such as aciclovir.

Diagnosis of viral eye infections

Viral isolation methods are difficult and are generally performed only by specialist virus laboratories. Fluorescent antibody tests can detect some viruses (e.g. herpes simplex and adenoviruses) in conjunctival scrapings.

OTHER EYE INFECTIONS

As we have seen, **keratitis**, or inflammation of the cornea, can result in permanent damage and vision impairment. Normally, the cornea is quite resistant to infection but factors such as trauma, contact lens wear and topical corticosteroid use can predispose to keratitis.

Keratitis can be caused by various fungi, viruses and protozoa, but bacteria are the most common cause. A wide variety of bacteria can be involved, including all the common causes of conjunctivitis. *Pseudomonas* spp. and the protozoan *Acanthamoeba* are important causes associated with contact lens use. *Acanthamoeba* is ubiquitous in soil and water (including tap water) and therefore commonly contaminates lens cases and solutions. Corneal thinning and perforation are potential threats of severe infection.

Blepharitis is predominantly caused by *Staphylococcus aureus*. Other possible causes include herpes simplex virus and the crab louse, *Phthirus pubis*. **Endophthalmitis** is an inflammation of the fluid behind the cornea and usually follows intraocular surgery when bacteria are exogenously introduced. **Retinitis**, inflammation of the retina, can occur following congenital infection or in immunocompromised patients. Cytomegalovirus retinitis is one of the more common AIDS-associated infections.

A summary of infections of the eye is presented in Table 16.4.

Table 16.4
Eye infections

TYPE OF INFECTION	COMMON CAUSES
• Bacterial conjunctivitis (inflammation of conjunctiva)	*Haemophilus influenzae* *Streptococcus pneumoniae* *Moraxella catarrhalis* *Staphylococcus aureus*
• Trachoma (chronic follicular conjunctivitis)	*Chlamydia trachomatis*
• Viral conjunctivitis	Adenovirus Herpes simplex virus types 1 & 2
• Keratitis (inflammation of cornea)	All causes of bacterial conjunctivitis *Pseudomonas* spp. Herpes simplex virus *Acanthamoeba*
• Blepharitis (inflammation of eyelid margin)	*Staphylococcus aureus*
• Endophthalmitis (inflammation of fluid behind cornea)	*Staphylococcus epidermidis* *Propionibacterium acnes* *Actinomyces* sp.
• Retinitis (inflammation of retina)	Cytomegalovirus Human immunodeficiency virus
• Preseptal cellulitis (cellulitis of eyelid)	*Staphylococcus aureus* Streptococci *Haemophilus influenzae*
• Orbital cellulitis (cellulitis of orbit)	*Staphylococcus aureus* Streptococci *Haemophilus influenzae*

- Undamaged skin provides an effective barrier against invasion by most microorganisms.
- The eye has a number of highly effective defences which generally keep it free of infection.

INFECTIONS OF THE SKIN

- Tissue damage is the most common factor leading to infection of the skin.
- In some systemic infections (e.g. measles, rubella and chickenpox), a skin rash may be the major manifestation of infection.

Bacterial skin infections

- *Staphylococcus aureus* is a common cause of skin infections.
- Infection can occur when the organism invades a hair follicle (folliculitis, furuncle or boil). A carbuncle occurs when boils discharge to adjacent areas of skin.
- Impetigo is a highly infectious, pyogenic infection caused by staphylococci, streptococci, or both.
- Scalded skin syndrome is caused by strains of *S. aureus* that produce a toxin called exfoliatin.
- Erysipelas is an infection that begins as a small, raised, rubbery lesion, and then develops into a bright red, swollen lesion with a sharply demarcated edge, followed by bullae that rupture and weep. It is usually caused by Group A streptococci.
- Cellulitis is an acute bacterial infection of the skin that spreads to subcutaneous tissues. It can be caused by streptococci, *Clostridium perfringens* and other anaerobes.
- Wound drainage and debridement of crusted lesions are often all that is necessary for minor bacterial skin infections.
- Impetigo and other streptococcal infections are highly contagious. They are usually treated with an oral antibiotic or intravenous antibiotics in severe infections.
- *Propionibacterium acnes* has been strongly implicated as a cause of acne.

Viral skin infections

- Rubella (German measles) is caused by a togavirus spread mainly by the airborne route from infected individuals. A rash is the main symptom of rubella.
- Congenital rubella syndrome results from infection of a developing foetus when the virus crosses the placenta from the mother's circulation.
- A rubella vaccine is a component of the MMR (measles-mumps-rubella) vaccine.
- Measles, or rubeola, is a highly infectious disease, spread mainly by respiratory secretions. Typical symptoms are fever, runny nose, dry cough, watery eyes and a dusky red, maculopapular rash.
- Measles encephalitis is the most serious complication of measles infection.
- Measles vaccine prevents major epidemics and is usually given in the form of the MMR vaccine.

- The varicella zoster virus (VZV) causes both chickenpox and shingles.
- Chickenpox is a highly infectious disease transmitted by the airborne route from respiratory secretions, or by direct contact with skin lesions.
- Warts are caused by human papillomaviruses (HPV), which attack skin and mucous membranes.
- Infection with herpes simplex type 1 virus usually involves the skin around the mouth or nose. Skin lesions (cold sores) usually begin as areas of tender erythema, followed by vesicular, pustular and finally, crusting stages.
- Herpes simplex type 2 virus predominantly involves the genitalia.
- During primary infection, herpes viruses enter sensory nerves and travel to the sensory ganglion, where they remain latent. The virus can be reactivated by many stimuli.
- Molluscum contagiosum is a common viral infection caused by pox viruses. The infection is characterised by clusters of small, flesh-coloured papular lesions.

Fungal skin infections

- The fungi that cause tinea (ringworm) are called dermatophytes. They belong to three genera: *Epidermophyton*, *Microsporum* and *Trichophyton*.
- The characteristic lesion of tinea is an annular, scaling patch of dry skin with a red, raised margin.
- *Tinea pedis* (athlete's foot) usually starts between the toes; *Tinea corporis* usually occurs on the trunk; *Tinea cruris* occurs in skin folds in the pubic region; *Tinea capitis* occurs on the scalp.
- *Candida albicans* is present among the normal flora of the digestive, respiratory and urogenital tracts of humans.
- Superficial infection of mucous membranes by *Candida albicans* appears as thrush – milky-white patches of inflammation.
- Tinea versicolor (pityriasis versicolor) is a skin infection caused by the yeast *Malassezia furfur*. The lesions are small, demarcated, scaling macules; on white skin the lesions are dark, and on dark skin they are lighter.

Arthropod infestations

- Scabies is caused by the mite *Sarcoptes scabiei* var. *hominis*. It is spread by close personal contact.
- The female scabies mite burrows in the epidermis, laying eggs; the typical scabies lesion is the burrow.
- Norwegian (crusted) scabies is characterised by formation of thick crusts on the face, scalp, hands, feet and pressure-bearing areas.
- Three species of lice infest different sites: *Pediculus humanus capitis* (head louse), *Pediculus humanus corporis* (body louse) and *Phthirus pubis* (crab louse). The major symptoms of pediculosis are itching and a maculopapular rash.

WOUND INFECTIONS

- Most wounds provide an excellent culture medium for bacteria.
- If a wound contains non-replicating microorganisms only, it is said to be *contaminated*. If there are replicating microorganisms adhering to the wound surface without causing any tissue damage, the wound is said to be *colonised*.
- Wound infection is the invasion of replicating microorganisms into the wound with evidence of tissue injury.
- Local signs of erythema, pain, oedema, odour and purulent exudate are suggestive of wound infection.
- Infections of surgical wounds are among the more common health-care-associated infections.
- The most common causes of postoperative wound infections are *Staphylococcus aureus*, *Escherichia coli*, other Gram-negative bacteria and various anaerobes.
- Burns wounds are highly susceptible to infection. *Staphylococcus aureus* and a variety of Gram-negative organisms are the most common causes of burn infections.
- Necrotising infections are infections of the soft tissue below the dermis. Necrotising fasciitis is the name for the inflammation that develops in this tissue.
- Most necrotising infections are caused by multiple organisms, especially *Bacteroides* spp., *Peptostreptococcus* spp., β-haemolytic streptococci and Gram-negative enterobacteria (e.g. *E. coli*, *Enterobacter*, *Klebsiella*, *Proteus*).
- Two major types of necrotising infections are caused by a single bacterial species: streptococcal gangrene (caused by Group A streptococci) and gas gangrene (caused by *Clostridium perfringens* or other clostridial species).

INFECTIONS OF THE EYE

- Infections of the eye most often involve the conjunctiva (conjunctivitis), but may also involve the cornea (keratitis) or eyelid (blepharitis).
- Infection may be confined to the conjunctiva, or may involve the cornea (keratoconjunctivitis) or the eyelid (blepharoconjunctivitis).

Bacterial conjunctivitis

- The most common causes of bacterial conjunctivitis are *Haemophilus influenzae*, *Streptococcus pneumoniae*, *Moraxella catarrhalis* and *Staphylococcus aureus*.
- Conjunctivitis is extremely contagious.
- *Neisseria gonorrhoeae* conjunctivitis can be acquired by babies during birth.
- *Chlamydia trachomatis* serotypes D to K cause conjunctivitis.
- Trachoma, caused by *Chlamydia trachomatis* serotypes A to C, is the leading cause of preventable blindness worldwide.

Viral conjunctivitis

- Adenoviruses cause most viral conjunctival infections.
- Epidemic keratoconjunctivitis (EKC) is caused by adenovirus serotypes 8, 19 and 37. EKC is highly contagious.
- Pharyngoconjunctival fever is a highly contagious disease caused by adenovirus serotypes 3 and 7.
- Ocular herpes infections are most often due to herpes simplex type 1 virus.

Other eye infections

- *Pseudomonas* spp. and the protozoan *Acanthamoeba* are important causes of keratitis associated with contact lens use.
- Endophthalmitis is an inflammation of the fluid behind the cornea and usually follows intraocular surgery.
- Retinitis, inflammation of the retina, can occur following congenital infection or in immunocompromised patients.

STUDY QUESTIONS

1. What are the characteristics of skin that make it such an effective barrier against infection?
2. What defences does the eye have to protect it from infection?
3. Name the common causes and describe briefly the clinical features of (a) a boil, (b) a carbuncle, (c) impetigo, (d) erysipelas and (e) cellulitis.
4. What are the important infection control considerations for patients with impetigo or erysipelas?
5. Why is the spread of rubella difficult to control in an outbreak?
6. What is the congenital rubella syndrome?
7. How is rubella prevented?
8. What serious complication can result from measles infection?
9. Why do outbreaks of measles infection still occur in Australia despite the availability of an effective vaccine?
10. What are the contraindications for the use of measles vaccine? Explain.
11. What infections are caused by the varicella zoster virus?
12. Explain the implications of latency of the varicella zoster virus.
13. What are the causative agents of warts and what is their link with cancer?
14. What are the common sites of infection of the herpes simplex 1 and 2 viruses?
15. How does the herpes simplex 1 virus cause recurrent infections?
16. What is a dermatomycosis and what are the causative organisms?
17. How is tinea diagnosed?
18. What is thrush, and what are the common predisposing factors for this infection?
19. What is scabies?
20. Why is Norwegian scabies potentially very contagious?
21. What is pediculosis and how is it transmitted?
22. Why are wounds so readily colonised by microorganisms?
23. What are the signs that indicate a wound is infected?

24. List the factors that can increase the risk of surgical wound infection.
25. List the procedures that are implemented to prevent infection of surgical wounds.
26. How should pus be collected and transported to the laboratory for diagnosis of wound infection?
27. How are wound infections treated?
28. What are the common causes of burns wound infections and what are their usual sources?
29. What specimens are appropriately collected for the laboratory diagnosis of infected burns?
30. List the procedures that help to prevent infection of burns wounds.
31. What are necrotising infections?
32. What pathogenic mechanisms are utilised by *Clostridium perfringens* to cause gas gangrene?
33. What is conjunctivitis and what are the common causes?
34. What is ophthalmia neonatorum?
35. What is trachoma and what causes this infection?
36. What specimens are appropriate for the laboratory diagnosis of conjunctivitis?
37. What is epidemic keratoconjunctivitis and how is it transmitted?
38. Define the terms: keratitis, blepharitis, endophthalmitis and retinitis.

TEST YOUR UNDERSTANDING

Case History 16.1   Impetigo
1. What is the most likely reason for Timothy developing impetigo?
2. What specimen(s) should be collected in this case?
3. What important infection control considerations are there in this case?

Case History 16.2   Congenital rubella
1. What does this case indicate about the effectiveness of the rubella vaccine?
2. Why was the woman not vaccinated once she was found to be antibody-negative?
3. How could the doctor's diagnosis of congenital rubella be confirmed?
4. Why are the effects of infection so severe in this infant?

Case History 16.3   Measles
1. What does this case indicate about the transmissibility of measles?
2. What is the most likely reason for this outbreak involving mainly young adults?
3. It is thought that a vaccination rate of at least 90% is required to provide herd immunity. What does this mean?

Case History 16.4   Conjunctivitis
1. Was it reasonable that Michael be sent home from school? Why?
2. What is the likely cause of his infection?
3. What treatment would most likely be prescribed for Michael?

Case History 16.5   Pharyngoconjunctival fever
1. What does this outbreak indicate about the transmissibility of adenovirus 3?
2. What the two major sources of infection in this case?
3. What would be the most useful approach for preventing the spread of infection in such an outbreak?

Further reading

Dwyer DE & AL Cunningham 2002, 'Herpes simplex and varicella-zoster infections', *Medical Journal of Australia*, 177, pp. 267–273.
(Reviews the pathogenesis, clinical features, diagnosis and management of herpes and varicella zoster infections.)

Gottlieb T, BL Atkins & DR Shaw 2002, 'Soft tissue, bone and joint infections', *Medical Journal of Australia*, 176, pp. 609–615.
(Reviews the clinical features, diagnosis and management of soft tissue, bone and joint infections.)

Klauss V, UC Schaller & AA Bialasiewicz 2002, 'Importance and epidemiology of infectious eye diseases', in Kramer A & W Behrens-Baumann (eds) 2002, *Prophylaxis and Therapy in Ocular Infections*, Basel, Karger.
(Reviews the common causes of eye infections.)

Majeski JA & JF John 2003, 'Necrotizing soft tissue infections: A guide to early diagnosis and initial therapy', *Southern Medical Journal*, 96(9), p. 905ff.
(Examines the bacteriology, diagnosis and management of necrotizing infections.)

Oliva M & H Taylor 2004, 'Conjunctival conditions', *Australian Doctor*, 11 June, pp. 39–46.
(Reviews the signs and symptoms, diagnosis and management of common eye infections.)

Ovington LG 2003, 'Bacterial toxins and wound healing', *Ostomy/Wound Management*, 49(7A suppl), pp. 8–12.
(Discusses the relationship between wound colonisation and wound healing.)

Wilson MA 2003, 'Skin and soft-tissue infections: impact of resistant gram-positive bacteria', *American Journal of Surgery*, 186(5A), pp. 35S–41S.
(Reviews the common causes, prevention and management of surgical site infections.)

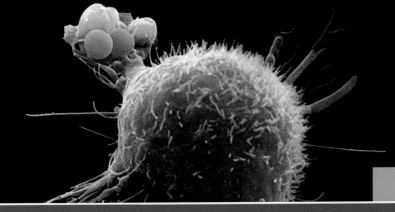

CHAPTER 17

Respiratory Tract Infections

[CHAPTER FOCUS]

- *What are the main defences that protect the respiratory system against infection?*

- *What are the main factors that predispose people to respiratory tract infections?*

- *What are the major types of upper respiratory tract infections and what are their common causes?*

- *How are upper respiratory tract infections diagnosed and treated?*

- *What are the major types of lower respiratory tract infections and what are their common causes?*

- *How are lower respiratory tract infections diagnosed and treated?*

- *What microorganisms cause chronic infection of the lower respiratory tract?*

- *How are chronic infections of the lower respiratory tract diagnosed and treated?*

Introduction

Thousands of litres of air pass into and out of the respiratory tract of a healthy adult each day. This air can contain up to thousands of microorganisms per cubic metre. It is not surprising, therefore, that respiratory infections are among the most common that afflict humans. Most of the microbes in air are harmless, but the respiratory tract is nevertheless a major route of entry into the body of potentially pathogenic microorganisms.

Respiratory pathogens may be expelled in enormous numbers as a result of coughing or sneezing. In addition, a number of potentially pathogenic microbes form part of the normal flora of the upper respiratory tract (see Table 17.1). These microbes are generally kept in check by other normal flora organisms, but they can cause infection if the host becomes more susceptible, or when they are transferred to another individual whose immunity is compromised in some way. Most pathogens that enter the body via the respiratory tract infect only the respiratory tract, but the respiratory system is also a route of entry for some organisms that infect other parts of the body (e.g. measles, mumps and rubella viruses).

To resist the constant threat of microbial invasion, the respiratory system has a number of important defence mechanisms for preventing organisms infecting the upper parts of the tract, and reaching and infecting the lower regions. These defences (summarised in Table 17.2) are responsible for keeping the lungs free of microorganisms and other foreign particles. The importance of these defences is clearly seen in individuals who have a defect in one or more of these mechanisms, or in whom some defences are bypassed, for example, by an endotracheal tube. The incidence of respiratory infection in such people is greatly increased.

A number of factors predispose people to respiratory infections. The most important are:

- *Young age.* Young children are much more susceptible because their immune system is not fully developed, and because their narrower airways are more easily obstructed.
- *Old age.* Pulmonary defences in the elderly are compromised by (1) reduced effectiveness of the cough reflex, due to loss of elastic recoil in the lung and reduced respiratory muscle strength, (2) a waning immune system, (3) other chronic diseases and their treatments, and (4) declining mobility.
- *Cigarette smoking.* Smoking inhibits ciliary action in the respiratory tract, increasing the risk of infection as well as its severity.
- *Chronic obstructive pulmonary disease (COPD).* The major types of COPD are asthma, chronic bronchitis and emphysema. Cystic fibrosis and bronchiectasis are less common but important forms. Lower respiratory infection is a common complication of COPD, due to factors such as reduced mucociliary clearance and diminished effectiveness of cough reflex because of reduced air flow and respiratory muscle fatigue.
- *Poor living standards.* Low socioeconomic standards, including pre-existing illness, poor health-care facilities and crowded living conditions, are major factors. Thus, chronic respiratory disease is very common in the children of many rural Aboriginal communities. This, in turn, contributes to the high prevalence of chronic airway disease seen in the adults of these communities.
- *Alcoholism.* Alcohol intoxication and liver disease interfere with virtually all respiratory tract defences, including cough reflex, ciliary motility, glottic reflex, and alveolar macrophage and NK cell activity.
- *Immunosuppression.* Immunosuppression can predispose a person to unusual and severe infections, the prime example being pneumocystosis (caused by *Pneumocystis jiroveci*) in people with AIDS. This organism is ubiquitous in nature, but rarely causes infection in immunocompetent individuals.
- *Cancer.* Pneumonia is one of the common causes of death in patients with malignancy. Respiratory tract defences may be compromised by the malignancy itself, by associated chronic diseases, or as a result of cancer treatments that cause immunosuppression.

Acute respiratory infections are major causes of illness throughout the world. They are the most common form of illness in developed countries, the most common reason for consultation of general practitioners, and a major reason for hospital admission of children. Although the respiratory system is a continuous tract from the mouth and nose to the lungs, it is convenient to consider it in two parts: the upper respiratory tract and the lower respiratory tract (see Figure 17.1).

In this chapter, we first consider infections of the upper respiratory tract. This region is colonised by normal flora organisms and infections there are generally not life-

---

Table 17.1
Normal flora of the upper respiratory tract

• Commonly present	Viridans streptococci
	Neisseria spp.
	*Moraxella catarrhalis**
	Staphylococcus epidermidis
	Corynebacteria (avirulent strains)
	Bacteroides spp.*
	Veillonella spp.
	*Candida albicans**
	Streptococcus mutans
	*Haemophilus influenzae**
• Occasionally present	*Streptococcus pyogenes**
	*Streptococcus pneumoniae**
	Neisseria meningitidis
	*Corynebacterium diphtheriae**
	*Klebsiella pneumoniae**
	Pseudomonas spp.*
	*Escherichia coli**

* Potentially pathogenic in the respiratory tract.

Table 17.2

Defences of the respiratory system

DEFENCE MECHANISM	ACTION
• Normal flora of upper respiratory tract	Inhibit the establishment of potential pathogens by blocking their adherence to the mucosal surface
• Nasal hairs	Trap large particles in air
• Mucus secretions	Trap particles in air and prevent organisms attaching to tissue surface
• Ciliated epithelium lining the larynx, trachea and bronchi	Moves mucus and particles trapped in it upwards away from the lungs, to be swallowed or expelled
	Together with mucus it is termed the mucociliary escalator
• Non-specific antimicrobial substances in secretions (e.g. lysozyme, lactoferrin)	Destroy microbes or prevent their establishment in the respiratory tract
• Secretory IgA antibodies	Present in secretions protecting against a variety of pathogens
• Cough and sneeze reflexes	Expel large particles and purulent or excessive secretions from central airways and larynx
• Alveolar macrophages	Phagocytosis of foreign materials and microbes that reach the lungs
• Tonsils and lymph nodes	Line the respiratory tract and provide specific humoral and cellular immunity against organisms that enter the tissues

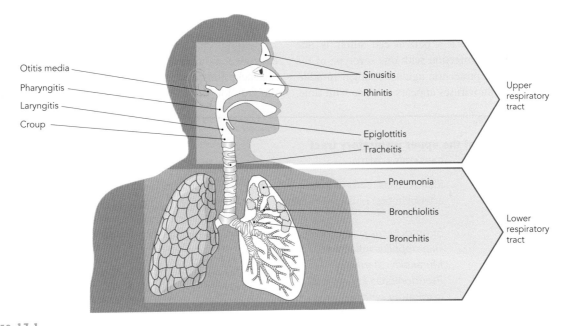

Figure 17.1

Possible sites of infection in the respiratory tract

threatening (although there are exceptions). In contrast, the lower respiratory tract, especially the lungs, is normally free of microorganisms and infections there are often serious. Pneumonia, especially in infants and the elderly, is one of the leading causes of death worldwide, and is still responsible for a large number of deaths in developed countries. While the incidence of upper respiratory tract infections is similar throughout the world, the incidence of lower respiratory infections, especially pneumonia, is more than ten times greater in undeveloped regions than in industrialised countries.

Most acute respiratory infections are caused by viruses, but the more severe diseases are generally caused by bacteria. Fungi and protozoa are important causes of pneumonia, but tend to occur mainly in immunocompromised people. The main reservoirs of respiratory pathogens are people with infections, although for some lower respiratory infections the source may be the normal flora of the upper respiratory tract. Respiratory infections are spread mainly via the airborne route through coughing and sneezing. In addition, some organisms can be readily transferred from the eyes and nose of infected people by hands or on contaminated fomites. A few diseases, such as Q fever and ornithosis, are acquired from animals. In the case of legionellosis, environmental sources are responsible (see pages 405–6).

Upper respiratory tract infections

The upper respiratory tract consists of the nose, throat (pharynx), sinuses, eustachian (auditory) tubes and middle ear. They are all closely interconnected, enabling infection to spread readily from one site to another. Generally, the epiglottis, larynx and trachea are also considered to be part of the upper respiratory tract. The majority of upper respiratory infections are due to viruses and are mostly self-limiting, mild infections. However, they do cause significant morbidity and carry a considerable economic burden in terms of time lost at work or school, visits to health-care providers and amount of treatments used. The infections of the upper respiratory tract are summarised in Table 17.3.

THE COMMON COLD

The common cold is normally a mild illness, lasting less than a week. It is mainly an infection and inflammation of the nasal passages (called **rhinitis** or **coryza**) and the oropharynx (**pharyngitis**). There are many different causes, but rhinoviruses are the most common, followed by coronaviruses (see Table 17.4). Rhinoviruses have great antigenic diversity, with over 100 serotypes found. The large number of colds that a person can suffer is due mainly to the fact that infection with one serotype of the virus may not confer protection against another. In addition, immunity to rhinoviruses appears to wane with time.

Table 17.4 **Causes of the common cold**	
VIRUS	TYPES INVOLVED
• Rhinovirus	More than 100 serotypes
• Coronavirus	Several types
• Parainfluenza virus	Types 1–4
• Respiratory syncytial virus	One type
• Influenza virus	Several types
• Adenovirus	Up to 10 types
• Other viruses	Many

Coronaviruses (see Figure 17.2) also show marked antigenic variation. Despite this, immunity to cold viruses does appear to accumulate, since colds occur most frequently in childhood and progressively less often in adulthood.

Colds generally occur more frequently in colder weather, but the exact reason for this is not known. The most likely explanations are that closer, indoor contact in winter promotes transmission and that people may, for some as yet unknown reason, be more susceptible in winter.

A cold is characterised by a blocked or runny nose with excessive nasal discharge and sneezing. A sore throat, headache and cough may also occur. People with colds are the only known reservoirs of cold viruses, and their nasal

Table 17.3 **Common infections of the upper respiratory tract**		
DISEASE	CAUSATIVE AGENT(S)	MODES OF TRANSMISSION
• Common cold	Rhinoviruses, coronaviruses, adenoviruses, plus other viruses	Respiratory secretions – airborne, via fomites
• Otitis media	*Streptococcus pneumoniae*, *Haemophilus influenzae*, *Moraxella catarrhalis*, *Pseudomonas aeruginosa*, respiratory syncytial virus parainfluenza and influenza viruses	Direct, as a complication of other upper respiratory infections
• Acute sinusitis	As for otitis media	As for otitis media
• Pharyngitis and tonsillitis	Adenoviruses, E-B virus, rhinoviruses, other viruses, *Streptococcus pyogenes* *Neisseria gonorrhoeae* *Candida albicans*	Respiratory secretions Genital secretions Part of normal flora, after antibiotic therapy or immunosuppression
• Diphtheria	*Corynebacterium diphtheriae*	Respiratory secretions – cases and carriers
• Acute epiglottitis	*Haemophilus influenzae*	Respiratory secretions – cases and carriers
• Laryngotracheitis (croup)	Parainfluenza viruses, respiratory syncytial virus, influenza virus	Respiratory secretions

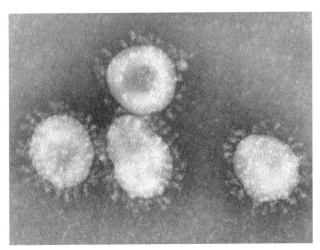

Figure 17.2
Coronavirus
One of the causes of the common cold.

secretions contain large numbers of virus particles. It has long been assumed that cold viruses are transmitted by coughing and sneezing, but it is now recognised they are also readily transmitted by hands and objects (e.g. door knobs, money, telephones) that have become contaminated with nasal secretions. Rhinoviruses are able to persist for some time on hands and objects because they are resistant to drying. Touching of the nose or eyes with contaminated fingers enables the viruses to enter the body. A person starts shedding the virus within 24 hours of infection and may continue to shed viruses for some time after resolution of symptoms.

The host response to cold viruses is the major cause of cold symptoms. Rhinoviruses first attach to specific receptors on respiratory epithelial cells, invade the cells and then spread to adjacent epithelial cells. They cause little damage to the epithelium, but induce excessive mucus production and the other symptoms of colds by stimulating the release and local action of inflammatory mediators. Coronaviruses have a similar effect on respiratory epithelium, although they can cause some damage to the cells lining the nose and trachea. Secondary bacterial infection of the paranasal sinuses and middle ear are possible complications of a cold when the sinuses or middle ear become blocked by the inflammatory exudate. Cold viruses have an important role in precipitating asthma attacks and exacerbating chronic bronchitis, especially in young children.

The common cold is usually diagnosed by clinical findings alone because the illness is generally mild and self-limiting with no effective treatment. Treatment with decongestants and analgesics may help to reduce symptoms. Antibiotic therapy for colds represents a misuse of these drugs, unless secondary bacterial infection is present. There is no definitive evidence that over-the-counter preparations such as vitamin C, zinc and Echinacea have any clinical benefit. There is no effective vaccine for the prevention of colds, essentially because of the large number of possible causes and the serologic diversity of the major causes.

MIDDLE EAR INFECTIONS

Infections involving the middle ear are called **otitis media**. They occur most often in infants and small children. It is thought that the diameter and shape of the eustachian tube in young children gives nasopharyngeal bacteria a greater opportunity to reach the middle ear. Blockage of the eustachian tube due to viral respiratory infection or allergy may interfere with normal mucociliary expulsion of upper respiratory bacteria (see Figure 17.3) The resultant proliferation of bacteria then causes further inflammation and blockage. Some children suffer from recurrent episodes of otitis media.

Otitis media can be caused by almost any bacterium present in the upper respiratory tract, but *Streptococcus pneumoniae* and *Haemophilus influenzae* are the most common causes, followed by *Moraxella catarrhalis*. Viruses, including respiratory syncytial virus, para-influenza virus and influenza viruses, are now recognised as having a significant role in the development of otitis media. Chronic middle ear infections tend to be caused by organisms such as *Pseudomonas aeruginosa*, *Proteus* spp. or *S. pneumoniae*. Otitis media can also be associated with swimming in contaminated water and with head trauma.

Some cases of otitis media are asymptomatic, but usually earache and fever are present. The eardrum becomes inflamed and swollen due to increased pressure in the middle ear. In severe cases perforation of the eardrum may occur. In some children, non-specific symptoms of fever, diarrhoea and vomiting occur. Diagnosis is usually based on the signs and symptoms in conjunction with a pneumatic otoscope. Laboratory diagnosis is not usually performed because of the pain associated with middle ear aspiration. Nasal administration of a vasoconstrictor, such as ephedrine, may be used to reduce congestion.

Antibiotic treatment of otitis media is a controversial issue. Most cases resolve spontaneously and research

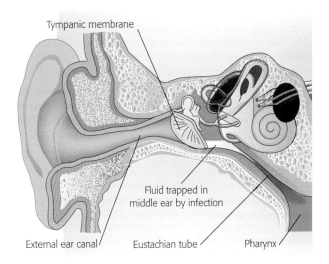

Figure 17.3
Middle ear infection
Accumulation of fluid due to inflammation may block the eustachian tube.

indicates that antibiotic treatment has only a slight advantage over no antibiotic therapy. In some countries (e.g. The Netherlands) symptomatic treatment alone is the standard, with antibiotics being used only if symptoms persist for more than two or three days. The drugs of choice are usually amoxycillin or cefaclor. Even with appropriate therapy, fluid can persist in the middle ear (called 'glue ear'), impairing hearing for weeks or even months. Perforation of the eardrum may also lead to later problems with hearing. Impaired hearing has often led to children being wrongly labelled as inattentive or disobedient, and can lead to poor speech development.

ACUTE SINUSITIS

The major causes of acute sinusitis are *S. pneumoniae* and *H. influenzae*. Viruses or environmental allergens or pollutants probably play a role in many cases of sinusitis by inducing inflammation and increased mucus production and congestion of the nasopharyngeal mucosa. Clinical features include facial pain, due to pressure caused by blockage and fluid accumulation in sinuses, a nasal discharge that is often purulent, and headache.

It may be possible to identify the causative bacteria by microscopy and culture of pus aspirated from the sinus, but sinus puncture is not often carried out. The patient is usually treated empirically with ampicillin or amoxycillin, plus an analgesic for the pain and a nasal vasoconstrictor to reduce congestion.

PHARYNGITIS AND TONSILLITIS

Cause, pathogenesis and clinical features

Pharyngitis, or an inflamed, sore throat, is a common condition that can be caused by many different organisms, although viruses are the usual causes (see Table 17.3). When the tonsils are affected it is called **tonsillitis**. A sore throat may be due to infection restricted to the throat, or may be one of the early symptoms of a cold, influenza or certain systemic infections. Apart from a sore throat, the patient may have a fever, chills, enlarged lymph nodes in the neck and a headache. Otitis media and sinusitis are possible complications.

Adenoviruses are particularly common causes of sore throat and may infect the conjunctiva as well, causing what is known as **pharyngoconjunctival fever**. Epstein-Barr (EB) virus causes a pharyngitis as part of the syndrome called infectious mononucleosis, or glandular fever (see Chapter 19). Other viral causes of pharyngitis include rhinoviruses, coronaviruses, herpes simplex virus and coxsackie A virus. Bacteria are less common causes of pharyngitis and tonsillitis, but the infections they cause can be more serious. The most important bacteria are:

- *Streptococcus pyogenes* (Group A streptococci), the cause of streptococcal sore throat
- *Corynebacterium diphtheriae*, the cause of diphtheria (see below)
- *Haemophilus influenzae* type b, the major cause of severe epiglottitis (see page 397)

- *Neisseria gonorrhoeae*, in pharyngeal gonorrhoea (see Chapter 21).

The yeast, *Candida albicans*, is an important cause of pharyngitis in immunosuppressed patients.

Acute pharyngitis caused by *S. pyogenes* is commonly referred to as a 'strep sore throat'. It occurs mainly in children. The oropharynx of humans is the natural reservoir of this organism. It can be found in low numbers in the throat and nose of normal people, and in large numbers in the throat of infected people. It is spread primarily by coughing and sneezing and can persist for long periods in dried mucus and dust. Although this organism causes less than 10% of cases of acute pharyngitis, it is important because of the possibility of serious complications (see below). Some strains of *S. pyogenes* also produce an erythrogenic toxin, which causes the erythematous skin rash characteristic of **scarlet fever**. (See Figure 7.8 on page 144). The toxin also causes the tongue to be reddened and enlarged, and it develops a strawberry-like appearance. A high fever is also characteristic.

Laboratory diagnosis and treatment

In most cases, the clinical condition of pharyngitis or tonsillitis is not serious enough to require a laboratory diagnosis and, because the vast majority are caused by viruses, no specific therapy exists. One viral infection, infectious mononucleosis, warrants identification and is diagnosed by serological means (see Chapter 19). Bacterial infections can usually be readily identified by culture of a throat swab (see Chapter 15). When bacteria are suspected, a laboratory diagnosis may be warranted because of the potential seriousness and because they can be treated with antibiotic therapy.

Possible sequelae of streptococcal sore throat

Two non-infectious complications of streptococcal sore throat occasionally occur. **Rheumatic fever** is a possible sequela of streptococcal sore throat in which antibodies, formed against antigens in the streptococcal cell wall, cross-react with the sarcolemma (muscle cell membrane) of human heart and other tissues. Rheumatic heart disease, representing damage to the heart valves by these antibodies, can result from repeated infections. **Acute glomerulonephritis** develops when antibodies combine with certain streptococcal antigens to form circulating immune complexes. If these complexes are deposited in glomeruli, local inflammation and kidney disease can result.

Rheumatic fever occurs in only a minority of people but is, nevertheless, a potentially serious consequence of streptococcal sore throat. It is a common disease in some rural Aboriginal communities in Australia where the rate of streptococcal infection is high. In susceptible people each episode of untreated streptococcal sore throat will lead to an episode of rheumatic fever. Therefore, prompt diagnosis and treatment of streptococcal sore throat in individuals with a history of rheumatic fever are essential. Penicillin or erythromycin is usually used for streptococcal sore throat. In severe cases, prophylactic antibiotics to prevent streptococcal infection may be warranted. Rheumatic fever is discussed in detail in Chapter 19.

In contrast, antibiotic treatment of streptococcal sore throat does not necessarily prevent post-streptococcal glomerulonephritis.

DIPHTHERIA

Cause, pathogenesis and clinical features

Diphtheria is an acute infectious disease caused by toxin-producing strains of *Corynebacterium diphtheriae*. The infection was once a major cause of death, especially in children, throughout the world, but is now rare in developed countries due to the availability of an effective vaccine which became freely available from about 1940 (see Figure 17.4). In developed countries it tends to occur now more often in adults, due to waning immunity, than in children. It is still common in many developing countries where the vaccine is not so readily available or administered.

Diphtheria has been almost eradicated in Australia with only one case (in 2001) reported since 1993, but the possibility of resurgence exists if population immunity drops to a low level.

The organism is usually transmitted by the airborne route from infected people or asymptomatic carriers. Once it is established in the respiratory tract, usually on the pharynx or larynx, it secretes a toxin that destroys the epithelial surface, forming an ulcer. A sore throat and fever are the first symptoms to develop after an incubation period of 2–5 days. The ulcer becomes covered by a greyish membrane (called a pseudomembrane), consisting of dead tissue cells, bacteria and inflammatory exudate. In severe cases the membrane can block the airway. If the larynx is infected, a life-threatening respiratory obstruction is more likely.

The bacteria multiply locally without invading deeper tissues or spreading to other sites in the body, but the toxin is absorbed into the bloodstream and then kills cells in the heart, kidneys and nervous system by interfering with protein synthesis. The toxin is highly potent – 10 μg is sufficient to kill a healthy adult. Cardiac failure and death can result from the action of the toxin on the heart.

C. diphtheriae can also infect the skin, but usually only occurs in people in the tropics with poor skin hygiene. The organism infects existing skin lesions, causing poorly healing ulcerations covered by a grey membrane. Non-toxigenic strains of *C. diphtheriae* have been shown to cause a variety of other infections such as pharyngitis, endocarditis and septic arthritis, mainly in people with underlying risk factors.

Diagnosis and treatment

Diphtheria is a life-threatening disease and has considerable public health importance. It therefore warrants urgent diagnosis and treatment. A diagnosis of diphtheria is confirmed by the isolation and identification of toxin-producing corynebacteria in a swab from under the membrane. Polymerase chain reaction (PCR) methods for detection of toxin production in cultures and directly on patient specimens have been developed. As soon as the diagnosis is suspected clinically, treatment with antitoxin, to neutralise the toxin, should be commenced. Penicillin or erythromycin is given in conjunction with antitoxin to eliminate the infection and prevent further toxin production. Diphtheria of the larynx may require a tracheostomy.

Close contacts should be tested for carriage of toxigenic *C. diphtheriae* and have their immunisation status checked. Non-immunised contacts should be given penicillin or erythromycin as a prophylactic measure, and be vaccinated.

Prevention

Diphtheria has almost disappeared from developed countries, due to immunisation of children with the diphtheria vaccine. However, the serious outbreak of diphtheria in Russia from 1991 to 1996, in which there were over 140 000 cases and 4000 deaths, emphasises the need for continued vigilance. The vaccine consists of formaldehyde-inactivated diphtheria toxin, which stimulates production of antitoxin. It is part of the standard childhood vaccination schedule and is incorporated in the diphtheria, tetanus and pertussis (DTPa) triple vaccine, recommended at 2, 4 and 6 months of age (primary course) with a booster dose at 4 years. Further boosters with the lower dose adult/adolescent formulation are recommended at 15–17 years and at 50 years. Travellers to some countries (e.g. the Russian Federation, the Ukraine and Baltic countries) should have current diphtheria vaccination.

ACUTE EPIGLOTTITIS

The epiglottis is a flap of cartilage that prevents food and fluids from entering the larynx. **Epiglottitis**, inflammation of the epiglottis, is most often seen in young children and is almost always caused by *Haemophilus influenzae* type b. It has a peak incidence in children 2–4 years old, and in

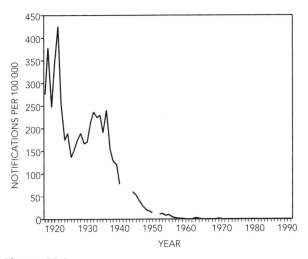

Figure 17.4

Annual rate of notifications of diphtheria in Australia, 1917–91

Source: Communicable Diseases Intelligence 17/11, 31 May 1993, © Commonwealth of Australia, reproduced by permission

Epiglottitis

Timothy, a 3-year-old, had been suffering from symptoms of a cold for two days. His crying woke his parents in the middle of the night and they observed that he was feverish and having some difficulty breathing. They immediately took him to the casualty department of the local hospital.

On examination, his epiglottis was red and swollen, confirmed by X-ray of the neck. A diagnosis of epiglottitis was made and Timothy was immediately taken to theatre to have an endotracheal tube inserted. Blood cultures were taken and treatment with cefuroxime was commenced. In four days he had completely recovered.

this group it is one of the more serious types of upper respiratory infection. The organism probably spreads from an initial focus of infection in the nasopharynx. Bacteraemia is usually present and the patient is usually toxic and febrile. A swollen, red epiglottis may be seen when the child's mouth is opened.

There may be respiratory distress because of obstruction of the airway. The infected child often adopts a characteristic posture with the neck hyperextended and the chin pushed forward, to maximise airway diameter. Forcing the child to adopt another posture is not advisable as this may precipitate complete airway obstruction. It is a rapidly progressive disease which can result in death within a few hours due to airway obstruction. Older children and adults may be affected, but usually only if immunocompromised. Airway obstruction is not a prominent feature in these older groups because of their greater airway diameter.

Young patients with epiglottitis must be treated as a medical emergency. An endotracheal tube is often inserted as a prophylactic measure and treatment with antibiotics is begun immediately. The clinical diagnosis is confirmed by isolating bacteria from blood and possibly the epiglottis. Extreme care must be taken when examining the throat, since the swollen epiglottis can be sucked into the airway and cause total obstruction. Treatment with antibiotics such as cefotaxime is usually effective.

Epiglottitis is the second most common infection caused by *H. influenzae* type b (Hib), after meningitis. Hib vaccines have been available in Australia since 1992 and have been part of the standard childhood vaccination schedule since 1993. The vaccines have resulted in a dramatic reduction in incidence of epiglottitis and other Hib disease. Hib vaccines are discussed in more detail in Chapter 20.

LARYNGOTRACHEITIS

Viral infections of the upper respiratory tract may spread downwards to involve the larynx and the trachea. **Laryngotracheitis** (inflammation of the larynx and trachea), or **croup**, is characterised by stridor (noisy respiration), hoarseness and a resonant cough that is often described as 'barking' or 'brassy'. These signs are due to partial obstruction of the larynx, due to oedema and spasm. In most cases, the symptoms become no more serious than this and recovery occurs within a week. However, in some children, respiratory failure can occur.

Croup is most common in children under four years old because of the narrowness of their larynx, and the ease with which it can be partially obstructed by inflammation. There is often a preceding cold, pharyngitis or cough. Some children suffer repeated episodes of croup, probably because they have hyperreactive airways. Laryngeal or tracheal infection in adults (**laryngitis** or **tracheitis**) causes hoarseness and a burning pain, usually without obstruction of the larynx.

Laryngotracheitis is usually caused by viruses, especially the parainfluenza group, and sometimes respiratory syncytial virus or influenza viruses. *H. influenzae* (epiglottitis) and *C. diphtheriae* (diphtheria) are rare causes. Croup can also be caused by the inhalation of a foreign body and subsequent airway obstruction.

The diagnosis of viral croup is based on clinical and radiologic examination. Patient management involves humidification to soften mucus and soothe the inflamed mucosa, and oxygenation to reverse hypoxaemia. Intubation or tracheostomy may be required if complete obstruction is likely. Antibiotics are administered if a bacterial cause is demonstrated.

Lower respiratory tract infections

In contrast to the upper respiratory tract, the lower respiratory tract is normally sterile and so infections involving it are potentially more serious. Lower respiratory tract infections include a spectrum of diseases ranging from acute bronchitis to pneumonia. The major syndromes discussed here are whooping cough, bronchitis, bronchiolitis, influenza and pneumonia. Chronic infections of the lower respiratory tract are dealt with later in the chapter (see page 408).

Pathogenic microorganisms may reach the lower respiratory tract in a number of ways:

- inhalation of organisms suspended in air (aerosols or dust)
- aspiration of oropharyngeal contents (sometimes gastrointestinal contents) when asleep, intoxicated or unconscious
- spread of infection from the upper respiratory tract
- via the bloodstream, from a primary site of infection elsewhere in the body.

PERTUSSIS

Causative agent and pathogenesis

Pertussis (**whooping cough**) is a severe, sometimes fatal, disease caused by the Gram-negative coccobacillus, *Bordetella pertussis*. It is a highly contagious disease, spread from person to person by respiratory droplets.

Its incidence in developed countries has been markedly reduced through immunisation, but in developing countries where immunisation is lacking infection rates are high.

Despite the availability of a vaccine, epidemics tend to occur every 3–5 years, and pertussis was at an epidemic level in Australia in 1993–94, 1997–98 and 2001–02 (see Figure 17.5). In 2001 almost 10 000 cases were notified. Highest rates occur in infants under one year and in 10–14-year-olds. Overall, the majority of infections occur in people over 10 years of age.

B. pertussis has specific adhesins that allow it to attach to the ciliated respiratory mucosa. It multiplies in the epithelial cells but does not invade further. The organism produces several toxins, which combine to produce the symptoms of disease. The exact activity of pertussis toxin is not clear, but it appears to enter phagocytes and impair their chemotaxis and killing power. It may also be partly responsible for the increase in respiratory secretions and mucus production that is characteristic of whooping cough.

Adenylate cyclase toxin also appears to inhibit vital functions of neutrophils such as chemotaxis, phagocytosis and killing activity, and may also be involved in inducing the inflammatory response. Tracheal cytotoxin is a cell wall component that specifically kills tracheal epithelial cells, thereby partially immobilising the mucociliary escalator and causing an accumulation of mucus in the airway. No exact role for pertussis endotoxin has been established but, like the endotoxin of other Gram-negatives, it may be involved in the production of fever and inflammation.

The major activities of *B. pertussis* toxins are illustrated in Figure 17.6.

Clinical features

After an incubation period of 7–20 days, there is an initial illness that resembles a cold, characterised by runny nose, infrequent cough and mild fever. This is the most infectious period. The cough, caused by an accumulation of mucus in the airway, gradually becomes more irritating and paroxysmal (abrupt, short attacks) over the next 1–2 weeks. A paroxysm is characterised by a series of short coughs followed by a 'whoop' – the characteristic sound produced by a gasp of air at the end of a coughing episode. The whoop represents the rush of air through the narrowed airway. The characteristic whoop may be absent in some patients, particularly in very young infants, older children and adults. Because of this the illness is often mistaken for other conditions such as a cold, influenza or asthma.

Frequent coughing episodes can cause exhaustion in a young child. The cough may persist for up to three months. A person with pertussis is infectious for up to three weeks from the onset of illness.

Possible complications include cerebral hypoxia, which can result in brain damage, bronchopneumonia and secondary pneumonia due to invasion of the damaged

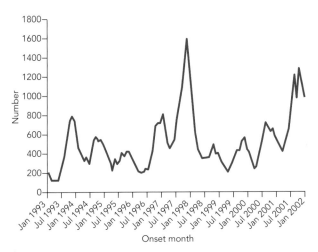

Figure 17.5

Notifications of pertussis in Australia, 1993–2001, by month of onset

Source: Australian Immunisation Handbook 2003, 8th edn, p. 206.

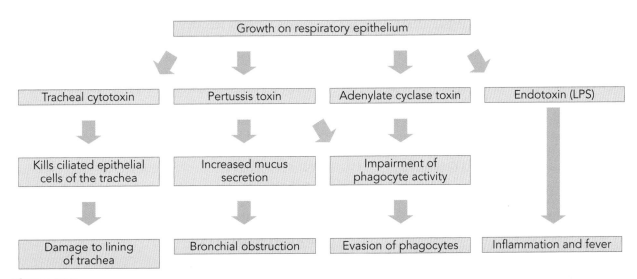

Figure 17.6

Proposed mechanisms of action of the toxins of *Bordetella pertussis*

respiratory tract by other bacteria (e.g. *Staphylococcus aureus*). Death, due to hypoxia, occurs in up to 3.5% of infected babies under six months of age. Infection in adults is often asymptomatic or mild. Adults can become infected if never immunised, or once their vaccine-induced immunity has waned.

Diagnosis

B. pertussis is extremely fastidious and difficult to culture. The optimal specimen for culture is a nasopharyngeal aspirate or swab. PCR testing on a nasopharyngeal swab or aspirate is the gold standard laboratory method for diagnosis of whooping cough. Serological testing for specific IgA antibodies in the serum of the patient may be useful in some circumstances.

Treatment

Supportive care, including oxygen and suctioning, is of prime importance. Antibiotics do not appear to reduce the severity or duration of infection. However, erythromycin reduces the numbers of organisms in the throat and is thus useful in helping to control the spread of infection. Erythromycin prophylaxis of close contacts of active cases may prevent infection or reduce the severity of subsequent infection. Infants are very susceptible prior to immunisation.

Prevention

The National Health and Medical Research Council of Australia recommends immunisation against pertussis

---

CASE HISTORY 17.2

Whooping cough (pertussis)

In late 1999, an outbreak of pertussis occurred in a small town in the north west of Western Australia. The first signs were on 24 November when a woman and her daughter presented to a local general practitioner with a persistent cough. Nasopharyngeal aspirates were collected and on 26 November *B. pertussis* was confirmed in both cases by PCR. An emergency pertussis clinic was established by the local Public Health Unit and people with respiratory symptoms were provided with appropriate antibiotic treatment or prophylaxis. Ultimately, 59 cases of confirmed or probable pertussis were identified from 124 households by school survey and clinical follow-up. Ages ranged from 5 months to 67 years, with children aged 9 to 11 years comprising 41% of cases. Missed diagnoses and a school camp in September attended by two symptomatic children appeared to facilitate the spread of infection.

From immunisation records, childhood vaccination coverage in the cases was estimated at 96%. All 21 cases of pertussis among the under 10 years age group were at least partially vaccinated.

Adapted from: Cordova SP, MT Gilles & MY Beers 2000, 'The outbreak that had to happen: *Bordetella pertussis* in north-west Western Australia in 1999', *Communicable Diseases Intelligence*, 24, pp. 375–379.

---

from two months of age, unless there are contraindications such as a current acute illness or significant reaction following a previous dose. The primary course consists of three doses, two months apart. Booster doses are recommended at 4 years and again at 15–17 years of age. Pertussis vaccine is usually combined with diphtheria and tetanus toxoids and administered as **DTPa** (called **triple antigen**) as part of the standard childhood immunisation schedule. Pertussis vaccine offers complete protection in only about 80% of people and protection wanes to almost zero after 12 years. Nevertheless, it has been very effective in reducing the number of infections (up to 90% reduction) in countries where uptake has been high.

In the past there have been major concerns about the possible side effects of the whole-cell pertussis vaccine, leading to its reduced uptake and subsequently an increase in incidence and some major epidemics (e.g. in the UK and Japan). It is hoped that public concern over pertussis vaccines will be alleviated by the acellular vaccines, which were introduced in 1997 and which produce fewer and milder side effects than the whole-cell vaccines. Greater public confidence in the vaccine should lead to increased uptake.

To reduce the side effects of vaccination further efforts are now being concentrated on the production of subunit vaccines containing only the 'protective' antigens. The difficulty has been to identify those antigens.

BRONCHITIS

Acute bronchitis represents an inflammation of the tracheobronchial tree, and is usually a result of the spread of an infection from the upper respiratory tract into the bronchi. Viruses are the most common causes, including influenza virus, respiratory syncytial virus, common cold viruses and adenoviruses. *Mycoplasma pneumoniae* can also be responsible. A dry or slightly productive cough lasting 1–3 weeks is the major feature. Treatment is mainly symptomatic. There is little evidence that antibiotics are effective, except when secondary bacterial infection occurs. In otherwise healthy individuals, there is usually a speedy recovery with few sequelae.

Chronic bronchitis is a condition in which there is a chronic or recurrent cough and excessive secretion of mucus. It appears to result from a combination of factors, which may include infection, cigarette smoking, inhalation of pollutants and a genetic predisposition. Infection with rhinoviruses or influenza virus may precipitate relapses, and bacteria such as *S. pneumoniae*, *H. influenzae* and *M. catarrhalis* may be involved in acute exacerbations. Further spread of bacteria into the lungs can result in pneumonia.

Antibiotics such as amoxycillin or cotrimoxazole are used for the treatment of associated bacterial infections.

BRONCHIOLITIS

Cause and epidemiology

Bronchiolitis is predominantly a disease of childhood, especially in children less than two years old. The bronchioles of a young child are narrow and, if their lining cells are swollen by inflammation, the passage of air to and from the alveoli may be severely restricted. Infection results in necrosis of the epithelial cells that line the bronchioles and the infection may spread into the lung tissue and cause pneumonia. Most of these infections are caused by respiratory syncytial virus (RSV), although other viruses (e.g. influenza and parainfluenza viruses) and *Mycoplasma pneumoniae* may be involved.

RSV is highly infectious and can cause community and hospital outbreaks in winter. It is a frequent cause of lower respiratory tract infections in infants, but rarely produces significant illness in adult contacts. Its surface spikes are fusion proteins (not haemagglutinins or neuraminidases) which fuse host cells to form **syncytia** (multi-nucleated masses of fused cells – hence the name, respiratory syncytial virus). The infection is transmitted by droplets and to some extent via hands. The only known reservoir is infected humans.

Clinical features

In children and adults the virus is restricted to the upper respiratory tract, causing a mild, common cold-type illness. However, infection in infants can be severe if the virus invades the lower respiratory tract. Typical symptoms include fever, coryza (rhinitis – inflammation of the nasal passages with nasal discharge), a cough and respiratory obstruction resembling asthma, possibly leading to respiratory distress and cyanosis, especially in infants with some other underlying disorder. Viral pneumonia can develop in some patients. Most cases begin to resolve within a few days but some children, even a year or two later, may continue to show depressed pulmonary function or wheezing. Recurrent infections are common although they are generally less severe.

Diagnosis and treatment

The diagnosis of bronchiolitis is based mainly on clinical appraisal. RSV-specific antigens in nasopharyngeal washings are detectable by immunofluorescence or ELISA. As bronchiolitis is caused mainly by viruses, treatment options are limited and, once symptoms have developed fully, viral replication and load have already begun to decline. The major concerns in the management of a patient with bronchiolitis are the maintenance of adequate hydration (e.g. parenteral fluids) and supplementary oxygen if necessary.

INFLUENZA

Influenza epidemics regularly occur worldwide and cause significant morbidity and mortality. Influenza viruses cause a range of clinical conditions that affect all levels of the respiratory tract.

Causative agents

The causative agents are the influenza viruses (myxoviruses), whose structure is shown in Figure 17.7. Influenza A viruses can infect a variety of animals and birds as well as humans, and cause epidemics and occa-

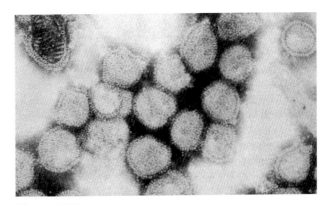

Figure 17.7
Electron micrograph of the influenza virus

sionally pandemics; influenza B viruses infect only humans and can cause epidemics but not pandemics.

The envelope of an influenza virus has two surface glycoprotein antigens, the haemagglutinin (H) and neuraminidase (N) spikes. Protective antibodies are made to both these antigens in infected people, but influenza viruses can vary these antigens over time by *antigenic drift* and *antigenic shift* (see Chapter 10). Antigenic drift represents small, constantly occurring mutations, affecting the H and N antigens. If the changes occur in areas where antibodies bind to these antigens, the antibodies may not bind as well, allowing the virus to reinfect communities repeatedly over time, even though the individuals have immunity from previous flu infections.

Antigenic shift is a sudden and unpredictable, major change in the H or N antigens, based on a reassortment or mixing of genes from different virus strains, leading to a new strain. The new strain develops from a mixing of genes from an animal or avian virus with a human virus. This results in completely different antigen structures, enabling the new strain to spread through populations in epidemic form. Only type A strains undergo antigenic shift. Major shifts have resulted in four major pandemics: Spanish flu (which killed up to 40 million people worldwide) in 1918, Asian flu in 1957, Hong Kong flu in 1968 and Russian flu in 1977.

Transmission of influenza is by droplet inhalation and fomites, and infectivity can be very high (up to 30% attack rate generally, and over 50% in epidemics). Influenza occurs throughout the world, typically during the coldest months of the year. This is largely because people spend more time inside buildings during cold weather and this favours virus transmission via aerosols and fomites.

Pathogenesis and clinical features

The virus enters the respiratory tract via droplets and attaches to sialic acid receptors on respiratory epithelial cells via the H spikes on its envelope. One to three days after infection, symptoms such as fever, chills, malaise and muscle pain develop, due mainly to cytokines liberated from damaged cells and infiltrating leucocytes. As the virus spreads, symptoms of runny nose, sore throat and dry

Influenza

On 17 August 1993 the Infectious Diseases Program of Health and Community Services, Victoria, was contacted by the director of nursing from a Melbourne metropolitan nursing home. She was concerned about an outbreak among residents and staff of a febrile illness with upper respiratory symptoms; approximately half the residents became ill over a two-week period.

Sera were collected from six acutely ill residents and four acutely ill staff, as well as from those who had been acutely ill during the previous five days. Convalescent sera were collected three weeks after the acute sera. All samples were tested for antibodies to influenza A and B. Seroconversion to influenza A virus was demonstrated in most cases.

The mean age of all residents was 83 years and, of staff, 43 years. There were 34 cases in total, of which 18 were staff and 16 were residents. The mean age of affected residents was 82 years, and the mean age of affected staff was 44 years. The index case (a member of staff) occurred on 6 August 1993, and there was a subsequent outbreak among residents that peaked on August 12. The last case occurred on August 29.

The mean duration of illness was 12 days, with a range of 3–28 days. Fever, malaise, cough, rhinorrhoea, muscle aches, headache and sore throat were the most commonly reported symptoms. There were three deaths, four hospitalisations for pneumonia or chest infection (with eventual recovery), and four cases with respiratory complications not requiring hospitalisation. All complications and deaths occurred in residents.

Influenza cases at the nursing home by date of onset and patient type

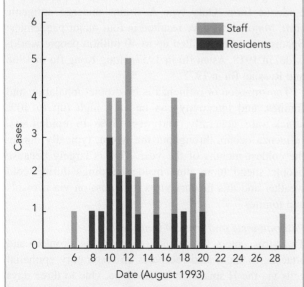

Source: MacIntyre R, C Mansell, P Lynch & J Rich, 'An outbreak of influenza A at a Victorian nursing home', *Communicable Diseases Intelligence* 18/2, 24 January 1994, p. 32.

cough may occur. Subclinical or mild infections resembling a cold are common. Recovery usually occurs within 1–3 weeks, although the infection can be severe enough to develop into bronchitis or pneumonia. Secondary bacterial infection may occur, especially in people with COPD (chronic obstructive pulmonary disease).

The life-threatening form of influenzal pneumonia, which caused millions of deaths in the 1918 pandemic, and which still occurs occasionally, is usually due to a mixed influenza virus and bacterial (e.g. staphylococcal) infection.

Mortality is highest in the elderly and the debilitated, especially in developing countries, and is usually due to secondary bacterial pneumonia or exacerbation of chronic cardiac or respiratory disease.

Diagnosis

A specific diagnosis can be made by serological means or by isolating the virus. Rapid diagnostic tests that detect viral antigen in respiratory samples have recently been developed. However, in most cases, these methods are impractical and unnecessary for an individual patient, but are important for public health authorities when following infection with a new virus strain.

Treatment and prevention

Rest, fluids and analgesics form the basis of treatment and recovery is usually within a week. Antibiotics are required if secondary bacterial infection occurs. Amantadine and rimantadine can be used prophylactically to limit outbreaks in elderly, non-immunised residents of institutions such as nursing homes. However, these drugs are effective only against influenza A and can cause neurological side effects, and viruses seem to become resistant to them fairly easily.

Zanamivir and oseltamivir are related drugs that can be used to treat influenza caused by either influenza A or B viruses. They act by inhibiting viral neuraminidase, which prevents viral infection of cells. The disadvantages of these drugs are that they are very expensive and are only effective if given within two days of development of symptoms.

When given before the epidemic season arrives, influenza virus vaccine offers partial protection, but only against those strains covered by the vaccine. The vaccines are made from inactivated viruses and are multivalent, directed against several strains of the virus. The composition of annual vaccines in Australia is decided by the Australian Influenza Vaccine Committee and is based on the anticipated spread of active influenza A and B viruses, according to worldwide surveillance coordinated by the World Health Organization. In this way we try to have the right vaccine ready when the epidemic strikes.

Vaccination is recommended for high-risk individuals such as the elderly and debilitated (e.g. residents of nursing homes and chronic care facilities), people with chronic cardiopulmonary disease, and health-care providers in facilities for the aged. Because of antigenic drift and the short duration of protection afforded by the vaccine, annual immunisation is necessary. A live, attenuated vaccine is currently being trialled.

PNEUMONIA

Pneumonia is an infection and inflammation of the lungs. It is a major cause of death throughout the world, especially in the elderly in developed countries, and in children and the malnourished living in crowded and unhygienic conditions. It is one of the most life-threatening types of infection in the immunocompromised. Worldwide, as many as five million people are thought to die each year from pneumonia.

A wide variety of microorganisms are capable of causing pneumonia. Bacteria and viruses cause most cases, but fungi (e.g. *Aspergillus* and *Pneumocystis jiroveci*) can also be responsible, especially in the immunocompromised. The common causative agents of pneumonia are listed in Table 17.5. The common causes of community-acquired infections are somewhat different from those that cause hospital infections. The cause also depends on a number of risk factors such as age, underlying disease and particular exposure to pathogens through occupation, travel or contact with animals.

Pneumonia is the most commonly fatal type of hospital-associated infection. As many as 15% of all deaths in hospitals may be attributed to a hospital-acquired pneumonia. Most of these occur in postsurgical patients or patients in intensive care.

Clinical features

Patients with pneumonia usually present with a fever, cough and chest pain. The cough is generally unproductive at first, but later may become purulent and sometimes blood-stained. As the disease progresses, the patient experiences increasing breathlessness and shallow, rapid breathing. Inspiratory rales (crackling sounds) are usually heard over the affected area of the lung. Some infections result in symptoms confined mainly to the chest, whereas others, such as Legionnaires' disease, have a much wider systemic involvement and the patient may present with mental confusion, diarrhoea and evidence of renal or liver dysfunction.

A chest X-ray confirms the presence and distribution of shadows in the lung, indicating consolidation. Severe pneumonia can quickly lead to respiratory failure, requiring ventilation and intensive care. Antibiotics have greatly reduced the mortality rate, but deaths still occur despite appropriate treatment.

Complications of infection include spread of the infecting organisms directly to extrapulmonary sites such as the pleural space, giving rise to empyema, or indirectly via the bloodstream to other parts of the body.

Pathogenesis

Microorganisms may reach the lungs by inhalation of fine, aerosolised particles or by the downward movement of mucus, which carries normal flora organisms or pathogens from the upper respiratory tract. Micro-aspiration of oropharyngeal and gastric secretions may also occur, especially in the critically ill, because of their supine position or use of nasogastric tubes. The mucociliary escalator normally functions to move mucus, foreign material and microorganisms trapped in it upwards away from the lungs, but this function can be impaired in people with an upper respiratory viral infection, and in those with damaged cilia due to inhalation of pollutants (e.g. cigarette smoke), alcoholism or the presence of a tumour or foreign body.

Sometimes, the lungs become infected by organisms that have spread, via the bloodstream, from another infected site in the body.

In response to infection or the action of microbial toxins, inflammation occurs, resulting in the filling of the affected alveoli – first with a serous exudate and then later with pus cells and sometimes red blood cells. Once the alveoli fill with infectious exudate, an overflow of the fluid occurs and there is a progressive spread of infection to adjacent alveoli.

Pneumonia has traditionally been classified into types according to differences in clinical signs and radiological

Table 17.5

Common causes of pneumonia: community-acquired versus hospital-acquired infections

COMMUNITY-ACQUIRED		HOSPITAL-ACQUIRED	
Organism	% of cases	Organism	% of cases
Streptococcus pneumoniae	15–40	*Pseudomonas aeruginosa*	15–30
Mycoplasma pneumoniae	10–20	*Staphylococcus aureus*	10–30
Haemophilus influenzae	5–10	*Klebsiella* species	5–15
Chlamydia pneumoniae	5–10	*Acinetobacter* species	5
Enteric Gram-negative bacteria	5–10	*Escherichia coli*	5–15
Influenza viruses	5–10	*Enterobacter* species	5–10
Legionella species	5	*Proteus* species	5
Staphylococcus aureus	< 5	*Streptococcus pneumoniae*	< 5
Moraxella catarrhalis	< 5	*Candida* species	< 5
Parainfluenza virus	< 5	*Legionella* species	< 5
		Moraxella catarrhalis	< 5

findings. **Lobar pneumonia** is an infection and consolidation (solidification of the tissue due to inflammatory exudate in the alveoli) confined to one or two lobes of the lung. Most cases are caused by *Streptococcus pneumoniae*. **Bronchopneumonia** is a more diffuse, patchy inflammation of the lungs with numerous small foci of consolidation occurring throughout the lungs. A large variety of bacteria such as *S. pneumoniae*, *Staphylococcus aureus*, *Mycobacterium tuberculosis* and *Haemophilus influenzae*, or viruses, can be responsible.

Outcomes common to both types of pneumonia are respiratory distress resulting from the interference with air exchange in the lungs, and systemic effects typical of any severe infection. A **pleural effusion** occurs if the inflammatory exudate enters the space between the lung tissue and pleural membranes. **Empyema** is the term used to describe infection of the pleural space, and **pleurisy** means an inflammation of the pleural membranes.

Bacterial causes

Pneumococcal pneumonia. The most common bacterial cause (approximately 30% of cases) of community-acquired pneumonia is *Streptococcus pneumoniae* (the 'pneumococcus'), a normal inhabitant of the upper respiratory tract of some people. Pneumococcal pneumonia is still a cause of significant morbidity and mortality throughout the world, and is an important infection and cause of death in patients post-splenectomy. The virulence of the organism is due to an extracellular polysaccharide capsule, which makes it resistant to phagocytosis (see Chapter 4).

There are at least 83 different serotypes of pneumococcus, but most infections are caused by a limited number of these serotypes. Pneumococcal pneumonia is a common complication of AIDS.

Usually, a chest X-ray is performed when pneumonia is suspected. This may indicate that infection and inflammation exist but laboratory investigations are required to identify the causative organism. Making a specific laboratory diagnosis of pneumonia is often a problem, because of the variety of causes. Blood and sputum culture are the main methods of diagnosing bacterial pneumonia, although they are not especially sensitive methods. More invasive techniques, such as transtracheal aspiration, bronchoscopy and broncho-alveolar lavage, and lung biopsy, may yield more useful results. However, collection of sputum and blood are relatively simple and non-invasive and are therefore most often done. Specimens should be collected before antibiotic therapy is started.

Sputum samples are best collected in the morning, because sputum tends to accumulate while the patient is lying in bed, and before breakfast, to reduce contamination by food particles and bacteria from food. It is critical that the specimen collected is truly sputum and free of oropharyngeal contamination, since some oropharyngeal flora can cause pneumonia and may be incorrectly identified as the cause.

Examination of a Gram-stained smear of sputum can give a presumptive diagnosis of pneumococcal pneumonia quickly if it demonstrates polymorphs and Gram-positive diplococci characteristic of *S. pneumoniae* (see Figure 17.8). Detection of pneumococcal antigen by agglutination of antibody-coated latex particles can be used both on sputum and urine specimens (antigen is excreted in the urine). Use of this technique means the result is available within an hour of receipt of the specimen, but antibiotic susceptibility tests cannot be performed unless the organisms are isolated.

First-line treatment of pneumonia before results are available is usually with amoxycillin and/or erythromycin, but treatment failure is possible because of the wide range of potential causes and their differing drug sensitivities. Increasing resistance of *S. pneumoniae* to a variety of drugs, including penicillin, is of great concern. Amoxycillin is currently the drug of choice for pneumococcal pneumonia. The patient with pneumonia may also require oxygen, and physiotherapy should be given if there is significant sputum. In the severely ill, direct suction with an endotracheal tube may be necessary. Even with appropriate antibiotic therapy, pneumonia can be fatal, usually because of rapidly progressive disease or because of its interaction with some other underlying disorder.

A polyvalent vaccine containing 23 of the most common or most virulent polysaccharide capsular antigen types of *S. pneumoniae* is available and recommended for people at high risk, especially individuals with asplenia and sickle-cell disease, other immunocompromised people (e.g. people with AIDS or Hodgkin's disease) and patients with CSF leaks. It is also recommended for people over the age of 65 and for those over the age of 50 in communities with high attack rates (e.g. some Aboriginal and Torres Strait Islander communities). Young children do not respond well to this vaccine and alternate types of vaccines (conjugate vaccines) are currently being trialled.

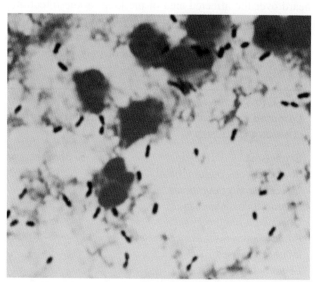

Figure 17.8

A Gram stain of a smear of sputum can provide a rapid presumptive diagnosis

This slide shows Gram-positive diplococci and pus cells suggestive of *Streptococcus pneumoniae* infection.

Staphylococcus aureus. Staphylococcal pneumonia is most common as a complication of viral respiratory infection such as influenza or measles. Intravenous drug users may develop a staphylococcal endocarditis and pneumonia, following use of a contaminated needle or syringe. Elderly people, the immunocompromised, and patients with diabetes or cystic fibrosis are also susceptible. Diagnosis is by sputum culture and possibly blood culture (as for pneumococcal pneumonia).

Gram-negative enterobacteria. Gram-negative enterobacteria, such as *Escherichia coli*, *Pseudomonas aeruginosa*, *Klebsiella* spp. and *Serratia marcescens*, are particularly associated with pneumonia acquired in hospital but can also cause community infections in alcoholics, the elderly and the immunocompromised. These organisms can colonise the upper respiratory tract of hospitalised people, especially after antibiotic therapy, and then be aspirated into the lower airways.

Ventilators and humidifiers provide the necessary moisture for these organisms to persist and are well recognised as potential sources of infection in hospitals. Mechanical ventilation is a major risk factor for patients in intensive care, because an endotracheal tube bypasses upper airway defences. These organisms can also infect the lungs via the bloodstream, from infectious foci in the genitourinary or gastrointestinal tracts. The endotoxins in the cell wall of these bacteria are potent inducers of inflammation.

The diagnosis of pneumonia caused by Gram-negative bacteria is based on culture of sputum and sometimes blood (see pneumococcal pneumonia for general principles). Appropriate antibiotic therapy is based on the culture results and sensitivity testing. Drug resistance is a problem in hospital-acquired infections, especially in Gram-negative enterobacteria.

Haemophilus influenzae. *H. influenzae* causes pneumonia, often as an exacerbation of epiglottitis, chronic bronchitis, brochiectasis, septicaemia or meningitis. In general, type b strains of *H. influenzae* cause most cases, but non-type b strains are also possible causes. *H. influenzae* mainly affects non-immunised children under the age of four years. Diagnosis is based on culture of blood and sputum (see pneumococcal pneumonia).

Infections caused by *H. influenzae* have classically been treated with ampicillin, but the emergence of resistant strains has led to increased use of third-generation cephalosporins (e.g. cefotaxime or ceftriaxone). Effective *H. influenzae* vaccines have been available in Australia since 1992 (see page 398) and have substantially reduced the incidence of all types of invasive disease caused by *H. influenzae*.

Pneumonia in cystic fibrosis. Several of the organisms described above are involved in recurrent or chronic lung infections in patients with cystic fibrosis (CF). The organisms most often encountered are *H. influenzae*, *S. aureus*, *S. pneumoniae*, *P. aeruginosa* and other *Pseudomonas* species.

Of these, *P. aeruginosa* is the most important, causing a chronic lung infection that is almost impossible to eradicate in most CF patients. Over time, the infection and, more particularly, the inflammation it induces lead to permanent lung damage and often death. The predisposition of CF patients to lung infections appears to be related to the production of overly viscid bronchial secretions, and the suppressive effect this has on mucociliary clearance.

Once established, the *Pseudomonas* protects itself against other defence mechanisms and antibiotics by growing in microcolonies coated with a film of alginate, a mucoid barrier through which many substances cannot pass.

Legionellosis. *Legionella pneumophila* (serogroups 1–6) and other species, particularly *L. longbeachae*, *L. bozemanii* and *L. micdadei*, cause a pneumonia referred to as **legionellosis (or Legionnaires' disease)**. *L. pneumophila* causes the majority of infections worldwide, although *L. longbeachae* tends to predominate in Australia. These aerobic, Gram-negative, rod-shaped organisms are widely distributed in warm, wet habitats, such as air-conditioning cooling towers, reticulated water supplies, spa baths and environmental sources (e.g. creeks, lakes, compost and soil). The organism is spread in airborne droplets from these sources.

Dispersion from cooling towers can lead to outbreaks of infection as occurred in the first recognised incident, involving 182 people (29 deaths) at a conference of the American Legion (war veterans) in Philadelphia in 1976. The high fatality rate in that outbreak was due partly to the delay (six months) in identifying the causative agent.

Person-to-person transmission of legionellosis does not appear to occur. In Australia there are, on average, fewer than 300 cases per year, with the highest rates of notification in the over-60 age groups (see Figure 17.9).

The incubation period of Legionnaires' disease is usually 2–10 days. Together with symptoms of pneumonia, there may be: systemic manifestations, including diarrhoea; abdominal pain; neurological signs, such as

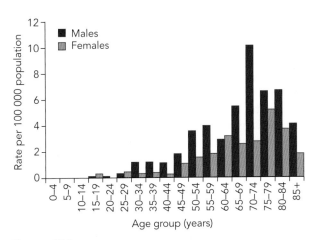

Figure 17.9

Notification rates of legionellosis in Australia, 2003, by age group and sex

Source: Communicable Diseases Intelligence, 29(1), 2005, p. 53, © Commonwealth of Australia, reproduced by permission

clouded consciousness and ataxia; and renal failure, with blood and protein in the urine.

The cough in Legionnaires' disease is usually only slightly productive, if at all. Fever is almost always present. The disease is more likely to affect the elderly, but other major risk factors are cigarette smoking, underlying respiratory disease (e.g. chronic obstructive pulmonary disease), immunosuppression (e.g. malignancy, corticosteroid use) and excessive alcohol intake. However, legionellosis can occur in apparently healthy people of all ages.

Pontiac fever is a mild form of *Legionella* infection, characterised by influenza-like symptoms and rapid recovery.

Hospital-acquired legionellosis can occur when water supplies in hospitals become contaminated, particularly when hot water lines are kept at low temperatures (less than 55°C). Below this temperature *Legionella* are able to survive and multiply in water supplies and can be spread from shower roses and taps, as well as from cooling towers. *Legionella* have also been isolated from humidifiers and vaporisers. An important factor in hospitals is the many people who are very susceptible and at high risk of infection. Mortality rates in the immunosuppressed can be very high.

The diagnosis of legionellosis is not straightforward. Culture of sputum is the definitive method but has the disadvantage of taking 3–5 days for growth to occur. There is a urinary antigen test that is fairly sensitive, but it is only specific for *L. pneumophila* serogroup 1. Fluoroquinolines or erythromycin usually provide effective treatment.

The contamination of cooling systems and hot water supplies by legionellae has been the subject of intense study and regulations are now in force to provide guidance for maintenance engineers (see Spotlight box, page 167).

Atypical pneumonia. A variety of microorganisms, including bacteria, viruses and fungi, cause what is sometimes referred to as an **atypical pneumonia**. It is so named not because it is uncommon but because of the diffuse, patchy nature of the infection and the insidious onset and non-productive cough. The major causes are *Mycoplasma pneumoniae*, *Chlamydia pneumoniae*, *Legionella* (see previous section) and *Pneumocystis jiroveci* in people with AIDS.

M. pneumoniae is transmitted in airborne droplets. It affects mainly the upper respiratory tract, but causes clinical pneumonia in 3–30% of infected people. It occasionally causes epidemics of pneumonia. *C. pneumoniae* is recognised as an important pathogen of both the upper and lower respiratory tracts, causing as much as 10% of community-acquired pneumonia.

Perhaps of greater significance is the possible role of *C. pneumoniae* in atherosclerosis. The organism has been shown to be present in coronary atherosclerotic lesions. However, a causal role for the organism in this disease has yet to be proven.

Mycoplasma can be cultured in the laboratory, but they are very slow-growing and can take up to two weeks to form visible colonies. Thus, diagnosis is usually based on PCR or serological tests. Culture of *Chlamydia* is also difficult, so PCR or serological tests are also used for infections caused by this organism. It is also possible to detect *C. pneumoniae* directly in a smear of sputum, using fluorescent-labelled antibodies (see Figure 17.10). Roxithromycin or tetracyclines are used for the treatment of mycoplasmal and chlamydial pneumonia.

Q fever. The bacterium *Coxiella burnetii* is the cause of **Q fever**, a pneumonia in which chronic infection of the liver, heart valves and other organs may occur. It was originally recognised in the 1930s in Australia, when it was found to be infecting workers in a Brisbane abattoir. It was given the name Q (for query) fever, because the cause was unknown until Sir FRANK MACFARLANE BURNET identified the causative agent as a rickettsia.

The organism is found in a variety of wild animals including kangaroos, and in goats and sheep and, especially, in cattle. It is spread from animal to animal via ticks. It is shed in the faeces, milk and urine of infected animals. Humans acquire Q fever mainly by consumption of unpasteurised milk or by occupational exposure, although non-occupational infection also occurs. Outbreaks have occurred in people working in the livestock industry, such as stockyard workers, abattoir and dairy workers, and meat packers.

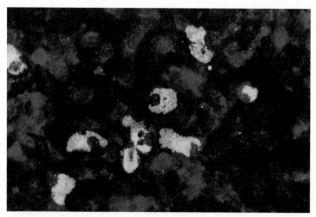

Figure 17.10

***Chlamydia pneumoniae* identified with a fluorescent-labelled antibody**

The organism is very resistant to drying and can survive for months in dust or on wool, animal hides and straw. Generally, there are 500–1000 notifications per year in Australia, with highest rates of notification usually in Queensland and New South Wales. *C. burnetii* is removed from milk by pasteurisation.

Many cases of Q fever are asymptomatic. When symptomatic, it has an incubation period of 1–4 weeks and produces an influenza-like illness of severe headache, fever and muscle pain lasting 1–2 weeks. Pneumonia or mild hepatitis may subsequently develop. The disease can also result in a fatigue syndrome that can last weeks, months or years. Endocarditis, which may occur years later, is one of the more serious possible complications.

Diagnosis of Q fever is usually by serological means. Treatment with tetracyclines is generally effective. A Q fever vaccine is available and recommended for those at risk (e.g. abattoir workers and veterinarians). Severe reactions to this vaccine can occur in individuals already immune, so it is essential that a person's immunity and skin sensitivity to the vaccine antigens is tested before immunisation.

Ornithosis. Sir Frank Macfarlane Burnet also identified *Chlamydia psittaci* in the 1930s, in Australian parrots. This bacterium causes a pneumonia called **ornithosis** (or **psittacosis**), mainly acquired by inhalation of dust particles from bird droppings, especially parrots, but potentially any bird. Sometimes, the birds themselves suffer from a diarrhoeal or respiratory illness. Infections in humans are found mainly in people who keep birds as pets. Person-to-person transmission is rare.

Ornithosis is notifiable throughout Australia, except in New South Wales. There are 100–150 cases reported per year, with no clear geographical or seasonal trend. Most cases are mild and self-limiting, but severe pneumonia occurs in some patients, with a need for prolonged hospitalisation.

Diagnosis of ornithosis is usually by serological testing or by antigen detection in sputum using a fluorescent antibody technique. Tetracyclines are generally effective in the treatment of ornithosis.

Melioidosis. **Melioidosis** is caused by the bacterium *Burkholderia pseudomallei* which is found in soil and surface water. It is a disease found mainly in tropical areas, including South-East Asia and northern Australia. Most cases in Australia occur in the wet season in the Northern Territory and Queensland. In the Northern Territory, 20–30 cases are reported each year.

Humans usually become infected via skin lesions in contact with contaminated soil or water or by inhalation of dust or aerosolised polluted water. Infection may be subclinical; the most common form of acute illness is pneumonia. The organism can spread via the bloodstream to almost any organ of the body. Abscesses can form in the skin, spleen, prostate and other organs. Severe illness and mortality are usually associated with other factors, such as alcoholism, diabetes and renal disease.

Laboratory diagnosis is by culture of sputum, blood, pus or other specimen from the likely site of infection. Growth can take up to 72 hours. Direct immunofluorescent microscopy of an appropriate specimen is only 70% sensitive, but provides a positive diagnosis in less than 1 hour. Ceftazidime is the drug of choice, followed by maintenance therapy with chloramphenicol, doxycycline and cotrimoxazole for three months to prevent relapse.

Viral causes

A number of viruses can cause pneumonia. Respiratory syncytial virus (RSV) is recognised as a major cause of pneumonia, especially in children and in adults with heart or lung disease. The *human metapneumovirus* was identified in 2001 as a cause of lower respiratory tract infection in the very young, in hospitalised children and in the elderly. RSV and metapneumovirus cause similar respiratory infections which range from a mild, self-limiting illness to respiratory failure.

Adenoviruses and influenza viruses are occasional causes of pneumonia, when they spread from their usual sites of infection higher up in the respiratory tract. Similarly, parainfluenza viruses occasionally cause pneumonia in infants when infection extends beyond the bronchioles.

Viruses tend to cause an interstitial pneumonia – that is, one that involves the interstitium of the lung. Some viruses do not themselves cause pneumonia but may, by damaging tissues and defences, predispose the patient to secondary bacterial pneumonia.

Severe acute respiratory syndrome (**SARS**) is a pneumonia caused by a new virus (thought to be a new type of coronavirus) that appeared in late 2002. The virus is thought to have originated in southern China and spread to 27 countries worldwide within a few months. In March 2003 the World Health Organization issued a global alert, recommending worldwide surveillance for this disease. By April 2003 there were about 3000 known cases. Mortality due to this disease is about 7%, occurring mainly in the elderly. SARS appears to be spread by respiratory droplets (coughing and sneezing) of an infected person, or by contaminated hands or objects.

People infected with the SARS virus display a range of symptoms. After an incubation period of 2–7 days a person may demonstrate virtually any combination of fever, chills, cough and breathing difficulties, headache, muscle ache, dizziness, diarrhoea and sore throat. The vague symptoms and the lack of a diagnostic test for the disease are partly why it was able to spread so quickly.

The measles virus can cause pneumonia in individuals with impaired immune defences or, under certain circumstances, cause enough damage to predispose the person to secondary bacterial pneumonia. In children in developing countries, secondary bacterial pneumonia is a frequent complication of measles infection. Cytomegalovirus does not normally cause respiratory illness, but in immunocompromised patients (e.g. transplant recipients and AIDS patients) it can give rise to an interstitial pneumonia.

Measles and cytomegalovirus infections are discussed more fully in Chapters 16 and 19, respectively.

A laboratory diagnosis of viral pneumonia is usually only undertaken for epidemiological or public health reasons. Virus culture of a suitable respiratory sample was the gold standard, but is a slow and highly specialised technique. Antigen assays have been developed for many of the pathogens, but they can be lacking in sensitivity and specificity. Molecular methods, especially PCR-based assays, are now the most common techniques being used and developed.

Chronic infections of the lower respiratory tract

TUBERCULOSIS

Tuberculosis, or consumption, as it was formerly called, has plagued the world since ancient times and is still one of the major diseases affecting humans. In the developing world it ranks as one of the most common causes of death due to a single infectious agent.

Incidence

According to the World Health Organization (WHO), one-third of the world's population has tuberculosis and in 1995 the WHO declared the disease a global emergency. Approximately 8–9 million new cases occur in the world each year, with 2–3 million deaths. The highest incidence is in Africa, South-East Asia, the eastern Mediterranean and the western Pacific. In developed countries, the incidence has declined significantly since the early 20th century (see Figure 17.11), although there was a disturbing trend of increased occurrence in the United States and some European countries in the late 1980s. Rates in these countries are now falling again, due mainly to increased investment in tuberculosis control measures.

In Australia, about 1000 cases of tuberculosis are reported each year. The notification rate in Australia has remained stable since 1986, and the overall rate of fewer than 6 cases per 100 000 population per year is one of the lowest in the world. The highest rates of infection are in the northern parts of Australia, reflecting the high incidence in Aboriginal and Islander populations. Other high-risk groups are migrants, especially those from China, Vietnam, Cambodia, other South-East Asian countries and the Philippines.

Figure 17.12 compares the notification rates of tuberculosis in indigenous Australians, non-indigenous Australians and overseas-born people.

Apart from its persistence worldwide, the other main concern with tuberculosis is the emergence of strains that are resistant to at least two of the standard anti-tuberculous drugs (isoniazid and rifampicin) – referred to as multi-drug-resistant tuberculosis (MDR-TB). Some strains of MDR-TB have been found to be resistant to as many as seven drugs. Currently, in Australia, less than 2% of isolates are multi-drug-resistant.

Cause and transmission

Tuberculosis is caused mainly by the rod-shaped, acid-fast bacterium *Mycobacterium tuberculosis* but other species of mycobacteria, *M. bovis*, *M. microti*, *M. canettii* and *M. africanum*, can also be responsible. Together, these organisms are referred to as the *Mycobacterium tuberculosis* complex (MTBC). The usual source of infection is a person with pulmonary or laryngeal tuberculosis, who can emit enormous numbers of mycobacteria when coughing. The organisms are passed on in aerosols, droplet nuclei or dust. They can survive for long periods in air and dust because of their waxy outer coat that allows them to resist drying.

Lung disease is the most common form of tuberculosis, but the organism may infect other sites (e.g. the lymphatic system, meninges, bones and joints) and sometimes cause disseminated infection. Generally, people with tuberculosis of other organs (e.g. bone marrow or kidneys) are unlikely to be contagious, except during surgery or autopsy procedures, when there may be contact with infected tissues or aerosolisation of organisms in the tissues. Overcrowding and inadequate ventilation increase the potential for tuberculosis transmission.

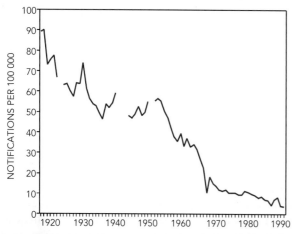

Figure 17.11

Annual rate of notifications of tuberculosis in Australia 1917–91
Source: Communicable Diseases Intelligence, 17(11), 31 May 1993, © Commonwealth of Australia, reproduced by permission

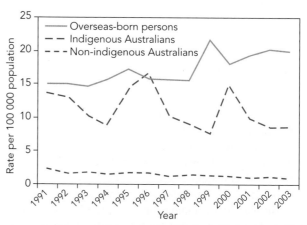

Figure 17.12

Tuberculosis notification rates in Australia, 1991 to 2003, by Indigenous status and country of birth
Source: Communicable Diseases Intelligence, 29(1), 2005, p. 56, © Commonwealth of Australia, reproduced by permission

Tuberculosis

In 1979 a 57-year-old man was admitted to hospital with fever and rapidly increasing breathlessness. He had been treated with cytotoxic drugs three months earlier, after a bronchial biopsy had shown that he had a small cell carcinoma in the left lung. There was some improvement initially but he soon became much more dyspnoeic, and radiotherapy to the upper part of his body was begun two weeks before his final admission to hospital.

Consolidation of the left lung was obvious on both physical examination and chest X-ray. No likely pathogens were isolated from sputum or blood cultures, and the patient died after three days of intensive treatment with antibiotics.

At autopsy on the following day, the primary tumour could not be found. Ten days later, routine histology of lung sections revealed numerous acid-fast bacilli. Miliary tubercules were also found in the spleen.

A group of 48 newly enrolled third-year medical students attended the autopsy demonstration on this patient. Following the usual practice at the University, these students were scheduled to have Mantoux tests during their first term, so that those with negative results could complete BCG vaccination before they began their clinical training in the hospitals.

One week after the autopsy, Mantoux tests were performed by the Student Health Service on all third-year medical students. It was found that 13 of the students who attended the autopsy were already Mantoux-positive, eight because of previous BCG vaccinations. Mantoux tests were repeated two months later and 13 of the 35 students who had previously tested negative had converted to positive.

That is, of the 35 Mantoux-negative students at risk:

- Twenty-two had no evidence of infection two months later. They were then vaccinated with BCG.
- Five had inadvertently received BCG soon after exposure. They were kept under clinical surveillance. All had normal chest X-rays in July 1981.
- Eight had presumptive evidence of infection. They were advised to take isoniazid prophylactically, and chest X-rays were taken after six months and two years.

Although some did not take isoniazid, seven of the eight remained well, with no evidence of active tuberculosis. One who had elected to take isoniazid developed a minimal radiological lesion in the upper zone of the right lung and acid-fast bacilli were detected in one gastric aspirate six weeks after exposure. Culture yielded *M. tuberculosis*. He was treated with standard therapy and the radiological lesion resolved.

Adapted from D Wilkins, AJ Woolcock & YE Cossart 1994, 'Tuberculosis: medical students at risk', *Medical Journal of Australia*, 160: 395.

M. tuberculosis grows very slowly, with a generation time of 20 hours or more, compared with 20–30 minutes for most bacteria.

Pathogenesis

In primary infection the organisms are engulfed by the alveolar macrophages. However, the bacteria can both survive and multiply in these cells because of their resistance to intracellular killing. The macrophages eventually carry the bacteria via the lymphatics to the local lymph nodes, where an immune response, predominantly cell-mediated immunity (CMI), is stimulated. The CMI response acts to prevent the spread of the bacteria by causing the release of lymphokines from sensitised T cells, which activate macrophages and increase their ability to destroy the bacteria. In addition, an infiltration of cells (lymphocytes, macrophages and epithelioid cells) to the sites of infection serves to contain the organisms within **tubercles**, or small granulomas.

A tubercle in the lung, plus the enlarged lymph nodes, is called the **Ghon** (or primary) **complex**.

After a time, the material within the granuloma becomes necrotic and caseous (cheesy). In people who are otherwise healthy, the tubercles may heal spontaneously, become fibrotic or calcified and persist as such for a lifetime. They will show up years later on a chest X-ray. However, in a small percentage of people with primary infection, particularly in the immunocompromised, the mycobacteria are not destroyed or contained within the tubercles. Instead, they invade the bloodstream and cause a potentially fatal disseminated disease (called **miliary tuberculosis**). Tubercles may then form in many organs, including the liver, spleen, kidneys and meninges.

In some people, the activated macrophages never completely eliminate these extremely hardy bacteria, even though the patients recover clinically from the primary infection. The bacteria can remain dormant within granulomas for many years because the macrophages have controlled their multiplication but not killed them.

Secondary tuberculosis occurs in a small percentage of people, often many years later; this is due to the reactivation of dormant mycobacteria. Factors influencing the reactivation of these bacteria include age, impaired immune function resulting from factors such as malnutrition, infection (e.g. AIDS), chemotherapy for treatment of malignancies, and corticosteroids for treatment of inflammatory diseases. Obviously, anything that compromises either T cell or macrophage function can lead to reactivation. Reactivation usually occurs in the apex of the lungs, fitting more closely the classical form of tuberculosis.

The pathogenesis of tuberculosis is illustrated in Figure 17.13.

Clinical features

Primary tuberculosis is completely asymptomatic in the majority of immunocompetent people (about 90%). In the asymptomatic there may be only a small lesion in the periphery of the lung and minor enlargement of draining lymph nodes.

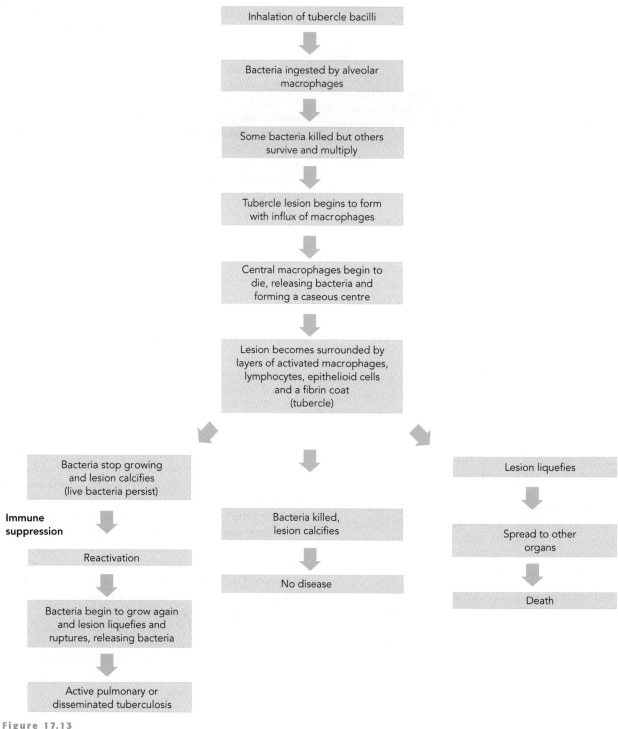

Figure 17.13
The pathogenesis of tuberculosis

In the symptomatic, the onset of symptoms is often insidious, infection proceeding for some time before the patient develops fever, weight loss and malaise, and becomes sufficiently ill to seek medical attention. Without treatment, pneumonia-like symptoms may develop, with a chronic cough productive of sputum which may be blood-stained. The infection can resolve spontaneously or the organisms may spread locally to cause pleurisy or bronchopneumonia, or via the bloodstream to cause meningitis or disseminated disease.

Factors that increase the probability of a person becoming symptomatic include co-infection with HIV, immunosuppression, alcoholism, renal failure and diabetes mellitus. HIV and tuberculosis are a lethal combination because each accelerates the other's progress in a person suffering from both diseases.

In miliary (disseminated) tuberculosis, numerous small granulomas (resembling millet seed, hence the name) develop in a variety of tissues. The prognosis is poor in this form of the disease.

Diagnosis

A diagnosis of tuberculosis is usually made by the clinical signs and symptoms, supported by chest X-ray findings and a positive tuberculin (Mantoux) skin test (see below). Confirmation is by demonstration of acid-fast rods in sputum stained by Ziehl-Neelsen's method (see Figure 17.14), and culture of *M. tuberculosis* from sputum. With microscopic examination of a smear of sputum, a result can be obtained within hours of receipt of the specimen by the laboratory. A positive smear also indicates that the patient is infectious.

Microscopy is important because *M. tuberculosis* can take up to six weeks to form visible colonies in culture. Culture enables drug sensitivity testing to be performed. New molecular methods that amplify and detect *M. tuberculosis* nucleic acids in specimens (e.g. PCR) have been developed and are useful supplementary tests to the standard microscopic and culture methods.

Tuberculin (Mantoux) skin test

A skin test is performed by intradermal injection of tuberculin, a purified protein derivative (PPD) of *M. tuberculosis*, and examination 48–72 hours later for a reddening and thickening (induration) of the skin at the site of injection. This is a delayed hypersensitivity reaction to the antigen (see Chapter 9). In general, if the diameter of induration is less than 5 mm it is considered to be negative. The interpretation of positive reactions is complex and dependent on many factors. A strongly positive reaction is suggestive of active or recent infection. A weak reaction may reflect past infection or vaccination. However, positive reactions can become negative when a person's cellular immunity is depressed by immunosuppressive therapy, other infection or by tuberculosis itself. The skin test is most useful as an indicator of infection if a baseline test before exposure is available for comparison.

Treatment

The basis of treating drug-sensitive tuberculosis is the use of three or four drugs in combination therapy (usually isoniazid, rifampicin, pyrazinamide and ethambutol).

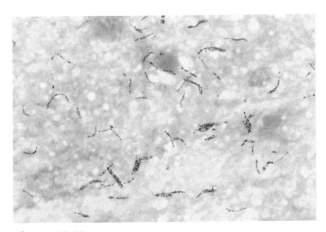

Figure 17.14

Ziehl-Neelsen stain of sputum
Acid-fast (pink) rods of *Mycobacterium tuberculosis* against a blue background.

M. tuberculosis rapidly develops resistance to anti-tuberculosis drugs, but this is minimised with combination therapy. Treatment is usually continued for at least six months after sputum tests become negative for tuberculosis bacilli, because the bacteria can remain hidden in intracellular locations for long periods and be difficult to reach with antibiotics.

With good compliance, the cure rate of drug-sensitive tuberculosis approaches 100%, usually without serious side effects of treatment. However, patient compliance for prolonged therapy can be difficult to achieve, especially after they start to feel well. Failure to complete the full drug treatment can result in incomplete elimination of the organism and the development of resistance. For this reason the WHO introduced the DOT (directly observed treatment) strategy in 1991, which includes the supervised administration of anti-tuberculosis drugs.

If the organism is multi-drug-resistant (i.e. resistant to at least isoniazid and rifampicin), a course of treatment with more toxic second-line drugs, such as ofloxacin, ciprofloxacin, ethionamide and kanamycin, is needed. Treatment for as long as 24 months may be required and the cure rate falls below 50% in the immunocompetent, and much lower in the immunosuppressed.

Prevention

Prevention of tuberculosis in areas of low prevalence is based on case finding and effective treatment, and contact tracing and chemoprophylaxis with isoniazid. The BCG (Bacille Calmette et Guerin) vaccine, a suspension of live, attenuated *M. bovis*, was developed in the 1920s by the French bacteriologists Albert Calmette and Alphonse Guerin of the Pasteur Institute. The BCG offers significant protection against tuberculosis in children but it has less certain protectiveness for adults (reported to be 0–80%). BCG vaccination is recommended for:

- children under the age of five who are going to live in countries of high incidence
- Aboriginal and Torres Strait Islander neonates in areas of high incidence
- neonates born to women with TB or leprosy (to protect against leprosy, see Chapter 20).

The general use of BCG in low-risk areas is no longer recommended because of its variable efficacy. Furthermore, in low-risk countries it is considered to be a disadvantage because it makes the interpretation of the tuberculin skin test difficult, and hence the ability to identify recent infection is lessened. A tuberculin test should be performed before vaccination with the BCG, and the vaccine is given only to those who are negative for the tuberculin test.

In hospitals, patients with active tuberculosis should be isolated from non-tuberculous patients in a well-ventilated room. Patients should be educated to cover their mouths when coughing or sneezing, and on the careful disposal of materials contaminated with sputum. Other people entering the room should wear a mask.

Certain health-care workers have a high risk of exposure, particularly staff of respiratory and chest clinics, high dependency or emergency departments, staff who work with tuberculosis or HIV-infected patients, mortuary staff, physiotherapists, most medical and nursing staff of public hospitals and microbiology laboratory staff. Such people, if Mantoux-negative, should have regular tuberculin skin tests. The use of BCG in these people is controversial and advice should be sought from local health authorities.

Rapid diagnosis and treatment of infected patients and properly implemented infection control procedures are important approaches, since the greatest risk in hospitals comes from undiagnosed cases. The incidence of *M. bovis* infections is controlled by pasteurisation of milk, and screening and eradication of infected cattle.

Atypical mycobacteria infections

Other species of *Mycobacterium* can cause tuberculosis-like illnesses. *M. avium* and *M. intracellulare*, often referred to as the *Mycobacterium avium* complex (MAC) or *M. avium-intracellulare*, are the most important of these but there are other species, including *M. kansasii*, *M. fortuitum*, *M. chelonei* and *M. scrofulaceum*. MAC has come to prominence as a result of the AIDS epidemic but, curiously, it is not very common in people immunosuppressed by factors other than the human immunodeficiency virus. It is also rare in immunocompetent people.

In people with AIDS, the gastrointestinal tract is often the primary site of infection, but disseminated disease is common in the later stages of AIDS. The diagnosis is difficult because MAC is ubiquitous in the environment (water, soil, dust) and is sometimes isolated from clinical specimens in the absence of infection. Blood culture is the most reliable method for diagnosis. These mycobacteria are atypical in being resistant to most anti-tuberculous drugs. Many of the drugs used to treat this infection are toxic.

FUNGAL PNEUMONIA

A variety of fungal spores is usually present in air, but these organisms are much less frequent causes of lower respiratory tract infection than bacteria and viruses. In the main, fungi are opportunistic pathogens and so most infections are seen in immunosuppressed patients. Given the increasing number of people who are immunosuppressed as a result of treatment (e.g. chemotherapy, corticosteroids, radiotherapy), infection (e.g. AIDS) and other diseases (e.g. cancer), the number of infections has also increased significantly over the last two decades. Several fungi can cause a chronic type of pneumonia.

Pneumocystis pneumonia

Pneumocystis jiroveci (formerly *Pneumocystis carinii*) is a ubiquitous organism that was originally classified as a protozoan, but is now recognised to be a fungus. This organism has come to prominence with the AIDS epidemic. It is a common infectious complication of HIV-infected persons who are either not receiving appropriate therapy or not responding to it. It can also infect other immunocompromised individuals, as well as infants and the elderly.

P. jiroveci infects the tissue surrounding the alveoli, in which a foamy exudate forms, containing large numbers of the thick-walled cyst form of the organism. Typical symptoms include fever, dyspnoea and cyanosis. Laboratory diagnosis is by microscopic demonstration of the organism in a specimen from the patient (Figure 17.15). Sputum is rarely positive, so lung biopsy or bronchial alveolar lavage may be necessary. The organism is usually sensitive to cotrimoxazole, but treatment frequently fails because of the associated immune deficiency. Strains resistant to cotrimoxazole have been isolated in other countries (e.g. the United States and in Europe).

Cryptococcal pneumonia

Cryptococcus neoformans is an encapsulated yeast that is widely distributed in nature. A number of serotypes exist, belonging to two subspecies: *C. neoformans* var. *neoformans* and *C. neoformans* var. *gatti*. Like other fungi, these organisms mainly cause infection in the immunocompromised, especially in patients with HIV infection. The major route of infection is the respiratory tract, where these organisms cause pneumonia. However, in most patients, the organisms quickly spread to the brain and thus the presenting symptoms often reflect a meningitis, rather than pneumonia. In lung infection, the organism can be observed in sputum. A microscopic examination of the specimen treated with India ink stain shows the yeast cell with its characteristic large capsule. Chapter 20, on central nervous system infections, has further information on *C. neoformans*.

Other causes

A number of other fungi can cause pneumonia. Exposure of immunosuppressed individuals to the widespread, airborne spores of *Aspergillus fumigatus* can result in pulmonary infection. Similarly, exposure to spores of *Rhizopus* and *Mucor* can lead to infection.

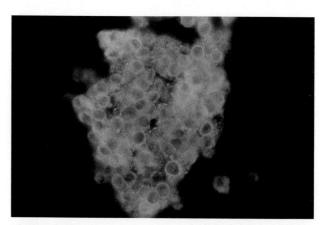

Figure 17.15

***Pneumocystis jiroveci* (fluorescent antibody stain)**
Found by microscopic examination of sputum, lung biopsy or bronchial alveolar lavage.

PARASITIC INFECTIONS OF THE LUNG

Various parasitic infections may involve the lung. Certain nematodes, namely *Ascaris* and some hookworms, transiently infect the lungs as their larvae migrate through the body on their way to the intestine. The tapeworm, *Echinococcus granulosis*, can infect the lungs and form hydatid cysts in the lung tissue. The cysts can become quite large and cause considerable respiratory dysfunction. These helminth infections are discussed more fully in Chapter 18.

SUMMARY

- Respiratory infections are among the most common that afflict humans.
- Respiratory pathogens may be expelled in enormous numbers by coughing and sneezing.
- Potentially pathogenic microbes are part of the normal flora of the upper respiratory tract.
- Factors that predispose people to respiratory infections include young age, old age, cigarette smoking, chronic obstructive pulmonary disease, poor living standards, alcoholism, immunosuppression and cancer.

UPPER RESPIRATORY TRACT INFECTIONS

- Most upper respiratory infections are due to viruses, and most are self-limiting, mild infections.
- Rhinoviruses are the most common causes of the common cold.
- Cold viruses are transmitted by coughing and sneezing, and by hands and objects contaminated with nasal secretions.
- Infections involving the middle ear are called otitis media. They occur most often in infants and small children.
- *S. pneumoniae* and *H. influenzae* are the most common causes of otitis media.
- The major causes of acute sinusitis are *S. pneumoniae* and *H. influenzae*.
- Pharyngitis, or sore throat, is a common condition caused by many different organisms.
- Adenoviruses are common causes of sore throat.
- Epstein-Barr (EB) virus causes a pharyngitis in the disease called glandular fever.
- The most important bacterial causes of sore throat are *Streptococcus pyogenes*, *Corynebacterium diphtheriae* (diphtheria), *Haemophilus influenzae* type b (epiglottitis) and *Neisseria gonorrhoeae* (pharyngeal gonorrhoea).
- *S. pyogenes* pharyngitis is important because of the possibility of the serious complications of rheumatic fever and acute glomerulonephritis.
- Diphtheria is an acute infection caused by toxin-producing strains of *Corynebacterium diphtheriae*.
- *C. diphtheriae* secretes a toxin in the respiratory tract that destroys the epithelial surface.
- Cardiac failure and death can result from the action of diphtheria toxin on the heart.
- Diphtheria vaccine is currently incorporated in the diphtheria, tetanus and pertussis (DTP) triple vaccine and the combined diphtheria and tetanus (CDT) vaccine.
- Epiglottitis is most often seen in young children and is almost always caused by *Haemophilus influenzae* type b.

- *H. influenzae* vaccine is part of the standard childhood vaccination schedule.
- Laryngotracheitis, or croup, is characterised by stridor, hoarseness and a resonant cough.
- Croup is most common in children under four and is usually caused by viruses, especially the parainfluenza group.

LOWER RESPIRATORY TRACT INFECTIONS

- Because the lower respiratory tract is normally sterile, infections involving it are potentially serious.
- Pathogenic microorganisms may reach the lower respiratory tract by inhalation, aspiration or spread of infection from the upper respiratory tract or via the bloodstream.
- Pertussis (whooping cough) is a severe disease caused by *Bordetella pertussis*.
- The incidence of pertussis in developed countries has been markedly reduced by immunisation.
- Immunisation against pertussis is recommended from two months of age and is part of the triple antigen vaccine.
- Acute bronchitis is an inflammation of the tracheobronchial tree.
- Viruses are the most common causes of acute bronchitis, including influenza virus, common cold viruses and adenoviruses.
- Bronchiolitis occurs mostly in children under two years and is caused mainly by the respiratory syncytial virus (RSV).
- The typical symptoms of bronchiolitis include fever, coryza, cough and respiratory obstruction.
- Influenza A viruses cause flu epidemics and occasionally pandemics. Influenza B viruses cause flu epidemics.
- Influenza viruses can vary their antigens by antigenic drift and antigenic shift.
- One to three days after infection with an influenza virus, symptoms such as fever, chills, malaise and muscle pain develop. Recovery usually occurs within 1–3 weeks.
- Influenza virus vaccine offers partial protection, but only against strains covered by the vaccine.
- Pneumonia is an infection and inflammation of the lungs and is a major cause of death throughout the world.
- Bacteria and viruses cause the vast majority of cases of pneumonia.
- Lobar pneumonia is an infection and consolidation confined to one or two lobes of the lung.
- Bronchopneumonia is a diffuse, patchy inflammation of the lungs, with numerous small foci of consolidation.
- Empyema is the term used to describe infection of the pleural space, and pleurisy means an inflammation of the pleural membranes.

- The most common bacterial cause of community-acquired pneumonia is *Streptococcus pneumoniae*.
- Staphylococcal pneumonia, due to *Staphylococcus aureus*, is a common complication of viral respiratory infection.
- Gram-negative enterobacteria often cause hospital-acquired pneumonia.
- *Haemophilus influenzae* can cause pneumonia, usually following epiglottitis, chronic bronchitis, brochiectasis, septicaemia or meningitis.
- *Pseudomonas aeruginosa* and other organisms cause chronic lung infections in patients with cystic fibrosis.
- *Legionella pneumophila* and other species of *Legionella* cause a pneumonia referred to as Legionnaires' disease (or legionellosis).
- The major causes of atypical pneumonia are *Mycoplasma pneumoniae*, *Chlamydia pneumoniae* and *Legionella*.
- The bacterium *Coxiella burnetii* is the cause of Q fever.
- *Chlamydia psittaci* is a bacterium that causes a pneumonia called ornithosis (or psittacosis), acquired by inhaling dust particles from bird droppings.

- Melioidosis is a type of pneumonia caused by the soil organism, *Burkholderia pseudomallei*.
- Respiratory syncytial virus is a major cause of pneumonia; adenoviruses and influenza viruses are occasional causes.

CHRONIC INFECTIONS OF THE LOWER RESPIRATORY TRACT

- Tuberculosis is caused mainly by *Mycobacterium tuberculosis*, but other species of mycobacteria can also be responsible.
- Lung disease is the most common form of tuberculosis, although in the immunocompromised the mycobacteria can invade the bloodstream and cause a potentially fatal disseminated disease.
- Pneumonia caused by *Pneumocystis jiroveci* is the most common infectious complication of AIDS.
- *Cryptococcus neoformans* is a yeast that can cause a lung infection, mainly in the immunocompromised.
- The tapeworm, *Echinococcus granulosus*, can infect the lungs and form hydatid cysts in the lung tissue.

STUDY QUESTIONS

1. List the major defences of the respiratory tract.
2. List the important factors that predispose people to respiratory infections.
3. What type of microorganisms are responsible for the majority of upper respiratory infections?
4. Why do people suffer repeatedly from the common cold?
5. What is otitis media and what are the common causes?
6. What are the common causes of pharyngitis?
7. Why is *Streptococcus pyogenes* an important cause of pharyngitis?
8. What is the cause of diphtheria and what are the major features of this disease?
9. Describe the treatment for diphtheria.
10. How is diphtheria prevented?
11. Why is acute epiglottitis a potentially life-threatening disease?
12. What is croup?
13. How do microorganisms gain access to the lower respiratory tract?
14. Name the cause and describe the pathogenesis of whooping cough.
15. Explain the importance of vaccination against whooping cough, and also describe the disadvantages.
16. What is acute bronchitis and what are the common causes?
17. What is bronchiolitis and what is the usual cause?
18. What is meant by antigenic drift and antigenic shift in influenza viruses?
19. How can people be protected against influenza and who should be protected?
20. What is pneumonia?
21. Distinguish between lobar pneumonia and bronchopneumonia.
22. Define the terms: pleural effusion, pleurisy, empyema.
23. What virulence factor enables *Streptococcus pneumoniae* to cause pneumonia?
24. What specimen(s) is/are commonly collected for the laboratory diagnosis of pneumonia?
25. What is Legionnaires' disease?
26. What are the major risk factors associated with Legionnaires' disease?
27. What is atypical pneumonia and what are the major causes?
28. What is Q fever and how is it acquired by humans?
29. What is ornithosis and how is it acquired by humans?
30. What viruses most commonly cause pneumonia?
31. What are the common clinical features of pneumonia?
32. What are the major aspects of patient management for a person with pneumonia?
33. In which groups in Australia is tuberculosis most commonly found?
34. What sites in the body does *Mycobacterium tuberculosis* infect?
35. Define the terms: tubercle, miliary tuberculosis, secondary tuberculosis.
36. How is tuberculosis diagnosed?
37. What is a Mantoux test and what does it detect?
38. How is tuberculosis treated?
39. What is the greatest risk factor for atypical mycobacteria infection?
40. What is the cause of pneumocystis pneumonia and what is the major risk factor?
41. In a patient with fungal pneumonia, what is the most likely predisposing factor?

Case History 17.1   Epiglottitis
1. Why did Timothy have an endotracheal tube inserted?
2. Why were blood cultures collected from Timothy?
3. *H. influenzae* typically causes infections in children less than four years old. Why is this age group so susceptible?

Case History 17.2   Whooping cough (pertussis)
1. Why is pertussis so easily transmitted from person to person?
2. Why is the early stage of pertussis difficult to diagnose?
3. What does this case illustrate about the effectiveness of pertussis vaccine?

Case History 17.3   Influenza
1. What evidence confirmed this as an outbreak of influenza?
2. How could this outbreak of influenza have been prevented?
3. Why is influenza infection so important in nursing home residents, and what makes staff infections so important?
4. Why does influenza vaccination have to occur annually?

Case History 17.4   Legionnaires' disease
1. Are the people involved in this outbreak typical of those usually affected by Legionnaires' disease?
2. How is Legionnaires' disease usually acquired?
3. Why are the sources of infection in Legionnaires' disease often difficult to identify?

Case History 17.5   Tuberculosis
1. What was the most likely means of transmission of infection in this outbreak of tuberculosis?
2. What are the advantages and disadvantages of BCG vaccination?
3. What infection control procedures are necessary to prevent the spread of tuberculosis in hospital?
4. What is it about tuberculosis that makes it so difficult to control in a population?

Further reading

Bastian I 2004, 'TB and not TB: Mycobacteriology in Australia in the 21st century', *Microbiology Australia*, 25(4), pp. 4–9.
(Reviews the importance of tuberculosis in Australia and current laboratory diagnostic methods.)

Fielding JE, K Yohannes, H Vally & JD Spencer 2004, 'Severe acute respiratory syndrome surveillance in Australia', *Communicable Diseases Intelligence*, 28(2), pp. 181–186.
(Discusses the impact of the global SARS epidemic in 2003 on Australia.)

Klig JE 2004, 'Current challenges in lower respiratory infections', *Current Opinion in Pediatrics*, 16, pp. 107–112.
(Reviews the causes, diagnosis and management of lower respiratory infections.)

Laver WG, N Bischofberger & RG Webster 1999, 'Disarming flu viruses', *Scientific American*, January, pp. 56–65.
(Discusses the genetics of influenza viruses and explains how the viruses cause epidemics.)

Musher DM 2003, 'Medical progress: How contagious are common respiratory tract infections?', *New England Journal of Medicine*, 348(13), pp. 1256–1266.
(Examines the modes and ease of transmission of respiratory tract infections.)

Soldatou A & EG Davies 2003, 'Respiratory virus infections in the immunocompromised host', *Paediatric Respiratory Reviews*, 4, pp. 193–204.
(Discusses the nature of respiratory infections in the immuno-compromised, and reviews current diagnostic and management approaches.)

West JV 2002, 'Acute upper airway infections', *British Medical Bulletin*, 61, pp. 215–230.
(Reviews the diagnosis and management of upper respiratory infections.)

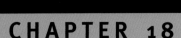

CHAPTER 18

Gastrointestinal Tract Infections

[CHAPTER FOCUS]

- ■ *What microorganisms cause acute diarrhoeal disease in humans?*

- ■ *What is the role of microorganisms in peptic ulcer disease?*

- ■ *What microorganisms cause typhoid and paratyphoid fevers?*

- ■ *What helminths are associated with gastrointestinal infections?*

- ■ *What viruses cause hepatitis?*

- ■ *What are the common modes of transmission of gastrointestinal infections?*

- ■ *What are the important clinical features of gastrointestinal infections?*

- ■ *How are gastrointestinal infections treated and how may they be prevented?*

Introduction

Intestinal infections are a major health problem throughout the world, but particularly in developing countries. Numerous microorganisms may enter the gastrointestinal tract in foods and beverages but, fortunately, relatively few microbes are capable of causing intestinal disease. To establish and cause infection, the microbes have to be ingested in sufficient numbers, and then be able to circumvent a variety of highly effective antimicrobial defences, which include:

- gastric acidity
- digestive enzymes
- bile salts
- intestinal motility
- the normal flora of the intestine (see Figure 18.1)
- specific immune defences provided by the lymphoid tissues of the GIT.

These defences are described in detail in Chapter 9. It should be noted that the gastrointestinal tract is a hostile environment for most microorganisms, the majority of which are killed by the acid of the stomach and do not even reach the intestine alive. Certain pathogens, however, have properties that enable them to survive these defences and ultimately cause disease.

Most intestinal pathogens remain localised in the gastrointestinal tract, multiplying and/or producing toxins there and causing local symptoms. There are some, however, that cause more generalised symptoms by invading intestinal tissues and then spreading to other parts of the body. Other microbes cause gastrointestinal disease by growing and secreting toxins (exotoxins) in the food before it is consumed. These diseases have a very short incubation period, because symptoms are produced soon after the preformed toxins are ingested and absorbed.

Most gastrointestinal infections manifest as an acute diarrhoeal disease. In this chapter we first consider the major causes of acute diarrhoeal disease, which include bacteria, viruses and protozoa. There are other types of gastrointestinal infection in which diarrhoea is not a major symptom, and these include *Helicobacter pylori* infections (gastritis and peptic ulcers) and helminth (worm) infections. Other infections discussed in this chapter are the enteric fevers, typhoid and paratyphoid fever, caused by bacteria that invade the GIT and spread to other parts of the body, and hepatitis, an infection of the liver caused mainly by viruses.

The terminology used to describe infections of the gastrointestinal tract can be very confusing. Some terms are used interchangeably and some terms are given different meanings by different authors. In this text, **food poisoning** (or **food-borne illness**) is used in a general sense to refer to any gastrointestinal disease related to the consumption of food, including microbial and non-microbial factors. A **gastrointestinal infection** is a disease of the gastrointestinal tract caused by the establishment and multiplication of microorganisms in the gastrointestinal tract. **Food intoxication** is used for diseases caused by the presence of preformed toxins (microbial or non-microbial) in food. Other terms in common use and their meanings as applied in this text are given in Table 18.1.

Acute diarrhoeal diseases

A range of microbial pathogens is capable of producing symptoms of diarrhoeal disease. They include those that multiply in the GIT, as well as those that secrete toxins in food (food intoxications). Gastrointestinal pathogens are acquired mainly by the faecal-oral route, from contaminated food, fluids or hands. The major symptom of infection is **acute diarrhoea**, a sudden disruption in bowel habits in which normally formed stools are replaced by more frequent, liquefied movements. Diarrhoea is the result of increased secretion of fluid and electrolytes into the lumen of the intestine, and represents a non-specific response of the intestine to a number of different factors, including infection, the action of toxins, sensitivity to drugs, and ischaemia. However, the most common causes are microbial infections due to bacteria, viruses or protozoa. Some helminths can cause diarrhoea but usually only in chronic infections.

Acute diarrhoeal infections can result in a wide range of illnesses, from a mild attack of loose stools lasting one to several days to a severe illness with considerable fluid loss, which can be fatal. Overall, they are extremely common throughout the world, second only to upper respiratory infections.

In developing countries, diarrhoeal diseases are a major cause of morbidity and mortality. It has been estimated

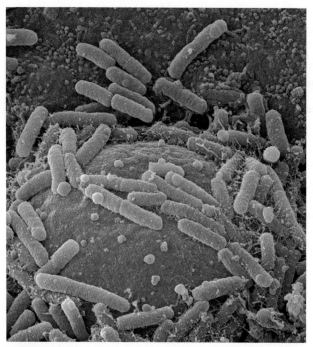

***Escherichia coli* in the intestinal tract**
This organism is a major part of the normal flora of the intestine.

Table 18.1

Common terms used to describe gastrointestinal infections

TERM	DEFINITION
Food poisoning or food-borne illness	Gastrointestinal disease related to the consumption of food containing pathogenic microorganisms or their toxins, or other non-microbial toxins
Gastrointestinal infection	A disease of the gastrointestinal tract caused by the establishment and multiplication of microorganisms in the gastrointestinal tract
Food intoxication	Gastrointestinal disease caused by the consumption of food containing toxins (microbial or non-microbial)
Gastroenteritis	Inflammation of the gastrointestinal tract, including the stomach and intestine
Gastritis	Inflammation of the mucosa of the stomach
Diarrhoea	A disruption in bowel habits characterised by more frequent passage of loose and watery stools
Dysentery	An inflammatory disorder of the gastrointestinal tract characterised by severe diarrhoea with blood and pus in the stools

that they may be responsible for up to 4.5 million infant and childhood deaths per year. Diarrhoeal disease also contributes to the malnutrition that is prevalent in the children of Third World countries. The magnitude of the problem of diarrhoeal disease in developed countries has declined with economic and public health improvements, but this type of disease is still a common complaint. In the latter context it is, however, usually mild and self-limiting, except in the very young, the elderly and immunocompromised patients.

Notification rates of diarrhoeal diseases (including those given in this chapter) generally underestimate the true incidence since many people with diarrhoeal disease do not seek medical attention and many cases are not identified by laboratory diagnosis.

EPIDEMIOLOGY OF ACUTE INFECTIOUS DIARRHOEA

Acute infectious diarrhoea is usually acquired through ingestion of pathogenic microorganisms. Common sources of the organisms include:

- food or water contaminated with faeces
- faecally contaminated hands
- food contaminated with faecal organisms spread by flies.

Many pathogens of the intestinal tract are able to survive for at least a short time in the environment and on the surface of fomites. Some can survive for long periods in polluted natural water courses.

The highest incidence of acute diarrhoeal disease is in areas of the world where there are poor facilities for sanitation and sewage disposal. Transmission is mainly via contaminated food or water. In developed countries, food-borne transmission is the most common, but acute diarrhoeal disease also occurs in international travellers, hospitalised people and immunocompromised people. Outbreaks sometimes occur in hospital nurseries and day-care centres. Certain microbes tend to be associated with each of these particular epidemiological settings (see Table 18.2).

Food-borne gastroenteritis

Most cases of food-borne gastroenteritis (inflammation of the gastrointestinal tract) are due to bacteria, but viruses and parasites can also be involved. Food-borne illness can occur when contaminated meats or seafood are eaten raw or are undercooked, or when food is improperly preserved, allowing significant multiplication of organisms in the food before its consumption. Generally, slightly contaminated food poses little risk if cooked properly and eaten fresh. Different foods tend to harbour certain types of organisms, as shown in Table 18.2.

Most cases of food-borne gastroenteritis are self-limiting, resolving in a few days with supportive care only. However, in certain situations, severe and even life-threatening disease can occur. Young children, the elderly and the immunosuppressed are particularly susceptible. Children can dehydrate very rapidly and may require hospitalisation and intravenous fluids.

Hospital nurseries

Many pathogens can cause diarrhoeal disease in neonates. Infants can become infected by bacteria or viruses during passage through the birth canal, or after birth from parents, siblings, hospital personnel or contaminated formula or water. Because of the immaturity of their immune system, they are highly susceptible to any pathogens encountered. Nursery outbreaks sometimes occur, often initiated by an asymptomatic infant shedding the organism.

Day-care centres

The incidence of diarrhoeal disease in children attending day-care centres has been reported to be up to twice that in children at home. Factors promoting spread include the presence of non-toilet trained children, oral exploration of objects, contamination of hands, close contact and lack of appropriate infection control measures. *Shigella* spp., *Giardia intestinalis*, rotavirus and *Cryptosporidium* have frequently been associated with outbreaks. These organisms typically require only a low inoculum in order to cause infection in infants.

Faecal-oral spread and environmental contamination

Table 18.2

Epidemiological associations with microbes that cause diarrhoea

EXPOSURE	COMMON ORGANISMS
• Food-borne:	
beef and pork	Salmonella, Staphylococcus aureus, E. coli Clostridium perfringens, Campylobacter, Yersinia
poultry	Salmonella, Staphylococcus aureus, Clostridium perfringens, Campylobacter
milk and cheese	Salmonella, E. coli, Campylobacter, Yersinia
vegetables	Clostridium botulinum, Salmonella, Shigella, Bacillus cereus
shellfish	Vibrios, norovirus, hepatitis A
water	E. coli, vibrios, Shigella, Giardia, Cryptosporidium
• Schools, nurseries and day-care centres	Shigella, rotavirus, Campylobacter, Giardia, Cryptosporidium, Salmonella, Aeromonas, Plesiomonas
• Travellers	E. coli, Shigella, Campylobacter, Giardia, Aeromonas, Salmonella, Entamoeba histolytica, Vibrio cholerae
• Hospitalised patients receiving antibiotics	Clostridium difficile
• Immunocompromised (e.g. AIDS)	Cryptosporidium, Isospora, Salmonella, Microsporidium

are the most common means of transmission. The most important interventions to prevent outbreaks of infection are good hygiene and handwashing practices.

Traveller's diarrhoea

This is the name given to acute diarrhoea that frequently occurs in people visiting a foreign country. Travellers may be exposed to unfamiliar organisms for which they have no specific immunity, and which may cause an episode of acute diarrhoea. Some pathogens are contracted by consumption of faecally contaminated food or water, especially when visiting countries with poor sanitation and sewage disposal, or by eating unwashed fruit and vegetables in areas where sewage is used as a fertiliser. Certain countries in Asia, the Middle East, Africa and South America are well recognised as destinations where there is a high risk of developing gastroenteritis. Enterotoxigenic *E. coli* is the predominant cause of traveller's diarrhoea; other common causes are shown in Table 18.2.

Traveller's diarrhoea is generally a benign, self-limiting disease, although some of the more virulent agents may cause severe illness, such as dysentery (e.g. *Shigella*) or a chronic diarrhoea (e.g. *Giardia*).

Hospitalised patients

People sometimes develop diarrhoea while in hospital. Mild diarrhoea is a common side effect of antibiotic therapy but a more serious form, also associated with antibiotic therapy, is due to the bacterium *Clostridium difficile*. Broad spectrum antibiotics can predispose a patient to a pseudomembranous colitis, caused by *C. difficile*, by altering the intestinal microbial flora that normally inhibit its establishment in the intestine.

People with AIDS

Almost all AIDS patients experience at least one episode of diarrhoea during their illness. The suppression of their immune system makes them susceptible to some unusual, opportunistic organisms, as shown in Table 18.2.

CLINICAL FEATURES OF ACUTE DIARRHOEAL DISEASE

It is difficult to differentiate between the causative agents of acute diarrhoea on the basis of signs and symptoms alone. Most acute diarrhoeal infections have an incubation period of 1–4 days, but shorter or longer incubations can occur (see Table 18.3). Most diarrhoeal infections are self-limiting, but the illness can be as short as one day or as long as three weeks, depending on the cause. Infectious diarrhoea can be divided into one of two syndromes based on the nature of the diarrhoea produced:

1. *non-inflammatory diarrhoea* – characterised by watery stools without blood, mucus or pus
2. *inflammatory diarrhoea (or dysentery)* – characterised by stools containing blood, mucus and pus.

In general, inflammatory diarrhoeas are more severe than the non-inflammatory types, although some cases of non-inflammatory diarrhoea can be very serious. The characteristics of these two forms of diarrhoea are summarised in Table 18.4.

Inflammatory diarrhoeas are caused by invasive microorganisms or by organisms that liberate toxins. Mainly the colon is affected, resulting in disruption of the mucosal lining. Damage to the colonic lining leads to the oozing of red cells, serous fluid and white cells into the lumen of the intestine. Typically, the patient has a small-volume, bloody diarrhoea, often with mucus. The patient also frequently complains of tenesmus (straining without passing stools), faecal urgency (inability to delay passing stools) and abdominal cramps. Also, the patient usually has a fever. Microscopic examination of the stool

Table 18.3
Diarrhoeal diseases: incubation period and duration of illness

PATHOGEN	INCUBATION PERIOD	DURATION OF ILLNESS
Staphylococcus aureus	1–6 hours	12–24 hours
Bacillus cereus	1–24 hours	12–48 hours
Clostridium perfringens	6–24 hours	12–24 hours
Norovirus	1–2 days	24–48 hours
Campylobacter spp.	1–4 days	3 days to 3 weeks
Salmonella spp.	1–2 days	2–7 days
Vibrio parahaemolyticus	1–2 days	1–3 days
Vibrio cholerae	1–3 days	5–7 days
Rotavirus	1–4 days	4–7 days
Enterotoxigenic *E. coli*	1–3 days	5–10 days
Shigella spp.	1–4 days	1–3 days
Yersinia enterocolitica	4–7 days	1–2 weeks
Cryptosporidium parvum	1–2 weeks	1–3 weeks
Giardia intestinalis	2 weeks	weeks to months

Table 18.4
The differences between inflammatory and non-inflammatory diarrhoea

CHARACTERISTIC	INFLAMMATORY DIARRHOEA	NON-INFLAMMATORY DIARRHOEA
Leucocytes in stools	Present	Absent
Blood in stools	Present	Rare
Mucus	Present	Rare
Stool volume	Small (normal)	Greatly increased
Abdominal pain	Severe – lower left quadrant	None to slight
Body temperature	May be elevated	Usually normal
Site of infection	Colon	Small intestine
Common causes	*Shigella, Salmonella, Yersinia, Campylobacter, Clostridium difficile*, invasive and enterohaemorrhagic *E. coli, Entamoeba histolytica, Vibrio parahaemolyticus, Aeromonas*	Viruses, *Vibrio cholerae, Giardia*, enterotoxigenic and enteropathogenic *E. coli, Staphylococcus aureus, Bacillus cereus, Clostridium perfringens, Cryptosporidium, Isospora, Cyclospora*

reveals the presence of numerous leucocytes. Some organisms may initially cause a watery diarrhoea before invading the mucosa, but later produce the typical inflammatory form when invasion occurs. The micro-organisms that usually cause an inflammatory diarrhoea are listed in Table 18.4.

Non-inflammatory diarrhoeas are caused by micro-organisms that primarily affect the small intestine. They may adhere to the intestinal epithelium, secrete toxins or even invade the cells, but they generally don't cause significant damage to the tissue. They produce diarrhoea by causing excessive secretion of fluids from the lining cells. Typically, the patient has a profuse, watery, non-bloody diarrhoea and often experiences nausea and abdominal cramping as well. In viral infections vomiting may be a major symptom. Leucocytes and red cells are not generally found in the stools, because of the absence of mucosal destruction and leakage of cells from the bloodstream. Typical causes are listed in Table 18.4.

BACTERIAL CAUSES OF ACUTE DIARRHOEA

Campylobacter

Campylobacter species are comma-shaped Gram-negative rods. Since the mid-1980s they have emerged as the most common causes of diarrhoea in humans in many developed countries. Currently, in Australia, about 14 000 cases are reported annually. Most commonly affected are children under four years old (see Figure 18.2). Several species are associated with human disease, but *C. jejuni* is by far the most common.

A large reservoir of *Campylobacter* exists in animals such as cattle, sheep, poultry and wild birds. Human infections are thus usually acquired by consumption of contaminated and poorly cooked foods of animal origin, especially poultry, red meat and milk.

Campylobacter enteritis is due to ulceration and inflammation of the mucosal surface in the jejunum, ileum and colon, suggesting an invasive process. Several toxins of

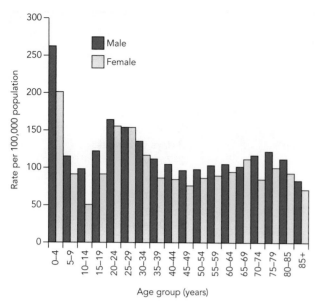

Figure 18.2

Notification rates of *Campylobacter* infections by age group and sex in Australia in 2003

Source: Communicable Diseases Intelligence, 29(1), 2005, p. 26, © Commonwealth of Australia, reproduced by permission

C. jejuni have been identified, but their role in the pathogenesis of infection has not been elucidated. Invasion and bacteraemia can occur, especially in neonates and debilitated adults. Some infected people excrete the organism asymptomatically. Guillain-Barre syndrome, characterised by neuromuscular paralysis, is now recognised as a rare post-infectious complication of *C. jejuni* infection.

Salmonella

In developed countries, salmonellae are second only to *Campylobacter* as a major cause of diarrhoea. In Australia

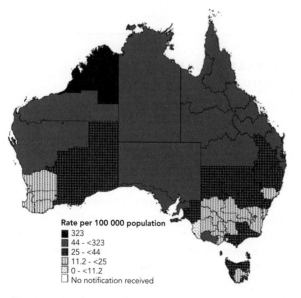

Figure 18.3

Notification rates of *Salmonella* infections in Australia, 2003, by statistical division of residence

Source: Communicable Diseases Intelligence, 29(1), 2005, p. 28, © Commonwealth of Australia, reproduced by permission

7000–8000 cases are reported annually. The highest rates of notification occur in children under four years of age and in the northern parts of the country (see Figure 18.3). There are numerous serovars (serotypes) of *Salmonella* that cause gastroenteritis, the most common being *Salmonella typhimurium*. Other serotypes commonly encountered in Australia include *S. virchow*, *S. saintpaul*, *S. chester* and *S. birkenhead*.

The major source of diarrhoea-causing salmonellae is the intestinal tract of animals. In developed countries the organisms are transmitted to humans mainly via contaminated foods, especially poultry and eggs, meats such as pork, lamb and beef, and dairy products. Typically, salmonellae are found contaminating poultry products and animal meats and cause infection when the food is improperly stored and/or cooked. Takeaway chickens and foods containing eggs, such as baby formulas, have caused outbreaks of infection. Salmonellae can also be transmitted from infected people and asymptomatic carriers to other people. Transmission by food handlers who are carriers and do not observe proper hygiene standards is particularly important.

Salmonellae invade the intestinal mucosa of the ileum and colon to produce disease. They replicate in the lamina propria, causing diarrhoea with blood and mucus. Most cases of salmonellosis are self-limiting diarrhoeal diseases. After clinical recovery, many patients become asymptomatic carriers for some weeks to months and continue to shed the organisms in faeces. In some cases, especially in the young, elderly and immunosuppressed, the organisms invade mesenteric lymph nodes from which they can spread via the bloodstream to cause arthritis, osteomyelitis, pneumonia or meningitis.

Escherichia coli

Some strains of *Escherichia coli* are harmless members of the normal GIT flora in humans and animals, but other strains possess virulence factors that enable them to cause infection in the intestinal tract. The strains that cause diarrhoeal disease have been classified into five main groups according to their pathogenic mechanism.

1. **Enterotoxigenic *E. coli* (ETEC)** bind to specific receptors on the intestinal cell membranes where they produce potent enterotoxins. The heat-labile toxin (LT) of ETEC is closely related to cholera toxin (see Chapter 10). LT, like cholera toxin, causes an increase in levels of cyclic AMP in intestinal epithelial cells, resulting in a massive outflow of water and electrolytes into the lumen of the intestine, manifested as profuse diarrhoea. In addition, ETEC have a heat-stable toxin (ST) that also causes diarrhoea by similar mechanisms. ETEC are a major cause of diarrhoea in children in developing countries, and of traveller's diarrhoea.

2. **Enterohaemorrhagic *E. coli* (EHEC)** include a number of different serotypes which have become recognised as important causes of gastrointestinal disease ranging from mild diarrhoea to a life-

threatening haemorrhagic colitis, and which can sometimes cause **haemolytic uraemic syndrome (HUS)**. This is a serious complication, characterised by a haemolytic anaemia (see Figure 18.4), uraemia and thrombocytopaenia, and renal failure, which can occur within the first few days of onset. Renal failure causes death in some patients. HUS can occur in any age group but is most common in children under four. Throughout the world *E. coli* O157 is the serotype most often associated with HUS, but other serotypes (e.g. *E. coli* O111) may also be responsible.

The main virulence factor of EHEC is Shiga toxin (also called Verotoxin or Shiga-like toxin), which causes destruction of the colonic epithelium and haemorrhage. It is very similar to the Shiga toxin that was first identified in *Shigella* (see later in this chapter). HUS occurs when Shiga toxin and probably other toxins together cause small blood vessel damage in various sites including the kidney. Red cells are fragmented when passing through these damaged vessels, resulting in anaemia. Platelets, which cluster in the vessels, are destroyed, causing a thrombocytopaenia.

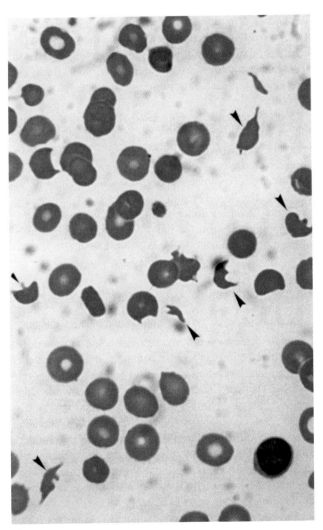

Figure 18.4

Smear of peripheral blood from a patient with haemolytic uraemic syndrome, showing red cell fragments (arrowheads)

The diagnosis of EHEC infections can be difficult because the organisms are rarely present in stools after the initial diarrhoeal phase. The need for treatment of HUS is urgent and may involve intensive care treatment, haemodialysis and prolonged hospitalisation.

Sporadic cases of HUS associated with EHEC have been reported in Australia, but the first outbreak due to a common source was recorded in South Australia in early 1995 (see Spotlight box, below). HUS only became notifiable in Australia in late 1998. Thirteen cases of HUS were notified in Australia in 2002. Large

---

> **SPOTLIGHT ON**
> ### Haemolytic uraemic syndrome
>
> In early 1995, 20 children were diagnosed with haemolytic uraemic syndrome (HUS) and treated at the Women's and Children's Hospital, Adelaide. There were 12 boys and 8 girls (aged 6 months to 12 years; median 5 years).
>
> Fourteen children had eaten the same brand of mettwurst, seven samples of which (taken from the homes of eight patients) were PCR-positive for Shiga toxins 1 and 2. The contaminated product was found in the family homes of three other patients, but consumption by the children could not be confirmed. In the other three children, there was no proven link with the mettwurst; possibly, human to human transmission was responsible in these cases. Faecal cultures from 18 children were PCR-positive for Shiga toxins 1 and 2. *E. coli* O111: H– was isolated from cultures obtained from 15 of these 18 children.
>
> Nineteen of the children had a prodromal illness characterised by abdominal pain and bloody diarrhoea. All children had evidence of haemotological and renal disease at presentation, and haemoglobin and platelet levels fell progressively during the days after diagnosis. Most of the children required substantial supportive treatment: renal dialysis in 18, repeated blood transfusion in all 20, and parenteral nutrition in 17. One child died and nine children suffered major non-renal complications. The children were hospitalised for a median period of 17.5 days (range 3–74 days). Five children have been left with a glomerular filtration rate (GFR) below 80ml/min per 1.73m^2 and must be considered at risk for progressive deterioration of renal function in the long term.
>
> In this outbreak of HUS, *E.coli* O111:H– was identified as the principal culprit, rather than the more commonly reported *E.coli* O157:H7. The source of this outbreak was a locally produced semi-dry fermented sausage (mettwurst) contaminated with various Shiga-toxin-producing *E. coli*. A coronial inquest found that inadequate processing by the manufacturer was a major contributor to the outbreak.
>
> *Source:* Henning, PH et al. 1998, 'Haemolytic-uraemic syndrome outbreak caused by *Escherichia coli* O111:H-clinical outcomes', *Medical Journal of Australia* 168, p. 552.

outbreaks have occurred in the United States and other developed countries. This organism has a low infectious dose (perhaps as low as 100 bacteria).

3. **Enteropathogenic _E. coli_ (EPEC)** were the first group of this species to be identified as intestinal pathogens. These organisms appear to adhere intimately to enterocytes and cause destruction of the microvilli at that site. EPEC is a leading cause of infantile diarrhoea in developing countries, but also occurs occasionally in developed areas of the world.

4. **Enteroinvasive _E. coli_ (EIEC)** cause a gastrointestinal disease that is similar to the dysentery caused by _Shigella_ spp. EIEC secrete toxins and actively invade epithelial cells of the large intestine and spread laterally to adjacent cells, causing cell death, ulceration of the mucosa and consequently inflammation. The inflammatory response causes an outpouring of pus, blood and mucus into the lumen.

5. **Enteroaggregative _E. coli_ (EAEC)** is a recently recognised group that appears to cause disease by releasing toxins that damage intestinal cells. EAEC cause acute and persistent diarrhoea, mainly in children in less developed countries, in travellers and the immunocompromised.

Cholera

Cholera is an acute infection of the gastrointestinal tract caused by the comma-shaped Gram-negative bacterium _Vibrio cholerae_. Cholera is endemic in South-East Asia, parts of Africa and much of Central and South America. Several pandemics of cholera occurred during the 19th century, originating in the Indian subcontinent. In Australia fewer than six cases are reported annually and these are almost always imported cases. However, _V. cholerae_ has been isolated from some coastal rivers in Queensland and one locally acquired case has been linked to this.

V. cholerae causes infection only in humans. Symptomatic people and asymptomatic carriers are the reservoirs of infection. The organism is able to survive for long periods in water and thus occurs most frequently in areas where clean drinking water and adequate sewage disposal are not available. Transmission via food (e.g. seafood) contaminated with human faeces also occurs. The disease is often associated with natural disasters (e.g. floods, earthquakes) as well as situations of social unrest and upheaval. More than 7000 people died from cholera in Rwanda in 1994, associated with the civil crisis in that country.

V. cholerae causes disease by secreting the cholera toxin. This toxin causes the levels of cyclic AMP in intestinal epithelial cells to increase, resulting in a massive outflow of water and electrolytes into the lumen of the intestine, manifested as profuse diarrhoea. Chapter 10 gives a more detailed description of its action. Many cases are mild or asymptomatic. In severe cases, the patient may lose up to 30 litres of fluid in a day, and the stools are primarily a mixture of water and mucus, having the classic appearance of 'rice water stools'. Without fluid and electrolyte replacement, mortality can be as high as 40–60%.

A live, attenuated vaccine for cholera, for oral administration, has recently been developed. Being a live vaccine it should be used with caution, especially in the immunocompromised, young children and pregnant women. This vaccine is not recommended by Australian health authorities or by the World Health Organization for routine use, even for travellers to cholera-endemic areas. Ensuring consumption of clean food and water is considered to be of greater importance.

Shigella

Shigella diarrhoea is also known as bacillary dysentery. There are four species – _Shigella sonnei_ causes mostly mild infections, _S. flexneri_ and _S. boydii_ usually cause moderate disease, and _S. dysenteriae_ is the most serious. _Shigella_ infections are most common in children under 10 years and are often reported in schools and day-care centres. Day-care staff and family members may also become infected. Shigellosis is more common in disadvantaged communities and is much more prevalent among Aboriginal children than other Australian children. About 500–800 cases of shigellosis are notified annually in Australia, although the annual notification rate has been gradually declining. Highest rates of notification occur in children under four years of age.

Shigella are strictly human pathogens, so the source of infection is always a symptomatic person or carrier of the organisms. Faecal-oral spread is the major mode of transmission. Prolonged excretion of _Shigella_ may occur in

---

CASE HISTORY 18.1

Cholera

The outbreak was first recognised on 17 April 2000. As of 26 June, 1596 cases of watery diarrhoea had been reported – a figure based on inpatient and outpatient records from the Pohnpei Hospital in the Federated States of Micronesia, together with data provided by community-based dispensaries. Nine deaths were associated with the outbreak. _Vibrio cholerae_ was isolated by the Pohnpei Hospital and confirmed as the Ogawa serotype. Of these suspected cholera cases, 954 met the World Health Organization case definition for cholera. The epidemic was consistent with an initial point-source outbreak at a large funeral at Kitti, followed by a mixture of person-to-person transmission and additional point-source outbreaks in a clockwise direction around the island.

Up to 27 June 2000, 368 (92%) of the 399 admissions to hospital and 625 (80%) of 777 outpatient and emergency department presentations with acute watery diarrhoea met the WHO case definition for cholera.

Adapted from _Communicable Diseases Intelligence_ 24(6): 179, 2000.

Shigellosis

In December 2000, the director of a child-care centre notified the Communicable Diseases Section of the Victorian Department of Human Services that approximately 15 children, some of their family contacts and a number of staff had recently been ill with gastroenteritis over a two and a half week period. At this time there were approximately 70 children attending the centre and 11 staff employed. The centre has three rooms; nursery/baby room (0–1 years), toddler (2–3 years) and kindergarten (4–5 years).

Sixty-seven probable cases of shigellosis were subsequently identified: 33 children (47% of children attending), four staff (37% of staff employed) and 30 household contacts. Two cases were hospitalised and there were no deaths.

The first case was in a child from the toddler room. Within four days after the onset of illness in the first case, cases were detected in all three rooms at the centre.

At least twice daily, clean-up procedures were carried out throughout the centre. Diluted household bleach was used as a sanitiser; spray bottles with the bleach were used to clean door handles, knobs and surfaces and the solution was made up twice daily. Hand washing was emphasised and posters were displayed in bathrooms. Staff supervised the hand washing of children and assisted those children too young to wash their own hands. Loose soap in the toilets was replaced with liquid soap dispensers, which were washed and refilled at various times throughout the day; paper towels were provided for hand drying.

The nappy changing area was cleaned and sanitised twice daily.

New admissions to the centre were not permitted during the outbreak.

This investigation identified 20 confirmed cases of *Shigella sonnei* biotype g and a further 47 probable cases in children and staff who attended the child care centre, and in their household contacts. The implementation of stringent clean-up procedures, enhanced hand washing and hygiene, and the support of staff and families at the child care centre was an effective strategy in controlling the outbreak.

Adapted from: Genobile D et al. 2004, 'An outbreak of shigellosis in a child care centre', *Communicable Diseases Intelligence* 28(2), pp. 225–229.

some patients for several weeks after recovery. Handwashing and good hygiene are considered to be the most important means of preventing transmission of these organisms.

Shigella are readily transmitted and highly virulent – as few as 10–100 organisms may cause disease. Their pathogenesis is due to their enteroinvasive properties as well as their secretion of the Shiga toxin. In the intestine, the bacteria are phagocytosed by colonic epithelial cells. They then lyse the phagocytic vesicle, multiply intracellularly and invade adjacent cells. The Shiga toxin acts by cleaving ribosomal RNA in colonic cells, halting protein synthesis and killing the cell. The Shiga toxin is also thought to damage endothelial cells and in some cases causes haemolytic uraemic syndrome similar to the enterohaemorrhagic *E. coli*.

Clostridium difficile (antibiotic-associated colitis)

Diarrhoea can arise whenever the normal intestinal flora is disrupted or altered. When antimicrobial drugs, particularly broad spectrum agents, are used in the treatment of infectious diseases, they can affect the normal flora as well as the pathogen. A change in the balance of the normal flora can lead to a mild diarrhoea. Since the late 1970s it has been recognised that antibiotic therapy can sometimes lead to much more serious gastrointestinal disease; this is characterised by severe diarrhoea and a form of inflammation in the colon that results in the formation of yellow-white raised plaques or pseudomembranes on the colonic mucosa.

The Gram-positive anaerobic rod, *Clostridium difficile*, is the cause of this pseudomembranous colitis, not the antibiotics. The normal colonic flora of adults and children over the age of 12 months effectively prevent colonisation by *C. difficile*, but antibiotics can disrupt the flora, allowing *C. difficile* to become established, multiply and produce disease. Infection with *C. difficile* may present in a variety of ways, ranging from mild diarrhoea without abdominal discomfort to the potentially life-threatening pseudomembranous colitis.

C. difficile spores are ubiquitous. The organism is able to survive for long periods in the hospital environment, because of its spores. It has been cultured from floors, toilets, bedding, mops and furniture and also from the hands of hospital personnel. Heavy contamination can be found in rooms that have been occupied by infected patients. Thus, transmission of the organism to an individual who is susceptible because of antibiotic therapy can readily occur. It is now recognised as an important type of hospital-acquired infection.

Although pseudomembranous colitis was initially related to clindamycin usage, almost all broad spectrum antibiotic agents have now been implicated in this disease; the main offenders are clindamycin, ampicillin, cephalosporins and aminoglycosides. While the use of antibiotics is recognised as the major predisposing factor, anything that disrupts the intestinal flora of the gut, including another gastrointestinal infection, can lead to *C. difficile* infection. The time from antibiotic exposure to onset of symptoms can range from one day up to eight weeks.

C. difficile produces two exotoxins, toxins A and B, which are the main pathogenic factors. Both toxins are cytotoxic for a number of cell types; they cause haemorrhage and induce a local inflammatory response with the activation of macrophages and mast cells, the mobilisation of neutrophils and destruction of the mucosa. A pseudomembrane, consisting of necrotic tissue debris, mucus and neutrophils and monocytes, forms over the mucosa (see

Figure 18.5). Perforation of the colon, abscess formation and vascular thrombi are possible late complications.

C. difficile infection should be considered in any patient receiving antimicrobial drugs who develops diarrhoea while in hospital. However, it should be noted that *C. difficile* is not found in a significant proportion of cases of antibiotic-associated colitis, suggesting a probable role for other, as yet unknown, causes.

Vibrio parahaemolyticus

Vibrio parahaemolyticus is a Gram-negative, halophilic (salt-loving) organism commonly found in seafood such as crabs, oysters and fish. In Japan and South-East Asia, where seafoods are often consumed uncooked, this bacterium is responsible for a large number of cases of food-borne illness. The mechanism of pathogenesis is still unclear, but there is evidence to suggest that the organism invades the epithelial cells of the small intestine. A number of other vibrios cause diarrhoeal disease, including *V. vulnificus*, *V. fluvalis* and *V. hollisae*.

Yersinia

Yersinia enterocolitica is a Gram-negative rod that is a member of the family Enterobacteriaceae. The organism is found in a large variety of animals, especially pigs and cows. As a result, many cases of yersiniosis are traced to meat and dairy products. *Yersinia* is also sometimes found in other domestic animals – transmission to humans from pet dogs has been reported. Faecal-oral spread between humans also occurs, enhanced by the possible faecal excretion of the organism for weeks after infection. Most infections occur in young children. In Australia, 200–400 cases of yersiniosis are reported each year.

The pathogenesis of *Y. enterocolitica* stems mainly from its ability to invade the mucosa of the terminal ileum and replicate in the Peyer's patches, producing an inflammatory diarrhoea. The disease may be confused with an appendicitis, especially in children. The organism also secretes an exotoxin, but its role in virulence is unclear. Another species, *Y. pseudotuberculosis*, is also associated with diarrhoeal disease in humans.

Clostridium perfringens

Clostridium perfringens is associated with diarrhoeal disease when a threshold number of bacteria are ingested in contaminated food, followed by *in vivo* secretion of an enterotoxin. This organism produces two different food-borne illnesses. Type A organisms cause a self-limiting diarrhoeal illness, which occurs in developed countries, and type C organisms cause a potentially life-threatening syndrome known as *enteritis necroticans* in underdeveloped tropical areas.

Type A clostridial food poisoning is typically associated with meat and poultry products in which there is a long delay between cooking and serving of the food. Clostridial spores, which are widely present in human and animal faeces and uncooked meats and vegetables, can survive cooking temperatures and can germinate and multiply when meat products are allowed to stand at 15–60°C for several hours or more. The food must be heavily contaminated for infection to occur. This food-borne illness is usually associated with situations where bulk food preparation occurs, such as in institutions and fast food outlets (see Case History 13.1, page 297).

Enteritis necroticans is usually due to the consumption of ß-toxin-producing type C strains of *C. perfringens* in undercooked pork. In healthy individuals this toxin is inactivated by trypsin and other intestinal proteases. However, people with malnutrition may have a deficiency in proteases; the toxin is not destroyed and can cause necrosis of the intestinal wall. It is traditionally associated with ritual pig-feasting by the natives of highland New Guinea, where it is known as 'pig-bel'. This syndrome has also been reported in countries such as Thailand, Nepal and China. *C. perfringens* also causes gas gangrene in wounds and soft tissue (see Chapter 16).

Other bacterial causes

Aeromonas spp. and *Plesiomonas* spp. are potential causes of diarrhoeal illness. They are most often associated with seafood or contaminated water.

VIRAL CAUSES OF ACUTE DIARRHOEA

Viruses are responsible for more cases of diarrhoeal illnesses in developed countries than any other organisms, and they particularly affect children under the age of five years. Rotaviruses are the most important in this age group, but enteric adenoviruses and caliciviruses (including Noroviruses) also cause disease in this and other age groups. Enteric viruses survive well in the environment and are somewhat resistant to sewage treatment processes and post-treatment chlorination.

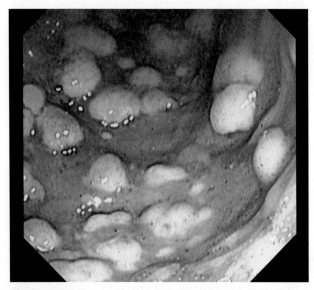

Figure 18.5

Pseudomembranous colitis
Photo taken through a colonoscope shows lesions in the wall of the colon.

Rotavirus

Rotaviruses (Figure 18.6), first identified in 1973 by the Melbourne scientists RUTH BISHOP and IAN HOLMES, are a

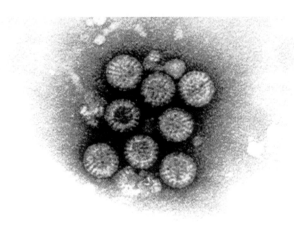

Figure 18.6

Rotavirus – wheel-shaped viruses that cause diarrhoea

major cause of gastroenteritis in infants. Rotavirus gastro-enteritis is a significant cause of death in young children in underdeveloped countries. In Australia, rotavirus is thought to be responsible for as many as 12 000 hospital admissions each year in the under five years age group.

Most infections occur in children under two years of age and are potentially life-threatening because of severe dehydration. Intravenous fluids may be urgently required. Older children and adults are less susceptible, presumably because of immunity developed early in life. Rotavirus infections in the day-care setting are common, generally attributed to faecal-oral transmission and contamination of fomites. Epidemics are sometimes seen in hospital nurseries.

Very large numbers of virus particles (>10^{12} particles per gram) are shed in faeces. Cross-infection readily occurs since the infective dose in a child is thought to be only 10–100 particles. The virus infects enterocytes at the villous tips in the small intestine, causing lysis of the cells and destruction of the villous tip epithelium, but there is no inflammation or loss of blood. Transport mechanisms in the intestine are disrupted and the loss of water and electrolytes results in a severe watery diarrhoea lasting 4–7 days.

Other viruses

Noroviruses (formerly known as Norwalk and Norwalk-like viruses) are important food-borne pathogens that can cause outbreaks of gastroenteritis. Infection is most common in older children and adults associated with contaminated food, or in institutions such as nursing homes or hospitals by person-to-person contact or in food. The foods most commonly implicated are poorly cooked or raw shellfish. For example, Sydney rock oysters have been implicated in a number of outbreaks of gastroenteritis, resulting in the introduction of compulsory purification of oysters in tanks of clean water. Contaminated drinking water and natural waters used for swimming have also been implicated. Norovirus is excreted in the faeces of infected people and shedding may continue in asymptomatic people for more than a year. The infectious dose is thought to be low, possibly less than 100 viruses.

Enteric adenoviruses (serotypes Ad40 and Ad41) cause

CASE HISTORY 18.3

Norovirus

On 26 February 1999 the Brisbane North Public Health Unit was notified of an outbreak of gastroenteritis in a nursing home. From the date the outbreak started (18 February) both staff and residents were affected. The home had a hostel section where the more ambulant residents lived and a nursing home section for those requiring more care.

Affected staff included domestic, administrative, catering and nursing personnel. An incubation period could be recognised for only one resident: he was absent from the nursing home when the outbreak started but developed symptoms within 48 hours of return. Most early cases occurred in the hostel section with subsequent spread to the nursing home. Analysis of food histories did not suggest any common food source and there were no reports of illness among food handlers just prior to the outbreak. Inspection of kitchen facilities did not reveal any major breaches of hygiene. Sixteen specimens were submitted and Norovirus genogroup 2 was detected by PCR from two specimens from two different cases.

The clinical and epidemiological features of the outbreak fit criteria for identifying Norovirus outbreaks, namely stool cultures negative for bacterial pathogens, mean or median duration of illness 12–60 hours, vomiting in ≥ 50% of cases and a mean or median incubation period of 24–48 hours.

Source: J Ward et al. 2000, 'Three nursing home outbreaks of Norwalk-like virus in Brisbane in 1999', *Communicable Diseases Intelligence* 24(8): 229.

gastroenteritis and are thought to be major causes of acute diarrhoea in paediatric patients. Adenoviruses appear to infect enterocytes, causing them to rupture, with the development of villous stunting.

Caliciviruses have been found to cause diarrhoea in children in day-care centres, typically affecting children aged three months to six years. Prolonged excretion of these viruses by symptomatic and asymptomatic individuals can make control extremely difficult.

Astroviruses mainly affect children under four years of age and are a common cause of diarrhoea in hospitalised children. The symptoms are similar to those of rotavirus, but less severe.

PROTOZOAL CAUSES OF ACUTE DIARRHOEA

The three main protozoal pathogens in diarrhoeal disease are *Giardia intestinalis*, *Entamoeba histolytica* and *Cryptosporidium parvum*. In most cases infection depends on contact with faecally contaminated material, infection flourishing where low standards of hygiene and sanitation, poverty and overcrowding exist.

Giardia intestinalis

The first intestinal parasite to be seen under a microscope was *Giardia intestinalis* (also called *G. lamblia* and *G. duodenalis*) when, in 1681, Anton van Leeuwenhoek peered through the simple microscope he had just made and saw the moving 'animalcules' in a preparation of his own faeces. *G. intestinalis* is a flagellated protozoan (Figure 18.7) now recognised to have a worldwide distribution.

In developing countries, infections are associated with overcrowding, poor sanitary conditions and poor water quality. In endemic areas, people often become reinfected within months of treatment. In developed countries, where prevalence rates range between 2% and 7%, faecal-oral transmission is most common and children are most likely to be infected. *Giardia* is readily spread in day-care centres, from child to child, and from children to other family members. In Australia, high rates of infection have been reported in some remote Aboriginal communities. A high prevalence of the parasite has also been found in domestic cats and dogs in Australia, but whether they act as a reservoir for human infection remains uncertain. Direct transmission of *Giardia* among homosexual men is increasingly being found.

Giardia has a simple life cycle with two forms: the flagellate trophozoite and the resistant cyst. The trophozoites live in the upper portion of the small intestine, attaching to the mucosa and rapidly multiplying there. Cyst formation occurs at regular intervals and they are passed out in stools. These resistant structures are the infective form and can survive for months in the environment when conditions are suitable. They are also somewhat resistant to chlorine, so can survive some water purification procedures.

Infection occurs when cysts are ingested, with as few as 10–25 being able to establish infection. Once in the small intestine they develop into the trophozoite form. Attachment of the parasite to the mucosa and resultant physical damage is thought to be part of the disease process, but the role of other factors such as toxins is unclear.

Many cases of giardiasis are asymptomatic but when illness occurs it is characterised by diarrhoea, nausea, a foul flatulence and fatigue. The incubation period is about 1–3 weeks. It is usually a self-limiting disease (resolving within a week) but may persist for months. Chronic infection is typically manifested as periodic episodes of these symptoms between periods without symptoms. In children in developing countries or from disadvantaged groups (e.g. Australian Aborigines), the major concern is the possibility of worsening malnutrition and retardation of growth and development.

Entamoeba histolytica

Entamoeba histolytica is an enteric protozoan with a worldwide distribution. It is thought to infect as much as 10% of the world's population. It is endemic in many areas, including Mexico, India and Africa, where as many as 50% of the high-risk population may be infected. Infection is transmitted by faecal contamination of food or drink by infected food-handlers or as a result of inadequate sanitation. Obviously, travellers to these areas are at high risk of infection.

Trophozoites of some low-virulence strains of *E. histolytica* live on the mucosal surface of the large intestine, frequently as harmless commensals. They replicate there, periodically forming resistant cysts that are excreted in faeces. These cysts can survive in the external environment and act as the infective stages. Most infected people are asymptomatic cyst passers or have only mild to moderate diarrhoeal symptoms. However, the trophozoites of some strains cause invasive disease, ulcerating the bowel wall and spreading via the bloodstream to remote sites, especially the liver, lung and brain.

Production of small, localised ulcers in the colon causes a mild diarrhoea, whereas the formation of deep, confluent ulcers leads to the classic inflammatory diarrhoea called **amoebic dysentery**.

Cryptosporidium parvum

Cryptosporidium parvum was first recognised as a cause of diarrhoea in humans in 1976. The advent of the AIDS epidemic focused attention on its capacity to produce disease and its widespread distribution. Prevalence rates of 1–3% of patients with diarrhoea is reported in developed countries, and 5–10% in Africa and Asia.

Cryptosporidiosis became nationally notifiable in Australia in 2001. In 2002, 3255 cases were reported, most occurring in children under the age of four. Transmission is possible by a variety of routes, including faecally contaminated food, water and hands, and from pets. A number of outbreaks in day-care centres have been reported, often with day-care workers and family contacts also being affected.

A massive outbreak, involving over 400 000 people, occurred in Milwaukee, USA, in 1993 due to contamination of the public water supply (see Spotlight box, page 121). The organism is also recognised as an important cause of traveller's diarrhoea and of outbreaks associated with swimming pools, especially when filters are not routinely checked.

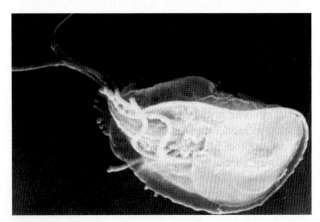

Figure 18.7

Giardia intestinalis
A flagellated protozoan that causes diarrhoea in humans.

Cryptosporidiosis

In November 1994 the supervisor of a child day-care centre in North Queensland advised the Tropical Public Health Unit in Cairns of an outbreak of diarrhoea in the centre. She was concerned that seven of the eight infants in the nursery (aged less than 15 months) had symptoms.

Faecal samples were collected from all eight infants in the nursery and *Cryptosporidium parvum* oocysts were identified in the faeces of all the symptomatic children. The asymptomatic child had been away from the centre during the previous two weeks. The children at the centre drank only boiled water. There was no paddling pool and no pets at the centre.

The diarrhoea persisted in all children for at least seven days, and for several weeks in some of them.

Comment

Cryptosporidium infection is commonly acquired via water-borne or zoonotic transmission, but in this outbreak these modes would seem to be unlikely.

Adapted from J Hanna & D Brookes, 'Cryptosporidiosis in a child day-care centre', *Communicable Diseases Intelligence* 19/1, 9 January 1995, p. 6.

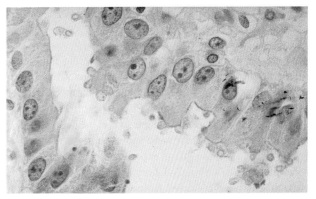

Figure 18.8

Cryptosporidium parvum
This section shows numerous *Cryptosporidium* at the luminal surface of epithelial cells.

Blastocystis hominis is a frequently identified protozoan in the gastrointestinal tract of humans, but the pathogenicity of this parasite remains uncertain. Some people with this organism and no other identifiable pathogen have mild diarrhoeal disease, but many are asymptomatic. No pathogenic mechanisms have been fully described.

FOOD INTOXICATIONS

These illnesses are characterised by the rapid onset of nausea, vomiting and abdominal pain, usually within 6–8 hours of ingestion of contaminated food. Fever and diarrhoea can occur but are less common. The major causes are the enterotoxins (see Chapter 10) of *Staphylococcus aureus*, and *Bacillus cereus* preformed in food. Thus, they are food intoxications, rather than infections. The fact that the toxins are preformed in the food is the reason why the incubation period is so short in comparison to infections. In these intoxications the organisms do not have to multiply in the intestine to produce disease; instead, the toxin must simply be absorbed.

Clostridium botulinum secretes a toxin that is absorbed in the intestine and enters the bloodstream, eventually reaching and acting on peripheral nerve synapses, causing a flaccid paralysis. Since the botulinum toxin blocks nerve transmission rather than causing gastrointestinal disease, botulism is discussed in Chapter 20.

Staphylococcus aureus intoxication

Foods rich in protein, salt and sugar (e.g. ham, creamy cakes, salads with mayonnaise), which have been inadequately refrigerated, favour the growth of staphylococci. If an enterotoxin-producing strain is involved, consumption of the food can result in gastrointestinal symptoms. Foods usually become contaminated by resident staphylococci in the nose or on the skin of food-handlers. Skin lesions colonised by staphylococci are a particularly dangerous source. Symptoms occur rapidly, typically 1–6 hours after consumption of the contaminated food.

There are more than six distinct enterotoxins produced by strains of *S. aureus*, with enterotoxin A the most commonly implicated. The exact mechanism of action of the enterotoxins has not been determined, but they cause

An important feature of *C. parvum* is its thick-walled oocyst, which is resistant to many disinfectants including hypochlorite (hence its association with swimming pool outbreaks). Another feature is its low infective dose (as low as 30 oocysts) and ease of transmission.

In the small intestine the organism invades the epithelial cells where it undergoes sexual reproduction, eventually forming oocysts that are excreted in faeces (see Figure 18.8). A watery diarrhoea occurs, on average seven days after ingestion of oocysts, and lasts one to three weeks. There may also be fever, abdominal pain, malaise and vomiting although many infections are asymptomatic. In young children the diarrhoea may persist for more than three weeks, and in immunodeficient hosts the disease may be severe and chronic, and sometimes fatal. Infected people can shed millions of oocysts in one gram of faeces.

Other intestinal protozoa

Isospora belli is another protozoan that, as a result of the AIDS epidemic, has been identified as an important cause of diarrhoeal disease. It is endemic in South America, Africa and South-East Asia and is probably transmitted by faecally contaminated food or water. Sporozoites invade the mucosa of the small intestine, destroying the microvilli. It can cause diarrhoea in travellers, but its highest prevalence is in immunocompromised people. Clinically, it is similar to cryptosporidial infection.

Protozoa of the genus *Cyclospora* have been confirmed as causes of diarrhoea in developing countries, and in travellers and people with AIDS. If untreated, symptoms can last for months.

Staphylococcal gastroenteritis

Six guests who had been to a noon wedding attended Casualty at the local hospital between 3 and 5 pm the same afternoon. All were complaining of diarrhoea, vomiting and abdominal cramps. Public health authorities were notified and the other 60 guests and the owner of the wedding reception venue were subsequently contacted.

Overall, 19 of the guests experienced gastrointestinal symptoms, all within 2–5 hours of the lunch. Faecal specimens were collected from each of the 10 people who ultimately attended the hospital. Enterotoxin-producing *Staphylococcus aureus* was cultured from four of these specimens.

An examination of the kitchen of the wedding reception house revealed a physically clean kitchen. None of the food served at the wedding remained for testing. The only food consumed by all the ill guests was cold chicken pieces, and it was assumed that this was the source of the staphylococcal food poisoning.

increased secretion of water and electrolytes in animal models and are thought to induce vomiting by stimulating enteric autonomic sensory neurons.

Bacillus cereus

Bacillus cereus is an aerobic, Gram-positive rod that is resistant to moderate cooking temperatures because of the production of heat-resistant spores. If the cooked food is allowed to cool for an extended period at room temperature, the spores germinate and the vegetative cells then produce a heat-stable enterotoxin in the food. Ingestion of preformed toxin in the food causes an acute onset of nausea, vomiting and abdominal pain without diarrhoea, within 1–6 hours. This emetic (vomiting-inducing) form of the disease is frequently associated with rice dishes, especially fried rice. The practice in restaurants of cooking a large amount of rice and allowing it to cool slowly over several hours, then flash frying it just before serving, is believed to be the major reason for the disease's association with this food in particular.

Less commonly, *B. cereus* causes another form of disease when vegetative cells, rather than toxin, are ingested and a different enterotoxin is formed in the intestine. This disease usually occurs 8–16 hours after ingestion of contaminated food, with diarrhoea and abdominal cramps the main symptoms. This form has been associated with a wide variety of foods.

LABORATORY DIAGNOSIS

Generally, it is not possible to distinguish between the different causes of diarrhoeal disease solely on clinical grounds. Information on the patient's recent food consumption and/or travel history is often helpful, but a precise diagnosis can only be achieved by laboratory investigations. For most patients with mild to moderate diarrhoea, the illness will be self-limiting and will require no evaluation other than a clinical one. However, for severe or persistent illness, or in the investigation of an outbreak, a definitive diagnosis is necessary. A number of laboratory tests can be used to provide such a diagnosis.

Microscopic examination of a stool specimen enables a differentiation to be made between inflammatory and non-inflammatory diarrhoeal disease. While this test indicates the pathological process occurring in the intestine and the likely causative agents, it does not identify the cause of infection.

Stool culture is the standard method for the diagnosis of most bacterial causes of diarrhoea. Fresh stool specimens (at least 5 g or 5 mL) should be sent immediately to the laboratory in a sterile, wide-mouth container with a firmly fitting screw lid. If transport is delayed, refrigeration is recommended. Special media are required for cultivation of some bacteria, such as vibrios and *Y. enterocolitica*, so the request form accompanying the specimen should provide adequate information about the patient's history and food consumption and an indication that such organisms are suspected. Testing for the Shiga toxin in a faecal sample should be performed when enterohaemorrhagic *E. coli* or haemolytic uraemic syndrome is suspected.

For suspected *C. difficile* infections, anaerobic culture on special selective media and the detection of toxin B in stool filtrate are the standard diagnostic procedures. In staphylococcal or *Bacillus* food intoxications, the organisms are often not present in faeces and are not able to be cultured, but culture of vomitus may be more productive. In all cases of bacterial food-borne illness, culture of the suspect food may be attempted, particularly in the investigation of an outbreak.

Culture of enteric viruses is not routine in diagnostic clinical laboratories. Laboratory confirmation of viral gastroenteritis has generally been based on the demonstration of viral particles or antigens in stools by serologic or electron microscopic means. However, these tests are not always available in routine laboratories and are not highly sensitive. Improved diagnostic methods, such as enzyme immunoassays for faecal antigens and reverse transcriptase-polymerase chain reaction (RT-PCR), have been developed for some viruses (e.g. Norovirus).

Diagnosis of protozoal infections usually involves the microscopic identification of cysts or trophozoites in stool specimens. Collection of three stool specimens on alternate days is recommended to improve the likelihood of organism detection. Highly sensitive and reliable ELISA and fluorescein-labelled antibody tests have recently been developed for detecting antigens or oocysts of some protozoa (e.g. *Giardia*, *Cryptosporidium*) in stools. A highly sensitive and specific stool antigen test for *E. histolytica* has recently been developed.

MANAGEMENT OF PATIENTS WITH DIARRHOEAL DISEASE

The major problem of infectious diarrhoea, irrespective of the cause, is loss of fluid and dehydration. Therefore, for any patient with acute diarrhoea, fluid and electrolyte replacement is essential and can be lifesaving in severe cases. In mild disease, oral intake of fluids is usually adequate but in cases of moderate to severe fluid loss, especially in young infants, intravenous hydration with isotonic fluids containing dextrose may be necessary.

Most patients with acute diarrhoea do not require specific antimicrobial therapy. In fact, antibiotic therapy should be avoided if possible, because in some cases it may prolong the carriage and excretion of an organism (e.g. *Salmonella*) by the patient, increasing the risk of transmission to others. Antibiotics may even increase the risk of severe complications (e.g. haemolytic uraemic syndrome) in people infected with enterohaemorrhagic *E. coli*. Also, the risk of increasing microbial resistance to antibiotics is not warranted in self-limiting diseases. There is no effective antimicrobial treatment for viral causes, and antibiotics are not warranted in food intoxications because disease is caused by preformed toxins, not multiplication of the bacterium in the intestine.

There are some situations, however, where antibiotic therapy is justified; for example:

- to reduce faecal excretion, environmental contamination and spread of infection (e.g. in *Shigella* infections)
- to resolve persistent infections (e.g. giardiasis)
- to resolve serious and life-threatening infections (e.g. amoebiasis and antibiotic-associated colitis)
- to hasten recovery in special groups (e.g. travellers).

In the case of *Shigella* infections, an antimicrobial agent such as ampicillin or cotrimoxazole may be administered to shorten the duration of symptoms and prevent the spread of infection. Because variable drug resistance in *Shigella* exists in different parts of the world, sensitivity testing should be done.

Antibiotic-associated colitis caused by *C. difficile* may be resolved by discontinuation of the antibiotic, but severe cases may require treatment with vancomycin or metronidazole. Relapse of disease often occurs with the termination of treatment, requiring a second course of the drug. Enteropathogenic *E. coli* can cause severe and protracted diarrhoea, especially in hospital nursery and paediatric ward outbreaks. When the organism is hospital-acquired, it may be highly resistant to antibiotics, making antibiotic sensitivity testing of the isolate necessary.

Although cholera is potentially fatal, most cases can be adequately treated with oral rehydration and electrolyte replacement. In severe cases, or to prevent transmission, doxycycline or amoxycillin are generally used.

Treatment of protozoal infections is often with metronidazole, because of its broad activity. For confirmed *G. intestinalis* infection, tinidazole or metronidazole is often used. Treatment of symptomatic *E. histolytica* infections is with metronidazole plus diloxanide furoate (an amoebicide). In cases of disseminated infection that do not respond to therapy, surgical drainage is usually required.

Cryptosporidial infections are generally self-limiting in immunocompetent people and do not require antimicro-bial treatment. Treatment of *Cyclospora* infections is with cotrimoxazole.

During a diarrhoeal illness, the patient's diet should also be modified. The intestinal tract has difficulty processing complex materials and starch foods are recommended. A number of non-specific drugs may be used to reduce the symptoms. Mostly, these are adsorbents (e.g. kaolin) to reduce the liquidity of stools, or anti-motility drugs (e.g. loperamide) to inhibit intestinal motility and enhance fluid absorption, thereby reducing the number of stools passed.

PREVENTION

Prevention of diarrhoeal disease essentially involves avoidance of the organisms. In the case of food-borne illness and traveller's diarrhoea, this means proper food processing, proper cooking of foods, the non-consumption of high-risk foods (especially raw) and beverages, and the sterilisation of drinking water where appropriate. In day-care centres, strict handwashing practice, good general hygiene, sanitary food preparation, use of disposable gloves when contact with faecal matter is possible, and exclusion of symptomatic children are important measures (see Chapter 14).

In hospitals and other institutions, people with severe diarrhoea are a potential source of infection for other patients. Standard precautions and strict handwashing after contact with these patients is essential. While the use of disposable gloves is strongly recommended, this *does not* obviate the need for strict handwashing practices.

Other gastrointestinal diseases

HELICOBACTER PYLORI INFECTION

The initial suggestions made in the early 1980s by BARRY MARSHALL and ROBIN WARREN in Western Australia that the spiral-shaped bacterium, *Helicobacter pylori* (Figure 18.9), might be responsible for duodenal ulcer were treated with great scepticism. However, much evidence has since accumulated and *H. pylori* is now recognised as a major cause of gastritis (inflammation of the stomach mucosa) and a major factor in the development of most cases of peptic (duodenal and gastric) ulcers (see Figure 18.10). It has also been established as a major contributing factor in gastric cancer and in a type of gastric lymphoma.

In developed countries, more than 25–50% of the population (especially those over 40 years) may be infected with *H. pylori*, but many cases are asymptomatic. The prevalence of infection is higher in lower socioeconomic groups and especially high in developing countries (up to 70–90%). How the organism is acquired is not clear, but it is probably by person-to-person contact. Iatrogenic transmission via contaminated endoscopes has been reported.

How *H. pylori* establishes in the hostile environment of the gastric mucosa and causes gastritis is not clearly known. Studies have indicated that motility and adhesins

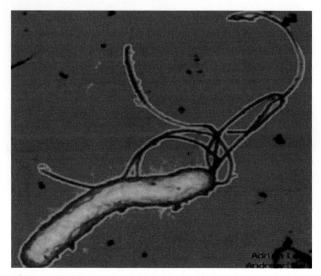

Figure 18.9
Electron micrograph of *Helicobacter pylori*

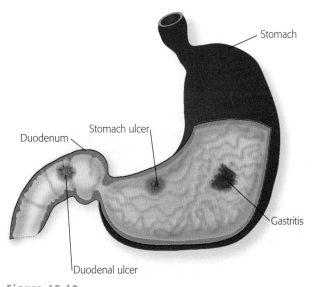

Figure 18.10
***Helicobacter pylori* diseases of the gastrointestinal tract**

are probably important in the organism's ability to colonise the gastric epithelium. The organism produces large amounts of the enzyme urease, which is important in its pathogenesis. By breaking down urea in the stomach this enzyme generates a 'cloud' of ammonia there; this neutralises the acid and thus protects the organism from the gastric acidity.

There are differences in pathogenicity between different strains of *H. pylori* such that some are able to cause gastric disease where others are not. Host factors, particularly the inflammatory response, are also involved in the production of disease. Only in some people is the inflammation induced by the bacterium severe enough to produce symptoms. Severe and prolonged inflammation of the gastric mucosa appear to be major requirements for ulceration and carcinogenesis. *H. pylori* appears to play an important role in the initiation of gastric cancer but other factors, such as diet, also seem to be involved.

The diagnosis of *H. pylori* infection is usually confirmed in one of two ways: by a urea breath test or by endoscopic biopsy. The non-invasive urea breath test has high sensitivity and involves the detection of radio-labelled carbon dioxide in the breath of an infected person after they have ingested an isotopically labelled solution of urea. Triple therapy with clarithromycin, amoxycillin and omeprazole (reduces gastric acidity) is effective in about 90% of cases. Drug resistance in *H. pylori* is an increasing problem, especially to clarithromycin. Treatment is not recommended for asymptomatic *H. pylori* infection. Considerable work is being undertaken to develop a vaccine.

ENTERIC FEVERS: TYPHOID AND PARATYPHOID

Causative agents and transmission

Salmonella typhi and *S. paratyphi*, types A, B and C, all cause enteric fevers (typhoid and paratyphoid fever) although *S. typhi* is responsible for the vast majority of infections. These species are restricted to humans and are usually spread via faecally contaminated food or water. Infections are most common in developing countries (especially Africa and South-East Asia) with poor standards of water supply and sewage disposal. Typhoid is particularly common in Indonesia and Papua New Guinea.

The World Health Organization estimates there are about 16 million infections worldwide each year, resulting in approximately 600 000 deaths. In Australia, fewer than 100 new cases of enteric fever are reported each year and most of these have been acquired overseas.

Pathogenesis

After ingestion, many of the salmonellae are killed by the acidity of the stomach but, if the infecting dose is high enough, some bacteria enter the small intestine. There they penetrate the intestinal mucosa, where they are ingested by macrophages. A major feature of these organisms is their ability to survive and actively multiply inside macrophages. They are transported by these cells to the mesenteric lymph nodes and eventually they reach the thoracic duct and then the bloodstream. Once in the blood they can seed many organs, especially the spleen, bones and liver. After further multiplication there is reinvasion of the blood, which marks the end of the incubation period and the beginning of clinical illness.

This second phase of bacteraemia leads to invasion of other organs, such as the kidney and gall bladder. The organism grows actively in the bile and enters the intestine for a second time. Most of the symptoms caused by *S. typhi* can be attributed to the inflammation induced by its lipopolysaccharide.

Clinical features

After an incubation period of 10–14 days, the early symptoms of fever, headache and respiratory symptoms (typically a dry cough) appear. Mild abdominal discomfort with either diarrhoea or constipation occurs. Without treatment, the fever increases in a stepwise fashion and the patient may eventually lapse into a stupor. Other common symptoms are rose spots (pink macular spots that blanch on pressure), bradycardia and splenomegaly. Without treatment, an uncomplicated infection lasts 4–6 weeks.

A serious complication is secondary invasion of the intestine from the gall bladder. In a small proportion of patients this can lead to inflammation and then perforation or haemorrhage of the intestine. Death occurs in approximately 15% of untreated cases.

Many patients continue to excrete *S. typhi* in the faeces for several weeks after recovery. In up to 3% of infected people, the organism persists in the gall bladder and kidneys, and bacteria can be shed, asymptomatically, in faeces and urine for years and sometimes permanently. Such chronic carriers are a major public health problem. In countries with inadequate sewage disposal it may mean continued contamination of water supplies.

In developed countries, chronic carriers can become a major hazard if they are employed in food handling. Mary Mallon ('Typhoid Mary'), a cook in New York City in the early 1900s, is the classic example. As a carrier, she caused many outbreaks of the disease and was ultimately imprisoned for life for refusing to stop working as a cook.

Laboratory diagnosis

The diagnosis of enteric fever relies on the isolation of *S. typhi* or *S. paratyphi* from the patient. Blood cultures are the standard method and generally become positive at the onset of symptoms and remain positive over the next two weeks (see Figure 18.11). Faeces and urine are also sometimes cultured, especially 2–4 weeks after onset of symptoms, when seeding of the kidneys and secondary infection of the intestine occurs. Asymptomatic chronic carriers are diagnosed by positive cultures from faeces and urine. Serum antibodies to the organisms can be detected by an agglutination test (the Widal test), but results can be unreliable and difficult to interpret. Enzyme linked immunoassays (ELISA) and polymerase chain reaction (PCR) tests have recently been developed for diagnosis of enteric fever.

Treatment and prevention

Fluoroquinolones (e.g. ciprofloxacin) are generally the most effective drugs for treatment of typhoid fever. They are more rapidly effective and result in lower carriage rates than traditional drugs used for treatment (chloramphenicol and cotrimoxazole). For chronic carriers, long-term therapy with ampicillin or ciprofloxacin may be effective but, if not, cholecystectomy (removal of the gall bladder – the site of carriage) may be warranted if the person is a risk to the community.

In developing countries, prevention of infection depends on good personal hygiene, adequate sewage disposal and a clean water supply. In the developed world, outbreaks of enteric fever are rare. Typhoid carriers are a particular concern and should be treated or excluded from employment that involves food handling. Vaccines against *S. typhi* are available, and are recommended for travellers to developing countries where typhoid is endemic, for close contacts of known carriers and for laboratory workers in high-risk situations.

LISTERIOSIS

Listeriosis is a food-borne disease caused by the bacterium *Listeria monocytogenes*. As the disease usually presents as a meningitis, it is discussed in Chapter 20.

Helminth infections of the gastrointestinal tract

The types and characteristics of helminths (worms) are described in Chapter 6. Briefly, there are three main groups:

- nematodes (roundworms)
- cestodes (tapeworms)
- trematodes (flukes).

The nematodes are further divided into roundworms, hookworms and threadworms (pinworms).

Parasitic helminths continue to be a major cause of morbidity in humans, particularly in the tropics and subtropics, and where there is poor sanitation. It has been estimated that more than half of the world's population could be infected with an intestinal helminth.

In Australia, helminth infections occur mostly in the northern (tropical) parts of the country and are predominantly due to nematodes. Intestinal nematodes are found particularly in northern Aboriginal communities with poor sanitation and inadequate medical facilities. Fortunately, some of the more serious helminth infections, such as schistosomiasis, river blindness and filariasis (elephantiasis), which are endemic in other parts of the world, do not occur in Australia. The common helminth infections in Australia are listed in Table 6.3 on page 124; all are nematodes except the beef tapeworm (*Taenia saginata*), the

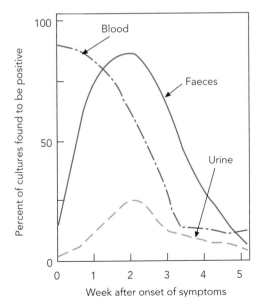

Figure 18.11

The isolation of typhoid bacteria from different specimens over the course of the disease

cause of hydatid cysts (*Echinococcus granulosus*), and the tapeworm, *Hymenolepis nana*.

The real incidence of helminth infections in Australia is difficult to determine. The most common is undoubtedly the pinworm (or threadworm) *Enterobius vermicularis*, which is found throughout the country. The least common is probably hydatid disease, of which there are 30–40 reports each year.

The helminths listed in Table 6.3 are acquired in two distinct ways. *Ancylostoma duodenale* and *Necator americanus* (the hookworms) and *Strongyloides stercoralis* infect humans by penetration of the skin by infective larvae, whereas all the others are acquired by ingestion of the infective eggs of the helminths. All specifically inhabit the bowel except for *E. granulosus* (liver and lungs) and *S. stercoralis*, which can spread from the bowel to cause disseminated infection.

In nematode infections, the severity of disease is largely a function of the number of worms in the body. Increasing the worm load generally requires repeated exposure to the infectious larvae or eggs, since all except *Strongyloides* do not multiply in the host. Thus, travellers and immigrants from non-endemic areas are likely to have mild, if any, symptoms, whereas residents of endemic areas are more likely to be reinfected frequently and to suffer a more severe disease.

ENTEROBIUS VERMICULARIS

In contrast to other nematodes, *Enterobius vermicularis* is prevalent in temperate as well as tropical regions. Tens of thousands of Australians are believed to harbour this worm, but it does not cause serious illness. Adult pinworms (approximately 1 cm in length) pass out of the anus at night, depositing eggs in the perianal area. Many people are asymptomatic but, when symptoms do occur, anal pruritis (itching), especially at night, is the classic sign. Transmission usually occurs directly from fingers contaminated by scratching, but the eggs are also light enough to be carried in dust. After hatching, the worms mature entirely in the intestine. Infestation usually lasts a maximum of six weeks.

The eggs of *Enterobius* are rarely present in faeces but can be identified by applying adhesive tape to the perianal skin when the patient wakes, followed by microscopic examination of the tape. Infections are effectively treated with mebendazole or pyrantel.

ASCARIS LUMBRICOIDES

Adult worms are 15–35 cm long, hence the common name of giant roundworm (Figure 18.12). The females lay an enormous number of eggs into the intestine (about 200 000 in a day) and these are passed in faeces. The eggs can remain infective in soil for many weeks or months, depending on the conditions. The infection is usually transmitted by the faecal-oral passage of eggs via contaminated hands.

After ingestion, the eggs hatch in the intestine, releasing the larvae. The larvae penetrate the gut wall and are

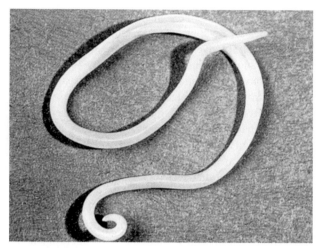

Figure 18.12

***Ascaris lumbricoides*, the giant roundworm**
Female worms can lay as many as 200 000 eggs in a day in the gut of an infected person.

carried via the blood through the liver to the lungs. From there they work their way up the bronchi and trachea and are swallowed, and once again enter the intestine. The adult worms live freely in the gut lumen, feeding on intestinal contents. Most people with a small worm load are asymptomatic or experience only mild abdominal discomfort. Most only become aware of their infection when they pass a worm in their stools.

In some cases, the migration of the larvae through the lungs can cause severe respiratory distress (pneumonitis). With large worm loads, especially in children, intestinal obstruction may occur. Even a single worm can cause harm if it migrates into the hepatobiliary tree and occludes the ducts, causing acute biliary colic, cholangitis and cholecystitis.

Diagnosis is based on the microscopic examination of faeces. The eggs of *Ascaris* and many other helminths are characteristic and readily recognised in a fresh stool specimen. Ideally, the specimen should be transported to the laboratory so that it can be examined within 30 minutes of collection, or else preserved with a fixative to maintain the egg structures. Three or more specimens may have to be collected in some cases, because of low numbers or intermittent shedding. A variety of antihelminthic drugs are available for treatment of intestinal nematodes (e.g. mebendazole, pyrantel).

HOOKWORMS

The hookworms *Ancylostoma duodenale* and *Necator americanus* are serious causes of long-term morbidity in developing countries, because of the anaemia and hypoproteinaemia that result from heavy infection. *A. duodenale* is very common in some Aboriginal communities and probably contributes to the iron deficiency and anaemia seen in many of these people. Adult hookworms (approximately 1 cm in length) attach to the intestinal mucosa by specialised mouth structures (Figure 18.13). They rupture capillaries and suck blood, and lay thin-

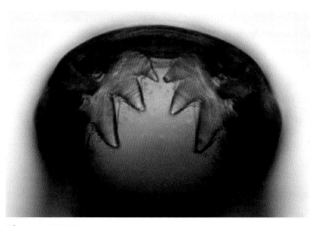

Figure 18.13

Ancylostoma spp.
This worm attaches to the intestinal mucosa by specialised mouth structures.

coated eggs that are passed in faeces into the environment. The eggs mature and hatch in soil, and infection of a new host takes place when larvae come into contact with the unprotected skin of a person (sometimes swallowed in the case of _Ancylostoma_). They penetrate the skin, migrate via the bloodstream to the lungs, climb the trachea and are swallowed with secretions, maturing into adult worms in the small intestine six weeks after initial infection.

Most people with light worm loads are asymptomatic. Heavy infections may cause abdominal pain, flatulence, a bloody diarrhoea and iron deficiency anaemia in children or in anyone with existing malnutrition. One of the main concerns of heavy infection is chronic blood loss. Untreated, severe infection in children can result in physical and mental retardation. Hookworm infections are diagnosed by microscopic visualisation of eggs in stool specimens. Treatment is with antihelminthic drugs such as albendazole, mebendazole or pyrantel.

STRONGYLOIDES STERCORALIS

The tiny adult worms (2–3 mm in length) dwell just beneath the intestinal mucosa, where they lay their eggs. These eggs hatch in the intestine and are passed in the faeces. _Strongyloides_ infection occurs when larvae in faecally contaminated soil or fomites penetrate the skin or mucous membranes. They then enter the bloodstream and break into the alveoli in the lungs. Like the hookworms, they ascend the bronchi and trachea, are swallowed and reach the small intestine where maturation is completed.

This worm, however, is unlike any other intestinal nematode in its ability to multiply in the host. In some cases, the internally generated larvae can then penetrate the intestinal mucosa or the perianal skin and migrate via the lungs back to the small intestine, in what is essentially an 'auto-infection cycle'. This cycle is most likely to occur in the immunocompromised, or in patients with malnutrition or other debilitating disease. Infection may persist for decades.

In uncontrolled infections larvae may infect other organs, including the urinary tract, liver and brain.

People with low worm burdens are often asymptomatic. With greater numbers of worms, there may be non-specific gastrointestinal symptoms of abdominal pain, intermittent diarrhoea and nausea. Heavy intestinal infection causes a persistent and profuse diarrhoea, with dehydration and electrolyte imbalance. Invasion of other body sites by large numbers of auto-infective larvae can be fatal. Asymptomatic immigrants from endemic areas such as South-East Asia, especially those with unexplained eosinophilia, are often found to be infected with _Strongyloides_. It is also found in some Aboriginal communities, and was common in Australian soldiers held in Asian prisoner of war camps.

Strongyloides infection is difficult to diagnose, but it can be done by finding larvae in fresh stools. Many stool specimens may have to be examined before larvae are found. Serological tests for _Strongyloides_ are available, but do not distinguish between past and current infection. Infections are usually treated with ivermectin or thiabendazole but eradication of the worm is not always achieved, especially in the immunosuppressed. Repeated, short courses of treatment may be necessary to keep the worm load at a low level.

HYDATID DISEASE

Hydatid disease is caused by the tapeworm _Echinococcus granulosus_. The parasite's definitive host is the dog but it can be transmitted to other animals, particularly sheep. Other dogs then become infected when fed on the viscera of infected sheep. Humans act as accidental hosts when the eggs of the parasite are ingested, usually as a result of contact with the fur or tongue of an infected dog. Young children of sheep-farming families are at greatest risk. Recent evidence indicates that the parasite is also found in certain wildlife species, such as dingoes, wallabies, kangaroos and foxes; these animals could therefore be additional sources of infection. Currently, in Australia, there are about 50 notifications of hydatid infection each year, with an average of three deaths per year.

After ingestion of eggs, the larvae emerge and migrate through the gut and into the bloodstream, and eventually localise in organs such as the liver, lungs and brain. In these organs they form fluid-filled sacs, called cysts (see Figure 18.14) which contain thousands of developing worms and can reach the size of a grapefruit. Residence within these sacs enables the worms to evade host defence mechanisms (see Chapter 10).

Symptoms result from the local pressure of the cyst on the organ. Bursting of the cyst can lead to seeding of other organs with the worms and, in some people, a life-threatening anaphylactic reaction to hydatid antigens.

Diagnosis of hydatid cysts is by radiologic demonstration of a cystic lesion, supported by positive serology. Treatment may be achieved with prolonged, high-dose albendazole, but surgical removal of the cysts is often necessary.

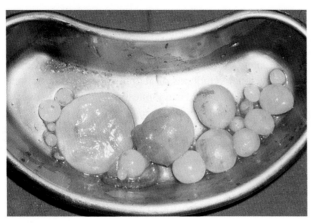

Figure 18.14

Hydatid cysts

Hydatid cysts are thin, fluid-filled sacs produced by the tape-worm *Echinococcus granulosus*. The worms hide from the body's defences by residing inside cysts.

TAENIA SAGINATA

The beef tapeworm attaches by its head to the intestinal mucosa. Most patients are asymptomatic or experience only mild abdominal discomfort. The most obvious sign of infection is the passing of white, motile proglottids, or long segments of a worm. Infections are diagnosed in a similar way to *Ascaris* infections. Treatment is usually with praziquantel.

TRICHURIS TRICHIURA

Adult worms are 3–4 cm in length. The worms remain within the large bowel, attaching to the epithelial layer. As with all intestinal worms, children are the members of the community most heavily infected with this parasite, acquiring eggs from contaminated soil or vegetation. Most infections are asymptomatic, but moderate to heavy worm loads, especially in children, can cause abdominal pain and diarrhoea, occasionally leading to prolapse of the rectum. Impaired nutrition and retarded growth of children may result. Infections are diagnosed and treated in a similar way to *Ascaris* infections.

HYMENOLEPIS NANA

Hymenolepis nana is a tapeworm (2–4 cm long) that causes an asymptomatic infection in most patients. In heavy infections it can cause diarrhoea, abdominal pain and loss of appetite. There are thought to be many millions of people worldwide infected with this parasite. Infections are diagnosed and treated in a similar way to *Ascaris* infections.

Hepatitis

The term **hepatitis** refers to injury and inflammation of the liver. Viruses are major causes of hepatitis but other microorganisms, alcohol, drugs and various other disorders (e.g. biliary obstruction) may also be responsible (see

Table 18.5). A number of important viruses, including cytomegalovirus, Epstein-Barr virus (infectious mononucleosis) and rubella virus, can infect the liver and cause hepatitis as part of a systemic infection. These are dealt with in Chapter 19. Here we focus on the viruses that infect mainly the liver. These are the hepatitis viruses A, B, C, D and E. Each of these belongs to a different virus family and they have little in common except the target organ they affect. The characteristics of the different hepatitis viruses are outlined in Table 18.6.

Viral hepatitis is a major cause of morbidity and mortality throughout the world. Hepatitis A virus (HAV) and hepatitis E virus (HEV) are spread mainly by faecal-oral means; the other three – hepatitis B virus (HBV), hepatitis C virus (HCV) and hepatitis D virus (HDV) – are spread principally by exposure to blood, although transmission via other body fluids, especially genital secretions for HBV, also occurs.

Hepatitis viruses produce acute inflammation of the liver. This may result in a clinical illness with variable features (see Table 18.7), including gastrointestinal symptoms such as anorexia, nausea and vomiting, fever, malaise and jaundice (yellowing of the skin and whites of the eyes). See Figure 18.15. In more serious cases, liver function can fail. Marked increases in serum concentrations of the liver enzymes, alanine aminotransferase (ALT) and aspartate aminotransferase (AST), are characteristic of acute viral hepatitis. Generally, the different types of hepatitis cannot be distinguished by their signs and symptoms. The patient's history and risk factors may indicate the likely type(s), but specific laboratory tests are required for a definitive diagnosis.

At present there is no completely effective treatment for

Table 18.5

Causes of hepatitis

Viruses
Hepatitis viruses A, B, C, D, E
Cytomegalovirus
Epstein-Barr virus (infectious mononucleosis)
Herpes simplex virus
Rubella virus
Yellow fever virus

Other infections
Syphilis
Tuberculosis
Toxoplasmosis
Q fever
Amoebiasis

Non-infectious causes
Biliary obstruction
Primary biliary cirrhosis
Drug toxicity
Drug hypersensitivity
Alcohol abuse

Table 18.6

Characteristics of hepatitis viruses

	HEPATITIS A	HEPATITIS B	HEPATITIS C	HEPATITIS D	HEPATITIS E
Family	Picornaviridae	Hepadnaviridae	Flaviviridae	(unclassified)	Caliciviridae
Genome	ssRNA	dsDNA	ssRNA	ssRNA	ssRNA
Mode of transmission	Faecal-oral	Blood; sexual; mother to child	Blood; sexual; mother to child	Blood; sexual	Faecal-oral
Incubation period	2–6 weeks	1–6 months	2–26 weeks	2–9 weeks	2–9 weeks
Acute mortality rate	0.2%	0.2%	0.2%	2–20%	0.2%
Infectious period	2 weeks before onset to 1 week after symptoms subside	Many weeks before onset to life in carriers	1 or more weeks before onset to life in carriers	Not known, but maximal just before onset	Not known
Chronicity	None	5–10%	50–70%	2–20%	None
Vaccine	Yes	Yes	No	No	No

Table 18.7

Common clinical features of viral hepatitis

- Jaundice
- Anorexia, nausea, vomiting
- Diarrhoea or constipation
- Abdominal pain
- Fever, malaise
- Myalgia, arthralgia
- Fatigue, weakness
- Anaemia
- Increased serum alanine aminotransferase (ALT)
- Increased serum aspartate aminotransferase (AST)

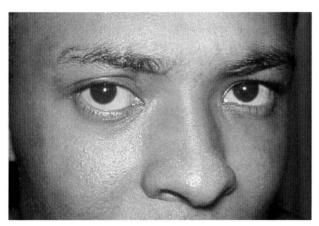

Figure 18.15

Jaundice caused by hepatitis A infection

acute viral hepatitis, although α-interferon plus other drugs have been used with limited success in chronic hepatitis B and C. Vaccines are currently available only for hepatitis A and B.

HEPATITIS A

HAV is a small RNA virus, belonging to the family of picornaviruses. The virus was first isolated in cell culture in 1979 and is still the only hepatitis virus that has been propagated *in vitro*. In Australia there are 2000–3000 notifications of hepatitis A annually. However, it is thought that a large number of asymptomatic (not notified) infections occur in northern parts of the country.

Transmission

Transmission of HAV is primarily by the faecal-oral route because it is excreted in large amounts in faeces. Peak infectivity from an infected person is in the two weeks before the onset of illness and for at least a week later. This is when the concentration of virus in faeces is highest. Transmission by other means, such as intravenous drug use and sexual contact (especially in homosexual men), is also possible. It is spread mainly from person to person by contact (hands) or by contamination of food or water. Once transferred to fomites from unwashed hands, the virus can persist on surfaces for several days.

Contamination of food or water can lead to sudden, explosive epidemics of hepatitis A. Poor personal hygiene, poor sanitation and close personal contact (e.g. household or sexual contact) facilitate transmission of the virus. Hepatitis A is endemic in many tropical and subtropical regions of the world and in most rural Aboriginal communities in Australia, with most infections occurring in young children. Because its spread is due primarily to poor hygiene, it was formerly referred to as 'infectious hepatitis'. It may also be transmitted via shellfish from polluted waters, especially if eaten raw.

HAV infection often occurs in institutional settings and has been reported in health-care workers caring for infected patients. In Australia there have been several

CASE HISTORY 18.6

Hepatitis A

On the 11 December 2003 the Central Sydney Public Health Unit (CSPHU) was notified of a case of hepatitis A in a man. The CSPHU interviewed the man, who reported working as a chef in a restaurant in a large community club in Central Sydney. His duties comprised food handling and preparation for one of the club's busy restaurants. He mentioned experiencing symptoms of a gastroenteritis-like illness while at work. Although he reported to regularly washing his hands between preparation tasks, he did not wear gloves and had not received specific training in food handling. The period he was infectious while working was from 22 November to 9 December 2003.

The club estimated that 1,000 patrons may have dined at the restaurant in the period that the case was infectious. Patrons were alerted to the risk of possible hepatitis A transmission through contaminated food served at the restaurant by a media release, an 1800 hotline, and through club staff calling restaurant patrons for whom there were booking details on record. A clinic was set up to provide advice and offer Normal Human Immunoglobulin (NIGH) to patrons who ate at the restaurant during the period that the case was infectious. At the clinic, a patron's eligibility for NIGH was assessed, based on the date they dined at the restaurant, previous history of hepatitis A infection, and immunisation. Patrons without a completed immunisation history or prior infection with hepatitis A, who were within 14 days of exposure, were offered NIGH.

Over five days, the clinic screened an estimated 1,166 people, 398 of whom did not qualify for the NIGH and 768 of whom were provided with NIGH.

By 31 January, four possible secondary cases emerged. Only one of these people had received NIGH; however, the exposure of that person was outside the two-week period for the administration of NIGH to be effective.

Adapted from: NSW Public Health Bulletin 2004, 15(3), p. 44.

reports of hepatitis in nursing staff, particularly in paediatric wards in hospitals in northern and central parts of the country, where there is a high incidence of infection among Aboriginal children. Failure to wear gloves when contact with faeces occurred, or omitting to wash hands thoroughly before eating, have been suggested as the major faults in these cases. Lack of good sanitation and hygiene can lead to outbreaks in schools, camps and day-care centres.

Outbreaks of hepatitis A among injecting drug users have been reported. These outbreaks are thought to be due to faecal contamination of drugs or injecting materials, or poor hygiene and close contact among abusers, rather than to blood-borne transmission. In recent years, there has been an increased incidence of hepatitis A among male homosexuals, possibly related to oral-anal sexual practices.

Pathogenesis and clinical features

After infection, the virus is believed to replicate initially in intestinal cells. This is followed by a brief period of viraemia (viruses in the blood) and then spreads to the liver. The incubation period ranges from 2 to 6 weeks, with an average of about 25 days. During this lengthy incubation period liver cells are damaged, possibly by immune mechanisms rather than direct viral action.

Hepatitis A varies considerably in its presentation. The illness is usually not apparent in children less than four years old, but it becomes progressively more severe with increasing age. When symptomatic, it is generally a mild to moderate disease with typical manifestations of fever, anorexia, nausea, vomiting, fatigue, liver pain and sometimes jaundice, due to impaired liver function. Complete recovery occurs in most cases in 4–6 weeks; there is no carrier state and chronic infection does not generally occur. However, shedding of the virus may continue for up to six months in asymptomatic neonates. Rarely, HAV causes a fulminant hepatitis with a high mortality rate.

Laboratory diagnosis

Since the clinical presentation of any type of hepatitis is not definitive, laboratory tests are required for the diagnosis. HAV is not routinely cultured and the other hepatitis viruses have not yet been cultured, so diagnosis of hepatitis in general is based on serological tests. The serologic tests for hepatitis virus infections are summarised in Table 18.8.

The standard method for diagnosing hepatitis A is by detection of anti-hepatitis A antibodies in the patient's serum. Anti-HAV IgM is usually detectable 25–30 days after infection and indicates current or recent infection. The anti-HAV test measures total antibody against HAV and includes IgM and IgG. IgG is present in the patient's serum for years after recovery and so a single anti-HAV titre does not differentiate between current and past infection. Therefore, with this test, a rise in titre in paired serum samples must be demonstrated to diagnose infection. Serum concentrations of liver enzymes are usually markedly increased during infection.

Treatment and prevention

As for many viral infections there is no specific cure for hepatitis A. Symptomatic treatment is all that is available. Prevention relies on good hygiene and the prophylactic use of gammaglobulin after suspected exposure. Normal human immunoglobulin (NIGH) is a pooled serum preparation from normal blood donors that contains antibodies to hepatitis A virus and other common diseases. NIGH must be given within 14 days of exposure to be effective. It is also recommended for close contacts of cases used to contain outbreaks of hepatitis A. Effective inactivated HAV vaccines have been developed and

Table 18.8
Serologic tests for the diagnosis of hepatitis

	HEPATITIS A	HEPATITIS B	HEPATITIS C	HEPATITIS D	HEPATITIS E
Antigens detected	HAAg	HBsAg, HBeAg	None available	None available	None available
Antibodies detected	Anti-HAV Anti-HAV IgM	Anti-HBs Anti-HBc Anti-HBc IgM Anti-Hbe	Anti-HCV	Anti-HDV Anti-HDV IgM	None available

licensed for use in Australia. Vaccination is recommended for high-risk groups including:

- travellers to endemic areas
- certain Aboriginal communities (especially in northern Queensland) and visitors to those areas
- workers in rural and remote indigenous communities
- nursing and medical staff in paediatric units, high-dependency units and emergency departments
- child day-care and preschool staff
- the intellectually disabled and their carers
- homosexual men
- injecting drug users
- people with chronic liver disease.

School-based outbreaks are often attributed to inadequate toilet facilities. Improvement of facilities and thorough handwashing are the most important interventions for preventing infections in schools.

HEPATITIS B

Hepatitis B is caused by a hepadna (hepatitis DNA) virus. The HBV has an outer coat containing an antigen called the *hepatitis B surface antigen* (HBsAg). This was formerly called the 'Australia antigen' because it was originally identified in the serum of an Australian Aborigine. The inner component is called the hepatitis core antigen (HBcAg) and inside this is the viral DNA (HBV-DNA) and the viral enzyme, DNA polymerase. Another hepatitis B antigen is the hepatitis Be antigen (HBeAg). The HBeAg is a secreted product of the core antigen and its presence in blood is indicative of active viral replication. The whole virus particle is called a *Dane particle*, named after the scientist who first saw it by electron microscopy. HBV has not been isolated or propagated in cell culture.

Hepatitis B has a worldwide distribution. There are thought to be 2 billion people infected throughout the world, including more than 400 million suffering with chronic hepatitis B. The virus is responsible for approximately 1.5 million deaths each year. High rates of chronic infection (up to 25%) are found in some populations, such as in some Asian and African countries, in some Pacific islands and in some Australian Aboriginal communities. It is not always clear when a person actually becomes infected with hepatitis B. In Australia, in 2002, 400 new

CASE HISTORY 18.7
Hepatitis B

A 27-year-old bank clerk went to Casualty at a local hospital because he had been feeling ill for several days. His illness was marked by fever, nausea and right abdominal pain. He thought he had flu, but noticed that morning that his eyes were quite yellow. He had never experienced any severe illness, although he recalled that he had experienced similar symptoms several years earlier. The symptoms then had been milder, so he hadn't seen a doctor. He admitted to using drugs occasionally, but said he never used a needle that someone else had used. He stated that he had a very active sex life, although he didn't have a permanent girlfriend.

Liver function tests revealed an AST (aspartate aminotransferase) level of 60 IU/L (normal range: 10–45 IU/L), an ALT (alanine transaminase) level of 56 IU/L (normal range: 5–45 IU/L), and a total bilirubin level of 27 μmol/L (normal: 0–18 μmol/L). Serology for hepatitis viruses was performed. Positive results were found for HBsAg and HBeAg, and the anti-HBc was negative.

cases of hepatitis B and almost 7000 cases for which the time of infection was not known, were reported.

Transmission

Hepatitis B virus can be found in the blood and body fluids of acutely infected people or carriers. Blood and blood products have the highest concentrations of HBV and are the most common sources of transmission, but other body fluids, especially semen, vaginal secretions, breast milk and serous fluids, can also transmit the virus. Since the number of infectious particles in blood can be extremely high (up to a million infectious doses per microlitre), very small amounts of blood can be infectious. The virus is fairly stable and can survive for days in dried blood. The virus has been found in saliva, urine and faeces, but infrequently and in lower concentrations. It is therefore only rarely transmitted via these body substances but it is important to recognise them as potential sources of infection.

Most cases in developed countries now occur in homosexual and bisexual males, injecting drug users, inmates in prison and people working in the sex industry. Babies born to mothers with hepatitis B have a high risk of infection. Perinatal transmission occurs as a result of the infant's exposure to infected blood or genital secretions during delivery or via breast feeding. Close personal contact (e.g. sharing of a toothbrush or razor) with an infected person has a low but important risk. Health-care workers may be exposed to HBV via needlestick injuries, or when contaminated blood comes into contact with mucous membranes (e.g. the splashing of blood into the eyes) or with skin cuts or abrasions. Doctors, nurses and dental workers are at particularly high risk. There has been much debate as to whether HBV is spread by mosquitoes or other biting insects. The evidence to date suggests that, if this does occur, it does so very infrequently.

Pathogenesis and clinical features

Replication of the hepatitis B virus in the liver results in cell damage but the virus does not directly kill hepatocytes. Much of the pathology is due to immune mechanisms, including destruction of infected liver cells by cytotoxic T cells. The virus replicates prolifically in the liver, but assembly of components to form complete virions is very inefficient. As a result, large numbers of virus particles are released into the bloodstream but only a small fraction of these are complete viruses (see Figure 18.16). Large amounts of antigenic viral components are released and these, and antibodies to them, can be detected in the blood in diagnostic laboratory tests.

The incubation period of hepatitis B is 4–26 weeks (average 75 days). Acute infection is symptomatic in approximately 50% of adults, but is usually asymptomatic in young children. Acute hepatitis B is clinically indistin-

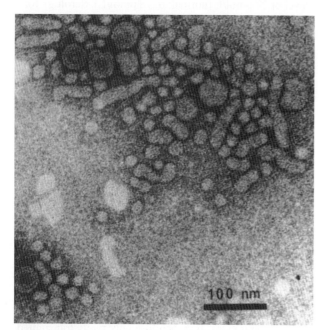

Figure 18.16

Hepatitis B virus

The complete virion (called a Dane particle – the larger, roughly circular particle) and different forms of HBsAg as seen in the serum of infected people.

guishable from other forms of hepatitis. Symptoms may include fever, jaundice, malaise, anorexia, nausea, abdominal pain, myalgia, arthralgia, skin rash and dark-coloured urine. A large proportion of cases are anicteric (without jaundice). As in most cases of hepatitis, serum levels of various enzymes are usually raised, especially alanine aminotransferase (ALT).

In otherwise healthy adults, 90% will spontaneously recover within six months of the onset of the illness. In 1% or less of patients, acute **fulminant hepatitis** occurs. This is a clinical syndrome in which there is severe impairment or necrosis of liver cells, liver failure and death in about 80% of those affected. Acute hepatitis B has a mortality rate of around 0.2%.

When people recover completely from acute HBV infection, they do so because of the destruction of all infected lymphocytes by primed cytotoxic T cells. However, in 5–10% of infected individuals, complete elimination of the virus does not occur and they develop chronic hepatitis, becoming chronic carriers of the virus. The risk of chronicity varies with age. Vertical transmission (from mother to baby) is very serious, because it is associated with an extremely high rate of chronicity. More than 90% of perinatally infected infants become chronically infected. For children infected at the age of 1–5 years the risk of chronicity is about 30%, and for children older than five years and adults the risk of chronicity is about 2%.

Many people with chronic hepatitis B infection are asymptomatic and may remain lifelong carriers of HBV without knowing it. However, at least 25% of people with chronic infection develop chronic active hepatitis and suffer a severe illness due to marked liver dysfunction. It is not known why some people are silent carriers, while others have active disease. Both forms are serious because both are associated with an increased likelihood of developing hepatic cirrhosis (fibrosis) and/or hepatocellular carcinoma later in life (10–30 years later), although patients with active persistent infection are much more likely to develop these sequelae. The cirrhosis occurs because of long-term inflammation of the liver.

The possible outcomes of hepatitis B infection are shown in Figure 18.17.

The mechanisms involved in oncogenesis have not been fully elucidated, but the integration of the viral DNA into the host cell's genome has been demonstrated. Hepatitis B is thought to be responsible for as much as 80% of all cases of liver cancer in the world, resulting in 1–2 million deaths per year.

Laboratory diagnosis

Diagnosis of hepatitis B is by examination of serum for evidence of various viral antigens and antibodies to those antigens (see Figure 18.17). HBsAg appears in the blood during the incubation period and implies ongoing infection, either acute or chronic. HBsAg levels generally fall and finally disappear during recovery, but HBsAg remains in the blood of carriers. Persistence of HBsAg in the blood for more than six months indicates **chronic hepatitis B**

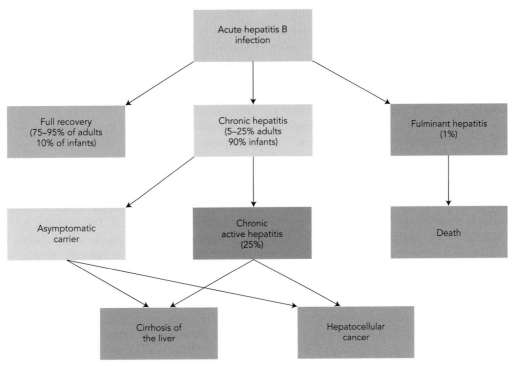

Figure 18.17
Possible outcomes of hepatitis B infection

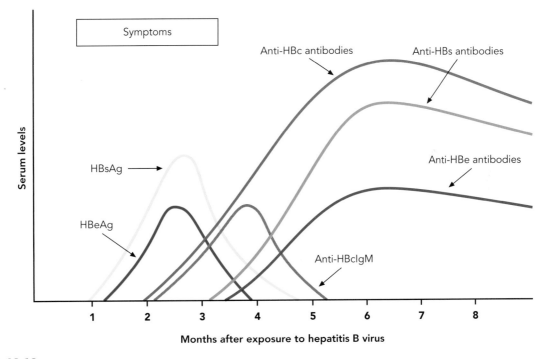

Figure 18.18
The typical course of acute hepatitis B infection and the associated serological events

infection. As HBsAg disappears, anti-HBs antibody becomes detectable. Anti-HBs antibodies are present for years in the serum of people who have fully recovered and are not carriers. Anti-HBs antibodies are the only serologic marker in people immunised with the hepatitis vaccine.

HBeAg is found in serum early during acute infection and in chronic infections. Detection of HBeAg indicates that there are large amounts of virus in the blood and thus high infectivity. HBeAg is not detected in serum that is negative for HBsAg, but HBeAg negativity in patients with detectable HBsAg may indicate low levels of viral replication. The appearance of anti-HBe antibody and disappearance of HBeAg signals a cessation of viral replication and resolution of disease.

HBV-DNA can be detected in serum during acute and chronic infection. It is considered to be the best evidence of viral replication and infectivity in patients and is often positive in patients with low-grade viraemia who are negative for HBeAg. The loss of HBV-DNA from serum indicates resolution of disease.

During the illness, antibodies to the core antigen, HBcAg, appear. These antibodies represent an immunologic response to infection but are not indicative of disease resolution.

The interpretation of the serologic tests for hepatitis B is summarised in Table 18.9.

Treatment and prevention

As with hepatitis A, there is no fully effective therapy for hepatitis B. Hydration and anti-nauseants are the basic forms of symptomatic treatment. Alpha-interferon, which appears to have both antiviral and immunomodulatory effects, has been used for the treatment of chronic hepatitis B with some success. In approximately one-third of patients with chronic HBV infection, treatment with α-interferon results in a suppression of HBV replication and clinical improvement, but discontinuation of the drug results in a relapse in some of these people.

A large number of possible side effects are associated with α-interferon use. The severity of side effects ranges from fever, chills, fatigue and muscle aches to vascular collapse, coma, cyanosis, congestive heart disease, bone marrow depression and severe depression. The drugs, lamivudine and adefovir dipivoxil, directly suppress HBV replication but rarely succeed in permanently curing infection.

Both passive and active immunisation are available for prevention of hepatitis B. Hepatitis B immunoglobulin (HBIG) is used to provide immediate post-exposure protection to unimmunised people following needlestick injury or high-risk sexual encounter, or to neonates born to HBsAg positive mothers. HBIG is prepared from plasma donated through routine blood bank collection and selected on the basis of containing high antibody titres to HBsAg. It should be administered within 72 hours of exposure.

The best way to prevent hepatitis B infection is with the HBV vaccine. This is a safe, effective vaccine consisting of genetically engineered HBsAg produced in yeast cells. Three doses of vaccine generally give good protection (efficacy around 95%) and vaccination is recommended especially for those frequently exposed to blood or blood products, such as surgeons, nurses, dentists and other health professionals, multiply transfused or dialysed patients and intravenous drug abusers. Vaccination of all babies at birth is now included in the standard childhood immunisation schedule, with boosters at 2, 4 and 6 or 12 months. It is essential that the vaccination schedule be completed for full protection.

Administration of both HBIG and HBV vaccine to neonates within 12 hours of birth is recommended if the mother is HBsAg positive, to prevent transmission of infection to the baby. Non-immune adults in high-risk groups should also be immunised. This includes household contacts, sexual partners of people with hepatitis B, injecting drug users, haemodialysis patients, people with chronic liver disease or hepatitis C, health-care workers, inmates and staff of long-term correctional facilities, and residents and staff in institutions for the intellectually impaired.

People with acute or chronic hepatitis B should be warned about the risk of infecting close contacts who are not immune. They should be made aware that some practices, like the sharing of toothbrushes or razors, carry a risk but that ordinary domestic, social and work contact carry negligible risk. Health-care workers should follow Standard Precautions to prevent cross-infection. Sensitive screening methods for detecting HBsAg are now employed by blood banks in Australia.

HEPATITIS C

The existence of a third hepatitis virus became apparent in 1975, when new diagnostic tests for hepatitis A and hepatitis B revealed that many cases of transfusion-associated hepatitis were not due to either HAV or HBV. The genome of the hepatitis C virus (HCV) was cloned in 1989 and viral proteins produced. Soon after, antibody assays were developed and HCV was established as the cause of 80–95% of cases of transfusion-associated non-A, non-B hepatitis. Australian blood banks began screening blood for anti-HCV antibody in early 1990. The virus itself has not yet been isolated. It is an RNA virus that is related to the flaviviruses. Six different HCV genotypes (designated 1 to 6) have been identified.

HCV has a worldwide distribution, with a very high prevalence in some countries in Africa (up to 18% of the

Table 18.9

Interpretation of serological assays for hepatitis B

	NO INFECTION PAST OR PRESENT	ACUTE INFECTION	CHRONIC INFECTION	PAST, RESOLVED INFECTION	PREVIOUS IMMUNISATION
HBsAg	–	+	+	–	–
Anti-HBc	–	+	+	+	–
Anti-HBc IgM	–	+	–	–	–
HBeAg	–	+	+/–	–	–
Anti-HBeAg	–	–	+/–	+/–	–
Anti-HBsAg	–	–	+/–	+	+

Hepatitis C

Between 1 July and 13 October 1998 HCV infection was diagnosed in four hospitalised patients. All these patients had undergone surgery in the same hospital 6–18 weeks earlier.

Following further investigations, a total of six surgical patients were subsequently found to have a hepatitis C viraemia (by detection of HCV-RNA in blood), but one of these (Patient 1) had almost certainly acquired the infection some years earlier through a transfusion of contaminated blood. None of the other five patients had a history of hepatitis, nor were they aware of any history of hepatitis in their families. All reported no other risk factors for HCV infection.

Testing of staff members revealed the presence of HCV antibodies in one anaesthesiology assistant. He had taken part in all six operations. At the end of February 1998 the assistant was HCV-negative, but had acute icteric hepatitis C in June 1998. Apart from occupational exposure, the anaesthesiology assistant had no known risk factors for HCV infection. The assistant was almost entirely responsible for the administration of general anaesthesia, including the preparation of narcotic drugs, the placement of venous and arterial catheters, the intubation of the patients and the subsequent artificial respiration. He usually did not wear gloves, because he claimed that they diminished his sense of touch and therefore impaired his work.

On questioning, he reported that during the time under investigation he had a wound on the medial side of the third finger of his right hand, sustained in the middle of April 1998. The wound initially bled repeatedly and he used a bandage for three or four days but not after that, although the wound was still weeping. Between 28 April and 9 June 1998, the assistant participated in 39 operations.

The available evidence suggested that Patient 1, who had chronic HCV infection, was the index patient. The anaesthesiology assistant contracted HCV from Patient 1 and subsequently transmitted the virus, during the incubation stage of his disease, to at least five patients.

Source: RS Ross et al. 'Brief Report: Transmission of Hepatitis C virus from a patient to an anaesthesiology assistant to five patients', *New England Journal of Medicine*, 343(25), December 2000.

population), South-East Asia and the Eastern Mediterranean. An estimated 3% of the world's population is infected with HCV, 200 million people are chronically infected and there are about 3 million new infections each year. In Australia about 0.5% of blood donors are found to be HCV-positive, and it has been estimated that around 200 000 Australians may be infected by the virus. It is difficult to determine rates of HCV infection accurately because many cases are asymptomatic but estimates range from 10 000 to 16 000 new cases annually. The highest number of infections occurs in people aged 15–44 years, with a preponderance in males.

Transmission

Transmission of HCV is predominantly via contaminated blood. Since 1990 blood banks have been able to screen blood donors for HCV, so injecting drug use is now the greatest risk factor in countries, such as Australia, where screening is routine. The prevalence of HCV among injecting drug users varies from 60–80%. A high proportion of prison inmates are seropositive, largely related to injecting drug use. Unsafe tattooing or body piercing also represents a risk. Occupational acquisition of infection after needlestick injury has also been reported.

Vertical transmission of HCV from mother to baby during pregnancy can occur, with the risk being greatest when the mother has a high viral load. It is thought that sexual transmission and perinatal transmission (from mother to baby after birth) of HCV can occur, but they are not common modes of infection. There appear to be other, as yet unknown, modes of transmission, because many cases occur in people with no known risk factor.

Pathogenesis and clinical features

The incubation period of hepatitis C appears to be quite variable, ranging from 14–180 days (average 50 days). Within 1–3 weeks of infection, HCV-RNA can be detected in blood. Most cases of HCV infection are asymptomatic. When symptomatic, the disease is usually mild and non-specific, with jaundice occurring in a minority of cases and liver enzymes only minimally to moderately elevated. The liver disease appears to be at least partly due to the host immune response in which T cells, attempting to kill virus-infected hepatocytes, cause damage and induce ongoing inflammation. Clinically, it is indistinguishable from other forms of acute viral hepatitis.

Despite the mild nature of acute infection, around 80% of cases progress to chronic infection. This is a much higher rate than occurs with hepatitis B infection. As with chronic hepatitis B infections, the majority of chronic infections are asymptomatic. In symptomatic cases, there are often only mild symptoms of fatigue, weakness and a tender liver. But whether asymptomatic or not, the virus causes relentless damage to hepatocytes and more than 20% of patients eventually develop, over 25–40 years, serious liver damage with symptoms ranging from disabling lethargy to cirrhosis and liver failure. Chronic HCV infection is also associated with an increased risk of hepatocellular carcinoma.

Laboratory diagnosis

Laboratory diagnosis of hepatitis C is based on the detection of antibodies in the serum of the patient. Unfortunately, the time from infection to seroconversion can be anywhere between two and nine months. This long 'window period' means that many cases of potentially infectious HCV may be missed by antibody tests. Direct demonstration of the virus itself is achieved by detection of viral RNA in serum, using the polymerase chain reaction (PCR) technique. PCR tests may be positive when antibody tests are negative, and a quantitative PCR test can provide information about the viral load in the bloodstream of the patient. PCR is also used to identify the specific HCV genotype.

When a diagnosis of hepatitis C is made the patient is usually advised to have a liver biopsy to determine the extent of their liver disease.

Treatment and prevention

Supportive care, as for other types of hepatitis, should be provided. Since acute HCV infection is asymptomatic and often undetected, specific treatment is rarely undertaken. Specific treatment for patients with chronic infection is recommended if progression to cirrhosis is likely. The current treatment regime is a combination of pegylated α-interferon and ribavirin, which achieves a sustained virological response (i.e. PCR-negative 6 months after completion of treatment) in 50–60% of cases. Treatment for genotype 2 or 3 infections must be maintained for 24 weeks, and for at least 48 weeks for all other genotypes. Treatment may not be recommended for patients in whom cirrhosis is unlikely to occur. Side effects of this treatment can be severe so regular clinical and laboratory monitoring are warranted.

There is no vaccine currently available for hepatitis C.

HEPATITIS D

In the late 1970s a new hepatitis virus was discovered in hepatitis B carriers in Italy. It was originally called the delta virus, but is now known as the hepatitis D virus. This virus has a very small RNA genome and is a defective virus – that is, it requires a coexisting, active hepatitis B infection to be able to complete its own replicative cycle. When it buds from the surface of an HBV-infected liver cell it is coated with the hepatitis B surface antigen, HBsAg, and it is this hepatitis B coat that enables it to attach to, and infect, other hepatocytes. Thus, a person cannot contract an HDV infection unless simultaneously infected with HBV (i.e. a co-infection) or unless already infected with HBV (i.e. an HDV superinfection).

HDV is found throughout the world but its highest prevalence is in Central and South-East Asia, the Middle East, Africa and South America. Hepatitis D is uncommon in Australia, with 20 notifications in 2002. It is estimated that 5% of HBV carriers worldwide are also infected with HDV, meaning that a total of 15 million people are infected with both viruses.

Blood and blood products are the major sources of HDV. People who are injecting drug users or who have received multiple blood transfusions are at highest risk. Perinatal transmission has been reported, but is rare. The incubation period varies from 2–9 weeks, being shorter in HBV carriers superinfected with HDV than when co-infection with both viruses occurs. When HDV super-infects a chronic carrier of HBV, the infection is usually severe and can lead to cirrhosis and hepatic failure, with high mortality. Chronic hepatitis develops in 1–3% of co-infections and in 70–80% of superinfections. Most patients with chronic HBV/HDV hepatitis develop hepatic cirrhosis and almost 25% of these die of liver failure.

Laboratory diagnosis is based on the detection of HDV-RNA by PCR. Serological tests are available for HDV antigen (HDAg) or for antibody to HDAg. Anti-HDV IgM levels are suggestive of acute infection. There is no fully effective treatment, other than physiologic support in rehydration and anti-nauseants. Limited success has been achieved with α-interferon, but this treatment has a low response rate and a high relapse rate. There is no HDV vaccine, but vaccination against hepatitis B prevents hepatitis D infection.

HEPATITIS E

Hepatitis E is caused by a small RNA virus that is a member of the calicivirus family. The virus is shed in faeces and spread by the faecal-oral route, but it appears to be less readily transmitted than HAV.

HEV appears to have a restricted distribution of Central and South-East Asia, Africa, the Middle East and Central America. It is best known for causing water-borne epidemics but is also responsible for a large proportion of sporadic hepatitis in countries where it is endemic. It is the cause of occasional cases of hepatitis in travellers to endemic areas. The first case of locally acquired HEV in Australia was reported in 1994 in the Northern Territory. Since then other cases have been reported, mainly in people returning from endemic areas.

The incubation period ranges from 2–9 weeks, with a mean of about 40 days. Clinically, HEV infection is similar to HAV infection. Hepatitis E is generally a mild to moderate disease (mortality rate of 1–3%), but initial illness may be severe and fatal when associated with the malnutrition or other medical problems that are typical of its Third World victims. It can also cause severe infection in pregnant women, in whom the mortality rate from severe liver disease can reach as high as 20% if infected in the third trimester. The virus is eliminated from the body on recovery and appears not to cause chronic infection or long-term sequelae.

Serological tests for antibodies to HEV are used to diagnose hepatitis E infection. HEV infection should be suspected in a patient who has travelled to an endemic region and exhibits signs of hepatitis, but who has negative test results for other hepatitis viruses. The risk of infection when travelling in endemic countries may be minimised by practising rigorous hygiene, drinking only appropriately treated water and care in food consumption. No effective therapy is currently available.

OTHER HEPATITIS VIRUSES

Up to 10% of transfusion-associated hepatitis and up to 5% of community-acquired infections cannot be attributed to a known virus. Other hepatitis viruses have thus been suggested. The hepatitis G virus may be responsible for some of these infections. This virus can be detected in blood using PCR methodology, but its role in causing liver disease has not been clearly established.

- The gastrointestinal tract (GIT) is a portal of entry into the body for numerous microorganisms.
- Food poisoning (food-borne illness) is a general term for any gastrointestinal disease related to the consumption of food.
- Gastrointestinal pathogens are acquired mainly by the faecal-oral route, from contaminated food, fluids or hands.

ACUTE DIARRHOEAL DISEASES

- The major symptom of gastrointestinal infection is acute diarrhoea.
- Most acute diarrhoeal infections have an incubation period of 1–4 days and are self-limiting.
- Infectious diarrhoea can be divided into non-inflammatory diarrhoea, characterised by watery stools; and inflammatory diarrhoea, characterised by stools containing blood, mucus and pus.
- The common bacterial causes of acute diarrhoea include:
  - *Campylobacter* species
  - Serovars of *Salmonella*
  - *Escherichia coli*
  - *Vibrio cholerae* (cholera)
  - *Shigella* species
  - *Clostridium difficile* (also causes pseudomembranous colitis)
  - *Vibrio parahaemolyticus*
  - *Yersinia enterocolitica*
  - *Clostridium perfringens*
- The common viral causes of acute diarrhoea include:
  - rotavirus
  - norovirus
  - enteric adenoviruses
  - caliciviruses
  - astroviruses
- Common protozoal causes of acute diarrhoea include:
  - *Giardia intestinalis*
  - *Entamoeba histolytica*
  - *Cryptosporidium parvum*
- Food intoxication is a disease caused by the presence of preformed toxins in food.
- Food intoxications are characterised by the rapid onset of nausea, vomiting and abdominal pain.
- The major causes of food intoxications are the enterotoxins of *Staphylococcus aureus*, *Bacillus cereus* and *Clostridium botulinum*.
- For any patient with acute diarrhoea, fluid and electrolyte replacement is essential.

OTHER GASTROINTESTINAL DISEASES

- *Helicobacter pylori* is a major cause of gastritis, a major factor in the development of duodenal and gastric ulcers, and has a role in gastric cancer.
- *Salmonella typhi* and *S. paratyphi*, types, A, B and C, cause typhoid and paratyphoid fevers.

HELMINTH INFECTIONS OF THE GASTROINTESTINAL TRACT

- Helminth infections are acquired either by penetration of the skin by larvae, or by ingestion of the eggs of helminths.
- The severity of the disease is largely a function of the number of worms in the body.
- The major helminth infections in humans are caused by:
  - *Enterobius vermicularis*
  - *Ascaris lumbricoides*
  - Hookworms (*Ancylostoma duodenale*, *Necator americanus*)
  - *Strongyloides stercoralis*
  - *Echinococcus granulosus*
  - *Taenia saginata*
  - *Trichuris trichiura*
  - *Hymenolepis nana*

HEPATITIS

- The term 'hepatitis' refers to injury and inflammation of the liver.
- Viruses are major causes of hepatitis, but other microorganisms, alcohol, drugs and various other disorders may also be responsible.

Hepatitis A

- Transmission of hepatitis A virus (HAV) is primarily by the faecal-oral route.
- The incubation period ranges from 2–6 weeks.
- Complete recovery occurs in most cases within 4–6 weeks, there is no carrier state and chronic infection does not generally occur.
- An effective HAV vaccine is available and recommended for high-risk groups.

Hepatitis B

- Blood and blood products are the most common means of hepatitis B virus (HBV) transmission, but other body fluids, especially semen, vaginal secretions and serous fluids, can also transmit the virus.
- Acute hepatitis B is clinically similar to hepatitis A, although usually more severe.
- Most healthy adults recover spontaneously within six months.
- In 5–10% of infected individuals, complete elimination of the virus does not occur; they develop chronic hepatitis and are chronic carriers of the virus.
- Chronic hepatitis is associated with an increased likelihood of developing hepatic cirrhosis and/or hepatocellular carcinoma.
- The HBV vaccine is now a part of the standard childhood immunisation schedule and is also recommended for adults in high-risk groups.

Hepatitis C

- Transmission of hepatitis C (HCV) is mainly via contaminated blood.

- Around 80% of cases of HCV progress to chronic infection.
- Most chronic infections are asymptomatic, but more than 20% of patients eventually develop hepatic cirrhosis and/or hepatocellular carcinoma.

Hepatitis D
- A person cannot contract an HDV infection unless simultaneously infected with HBV, or already infected with HBV.
- Blood and blood products are the major sources of HDV.

- There is no HDV vaccine, but vaccination against hepatitis B prevents hepatitis D infection.

Hepatitis E
- Hepatitis E virus (HEV) is shed in faeces and spread by the faecal-oral route.
- Clinically, HEV infection is similar to HAV infection.
- HEV can cause severe infection with high mortality in pregnant women.

STUDY QUESTIONS

1. What is the physiological basis of diarrhoea?
2. What microorganisms are commonly associated with outbreaks of diarrhoeal disease in day-care centres?
3. Describe the differences between inflammatory and non-inflammatory diarrhoea.
4. How are *Salmonella* diarrhoeal infections usually acquired?
5. How do enterotoxigenic *E. coli* cause diarrhoea?
6. What is haemolytic uraemic syndrome and what is the major cause?
7. Why is cholera a potentially fatal disease?
8. Why is cholera vaccine no longer recommended for routine use in travellers?
9. What is bacillary dysentery?
10. Why is shigellosis so readily transmitted from person to person?
11. What is the basis of antibiotic-associated colitis?
12. List the viruses that commonly cause diarrhoea and indicate their usual sources.
13. What is amoebic dysentery?
14. What characteristics of *Cryptosporidium parvum* enable it to survive so well in water?
15. What is a food intoxication?
16. How are diarrhoeal diseases usually diagnosed?
17. What are the major aspects of treatment of a patient with diarrhoea?
18. What important diseases are thought to be caused by *Helicobacter pylori*?
19. How is *Helicobacter pylori* infection diagnosed?
20. What important virulence factor is possessed by *Salmonella typhi*?
21. Explain how *Salmonella typhi* causes the symptoms that are commonly associated with typhoid fever.
22. What specimens are required for the laboratory diagnosis of typhoid fever?
23. What are the typical symptoms of *Enterobius vermicularis* infection and how is the infection diagnosed?
24. What specimens are required for the laboratory diagnosis of worm infestation of the intestine?
25. Describe the life cycle of *Ascaris lumbricoides*.
26. Describe the life cycle of hookworms.
27. What is the major difference between *Strongyloides stercoralis* and other nematodes that cause intestinal infection?
28. What is the cause of hydatid disease? Describe its main features.

29. Define hepatitis and list the possible causes.
30. Draw up a table to show the cause, common modes of transmission, important diagnostic tests, treatment and prevention of each of the five major types of viral hepatitis.
31. In which types of viral hepatitis is chronic infection possible, and what are the major problems associated with chronic viral hepatitis?

TEST YOUR UNDERSTANDING

Case History 18.1   Cholera
1. What does this outbreak indicate about how cholera can be transmitted?
2. In cholera outbreaks what factors/conditions would lead to high fatality rates?
3. Why is vaccination against cholera currently not recommended for travellers to endemic countries?

Case History 18.2   Shigellosis
1. What is the usual means of transmission of *Shigella*?
2. Why was this organism transmitted to so many people in this outbreak?
3. Why does this organism predominantly affect children?

Case History 18.3   Norovirus
1. What is the likely means of transmission of infection in this outbreak?
2. What measures would have reduced the infection rate in this outbreak?

Case History 18.4   Cryptosporidiosis
1. What are the possible means of transmission of *Cryptosporidium* in this outbreak?
2. What features of *Cryptosporidium parvum* enable it to be transmitted so easily?
3. What action could be taken to prevent further spread of the organism in this situation?

Case History 18.5   Staphylococcal gastroenteritis
1. Apart from the isolation of *S. aureus* from some of the stool specimens, what other information supports the diagnosis of staphylococcal food poisoning?
2. What are the possible sources of contamination of the chicken?
3. What treatment would you expect the affected people to receive?

Case History 18.6   Hepatitis A

1. What is the most likely way that the food became contaminated with hepatitis A virus?
2. Why is there not a carrier state normally associated with hepatitis A infection?
3. Why is NIGH usually ineffective if given more than two weeks after exposure to the hepatitis A virus?

Case History 18.7   Hepatitis B

1. What do the test results in this case indicate?
2. How do you think this patient contracted the disease?
3. What infection control measures should hospital staff observe when attending this patient?

Case History 18.8   Hepatitis C

1. Is transmission of HCV in this case consistent with the normal modes of transmission of HCV? Explain.
2. How could this outbreak have been prevented?
3. What makes hepatitis C a serious disease?

Further reading

De Luca, A & G Iaquinto 2004, '*Helicobacter pylori* and gastric diseases: a dangerous association', *Cancer Letters* 213, pp. 1–10. (Reviews the pathogenesis of gastric diseases that are associated with *Helicobacter pylori* infection.)

Khuroo, MS 2003, 'Viral hepatitis international travelers: risks and prevention', *International Journal of Antimicrobial Agents* 21, pp. 143–152. (Describes the modes of transmission, risk to travellers and prevention of infection of the five hepatitis viruses.)

Koopmans, M & E Duizer 2004, 'Foodborne viruses: an emerging problem', *International Journal of Food Microbiology* 90, pp. 23–41. (Describes the epidemiology and diagnosis of foodborne viral diseases.)

Kucik, CJ, GL Martin & BV Sortor 2004, 'Common intestinal parasites', *American Family Physician* 69(5), pp. 1161–1168. (Describes the organism characterisitics and diagnosis of the major protozoal and helminth infections in the world.)

Lavanchy, D 2004, 'Hepatitis B virus epidemiology, disease burden, treatment, and current and emerging prevention and control measures', *Journal of Viral Hepatitis* 11, pp. 97–107. (Reviews the transmission, clinical features, treatment and prevention of hepatitis B.)

Robins-Browne, RM & EL Hartland 2002, '*Escherichia coli* as a cause of diarrhea', *Journal of Gastroenterology and Hepatology* 17, pp. 467–475. (Reviews the different types of *Escherichia coli* that cause diarrhoeal disease.)

Thielman, NM & RL Guerrant 2004, 'Acute infectious diarrhea', *New England Journal of Medicine*, 350, pp. 38–47. (Reviews the major causes and treatment of infectious diarrhoea.)

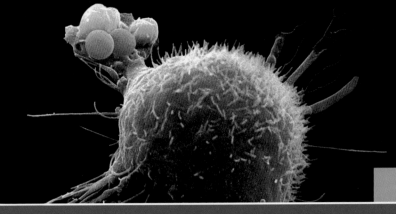

CHAPTER 19

Cardiovascular and Multisystem Infections

[CHAPTER FOCUS]

■ *What microorganisms commonly cause cardiovascular and multisystem infections in Australia and other countries?*

■ *How are cardiovascular and multisystem diseases usually transmitted?*

■ *What are the important clinical aspects of the common cardiovascular and multisystem infections?*

Introduction

The circulating blood can normally be considered sterile, although low numbers of bacteria may briefly circulate in a healthy person until phagocytes remove them. When large numbers of microorganisms enter the bloodstream from a wound or other focus of infection, they are easily disseminated through the body. In this way, they reach other body organs, where they may cause serious and often life-threatening diseases. Infections of the bloodstream and/or multiple organs are called **systemic infections**. A wide variety of microbes can cause such infections. Bacteria and viruses are most common, but protozoa are responsible for some serious infections throughout the world, the most notable being malaria. A number of fungi can cause systemic infections, but usually only in an immunocompromised host. Helminths also cause some important systemic infections, such as filariasis (elephantiasis) and schistosomiasis.

The terms used to signify microorganisms in the bloodstream often have a prefix that reflects part of the name of the microorganism, or the type of microorganism, plus the suffix *-aemia*. Thus, **viraemia** denotes the presence of viruses in the blood. Similarly, **fungaemia**, **parasitaemia** and **meningococcaemia** mean the presence of fungi, parasites (protozoa or helminths) and meningococci, respectively, in the bloodstream.

However, there is often some confusion over the usage and meaning of the terms 'bacteraemia' and 'septicaemia' because they are frequently used interchangeably. **Bacteraemia** literally means the *presence* of bacteria in the bloodstream. It may be manifested by the whole range of conditions from asymptomatic to seriously ill. Bacteraemia is in fact a fairly common occurrence in all people, since low numbers of bacteria often spill into the bloodstream when minor trauma to skin (e.g. cuts, abrasions) or mucous membranes (e.g. teeth cleaning, chewing) occurs. **Septicaemia** is a serious clinical syndrome resulting from the presence of bacteria in the bloodstream; it thus represents a bacteraemia with severe clinical manifestations.

Systemic bacterial infections

SEPTICAEMIA

The bloodstream is a relatively inhospitable place for microorganisms, even though it contains oxygen, water and an abundance of nutrients, has an approximately neutral pH and the right temperature for many organisms to multiply. First, it is constantly moving and thus it is difficult for microbes to colonise a surface and multiply. Second, it contains a variety of antimicrobial defence mechanisms, in particular the phagocytic leucocytes, antibodies and complement (see Chapter 9). Third, the blood recirculates through the spleen and liver, where sinusoids are lined with more phagocytic cells and where the blood flow slows, enhancing their phagocytic activity. Thus, microbes are usually quickly cleared from the bloodstream.

However, some pathogenic organisms are able to persist in the blood and be transported by it. In the majority of such cases the organisms enter the bloodstream from a primary focus of infection in organs such as the lungs, gastrointestinal tract or kidneys, or from an infected wound. Intravascular catheters are important causes of infection. These devices are readily colonised by microorganisms, which can ultimately lead to infection of surrounding tissue and the bloodstream. The use of intravenous catheters is very common, not only in hospitalised patients, but increasingly in patients receiving intravenous therapy at home.

For microorganisms to cause septicaemia, at least one of the following conditions must exist:

- the organisms have to be released, either continuously or intermittently, in large enough numbers to overwhelm the defence systems; or
- there is some anatomical defect that facilitates the colonisation of a site (e.g. a damaged heart valve); or
- the organisms have some protective mechanism that helps them to evade the defences of the blood (e.g. an antiphagocytic capsule or a coagulase enzyme); or
- there is some impairment in the body's defences (e.g. hypogammaglobulinaemia resulting from cancer therapy; or neutropenia due to chronic infection).

The last two conditions simply mean that fewer bacteria will be needed to produce septicaemia. While bacterial multiplication in the blood may occur, it is not a requirement in septicaemia. The common causes of septicaemia are shown in Table 19.1.

Clinical features

The clinical manifestations of septicaemia are extremely variable. Usually, the patient has a high, spiking fever, often with alternating severe shaking chills and sweats. These symptoms are often intermittent, interspersed with periods of improvement. Shock, manifested by low blood pressure and vascular collapse, is also common. **Endotoxic (septic) shock** is a severe, life-threatening form of septicaemia caused by the endotoxin (the lipid-A component of lipopolysaccharide) of Gram-negative bacteria.

Table 19.1	
Common causes of septicaemia	
HOSPITAL ACQUIRED	COMMUNITY ACQUIRED
Staphylococcus aureus	*Escherichia coli*
Coagulase negative staphylococci	*Staphylococcus aureus*
Escherichia coli	*Streptococcus pneumoniae*
Pseudomonas aeruginosa	*Klebsiella pneumoniae*
Enterobacter spp.	Group B streptococcus
Enterococci	*Pseudomonas aeruginosa*

Septicaemia

A 49-year-old man had a Hickman catheter surgically inserted for total parenteral nutrition. Six days after surgery it was noticed that the catheter entry site had become inflamed. He had a temperature of 39.8°C, a high respiratory rate and rapid pulse. Blood cultures were collected and two out of three sets grew *Staphylococcus epidermidis*.

Diagnosis

The diagnosis of septicaemia is made by the demonstration of bacteria in the blood, usually by blood culture (see Chapter 15). Indirectly, the diagnosis may sometimes be made by the demonstration of a focus of infection somewhere in the body. The bacteria causing septicaemia may be difficult to culture from a sample of blood for a number of reasons.

1. The organisms, although causing severe infection, may be present in the bloodstream only in low numbers. In addition, the amount of blood collected for culture (around 10 mL) is a small sample size of the total blood volume of 5–6 litres.
2. The organisms may be only transiently present in the bloodstream, particularly if they are shed intermittently from the primary focus of infection. In these circumstances, after each shower of organisms into the bloodstream bacterial numbers will gradually be reduced by the body's defence mechanisms. Thus, they may be present in large numbers for only a short time after release.
3. Some septicaemia-causing bacteria are difficult to grow or are very slow-growing *in vitro*.

To maximise the chance of isolating the causative agent, three samples of blood for culture are usually taken from a patient over a 24–48 hour period. The best time to take a sample is when the patient is experiencing a febrile episode, as this generally represents a showering of bacteria into the bloodstream from the focus of infection.

Culture of a catheter tip (see Chapter 15) may be helpful if it is thought to be a possible source of the infection.

Treatment

Treatment involves the administration of an appropriate antimicrobial drug. Because of the potential severity of the disease, antimicrobial therapy is usually commenced at the first clinical suspicion. A broad spectrum agent is used and then modified, if necessary, once the identity of the causative agent and its antimicrobial sensitivity are known. It is preferable that blood for culture be collected before commencement of antibiotic therapy (see Chapter 15). Location and treatment of the primary focus of infection are also necessary; if it is an abscess it may require surgical drainage. The patient may also require symptomatic treatment for systemic complications, such as hypotension.

RHEUMATIC FEVER

Incidence

Rheumatic fever is a non-suppurative (not pus-forming) complication of *Streptococcus pyogenes* sore throat. It is a non-suppurative disease because it is not a direct infection. It affects only a small percentage of people, following a streptococcal sore throat or, less commonly, scarlet fever. Its highest incidence occurs in 5–15 year olds. Rheumatic fever is still a major cause of cardiovascular disease in the Third World, where poverty, overcrowding and poor hygiene are important factors. In Australia and other developed countries, the incidence of rheumatic fever has generally been declining for several decades, except in socioeconomically deprived communities. In some Aboriginal communities the incidence is estimated to be 200–300 per 100 000 population. Similarly, the disease is much more common in New Zealand's indigenous population than in non-Maori people.

Clinical features and pathogenesis

Onset of rheumatic fever usually occurs 2–4 weeks after a streptococcal sore throat. Without treatment, the susceptible person can suffer recurrence of rheumatic fever after each episode of streptococcal sore throat, with a 2–4 week latent period each time. The major diagnostic criteria of rheumatic fever are:

- carditis, manifested usually by sinus tachycardia (fast heart rate), a heart murmur, chest pain or extra heart sounds
- acute migratory polyarthritis, mainly of large joints
- chorea (sudden, involuntary, irregular movements)
- subcutaneous nodules near joints
- erythema marginatum, a distinctive macular rash.

An acute attack of rheumatic fever lasts up to three months. If untreated, rheumatic fever can result in scarring and deformation of the valves and heart failure, which is known as **rheumatic heart disease**. Valve damage and disruption to normal blood flow around the valve can predispose it to colonisation by bacteria and, hence, endocarditis. This is discussed in the next section.

The development of rheumatic fever is thought to be due to cross-reactivity between antigens of certain streptococci and heart tissue antigens. Thus, antibodies produced against the streptococcus (while it is infecting the throat) cross-react with heart tissue, causing inflammation and damage. Certain strains of *S. pyogenes* have M-proteins that have an antigenic similarity to cardiac myosin and sarcolemma membrane proteins.

Genetic factors also seem to be important, since people with certain MHC types (see Chapter 9) have a much greater risk of rheumatic fever than people who lack those types.

Diagnosis

Diagnosis of rheumatic fever is made by correlation of clinical findings (especially major criteria) with certain laboratory findings indicating recent streptococcal infection, such as a positive throat culture, or high or rising antibody titres. Multiple serological tests are often performed, including an anti-streptolysin-O titre (ASOT), and anti-DNAse and anti-hyaluronidase tests.

Treatment and prevention

Antibiotics (e.g. penicillin or erythromycin) are given to remove the remaining microorganisms, and aspirin or other anti-inflammatory drugs are used to reduce pain and inflammation. Prompt antibiotic treatment of *S. pyogenes* throat infections in people known to be susceptible to rheumatic fever can prevent further attacks. Antibiotic cover is required for 10 days. In high-risk groups, such as some Aboriginal communities, treatment of sore throat in all members may be warranted. Continuous, prophylactic use of antibiotics may be prescribed for people known to suffer severe attacks of rheumatic fever.

INFECTIVE ENDOCARDITIS

The wall of the heart consists of three layers. The innermost layer is called the endocardium. It is a layer of epithelium covering the heart muscle and the valves, and is in direct contact with the blood. **Infective endocarditis** is an inflammation of the endocardium, initiated by an infectious agent. It often presents as a pyrexia of unknown origin (PUO) and is a fatal disease if untreated. It may occur as an acute, rapidly progressing disease which, in the pre-antibiotic era, invariably resulted in death within a few weeks. In addition, a chronic form exists. In more than 60% of patients there is a pre-existing heart condition such as congenital heart disease, mitral valve prolapse, valvular damage from rheumatic fever, or a prosthetic heart valve.

Causative organisms and pathogenesis

Infective endocarditis can be caused by a wide variety of bacteria. Although in most cases a pre-existing heart condition is present, in some cases there is no apparent defect. On abnormal or damaged valves, oral streptococci (e.g. *Streptococcus sanguis*, *S. milleri* and *S. oralis*) and staphylococci (especially *Staphylococcus aureus*) are the most common causes. The oral bacteria can enter the bloodstream through minor abrasions such as those caused by chewing, teeth cleaning or flossing, or following dental procedures or dental surgery. They then colonise the heart valves.

On prosthetic valves, staphylococci (especially *Staphylococcus epidermidis* and *Staphylococcus aureus*) are a major cause of early endocarditis; that is, occurring less than two months after implant surgery. These organisms are probably introduced during surgery. Late valvular endocarditis (more than two months after implant) can be caused by a wide range of organisms, including streptococci and Gram-negative bacteria. Overall, 1.5–3% of patients with a prosthetic valve implant develop an endocarditis within a year.

Intravenous drug users may develop an endocarditis caused by microorganisms they inject into themselves in unsterile procedures. In this group *Staphylococcus aureus* is most common, followed by oral streptococci and Gram-negative bacteria (e.g. *Pseudomonas*). Fungi, such as *Candida*, *Aspergillus* and *Mucor*, are also found occasionally as the cause of endocarditis in IV drug users. Polymicrobial infections (infection caused by more than one organism) may also occur. Iatrogenic endocarditis is an increasingly important type. Predominant causes are staphylococci and enterococci, associated with IV catheters, haemodialysis and other medico-surgical procedures. Table 19.2 summarises the causative agents of endocarditis.

It is a complex process and in many cases its development depends on prior endocardial damage. On damaged or abnormal valves, collagen in the endothelial basement membrane is exposed and this stimulates the deposition of fibrin and platelets on the membrane. The valve abnor-

---

Table 19.2

Common causative agents of endocarditis in different groups of patients. For each category the organisms are listed in decreasing order of frequency

Abnormal/damaged valve	Oral streptococci
	Staphylococcus aureus
Prosthetic valve (< 2 months after implant)	Coagulase negative staphylococci
	Staphylococcus aureus
	Gram-negative (enteric) bacteria
	Oral streptococci
	Fungi (mainly *Candida albicans*)
Prosthetic valve (> 2 months after implant)	Oral streptococci
	Coagulase negative staphylococci
	Gram-negative (enteric) bacteria
	Staphylococcus aureus
IV drug abuser	*Staphylococcus aureus*
	Oral streptococci
	Gram-negative (enteric) bacteria

mality and these fibrin-platelet clumps cause a disturbance to the normal smooth flow of blood through the valve, resulting in turbulence. In turbulent flow, bacteria are given the opportunity to attach to surfaces, particularly to the deposited fibrin, via specific adhesins or sticky polysaccharides secreted from the cell.

Having attached, the bacteria are able to multiply and attract monocytes which release cytokines. The bacteria and cytokines cause further platelet and fibrin deposition. Colonies of bacteria thus become sandwiched between layers of fibrin and platelets. This growing clump of bacteria, fibrin and platelets is called a **vegetation** (see Figure 19.1). The clumps of fibrin and platelets provide some shelter for the bacteria against body defences in the blood. These lesions can develop anywhere on the endocardium, but usually occur on heart valves or surrounding structures.

Vegetations vary in size and can grow to several centimetres. With increasing growth of the vegetations, there will be increasing destruction to underlying tissues and increasing valvular dysfunction, with the possibility of cardiac distress and congestive heart failure. Also, septic emboli (pieces of vegetations containing bacteria) may eventually break off and be carried to other organs, where they can infect and/or occlude blood vessels, causing inflammation and necrosis.

Clinical features

The signs and symptoms of infective endocarditis are extremely variable because they can reflect one or more of the following:

- damage and deformation of heart valves
- embolisation of vegetations with necrosis in remote tissues
- deposition of antigen-antibody complexes in blood vessels in the skin, the glomeruli or joints.

Typical clinical manifestations, then, are fever and heart murmur, often with anorexia, malaise, chills, nausea,

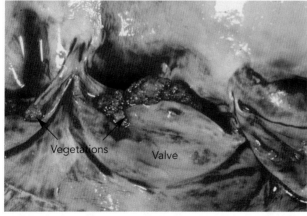

Figure 19.1
Infective endocarditis
The pathological feature of this disease is the development of vegetations (clumps of fibrin, platelets and bacteria) on the heart valve.

vomiting and night sweats. Splinter haemorrhages in the nail bed, skin lesions and signs of glomerulonephritis or synovitis may also occur. Death is usually due to congestive heart failure secondary to valvular dysfunction.

Diagnosis, treatment and prevention

Untreated endocarditis results in death, so an accurate diagnosis is required. Blood culture is the key to the laboratory diagnosis. The isolation of the causative agent is necessary so that antibiotic sensitivity results can be obtained and appropriate therapy provided. Blood cultures should be collected before commencement of antibiotic therapy. Bacteria tend to be released from vegetations at a fairly constant rate, resulting in a more or less continuous bacteraemia. In some cases of endocarditis blood cultures are negative, which may be due to:

- commencement of antibiotic therapy before collection of blood for culture
- infection by slow-growing or fastidious organisms (e.g. *Haemophilus* spp.)
- causation by unusual organisms not isolated by standard procedures (e.g. *Aspergillus, Coxiella burnetii*)
- non-infectious causes.

An echocardiogram provides supporting evidence of an abnormality of a valve or associated structure.

Prolonged, high-dose antibiotic therapy (4–6 weeks) is often necessary for infectious endocarditis because the organisms within vegetations are afforded a degree of protection from antibiotics. Even with treatment with a drug to which the organism is sensitive, infective endocarditis has a mortality rate of 10–20%. Empirical therapy, before culture results are available, usually includes a combination of drugs like penicillin, flucloxacillin and gentamicin, or vancomycin plus gentamicin if the infection was acquired in hospital. This would then be modified once culture and sensitivity results become available.

Prevention is based on the use of prophylactic antibiotics in people known to have a heart defect, who are to undergo any procedure that could lead to the introduction of bacteria into the bloodstream. Protection of such people during dental surgery is particularly important because of the common involvement of oral streptococci in endocarditis.

OSTEOMYELITIS

Cause and pathogenesis

Osteomyelitis is an inflammation of bone caused by infectious microorganisms. The organisms reach the bone either from the blood or externally, and thus the infection may be categorised according to the mode of entry of the microbe.

1. *Haematogenous osteomyelitis* is caused by organisms that are carried by the blood to the bone tissue, generally from a site of infection elsewhere in the body. Intravenous drug abusers may also develop haematogenous osteomyelitis from the use of contaminated needles.

2. *Exogenous osteomyelitis* is caused by organisms introduced directly from outside the body – for example, through a compound fracture (fracture in contact with an open wound), penetrating wound or surgery. Often the organism first infects adjacent soft tissue before spreading to the bone.

Haematogenous osteomyelitis most commonly affects the growing ends of long bones (e.g. the tibia and femur) and thus most often afflicts children and adolescents. The vulnerability of these bones is due to the anatomy of their vascular supply. A slow blood flow in the large-diameter vessels in these bones facilitates the colonisation and growth of bacteria. The most common cause is *Staphylococcus aureus*, but other organisms such as Group B streptococci, *Haemophilus influenzae* and *Mycobacterium tuberculosis* may also cause this infection. Haematogenous osteomyelitis is rare in adults and most often affects the spine.

Staphylococcus aureus is also the most common cause of exogenous osteomyelitis, but there can be other causes, depending on the circumstances of the trauma and the area of the body involved. For instance, in one recent report, *Pseudomonas* osteomyelitis occurred in a number of children who had suffered penetrating foot injuries. This organism was thought to be inhabiting their sneakers.

Clinical features, diagnosis and treatment
Haematogenous osteomyelitis in a child is usually manifested by a sudden onset of high fever, chills, nausea and progressive pain over the infected bone. In adults a more insidious and vague onset of fever, malaise and anorexia is usual. In exogenous infections, signs and symptoms of soft tissue infection usually predominate.

A variety of imaging methods, such as plain radiographs and ultrasonography, are used to provide confirmation of osteomyelitis and assessment of degree of tissue damage. Blood culture or bone biopsy (if blood culture negative) may identify the causative organism and its antibiotic sensitivity. However, the causative organism is isolated in only 60–70% of cases.

Treatment requires immediate intravenous antibiotics, usually starting with a broad spectrum drug, such as flucloxacillin, and then adjustment when culture and sensitivity results become available. Antibiotic therapy is

usually maintained for 4–6 weeks. Chronic infection can develop when bone necrosis occurs. Necrotic bone tissue presumably shields the bacteria from body defences and acts as a continuous source of infection. In this situation, surgical intervention for debridement and drainage as well as prolonged antibiotics may be necessary.

LYME DISEASE

Causative agent and transmission
Lyme disease is caused by the spirochaete *Borrelia burgdorferi* and occasionally by another species, *B. garinii*. The disease was first identified in 1975 in a cluster of 39 children and 12 adults with a distinctive skin rash in the village of Old Lyme in Connecticut, in the United States. It is now the most common vector-borne disease in North America, with approximately 20 000 cases per year being reported, and the number of cases is rising. It is also common in many areas of Europe and has been identified in several other northern hemisphere countries. The real incidence of Lyme disease in Australia is unknown, but there have been sporadic reports of Lyme disease-like illness in eastern coastal areas since 1982.

Borrelia burgdorferi is a micro-aerophilic spirochaete, 20–30 μm long and approximately 0.25 μm wide. In the United States the natural cycle of infection takes place in white-footed field mice and deer. It is transmitted in these animals and to humans by ticks of the genus *Ixodes* (see Figure 19.2). In the United States, *I. dammini* and *I. pacificus* are the major tick species involved, whereas in Europe it is *I. ricinus* and in Asia *I. persulcatus*. Lyme disease is found mainly in certain forested areas of these parts of the world.

These species of tick have not been found in Australia and *B. burgdorferi* has been difficult to find in Australian ticks that bite humans. While clinical and serological evidence suggests that the disease may occur in this country, the source and the vector are at present unclear. Seabirds, bandicoots and macropods have been suggested as possible sources.

CASE HISTORY 19.2
Osteomyelitis
Thomas, a 13-year-old boy, injured his lower left arm in a rugby match at school. The injury occurred when he fell heavily on the arm while being tackled. The next day his arm became extremely painful and was hot and swollen. He was taken to the family doctor who recorded his temperature at 39.4°C. The doctor also noticed several small boils on his chest, some of which had been broken.

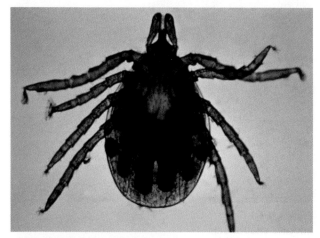

Figure 19.2
Nymphal stage of an *Ixodes* tick
This tick transmits Lyme disease.

Pathogenesis and clinical features

The spirochaete is injected into the skin of humans while the tick is feeding and then travels via the blood or lymph to virtually anywhere in the body. It seems to favour synovial tissue, skin and the nervous system. The course of Lyme disease is variable, ranging from no symptoms or only localised skin manifestations to severe and chronic disease with multiple symptoms. After a variable incubation period, mostly about a week, the full disease progresses in three stages.

Stage 1 is found in 50–80% of infected people and is characterised by **erythema migrans**. This is a unique skin lesion which begins as a red macule, usually, but not always, at the site of the tick bite; it then expands to form an erythematous annular lesion, often with a clear centre, giving it a 'bulls-eye' appearance. However, erythema migrans is not common in infections acquired in Australia. The skin lesion may be accompanied by local lymphadenopathy and minor flu-like symptoms. In untreated cases this stage resolves in several weeks.

Stage 2 follows within weeks to months and represents disseminated disease. Manifestations may include secondary annular skin lesions in other sites, neurologic disorders (e.g. lymphocytic meningitis, facial palsy, mental deterioration), cardiac disorders (e.g. myocarditis and atrioventricular block, causing palpitations and fainting) and recurrent, brief attacks of arthritis. Patients may be quite ill with debilitating malaise and fatigue.

Stage 3 occurs after a latent period of a year or more and represents chronic disease of the skin, nervous system and joints. Arthritis is the most common late sign. There is also some evidence that psychiatric disease (i.e. mental illness) may be a manifestation of this stage of the infection. This stage may persist for years. These late manifestations are thought to be due to chronic infection and/or autoimmune reaction. Stages 2 and 3 are seen in 10–15% of untreated patients.

Diagnosis

Lyme disease is difficult to diagnose. It is most straightforward in patients with typical clinical features (especially erythema migrans) and a history of tick bite in an endemic area. However, often the clinical picture is atypical or non-specific and exposure history is vague. Laboratory tests may be helpful but have significant limitations. Culture of biopsy material from skin lesions provides a definitive diagnosis, but it is slow (requiring up to eight weeks) and has low sensitivity. PCR (polymerase chain reaction) testing is superior to culture, especially in the later stages of the disease. Antibody tests are commonly used but false negative and false positive results are possible.

Treatment and prevention

Early-stage Lyme disease is usually effectively treated with doxycycline, amoxycillin or ceftriaxone. Ceftriaxone is usually preferred in more established infections. Chronic arthritis and other late manifestations may not respond to antibiotic therapy because of their immuno-logical basis. Prevention is based mainly on avoidance of tick bites, and an effective vaccine has been licensed in the United States.

RICKETTSIAL INFECTIONS

Causative organisms and incidence

Rickettsiae are named after Howard Ricketts who first identified them as the causes of typhus and Rocky Mountain spotted fever in the United States. The rickettsiae are Gram-negative rod-shaped bacteria. They have the unusual characteristic for bacteria of being strictly intracellular parasites – that is, like viruses, they can multiply only inside host cells. Another characteristic feature of these organisms is that they all multiply in arthropods such as ticks, lice, fleas or mites.

By far the most common rickettsial infection in Australia is Q fever, caused by *Coxiella burnetii*. It is most often transmitted by aerosol from faeces, milk and hides of infected sheep and cattle. Thus, farmers, meat-workers and animal transporters are most commonly affected. The primary site of infection is the lung, hence Q fever is discussed more fully in Chapter 17 which deals with respiratory system infections.

Of the arthropod-borne infections, scrub typhus and Queensland tick typhus – caused by *Orientia tsutsugamushi* and *Rickettsia australis* respectively – are the most common. On average, fewer than ten cases of all forms of typhus occur in Australia per year. Worldwide, a variety of species can cause human infection, as shown in Table 19.3. Generally, infections caused by *Rickettsia* are not very common but are important because they can be fatal.

Pathogenesis and clinical features

The classic rickettsial diseases are very similar in many respects. After introduction through the skin the organisms disseminate through the bloodstream, localising in small blood vessels in many organs, including the skin, brain and heart. They invade and damage the endothelial cells of these vessels, causing them to leak. The resultant haemorrhages and surrounding tissue necrosis produce the typical clinical features of rickettsial infections: skin rash (except in Q fever), severe headache and fever (often with rigors). Other possible symptoms include a local lymphadenopathy in the region of the arthropod bite, myalgia, and liver and spleen enlargement. The disease can be mild to fatal, with death usually resulting from shock and cardiorespiratory failure.

Laboratory diagnosis and treatment

Rickettsiae can be isolated from patient blood, but require highly specialised cell culture techniques. A serological diagnosis on paired serum samples is currently the preferred method. A PCR test is available for some species. Rickettsiae are hazardous organisms, so careful handling of patient blood should be observed. Skin contact with patient blood and its aerosolisation should be avoided. Prompt treatment with doxycycline or chloramphenicol is effective.

Table 19.3
Features of selected rickettsial infections

DISEASE	CAUSATIVE ORGANISM	DISTRIBUTION	VECTOR
Spotted fevers			
• Rocky Mountain spotted fever	*Rickettsia rickettsii*	Western hemisphere	Ticks
• Boutonneuse fever	*R. conorii*	Mediterranean, Africa, India	Ticks
• Queensland tick typhus	*R. australis*	Australia	Ticks
Typhus fevers			
• Epidemic typhus	*R. prowazekii*	South America, Africa	Lice
• Murine typhus	*R. typhi*	Worldwide	Fleas
Scrub typhus	*Orientia tsutsugamushi*	Asia, Australia, Pacific Islands	Mites

LEPTOSPIROSIS

Leptospirosis is caused by *Leptospira interrogans*. This highly coiled spirochaete, 5–15 μm long, has the ends of the cell bent into a hook, giving the cell the appearance of a question mark – hence the name *interrogans* (see Figure 19.3). Leptospirosis is a notifiable disease in Australia where the annual incidence is 100–300 cases. The most common strain (serotype) in Australia is *L. interrogans* var. *hardjo*.

The bacteria infect dogs, cats, cattle, sheep, pigs and many wild mammals such as rats, causing a chronic kidney infection. Infected animals excrete large numbers of bacteria in urine and humans usually become infected by skin or mucous membrane contact with water, soil, vegetation or food contaminated with urine. Australian cases are often associated with occupational exposure, particularly among meat-workers, farmers and stock-transporters. The bacteria enter through skin abrasions or mucous membranes, reach the bloodstream and then are carried throughout the body. Many infections are asymptomatic, but in some a febrile, flu-like illness occurs after an incubation period of

1–2 weeks. In most of the cases (about 90%) an uneventful recovery takes place within several weeks.

A severe form, called Weil's disease, represents infection of the liver and kidneys, and is characterised by hepatitis, jaundice, uraemia and bacteriuria. Pulmonary haemorrhage may also occur. Mortality can be as high as 20% in people with this form of the disease.

Bacteria may be isolated from blood, urine and CSF, with blood culture during the first week of the disease being the most reliable method. Highly sensitive serological methods are available, and are generally the main ways by which infection is diagnosed.

Penicillin or doxycycline may be effective, especially if given within the first week of illness. Patients with serious complications, especially kidney failure, require supportive care. An animal vaccine is available, but not one yet for humans.

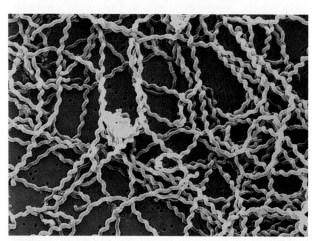

Figure 19.3

Leptospira interrogans
An electron micrograph of this hook-shaped spirochaete which causes urinary tract infections in animals and systemic infections in humans.

CASE HISTORY 19.3

Leptospirosis

After holidaying in Vanuatu, a 24-year-old man presented to an emergency department with chest pain and chest wall tenderness. He had previously been in good health. Two weeks earlier he had returned from a 10-day holiday in Vanuatu, where he had cut his foot on coral. After injuring his foot, he had swum in a freshwater river.

He was admitted to hospital with an initial diagnosis of musculoskeletal chest pain of unknown origin. Over the next few days his condition deteriorated. He initially developed an erythematous rash, vomiting, diarrhoea and a mild headache, and subsequently acute renal failure, jaundice, respiratory failure and myocarditis. Over his period of hospitalisation he was given a number of antibiotics and supportive therapy. On day 8 he suffered a cardiac arrest from which he could not be resuscitated.

Adapted from FM O'Leary et al., 'Fatal leptospirosis presenting as musculoskeletal chest pain', *Medical Journal of Australia*, 180, p. 29, 2004.

TOXIC SHOCK SYNDROME

Toxic shock syndrome is caused by certain strains of *Staphylococcus aureus* that produce a particular toxin called toxic shock syndrome toxin 1 (TSST-1). The disease came to prominence when outbreaks occurred in women, associated with their use of super-absorbent tampons. The tampons were sometimes left in place for too long and caused abrasion of the vaginal wall, providing appropriate conditions for infection. It is now recognised that toxic shock syndrome can result from any infection in men, women or children caused by strains of *Staphylococcus aureus* that produce TSST-1 or certain enterotoxins. Also, some strains of group A streptococcus (*Streptococcus pyogenes*) that produce certain exotoxins can cause a toxic shock syndrome, similar to the severe scarlet fever syndrome frequently described in earlier literature. These staphylococcal and streptococcal toxins cause widespread tissue injury and shock because they act as superantigens (see Chapter 10).

Toxic shock syndrome is a potentially life-threatening condition (even with treatment) characterised by fever, shock and a red, sunburn-like rash. In one or two days the skin starts to peel off in sheets, particularly on the palms and soles of the feet. Other parts of the body are usually involved, such as the gastrointestinal system (vomiting, diarrhoea), muscles (myalgia), central nervous system (disorientation) and mucous membranes (vaginal or conjunctival hyperaemia). Death, when it occurs, is usually due to shock. Patients should be examined for a focus of infection. Vigorous antibiotic therapy is warranted. If related to tampon usage, advice to the patient on proper, hygienic usage should be provided by the health professional.

ANTHRAX

Anthrax is a zoonosis (an animal disease that can be transmitted to humans) that is acquired primarily from herbivores, especially sheep, goats and cattle. It is caused by *Bacillus anthracis*, a large, spore-forming, Gram-positive rod. Its spores are extremely resistant to adverse environmental conditions and can remain dormant in soil for many years. Human infection mainly comes from direct contact with infected animals (skins or carcasses), inhalation of spores present in aerosolised animal products (e.g. milk) or ingestion of infected meat. The cases of anthrax in the United States in 2001, resulting from the deliberate release of anthrax spores in letters, illustrates the ease with which the disease is transmitted. Anthrax is generally not a major problem in developed countries. Following the events of 2001, anthrax became a notifiable disease in Australia. No cases were notified in 2002. The last reported human case was a knackery worker in 1997. Outbreaks of anthrax still occur in livestock (cattle and sheep) in Australia, despite the availability of an animal vaccine.

There are two major forms of anthrax: cutaneous and pulmonary. In cutaneous anthrax a cut or skin abrasion is

---

In early October 2001 a 63-year-old man in Florida died of anthrax. The discovery of anthrax spores in an envelope on his work desk led to a fear of 'suspicious white powders' and the prospect of further terrorist activity. The postal delivery of anthrax spores around this time led to the infection of 22 people, of whom five died.

Anthrax scares occurred throughout the world during October and November 2001. Announcements were made declaring that anthrax had been found in postal items in Kenya, the Bahamas, Greece, Brazil, Russia, India and Pakistan, but all were retracted after further testing.

Between 11 October and 16 November approximately 900 'white powder' incidents were reported by members of the public to emergency services in New South Wales. Police reported that over 1500 people may have been exposed to these substances. Samples from 535 incidents were received for testing at the NSW Police Forensics Services Group laboratory. Anthrax spores were not found in any sample and no incidents of exposure to anthrax were identified in New South Wales, or elsewhere in Australia.

Adapted from A Leask, V Delpech & J McAnulty, 'Anthrax and other suspect powders: initial responses to an outbreak of hoaxes and scares', *NSW Public Health Bulletin*, 14(11–12), 2003, p. 218.

---

the usual site of entry, where the spores germinate and the bacteria multiply and produce a number of toxins. Host defences are inhibited by the organism's antiphagocytic capsule. In 1–2 days a papular lesion develops, surrounded by a ring of vesicles. Eventually it ulcerates and becomes black and necrotic (Figure 19.4). In a minority of cases, septicaemia and severe toxaemia can occur, with generalised toxic effects. This form of anthrax has a mortality rate of 10–20% if untreated. Pulmonary anthrax ('woolsorter's disease') is the most serious form of anthrax, but is rare in developed countries. Inhalation of spores leads to multiplication in the lungs, pulmonary oedema and haemorrhage, and septicaemia. The mortality rate in this systemic form is around 90%, even with treatment.

Anthrax is best diagnosed by culture of organisms from skin lesions or blood. Treatment with antibiotics (e.g. benzylpenicillin or ciprofloxacin) does not alter the course of the infection but, if given early, reduces the risk of systemic symptoms in cutaneous anthrax. Animal vaccination greatly reduces the incidence of human disease. Contaminated materials should be incinerated or carefully sterilised or disinfected. Infected animals are killed and the carcasses cremated or deep buried and covered with anhydrous calcium oxide (quicklime). Human vaccines are available in Australia but are not registered for general use. Use in high-risk persons is authorised by the Therapeutic Goods Administration. Prophylaxis for

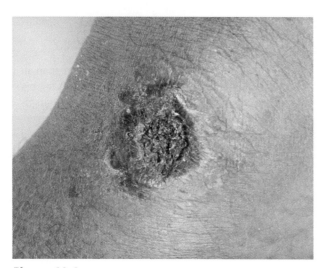

exposed, non-vaccinated people is with antibiotics such as doxycycline or ciprofloxacin.

BRUCELLOSIS

Cause and incidence

Human brucellosis was first described in 1860 among British soldiers in Malta, where it became known as **Malta fever**. It is also sometimes called **undulant fever** because of the rising and falling nature of the fever. The disease is caused by three species of the genus *Brucella*: *B. melitensis*, *B. abortus* and *B. suis*. These small, Gram-negative coccobacilli are primarily animal pathogens but cause disease in humans after contact with infected animals or their products.

Brucella melitensis is found mainly in sheep and goats. It causes the most serious infections in humans and has the most severe complications. The disease is endemic in Mediterranean countries, the Middle East, South America and areas of Europe, Asia and Africa. *Brucella abortus* is acquired mainly from cows. Infection with this species can lead to abortion (hence 'abortus') in animals. It has a worldwide distribution except in certain developed countries which have succeeded in eradicating the organism. Australia was declared free of bovine brucellosis in 1989, as a result of the National Brucellosis and Tuberculosis Eradication Campaign instituted in 1970. *Brucella suis* infects pigs and occasionally other animals such as horses, cows and dogs. It occurs mainly in South America and South-East Asia. Between 10 and 50 cases of brucellosis are notified per year in Australia, most occurring in Queensland among wild boar hunters. The organism is rare in domestic pigs.

Transmission

Brucellosis is highly communicable. Transmission from animals to humans occurs by direct contact with infected tissues or animal products, or via dust or aerosols. The organisms enter the body via abrasions in the skin, via the conjunctivae or the gastrointestinal tract or, most commonly, via the respiratory tract. Infection usually occurs in people consuming unpasteurised milk products, and in farmers, abattoir workers and hunters. Pig hunters are often heavily exposed to blood and body fluids during butchering of the animals. There is also a high risk of laboratory-acquired infection by aerosol transmission from an infected specimen. Appropriate infection control procedures must therefore be used when collecting and processing a specimen from a person suspected of having brucellosis.

Pathogenesis and clinical features

Inside the host, *Brucella* enter the lymphatic system and then the blood, causing an acute bacteraemia. They are facultative intracellular parasites and thus multiply within phagocytes in the spleen, liver, bone marrow and other lymphoid tissues. Granulomatous inflammatory reactions and necrosis of tissues may occur, with enlargement of affected organs. Often the infection is subclinical, but in clinical cases the onset of symptoms is gradual and begins one or more weeks after contact. Typical presenting symptoms are night drenching sweats, chills and fever, disabling lethargy, malaise, headache, myalgia and arthralgia. Anorexia and substantial weight loss may occur. Complications such as splenic abscesses, endocarditis, septic arthritis, osteomyelitis and meningitis are possible, especially if diagnosis and treatment are delayed for more than a month after onset of symptoms.

Diagnosis

Diagnosis of brucellosis is by serological tests or culture. Antibody titres are often high and stable at presentation, and thus a diagnostic fourfold increase may not be detected in paired sera. Isolation of the causative organism from blood or bone marrow may be attempted, but is not always successful.

Treatment and prevention

Treatment is with an antibiotic such as doxycycline or ampicillin in combination with a second drug such as

---

CASE HISTORY 19.4
Brucellosis

A 25-year-old Turkish-born woman travelled to Turkey in 1990 where she resided for 11 months. In 1991 she presented to Casualty at a hospital in Sydney with a number of health problems including a vaginal discharge. Blood cultures yielded *Brucella melitensis* biotype 1.

At the microbiology laboratory where the culture was made, staff were scanned for *Brucella* infection. One member, who was asymptomatic, was positive on blood culture. This young woman subsequently miscarried and *B. melitensis* biotype 1 was cultured from placental material.

Adapted from RE Everett, '*Brucella melitensis* in humans', *Communicable Diseases Intelligence* 17/18, 6 September 1993, p. 407.

rifampicin. Because of the organism's intracellular location, it can be difficult to eliminate completely and relapses are common. A prolonged course of therapy for at least six weeks is necessary. At present there is no effective human vaccine. Prevention is based on (1) pasteurisation of dairy products, (2) animal vaccination, (3) education of workers at risk of occupational exposure and (4) the use of protective clothing by at-risk workers.

PLAGUE

Cause and incidence

Few diseases have ravaged the human population throughout time in the way plague has done. Some authorities believe that the first historic mention of the disease is in the Book of Samuel, which describes an epidemic of 'emerods' (buboes?) among the Philistines. Several great pandemics of plague have been recorded. The Black Death, as it was known in the Middle Ages, killed an estimated one-quarter of the population of Europe in the 14th century. The Great Plague of 1665–66 was restricted largely to London and caused more than 75 000 deaths. Even as recently as the beginning of the 20th century, the disease was responsible for 10 million deaths in India alone, in a great pandemic affecting central Asia. Epidemics still occur, especially when preventive measures are not followed – for example, in war-torn Vietnam during the 1960s, as many as 10 000 deaths a year were due to this disease. Nowadays, most cases are restricted to some parts of Asia (e.g. Myanmar, Vietnam, China) and Africa (e.g. Madagascar, Zaire, Uganda). In Australia, as in other developed countries, the disease is rare. The last case recorded in this country was in 1923.

The causative agent of plague is *Yersinia pestis*, a small Gram-negative rod belonging to the family *Enterobacteriaceae*. The organism infects wild rodents, especially rats, and is transmitted from animal to animal and animal to human by flea bites. In epidemics, massive numbers of rats die of the disease and the fleas, deprived of their natural hosts, feed voraciously on humans instead.

Pathogenesis and clinical features

Yersinia pestis possesses a number of virulence factors including an antiphagocytic capsule, a coagulase, endotoxin and various other protein toxins. The organism multiplies rapidly and is able to survive within macrophages. It spreads via the lymphatics to regional lymph nodes. Within 1–7 days of the flea bite a haemorrhagic inflammation causes these nodes to form very large and tender **buboes** (enlarged lymph nodes), hence the term **bubonic plague**. They are most frequently found in the armpit or groin. If the organisms move into the circulatory system, infection, haemorrhage and necrosis occur in many parts of the body, including the skin, lungs, liver, spleen and CNS. The haemorrhages and resultant cyanosis turn the skin black, hence the name 'Black Death'. Fifty per cent of untreated cases of bubonic plague die.

Pneumonic plague occurs when the organism invades the lungs. One to six days after exposure symptoms including fever, chills, headache and myalgia develop, followed by cough, dyspnoea and chest pain. Unlike the bubonic form of the disease, it can be transmitted from person to person via droplets expelled during coughing (see Figure 19.5). The mortality rate is nearly 100% if treatment is delayed more than 24 hours after the onset of symptoms.

Diagnosis, treatment and prevention

Yersinia pestis can be found in fluid aspirated from buboes or in sputum. The organisms can be identified by direct microscopic examination of stained smears or by culture. Antibiotics used for the treatment of plague include streptomycin, gentamicin or doxycycline. Prevention is based on the following:

- rodent and flea control
- strict isolation of infected patients
- quarantine and fumigation of infected ships
- vaccination of workers in endemic areas (boosters are required every six months).

Systemic viral infections

HUMAN IMMUNODEFICIENCY VIRUS INFECTION AND AIDS

In 1981 a new syndrome, subsequently called the **acquired immunodeficiency syndrome (AIDS)**, was first recognised among homosexual men in the United States. It was characterised by the appearance of rare and fatal infections and rare types of cancer. It first appeared in Australia in 1982; by the mid-1980s it was obvious that the disease had spread, largely unnoticed, throughout the world. In 1983 the causative agent was isolated from blood lymphocytes and became known as the human immunodeficiency virus (HIV). The course of the disease varies from person to person but it is estimated that, of untreated people, up to 30% will develop AIDS within five years, and almost all will eventually develop AIDS and die from it. With appropriate treatment, however, the course of the disease is significantly altered.

Causative agents

Two serotypes of HIV have been identified: HIV-1 and HIV-2. The most common cause of AIDS throughout the world is HIV-1. However, HIV-2, which was found initially only in West Africa and predominates there, has been reported to have caused sporadic cases in East Africa, Europe, Asia and Latin America. A very small number of cases of HIV-2 infection have so far been diagnosed in Australia, the first in 1992. The transmission of HIV-2 and the clinical features of infection are similar to those of HIV-1. In this book, HIV will be used to refer to both HIV-1 and HIV-2 unless stated otherwise.

The structure of HIV is shown in Figure 19.6. It is a roughly spherical particle comprising an outer envelope of a bilayer of lipid molecules, originally from the cell membrane of a human cell. The envelope is studded with numerous 'spikes', which are thought to consist of two

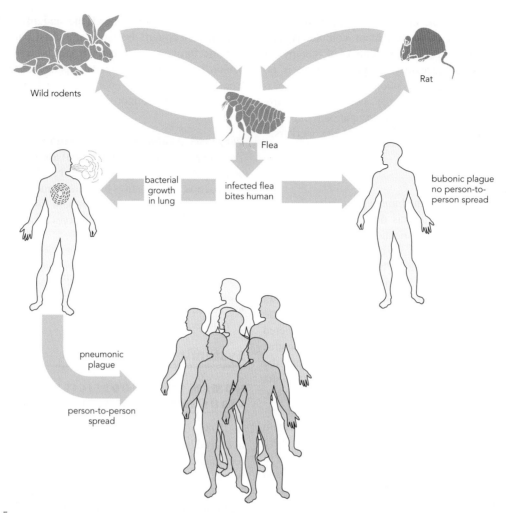

Figure 19.5

The epidemiology of plague

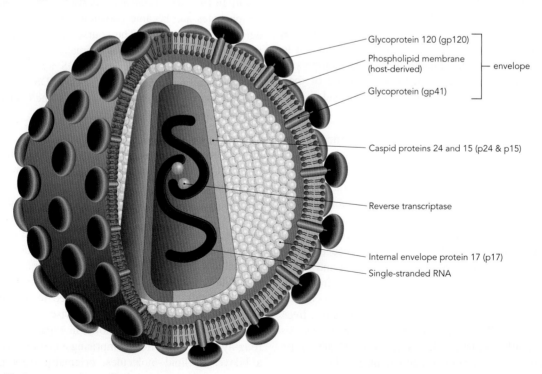

Glycoprotein 120 (gp120)
Phospholipid membrane (host-derived)
Glycoprotein (gp41)
envelope

Caspid proteins 24 and 15 (p24 & p15)

Reverse transcriptase

Internal envelope protein 17 (p17)
Single-stranded RNA

Figure 19.6

The structure of the human immunodeficiency virus (HIV), the causative agent of AIDS

glycoproteins – gp120, which projects out from the envelope, and gp41, which is embedded in the envelope. Beneath the envelope is a layer of protein called p18, which in turn surrounds the capsid (p24 antigen). Since HIV is a retrovirus, its genetic core is in the form of RNA. Inside the capsid there are two single-stranded molecules of RNA. Attached to the RNA are molecules of the enzyme, **reverse transcriptase**, which transcribes the viral RNA into DNA once the virus is inside its host cell. HIV has two other critical enzymes: an **integrase**, which integrates the viral DNA into the host cell DNA, and a **protease**, which cleaves newly produced viral proteins for a proper assembly of new viruses.

Incidence

There are around 40 million cases of HIV infection worldwide, and since the epidemic began there have been more than 20 million deaths. In 2003 there were an estimated 5 million new cases. The vast majority (90%) of people currently infected live in sub-Saharan Africa or in the developing countries of Asia. Currently in Australia there are an estimated 14 000 people with HIV infection. About 150–300 new cases occur annually.

Transmission

Characteristically, in developed countries most HIV infections have occurred in men, primarily as a result of homosexual intercourse or intravenous drug use. However, the difference in numbers of men and women infected is narrowing as transmission by heterosexual intercourse becomes more common. In the Caribbean and some parts of Asia and Africa, transmission has largely been through heterosexual relations and males and females are more or less equally affected. In Australia, sexual contact between men is the major means of transmission (see Figure 19.7). Very low rates of transmission occur through injecting drug use or heterosexual contact. Occupationally acquired infection in health-care workers, due mainly to needlestick injury, is well documented and a definite risk.

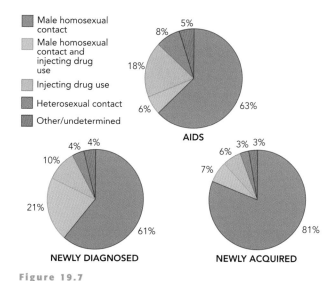

Figure 19.7

AIDS, HIV infection and newly acquired HIV infection, in Australia 1999–2003, by exposure category

Overall, it has been established that HIV is transmitted in three ways:

- through sexual intercourse
- through blood or blood products
- from mother to child.

It has been clearly established that prior genital ulcer disease (any genital infection causing ulceration of genital skin) substantially increases susceptibility to HIV. Thus, a person with syphilis, herpes or chancroid is much more likely to be infected by a sexual partner with the HIV virus than people without these diseases.

The transmission of HIV from mother to child may occur during pregnancy, at delivery, or through breast feeding. Breast feeding is a major way in which children are infected in developing countries. Without any intervention the risk of transmission of HIV infection from infected mother to baby is at least 30%, but this risk drops to under 5% with the use of anti-HIV drugs in the mother.

Pathogenesis

HIV disease results from chronic infection of cells bearing the CD4 antigen. The gp120 envelope protein of the virus can bind tightly to this antigen (Figure 19.8), making several types of immune system cells vulnerable. Helper T lymphocytes (T4 lymphocytes) are the main targets, but activated antigen-presenting cells (dendritic cells, monocytes and macrophages) are also infected. Macrophages may be responsible for transporting the virus to different parts of the body, including the brain. The gp41 protein of the virus attaches to a co-receptor that enables the virus to fuse with the cell membrane and then enter it.

When the virus enters a cell, it uncoats and then, like all retroviruses, transcribes its RNA into DNA using its **reverse transcriptase** enzyme (see Figure 19.9). The DNA is then converted into double-stranded DNA and integrated into the host cell genome using the **integrase** enzyme. Once the viral DNA is integrated, the cell is transformed into a factory for production of more viruses. HIV can replicate at a remarkable rate in an untreated person – around 10 billion virions a day! Complete viruses are released from the surface of infected cells by budding, and they can then infect other target cells. In some cells the HIV DNA is dormant for a time, possibly for decades. Later it may become activated and direct the synthesis of new viral RNA and viral proteins. This long latency period creates a problem with respect to treatment (see later section).

It is well recognised that the HIV causes immunosuppression by infecting and killing or suppressing T4 lymphocytes. The depletion/inhibition of T4 lymphocytes greatly diminishes the ability of the host to produce adequate amounts of antibodies or lymphokines, since functional T4 cells are needed for the initiation of immune responses (see Chapter 9). The patient thus becomes more susceptible to infections and cancers that the healthy immune system would deal with effectively. However, it is recognised that the immunosuppression caused by HIV is

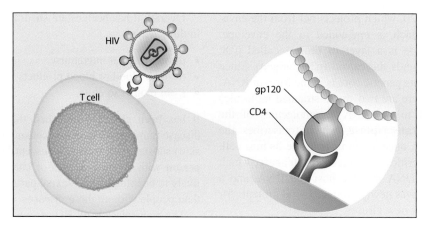

Figure 19.8

Binding of the HIV gp120 protein to the CD4 receptor of the human T lymphocyte

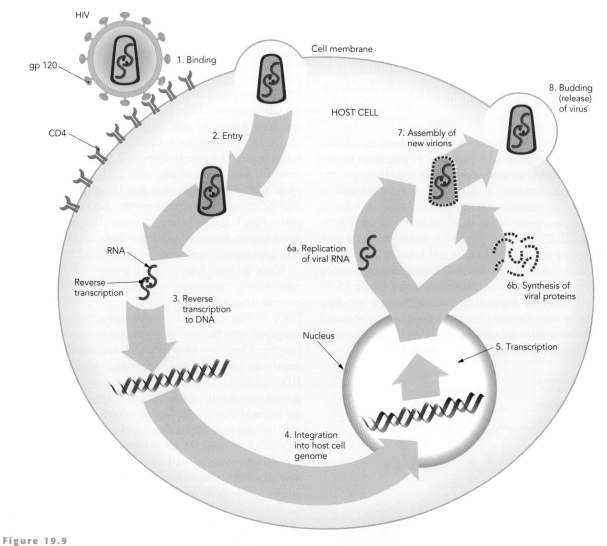

Figure 19.9

Replication cycle of HIV

a complex process, with the virus causing damage to the immune system in a number of ways, including:

- the direct killing of infected T4 cells by the virus
- the destruction of virus-infected immune cells, including T4 cells, by killer T cells

- the prevention of T4 cells responding to foreign antigens through the blocking of cell receptors (CD4) by detached viral proteins gp120 and gp41
- the release of a soluble suppressor factor by infected T4 cells

- the infection and killing or disrupting the function of other cells with the CD4 receptor, especially antigen-presenting cells
- virus-initiated autoimmune response to CD4 receptors and subsequent destruction of cells bearing those antigens.

In addition to immune system damage, the virus attacks the nervous system directly. It has been suggested that infected monocytes carry the virus into the brain. These infected cells are then thought to attack the myelin sheath that coats nerve cells. Damage to the central nervous system also occurs as a result of secondary infection by other microorganisms. The pathogenesis of AIDS is summarised in Figure 19.10.

The immune response to HIV typically (but not always) begins 2–4 weeks after infection. Neutralising antibodies are usually found, as well as a cell-mediated immune response. As the immune response gathers pace, the virus and its components become undetectable and any early clinical manifestations disappear. However, the immune mechanisms do not completely clear the virus, probably because of the weakness of the immune response and dormancy of the virus in some cells. Furthermore, the virus undergoes a high rate of mutation while it is causing infection, changing its antigens and thus allowing it to evade host responses. In fact, a number of different antigenic variants of the virus can often be isolated from a single person. These antigenic variants may evade host defences produced to previous antigenic types.

Clinical features

Current treatment regimes (see later section) significantly alter the course of HIV infection. Highly active antiretroviral therapy (HAART) slows the development of the disease and markedly increases patient survival time. The 'natural' course of the disease – that is, without treatment – is described here.

A wide spectrum of clinical manifestations is possible in an HIV-infected person. The first sign of infection usually occurs 1–3 weeks after infection and is an acute 'mononucleosis-like' illness with fever, headache, pharyngitis, nausea, mild CNS symptoms, mucocutaneous ulcers and a maculopapular rash. A lymphadenopathy may develop in the second week. These symptoms of acute infection occur in only 50–70% of infected people. At this time, substantial viral replication occurs and, as a result, pronounced depression in T4 lymphocyte numbers. Shortly after acute infection most patients undergo seroconversion – that is, produce antibodies. The symptoms subside within a few weeks and there follows a variable period of three years or more of reasonably good health.

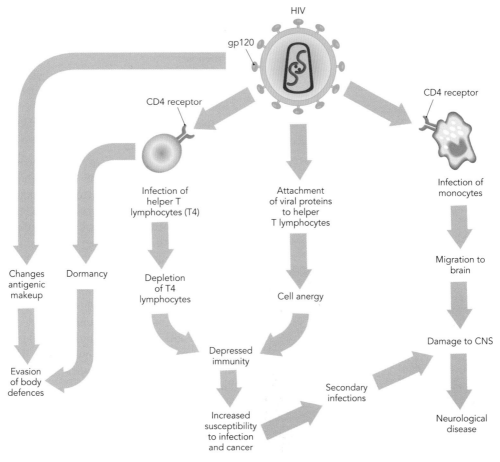

Figure 19.10

The pathogenesis of AIDS

During this stage the rate of viral replication is at a lower and relatively stable level. The T4 cell count generally remains above 500 per μL of blood.

Apparent good health continues because T4 levels remain high enough to prevent infections by other organisms. But over time T4 levels gradually fall. An intermediate phase of T4 cell depletion (200–500 per μL) can be manifested by a variety of minor infections such as pharyngitis, sinusitis, gingivitis, tinea, seborrhoeic dermatitis, warts, reactivation of herpes zoster and oral candidiasis, and symptoms like chronic diarrhoea, fever and weight loss. These infections may persist or increase in severity as the T4 cell count drops towards 200 per μL.

Advanced immune depletion (T4 cell count falling below 200 per μL) heralds the likelihood of developing an AIDS-defining infection or malignancy. At this stage the person is said to have AIDS. The common AIDS-defining diseases are listed in Table 19.4.

The microorganisms that cause secondary infections in people with AIDS are typically opportunistic pathogens; that is, they have low pathogenicity and only rarely cause infection in the general population. The most common secondary diseases in AIDS patients are *Pneumocystis jiroveci* pneumonia and Kaposi's sarcoma (see Figure 19.11), but many other diseases can occur including disseminated mycobacterial infections, toxoplasma encephalitis, cryptococcal meningitis, cytomegalovirus retinitis and non-Hodgkin's lymphoma (see Table 19.4). Once such diseases appear, death usually occurs in a year or two.

Infection with HIV can result in a large number of neurological manifestations throughout the course of the disease. These result from direct infection by HIV of the nervous system, secondary opportunistic infections and neoplasms involving the central nervous system, or a combination of these. Some of the more common manifestations are aseptic meningitis, peripheral neuropathy, recurrent seizures and the AIDS dementia complex (also referred to as HIV encephalopathy, HIV encephalitis, HIV dementia). The AIDS dementia complex is characterised by progressive cognitive dysfunction and motor and behavioural disorders.

Progression from HIV infection to AIDS occurs in approximately 50% of untreated people within 10 years. It was once thought that almost all untreated people would eventually die of AIDS. However, there is increasing evidence that some infected people do not develop clinical disease for an extended period of time. The lack of disease progression may be due to lower pathogenicity in certain strains of HIV.

The progress of the disease can be assessed by counting the number of T4 cells in blood and by assaying the viral load in the blood. Monitoring progress of the disease is useful for the following reasons:

- to provide the patient with a short- and long-term prognosis
- to help to determine the most appropriate time to begin treatment and chemoprophylaxis for opportunistic infections
- to monitor the effectiveness of anti-HIV treatment.

Laboratory diagnosis

The laboratory diagnosis of HIV infection most often involves the detection of anti-HIV antibodies in serum. Antibodies are usually detected in the first 2–4 weeks of infection, although in some people a 'window period' of three months or more occurs between infection and antibody production. ELISA (enzyme linked immunosorbent assay, see Chapter 15) is the most frequently used screening test for anti-HIV antibodies. Recently, several simple/rapid assays have been developed that allow a screening result to be obtained within hours, and without the need for elaborate laboratory equipment. Confirmation of positive results is done with more specific assays, such as the Western blot or Line immunoassay. This test detects and identifies specific antibodies against certain protein components of the virus.

One of the problems with these antibody tests is that the antibody-negative (window) period may be as long as several months in some infected people; so the diagnosis in these cases would be delayed. Also, the significance of antibodies in neonates born to HIV-infected mothers is not always clear. Antibodies passively transferred from

Table 19.4	
Percentage of people with AIDS who have specific AIDS-defining illnesses	
AIDS-DEFINING ILLNESS	PERCENTAGE
Pneumocystis jiroveci pneumonia (PCP)	35
Kaposi's sarcoma (KS)	15
Oesophageal candidiasis	10
HIV wasting disease	6
Atypical *Mycobacterium* infection	5
Cytomegalovirus	< 5
HIV encephalopathy	< 5
Cryptococcosis	< 5
Non-Hodgkin's lymphoma	< 5
Cerebral toxoplasmosis	< 5
Herpes simplex virus	< 5
Cryptosporidiosis	< 5

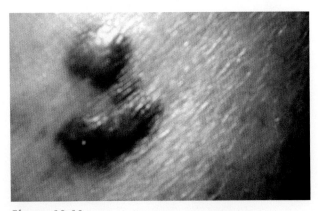

Figure 19.11

The purplish skin lesions of Kaposi's sarcoma

mother to foetus can remain in the infant's circulation for more than 12 months, making a serological diagnosis of infection very difficult.

As a result, a number of other diagnostic tests for HIV infection have been developed to supplement the antibody-detection methods. Assays for the detection of viral antigens in serum (e.g. HIV-1 p24 antigen test) are useful, since HIV antigens can, in some cases, be detected during the window period, in advanced disease when antibodies may not be detectable, and in infected neonates. As stated earlier, tests for detecting and assaying viral load in blood are now available. A polymerase chain reaction (PCR) test for HIV RNA is particularly useful because it can detect levels as low as 300 copies of RNA per millilitre of plasma and can quantitate the amount of viral RNA present. This test is the most accurate predictor of HIV disease progression.

Treatment

There has been substantial progress in the use of chemotherapeutic agents for treatment of HIV infection. The drugs that have been developed can be grouped into three main types.

1. The nucleoside reverse transcriptase inhibitors (e.g. zidovudine (AZT), lamivudine) compete with nucleosides during reverse transcription of viral RNA into DNA, thereby terminating reverse transcription before it is complete.
2. Non-nucleoside reverse transcriptase inhibitors (e.g. nevirapine) target the same viral enzyme and bind directly to it, changing its conformation and reducing its function.
3. The protease inhibitors (e.g. ritonavir) target the protease enzyme that the virus uses for splitting of viral proteins in the final stages of assembly of new virus particles.

All these drugs are designed to prevent viral multiplication inside target cells. Some of the drugs in current use are listed in Table 19.5.

Each of these drugs has some activity in HIV infection, but their effectiveness usually wanes with time as the virus develops increasing resistance to them. A major advance in the treatment of HIV infection came with the practice of using three of these drugs in combination. Combination therapy, called 'highly active antiretroviral therapy' (HAART), involves the use of several drugs together. The combination is typically a protease inhibitor plus at least two drugs from the other two classes. HAART has led to substantial reductions in morbidity and mortality related to HIV infection. The effectiveness of treatment is variable, but in many people there is a marked decrease in viral load, a significant improvement in T4 count, a reduced rate of disease progression, decreased incidence of AIDS-related opportunistic infections and increased survival time. Also, drug resistance is less likely to arise when combination therapy is used. This therapy prevents viral replication but does not appear to eliminate HIV from the

body. Dormant HIV DNA in cells is not affected by the drugs and, therefore, once therapy is stopped it is possible that a reactivation of the virus can occur. For this reason, combination therapy must be continued for years, perhaps indefinitely.

The effectiveness of therapy is monitored by measuring HIV viral load in plasma and the T4 cell count.

When combination therapy fails it is usually due to incomplete patient compliance and/or development of viral drug resistance. Non-compliance is a common problem because side effects of the drugs can be unpleasant to severe, and the daily requirement of taking as many as 16 or more pills is difficult for some people to maintain over a long period. Drug resistance most often develops as a result of non-compliance or in patients who have received single drug therapy (before HAART). Unfortunately, drug therapy is not widely available in underdeveloped countries, where it is needed most, due to cost.

Prevention

Numerous measures have been introduced to reduce the spread of HIV infection in the community. In Australia, preventive measures that have been adopted include:

- screening of blood donors for HIV and discouragement of people in high-risk groups from donating blood
- heat treatment of blood products (e.g. factor VIII for haemophiliacs)
- public education programs encouraging safe sex practices (e.g. use of condoms) and discouraging promiscuous behaviour
- public education programs about the dangers of sharing needles, and programs for the free distribution of clean needles and syringes
- drug therapy at the time of delivery, caesarean birth and formula feeding of the baby to reduce risk of transmission from mother to baby.

Table 19.5

Antiretroviral drugs

Nucleoside reverse transcriptase inhibitors
- abacavir
- didanosine
- lamivudine
- stavudine
- zalcitabine
- zidovudine (AZT)

Non-nucleoside reverse transcriptase inhibitors
- delaviridine
- efavirenz
- nevirapine

Protease inhibitors
- indinavir
- nelfinavir
- ritonavir
- saquinavir

To reduce the chance of infection in health-care staff, measures include:

- adoption of Standard Precautions procedures (see Chapter 13) in health-care institutions
- elimination of the practice of resheathing needles
- disposal of sharps in rigid containers
- use of gloves and masks by certain health professionals (e.g. dentists)
- use of disposable mouthpieces, resuscitation bags and other devices for resuscitation.

Post-exposure prophylaxis with antiretroviral drugs, if given early enough (within 72 hours of exposure), significantly reduces (by about 80%) the risk of infection following occupational exposure to HIV.

Despite intensive and ongoing efforts to develop a vaccine, none is yet available. The ability of the virus to mutate rapidly and the inability of the immune system to halt HIV infection pose serious obstacles to the development of useful vaccines.

ROSS RIVER VIRUS INFECTION

Cause, incidence and transmission

Ross River fever is the most important arbovirus (**ar**thropod-**bo**rne **virus**) infection in Australia. It is caused by the Ross River virus, an alphavirus of the family *Togaviridae*. The disease was first described in 1928 as an 'unusual epidemic' in Narrandera, New South Wales. It was later called **epidemic polyarthritis**, a term that is now used to describe infections caused by several different viruses. Isolation of the virus was first achieved in 1963 from a mosquito caught on the Ross River in Northern Queensland.

A less common virus that can also cause epidemic polyarthritis in Australia is the Barmah Forest virus, which causes a disease similar to the Ross River virus and is also spread by mosquitoes.

Annual notifications of Ross River virus infection in Australia are variable, ranging from 1500 to 8500 per year (see Figure 19.12). The highest rates of notification occur in the northern parts of the country (see Figure 19.13). Being a mosquito-borne disease, it predominates in regions with a

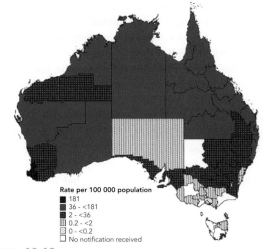

Figure 19.13

Notification rates of Ross River virus infection in Australia in 2003, by statistical division of residence
Source: Communicable Diseases Intelligence, 2005, 29(1), p. 46, © Commonwealth of Australia, reproduced by permission

warmer climate and higher rainfall, although it does occur throughout the country, including Tasmania. Although infection has been mainly in rural areas, a significant number of cases now occur in the major metropolitan areas of Australia. There are clusters of cases of Ross River virus infection every summer, but when mosquitoes reach plague proportions significant outbreaks may occur. The virus has been isolated from more than ten different species of mosquito from different regions in the country, explaining its country-wide incidence. There is concern that, with global warming, expanding mosquito populations could increase the incidence of this and other mosquito-borne diseases.

Clinical features, diagnosis and treatment

The intensity of Ross River virus infection varies considerably, with only approximately 30% of people seeking medical advice. Symptoms usually start to appear 3–21 days after being bitten by an infected mosquito. The main manifestation is arthritis, with morning joint stiffness, although a maculopapular rash, lethargy and flu-like symptoms are also common. The symptoms wax and wane, usually lasting a few weeks. The arthritic symptoms

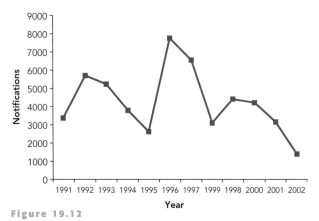

Figure 19.12

Notifications of Ross River virus infections in Australia, 1991 to 2002
Source: Communicable Diseases Intelligence, 2004, 28(1), p. 51, © Commonwealth of Australia, reproduced by permission

SPOTLIGHT ON
Ross River virus

In 2002, Tasmania reported 117 cases of Ross River virus (RRV) infections. This was the largest number of infections ever recorded for the state in a year. Thirty-seven of the cases had lived in, or visited, the Sorell Municipal Area, 25 km east of Hobart. In early 2002 a combination of spring tides and high summer rainfall created extensive salt marshes in the Sorell region, resulting in high densities of the mosquito *Ochlerotatus camptorhynchus*. This mosquito is a recognised vector for RRV. This is the furthest south that RRV has been found in Australia.

and lethargy sometimes persist for more than three months. Complete recovery may take 12 months or more, but there is no residual damage to joints. Symptomatic adults may not be able to work for a month or more, particularly if their work involves heavy physical activity.

Laboratory diagnosis of the disease is by serology. Detecting a fourfold increase in paired sera is the definitive method. Detection of specific IgM antibody in a single serum sample may provide a positive diagnosis, but does not absolutely indicate recent infection. At present, only symptomatic treatment (e.g. an anti-inflammatory drug for arthritis) is possible. Prevention is based on avoidance of mosquito bites, especially during epidemics.

DENGUE FEVER

Cause, incidence and transmission

Dengue virus is a flavivirus with four different serotypes. **Dengue fever** is a globally important infection, especially in tropical areas, and to a lesser extent the subtropics. Globally, there are an estimated 50–100 million cases per year. In Australia fewer than 200 cases are usually reported each year except when epidemics occur; several hundred cases may be reported in epidemic years (such as 1992, 1993 and 1998). The majority of cases are reported in Queensland. Dengue is only locally transmitted in northern Australia; all other cases are acquired overseas. The mosquito *Aedes aegypti* is the principal human vector.

Clinical features and complications

After an incubation period of 8–10 days, the disease is characterised by high fever, headache and a rash. Severe muscle and joint pain is also common, hence its other name, 'breakbone fever'. Except for its painful symptoms, dengue fever is a relatively mild and self-limiting disease that usually lasts about 10 days. A much more serious form of dengue, called **dengue haemorrhagic fever**, is characterised by high fever, bleeding from the gums, skin and gastrointestinal tract, and sometimes circulatory failure, shock and death.

The pathogenesis of dengue haemorrhagic fever is shown in Figure 19.14. After dengue virus infection, antibodies specific for the particular serotype are formed. If subsequently infected with a different serotype, it is thought that the preformed antibodies bind to the virus, but fail to neutralise it. The antibodies actually enhance viral infection of monocytes, by first binding with the virus and then attaching to Fc receptors on the monocyte membrane. Increased infection of monocytes is thought to induce an increased release of cytokines, leading to vascular damage and shock. Thus, dengue haemorrhagic fever becomes a possibility when dengue already exists in a region and subsequently a different serotype is introduced there.

Diagnosis, treatment and prevention

Diagnosis is often based on clinical and epidemiological grounds. Epidemics of dengue tend to be focal in nature, affecting the population in a fairly circumscribed geographical area. A serological diagnosis is most common, and there are several tests available for the detection of either the virus or specific antibodies. Confirmation may

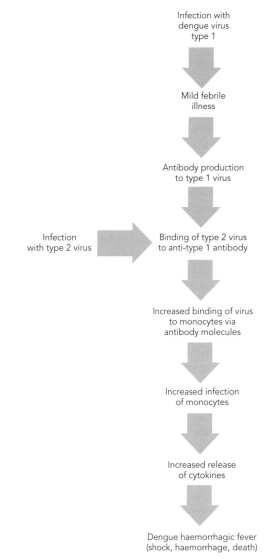

Figure 19.14

The pathogenesis of dengue haemorrhagic fever
There are four serotypes of dengue virus – types 1 and 2 have been used in this example.

be sought with a reverse transcriptase polymerase chain reaction (RT-PCR) or virus isolation. No specific antiviral therapy is currently available, although with intensive supportive therapy mortality is significantly reduced. No effective vaccine for dengue exists. One of the problems with vaccine development is that antibodies produced to a vaccine may predispose the individual to dengue haemorrhagic fever. Prevention is therefore based on mosquito control programs and disease surveillance.

INFECTIOUS MONONUCLEOSIS

Cause, incidence and transmission

Infectious mononucleosis, or **glandular fever**, is caused by a herpes virus called Epstein-Barr virus (EBV). In less developed parts of the world it is usually acquired in early childhood, whereas in developed countries a higher incidence occurs in teenagers and young adults (see Figure 19.15). The usual route of infection is by transfer of saliva – for example, by sharing drinking vessels or eating implements, or by kissing – it is sometimes referred to as

SPOTLIGHT ON
Dengue fever in East Timor personnel

Dengue fever, although not endemic in the region, is an important public health concern in north Queensland because *Aedes aegypti*, the mosquito vector, is present. Any importation of dengue (via a viraemic individual) could potentially result in local transmission and initiate an outbreak.

In late 1999 the Tropical Public Health Unit (TPHU) was informed that personnel who had been in East Timor would soon be returning in considerable numbers to Townsville. The majority had been serving as part of the Australian Defence Force. Because cases of dengue fever had been reported in East Timor in 1999, a high level of importation of dengue into Townsville early in 2000 was anticipated.

A number of measures were introduced aimed at preventing local transmission and, hence, an outbreak of dengue fever. Defence Force medical staff were familiarised with the notification procedures with emphasis on early notification. Notification was requested for any person developing a dengue-like illness within 12 days before, or 14 days after, arriving in Townsville from East Timor. Medical practitioners in Townsville were also alerted to the situation and reminded of the need for urgent notification of suspected cases. TPHU staff obtained a history from each suspected case of dengue. To reduce the possibility of local transmission of dengue, patients were provided with information on mosquito bite avoidance during the day, and advice on measures to reduce mosquito breeding around the home.

Mosquito control measures were undertaken including inspections and source reduction at Defence Force bases and around other high risk areas (e.g. hospitals). Additional mosquito control measures were undertaken if a case, suspected or confirmed, had apparently been viraemic in Townsville. Larval control involved source reduction in premises within 200 metres of any residence (and other premises) where the case had spent significant amounts of time while viraemic. Adult *Aedes aegypti* control involved interior insecticide spraying of premises within 100 metres of the case.

Approximately 2000 personnel returned from East Timor to Townsville in the first few months of 2000. Over a five-week period there were seven confirmed importations of dengue fitting the 'viraemic' time interval described to be of public health importance. Despite this intense period of multiple importations into the area, no subsequent local transmission of dengue occurred in Townsville.

Source: Hills S et al., 2000, 'Public health implications of dengue in personnel returning from East Timor', *Communicable Diseases Intelligence* 24(12), p. 365.

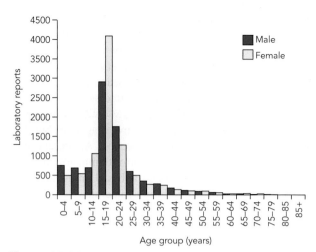

Figure 19.15

Notifications of Epstein-Barr virus infections in Australia, 1991 to 2000, by age and sex
Source: Communicable Diseases Intelligence, 2002, 26(3), p. 347, © Commonwealth of Australia, reproduced by permission

the 'kissing disease'. The virus may be shed intermittently in saliva for many years after infection.

Pathogenesis and clinical features

After entering the body via the oropharynx, the virus invades a number of organs such as the lung, parotid glands and various lymphoid organs, where it specifically infects B lymphocytes. The virus causes B cell proliferation, which may account for the excess of lymphocytes in the infected person. It is also thought to interfere with B cell and T cell interactions. After an incubation period of 5–6 weeks, mild symptoms of fever, headache, fatigue and malaise develop, which gradually worsen. Most patients develop a sore throat several days later, and after about a week the illness reaches its peak. The tonsils may be coated with a whitish-grey exudate and there may be inflammation of the rest of the pharynx. Palatal petechiae, swollen cervical and axillary lymph nodes, splenomegaly and hepatitis are also common. The virus establishes a lifelong latency in B cells.

Diagnosis and treatment

The clinical diagnosis of infectious mononucleosis is complicated by the fact that it resembles other systemic diseases like toxoplasmosis and cytomegalovirus infections. The name 'mononucleosis' refers to lymphocytes with abnormal morphology, and these can usually be found in a differential white cell count. Serologic tests for antibodies provide the most specific diagnosis. Bed rest and symptomatic treatment are the basis of management of the disease. No vaccine is available.

Complications

The Epstein-Barr virus has been implicated in a number of different malignancies. Its association with Burkitt's lymphoma, B cell lymphomas in immunodeficient patients, Hodgkin's disease and nasopharyngeal carcinoma is well recognised. However, its part in the development of these tumours is not fully understood. The virus has also been implicated in **chronic fatigue syndrome**. People with this condition often have a history of an initial viral-like illness. Excessive fatigue, to the extent of having difficulty in performing routine tasks, and general malaise are the main complaints. Other non-specific symptoms include fever, muscle weakness and headaches. Patients often complain of great debility, worsened by physical exertion, but otherwise may be quite well. Symptoms may last for three months or more. It is likely that other viruses, such as other herpes viruses, are also responsible for this condition.

Laboratory investigations in chronic fatigue syndrome are often remarkably normal, so diagnosis is usually based on clinical grounds and the exclusion of other causes. Bed rest is essential, together with symptomatic treatment. Attempts to exercise back to health are not recommended.

CYTOMEGALOVIRUS INFECTION

The majority of cytomegalovirus (CMV) infections occur in childhood and are often asymptomatic. In older children and adults, a mild malaise, fever, myalgia and lymph node inflammation may occur. The virus is not fully cleared from the body and establishes a lifelong, latent infection.

Transplacental transmission of CMV to the foetus may occur from a mother experiencing a primary or a reactivated infection. This leads to spread of the virus to multiple organs and a severe illness characterised by one or more of the following in the neonate: low birth weight, microcephaly, hepatosplenomegaly, growth retardation, impaired vision, hearing loss and haemolytic anaemia. Mortality among symptomatic neonates may be as high as 30% within the first few months of life. Some babies infected *in utero* may not show signs of infection at birth, but later develop mental or sensory disorders representing the neurological damage that the virus has caused.

CMV is also responsible for severe disseminated infections in the immunocompromised – such as people with AIDS, cancer patients (especially those with leukaemia or lymphoma) and organ transplant recipients. Infections in these patients may be due to primary infection by the virus from an exogenous source, or to the reactivation of latent virus. The virus may infect any organ but most often causes pneumonia, encephalitis, hepatitis or a sight-threatening retinitis.

CMV has been found in most body fluids, including saliva, urine, blood, breast milk, semen and cervical secretions, and thus can be transmitted in a variety of ways. It is usually spread by close contact but also by blood transfusions, organ transplants and during sexual intercourse. Shedding of the virus may occur intermittently for many months after infection, adding to its transmissibility.

PCR assays have become the routine methods for diagnosis of CMV infections. Blood or urine are most commonly tested. Culture of the virus from a body fluid may take up to six weeks and is thus too slow for clinical use. Serological testing on paired sera, taken two weeks apart, may be performed, but is not a useful method for immunocompromised patients.

Ganciclovir, foscarnet or cidofovir have been used in CMV-infected patients with some success. Pregnant health-care workers should be informed of the risk of infection and should not have contact with known cases. There is no vaccine for CMV registered in Australia.

FIFTH DISEASE (SLAPPED CHEEK DISEASE OR *ERYTHEMA INFECTIOSUM*)

Fifth disease is a common cause of rash in childhood caused by parvovirus B19. In children it is a mild illness characterised initially by flu-like symptoms with pyrexia, headache, myalgia and chills, and about a week later the typical rash on the cheeks, giving the slapped cheek appearance. The rash may then extend to the trunk and limbs and may fade and reappear over several weeks. In adults, especially women, infection is more often characterised by an arthralgia that can affect any joint but usually the wrist, hand, knee and ankle. Transmission is by the respiratory route and maximal infectivity is in the week before the rash appears. Epidemics are thought to occur in Australia every 2–3 years, although the majority of infected children are asymptomatic in outbreaks. Foetal infection is largely benign, but is occasionally severe, especially if infection occurs in the first 20 weeks of gestation. Foetal death occurs in a small percentage (< 1%) of cases. Diagnosis of fifth disease is generally by detection of specific IgM antibodies in serum. There is no specific treatment for fifth disease, and symptomatic treatment is only occasionally warranted.

HAND, FOOT AND MOUTH DISEASE

Hand, foot and mouth disease has a worldwide distribution, occurring in sporadic and epidemic forms. Children under 10 years are most commonly affected. Outbreaks have been reported in Malaysia, Singapore, Taiwan and Australia, most often occurring in schools and child care centres. A number of viruses cause this disease, including coxsackie A virus (A16), enterovirus 71 (EV71) and a number of other coxsackie A and B virus subtypes.

Hand, foot and mouth disease usually begins with a fever, sore throat and anorexia. One to two days later, vesicles begin to appear on the gums, palate and tongue. These painful lesions eventually blister and may ulcerate. A papular-vesicular skin rash on the palms, fingers (see Figure 19.16), toes, soles of the feet and buttocks is also characteristic. Meningoencephalitis is a rare feature of the illness, although in some outbreaks it is common. This more serious form of the disease may be associated with significant morbidity and mortality. Generally, however, hand, foot and mouth disease is a self-limiting illness that lasts one to two weeks.

The disease is highly infectious. The virus is shed in faeces and saliva, and from skin blisters of infected people. So transmission is usually by direct contact or droplet spread. The virus can be transmitted to the foetus, particularly if the mother is infected late in pregnancy. Foetal infection may be severe, including meningoencephalitis, cardiomyopathy and hepatitis.

Diagnosis is usually based on clinical findings. Virus

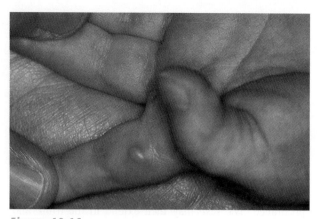

Figure 19.16

Hand, foot and mouth disease
A distinctive blister on the finger.

isolation or PCR testing of appropriate specimens may be undertaken, but are rarely warranted. Symptomatic treatment (e.g. providing relief for painful oral lesions) is usually all that is required. Antiviral drugs may be used in severe infections but there is little evidence of their effectiveness.

YELLOW FEVER

Yellow fever virus is a flavivirus restricted to parts of Central and South America and Africa, where it is endemic. It is transmitted to humans by the mosquito *Aedes aegypti*. It causes an acute disease characterised by sudden onset of fever, vomiting and prostration 3–6 days after infection. Progression to extensive haemorrhagic manifestations and jaundice (yellowing of the skin), leading to coma and death occurs in about 15% of infected people. Mortality in non-indigenous people may be as high as 50%. There is no specific treatment.

No case of yellow fever has been recorded in Australia, but the *A. aegypti* mosquito is present in North Queensland. So quarantine precautions to prevent introduction of the virus into Australia are very important.

Preventive measures include protection from mosquito bites, and vaccination. The vaccine contains a live, attenuated strain of the virus and is highly effective. It is recommended for travellers to high-risk areas, and in some countries it is mandatory for visitors. Any person over the age of 12 months who is not immunocompromised, but who has been in or passed through an infected area six days before arrival in Australia, must have a current International Certificate of Vaccination against yellow fever. This is aimed at preventing the introduction and establishment of the disease in this country, where the *Aedes* vector mosquito is widespread.

HAEMORRHAGIC FEVERS

Haemorrhagic fevers have received substantial attention in recent years. They are caused by a number of different viruses, including the dengue fever virus and yellow fever virus described above. Other viruses that have been associated with the haemorrhagic fever syndrome include

Lassa fever virus, Hantaan virus (Korean haemorrhagic fever), Marburg virus and Ebola virus. These viruses tend to have a specific geographical distribution (e.g. Africa for the Marburg and Ebola viruses). Humans are not the natural reservoir of haemorrhagic fever viruses. The normal hosts are animals (especially rodents) or insects (e.g. mosquitoes). Humans are infected when they come into contact with infected hosts, although some types can spread from human to human by secretions, blood or tissues (e.g. Ebola and Marburg viruses). The natural hosts of the Ebola and Marburg viruses are not presently known.

Although these viruses differ in terms of their sources, modes of transmission or mechanisms for producing disease, they are grouped together on the basis of some common clinical manifestations. Typically, patients suffer from fever, malaise, myalgia, prostration, multisystem involvement, and widespread haemorrhage due to endothelial cell damage. Severely affected patients may show signs of bleeding under the skin or from body orifices like the mouth, eyes or ears. Severe infection can lead to shock, nervous system malfunction and death.

Ebola virus (see Figure 19.17) is a member of the filovirus family. The natural reservoir of the virus is not known, but in outbreaks the main form of transmission is person-to-person contact via body fluids (e.g. blood, semen, saliva, mucus). There is no known treatment for Ebola haemorrhagic fever, apart from supportive therapy, and it has a fatality rate of 50–90%. In recorded outbreaks, health-care workers have often been infected (see Spotlight box, page 471). Marburg virus is related to the Ebola virus and has a 20–50% fatality rate.

Systemic fungal infections

The frequency of disseminated (systemic) fungal infections has increased substantially in recent years. The majority of these infections occur in immunocompromised

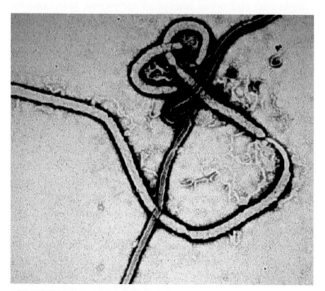

Figure 19.17

Ebola virus
A transmission electron micrograph.

An outbreak of Ebola haemorrhagic fever occurred in Uganda between October 2000 and January 2001. The last reported case was a woman who fell ill on 11 January 2001 and was cleared of infection on 16 January. On 8 February the World Health Organization indicated that the outbreak was probably over, given that no new cases had been reported in the previous 21 days, which is the maximum incubation period for the disease. The outbreak was centred around the northern district of Gulu. In all there were 426 cases, with 173 deaths. At least 14 medical/nursing staff were among the fatalities. The original source of infection is unknown, but person-to-person transmission occurs via blood, semen, saliva and other body fluids. The heavy demands on health-care workers during the outbreak undoubtedly meant that infection control procedures were not fully observed. The spread of the virus in the community may have been aided by the nature of traditional funerals in many parts of Uganda. At these funerals, the body of the deceased is washed and mourners later dip their hands in the water.

hosts, reflecting the impact of organ transplantation, intensive cancer chemotherapy and the HIV epidemic. The most commonly occurring infections are candidiasis, aspergillosis and cryptococcosis.

Candidiasis is the most frequent fungal infection among immunocompromised patients. Unlike the other opportunistic fungi, *Candida* spp. are part of the endogenous flora of humans. *Candida albicans* is the most common species causing infection, but non-albicans species, which are relatively resistant to antifungal agents, have emerged in the last decade as significant pathogens. The latter include *C. tropicalis*, *C. glabrata*, *C. parapsilosis*, *C. krusei* and *C. lusitaniae*. Disseminated candidiasis occurs primarily in organ transplant recipients and neutropenic patients.

Invasive aspergillosis has emerged as an important infection. Most infections occur in patients with neutropenia or in those receiving adrenal corticosteroids, which interfere with macrophage function. Several species are pathogenic, but *Aspergillus fumigatus* is the predominant cause. Most infections are acquired by inhalation of spores and therefore involve the lung. Haematogenous dissemination occurs in around 40% of infections, and the central nervous system is a common secondary site of infection, resulting in irreversible cerebral infarction. The gastrointestinal tract may also be involved, especially the oesophagus and large bowel, which may lead to perforation or massive haemorrhage.

Cryptococcus neoformans is found in the environment worldwide, especially associated with the excreta of pigeons and some other birds. Serotypes A and D (*C. neoformans* var. *neoformans*) cause most infections in immunocompromised hosts, particularly in AIDS patients, but patients with chronic lymphocytic leukaemia, Hodgkin's disease, sarcoidosis, diabetes mellitus and organ transplantation are also susceptible. *C. neoformans* is acquired by inhalation of organisms into the lung. In the absence of adequate host defences the organism disseminates and meningoencephalitis is the most common infection. Other sites of infection include the skin, bone, prostate, liver and eye.

Diagnosis of disseminated fungal disease is difficult. Signs and symptoms are non-specific, colonisation is difficult to distinguish from invasion, and blood cultures are often negative. Amphotericin B has been the mainstay of therapy, but it is not always effective. Treatment failure is usually related to the severity of the patients' underlying diseases, poor organ function, impaired host defences or inadequate dosing (due to the drug's toxicity). Azoles (e.g. fluconazole, voriconazole) are a group of newer antifungal drugs that are less toxic and at least as effective as amphotericin B.

Systemic protozoal infections

Although only a few protozoa cause systemic infections in humans, some are very important in terms of the number of people affected and the severity of the disease they cause. Malaria, in particular, continues to be a major problem in many areas of the world.

MALARIA

Incidence

Current estimates suggest there are 300–500 million cases of malaria each year, with an annual death toll of 2–3 million, mainly in children. Malaria occurs over most of the tropical and some subtropical regions of the world. The vast majority of infections and deaths occur in Africa, India, Brazil, Afghanistan, Sri Lanka, Thailand, Indonesia, Cambodia and China. For more than 30 years the World Health Organization (WHO) has been trying to control malaria. In 1998 the WHO, the United Nations Children's Fund (UNICEF), the United Nations Development Program (UNDP) and the World Bank formed the Roll Back Malaria Partnership. Despite the efforts of these formidable organisations, the worldwide malaria problem has not significantly improved, mainly because of increasing drug resistance, increasing resistance of vector mosquitoes to insecticides, deterioration of national control programs and migration and tourism. Malaria hits the poorer countries the hardest, where expensive drugs are least likely to be affordable. The extent of the problem is clearly illustrated in the Spotlight box on malaria on the next page.

Although Australia was certified free of indigenous (endemic) malaria by the WHO in 1981, environmental conditions in areas of Australia north of latitude 18°S (Townsville to north of Port Hedland) favour the transmission of the disease if the parasites are reintroduced. The malaria-receptive zone coincides with the distribution of the most important malaria vector in Australia – the

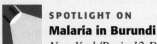

SPOTLIGHT ON
Malaria in Burundi
New York/Paris 12 December 2000

Burundi is currently suffering a malaria epidemic of unprecedented proportion; more than six of the country's 16 provinces are affected. More than 720 000 cases were registered in the country in November, including 60 435 new cases in the province of Kayanza (which has a population of approximately 510 000 people) and more than 46 000 in the area of Musema, the most affected part of the province. The mortality rates are alarming. A survey carried out by Doctors Without Borders/ Medecins Sans Frontieres (MSF) in this sector between 13 October and 6 December 2000 evaluated the mortality rate of children under five at 3.8 for 10 000 people per day, well above the emergency threshold of 2 for 10 000 per day. The figures show that 1000 people died from malaria during this period, half of them children under five.

In collaboration with the Burundian health authorities, MSF is working in three provinces that have been particularly affected – Kayanza, Ngozi and Karuzi – that is, a total population of 1.4 million people. The teams diagnose and treat patients as well as provide drugs and materials to 16 health centres in these provinces. 'Our teams are faced with a huge influx of people presenting signs of malaria,' explains Colette Gadenne, head of mission for MSF in Burundi. 'In the health centre of Muhanga alone, there are up to 600 patients a day. The Burundian medical staff is overwhelmed and many centres have run out of anti-malarial drugs.'

Since the beginning of the epidemic, it is mainly adults who come to the health centres. 'Many children may have died from lack of timely treatment,' adds Colette Gadenne. Eight mobile teams have been set up around 20 sites to improve access to health care in the provinces of Kayanza, Ngozi and Karuzi. Each team treats a minimum of 200 patients a day. A vector control program has also been set up in Kayanza: 9000 houses spread over 27 hills are to be sprayed with insecticide in December by a team of over 100 people. Two thousand houses will likewise be sprayed in the province of Karuzi and 15 000 impregnated mosquito nets will be distributed.

There is great concern at the renewed outbreaks of malaria in Burundi: last year there were over 2 million cases (for 6 million inhabitants), compared with 200 000 cases ten years ago. The current epidemic has erupted in medium to low endemic areas. The population is therefore less immune, which explains the explosion of the number of cases and the high mortality. The development of planting in marshland in which vector mosquitoes proliferate, the stopping of vector control programs and the probable resistance to chloroquine may explain this epidemic.

The protocols adopted are chloroquine/fansidar for simple cases of malaria and quinine for severe malaria. However, in the context of this epidemic, MSF requests the support of the World Health Organization (WHO) and its Roll Back Malaria Department in the use of combination therapies based on artemisinine derivatives. These associations could offer more effective and more rapid treatment and are better adapted to control the epidemic.

MSF has been present in Burundi since 1992. The MSF teams have been reinforced to cover this epidemic. There are currently 24 volunteers and 400 national staff working in three provinces.

Source: Medecins Sans Frontieres, press release, December 2000.

---

mosquito species *Anopheles farauti*. Therefore, malaria can be locally acquired in Australia, but is rare. The great majority of cases are imported from overseas. The highest-risk countries for travellers arriving in or returning to Australia are the Solomon Islands, Papua New Guinea, Africa and India. About 400–1000 notifications of malaria are made in Australia each year.

Causative organisms and transmission

The protozoa that cause malaria are sporozoans belonging to the genus *Plasmodium* (see Figure 19.18). There are four species that cause human malaria: *Plasmodium falciparum*, *P. vivax*, *P. malariae* and *P. ovale*. Falciparum and vivax malaria are the most common. Both cause significant morbidity, but only *P. falciparum* causes significant mortality. The protozoa are transmitted to humans by species of *Anopheles* mosquitoes. Malaria can also be transmitted by blood transfusion or needlestick injury, although these modes of transmission are rare in non-endemic regions.

A knowledge of the life cycle of these parasites helps in understanding the clinical features of the disease and the

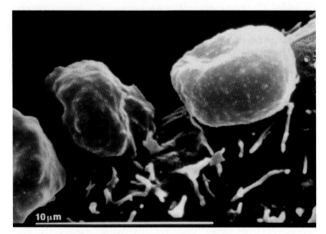

Figure 19.18

Electron micrograph of *P. falciparum* infected red cells adhering to host cells

problems of controlling it. Sporozoites in the saliva of an infected *Anopheles* mosquito are injected into the bloodstream when the person is bitten (see Figure 19.19). They enter the liver and infect parenchymal cells where enormous replication and development into the merozoite form occur over the next several days to weeks. The liver cell ruptures, releasing tens of thousands of merozoites into the bloodstream, where, after a few minutes, they invade red blood cells. Some species, especially *P. vivax*, but not *P. falciparum*, may remain in the liver as dormant hypnozoites, which some weeks or months later reactivate to cause relapses. Up to and including the liver stage of the infection the patient remains well, but symptoms begin once the merozoites invade red blood cells.

Over a 48- or 72-hour period, depending on the species of the parasite, the merozoite matures into a trophozoite; this reproduces asexually, forming many more merozoites which are again released into the bloodstream after rupture of the red cell. The number of parasites continues to increase as 48- or 72-hour cycles of red cell invasion, multiplication and release are repeated. This may continue for some months or even years.

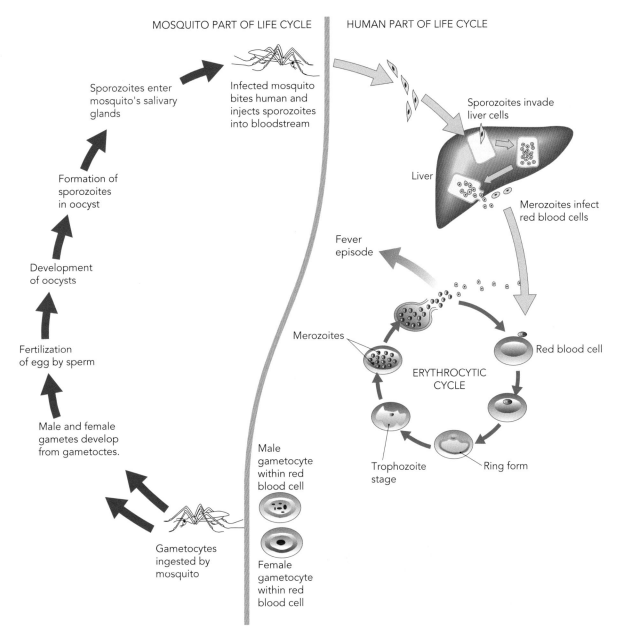

Figure 19.19

Life cycle of the malaria parasite, *Plasmodium*

Female *Anopheles* mosquito bites human, transmitting sporozoites from its salivary glands. In the liver the sporozoites multiply and become merozoites, which are shed into the bloodstream. The merozoites enter red blood cells and become trophozoites, which eventually form many more merozoites. Merozoites are released by rupture of the red blood cells, accompanied by chills, high fever and sweating. They can then infect other red blood cells. After several such asexual cycles, gametocytes (sexual stages) are produced. A mosquito bites the infected human and ingests blood cells containing gametocytes. In the mosquito the gametocytes form a zygote, which gives rise to more infective sporozoites in the salivary glands of the mosquito. These can infect another person when the mosquito bites again.

Some merozoites enter the sexual reproductive phase within red blood cells to form male and female gametocytes, which are taken up by a mosquito when feeding. Gametocytes unite in the stomach of the mosquito to form zygotes, which become sporozoites as they move to the salivary glands. Sporozoites are then injected into a new host when the mosquito feeds. This sexual phase in the mosquito is essential for completion of the life cycle of the protozoan.

The gametocytaemic phase in humans is important because it is the means by which malaria may be introduced or reintroduced into a non-endemic area. Immigrants or travellers with established infection and gametocytes in their blood can infect local mosquitoes, which may then cause indigenous spread of malaria.

Pathogenesis and clinical features

The clinical features of malaria are often vague and non-specific, and depend on the age and immune status of the patient. One to three weeks after infection by a mosquito there is usually a feeling of malaise, often accompanied by headache and muscular discomfort. The most characteristic feature is fever, which is thought to be due to the release of pyrogens (see Chapter 9) from ruptured red cells. If the cycle of red cell infection and rupture remains regular and synchronous, a characteristic pattern of recurrent chills followed by fever, drenching sweats, headache, muscular pain and vomiting occurs every 48 or 72 hours, depending on the causative species. Each symptomatic period tends to last for several hours.

The pattern of intermittent illness and well-being is usual in **benign malaria** – that is, infection caused by *P. vivax*, *P. ovale* and *P. malariae* – but less common in **falciparum malaria**. Without treatment, and if reinfection does not occur, benign malaria is normally self-limiting, resolving over a period of weeks or months, although relapses may occur. These relapses occur in vivax and ovale malaria when reactivation of dormant parasites in the liver occurs.

Falciparum malaria is a far more severe form, presumably because this species infects a larger number of red cells. It is also thought to cause aggregations of red cells that obstruct small vessels, especially in the heart, resulting in cardiac dysfunction. The progress to severe disease can be rapid, particularly in children (see Figure 19.20). A patient with falciparum malaria may present with irreg-

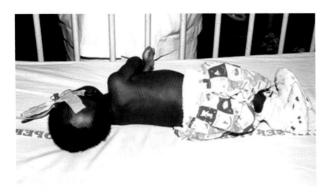

Figure 19.20

A child with severe malaria

ular fever and symptoms of gastrointestinal, respiratory or urinary tract infection. The symptoms are more persistent and there is often involvement of the brain. Liver impairment, kidney failure and severe anaemia are also common. In cerebral malaria there may be gradual progression from periods of confusion to coma. Even with treatment, mortality can be as high as 20%. Acute renal failure is also a major cause of death in falciparum malaria. An ominous sign is 'blackwater fever' (black urine) which is due to the excretion of large amounts of haemoglobin breakdown products in urine.

Diagnosis

Laboratory diagnosis is necessary because of the varied clinical features of malaria. The main means of diagnosing the disease is by microscopic examination of a blood film. In a positive film, a ring form of the parasite is seen within the red blood cell. Repeated blood samples should be collected if the first sample is negative, particularly if the symptoms persist and the patient has returned from an endemic area. PCR methods have been developed and are highly sensitive. They are important in epidemiological studies but have yet to gain a place in clinical diagnosis.

Treatment and management

Increasing resistance of *Plasmodium* spp. to antimalarial drugs is a very serious problem and one of the major reasons for the rising incidence of malaria throughout the world. Chloroquine is one of the safest antimalarials and is the drug of choice for benign malaria, although some resistance has been reported. It is also the drug of choice for sensitive *P. falciparum* infections, but unfortunately most strains throughout the world are resistant. Quinine sulphate plus either fansidar (a combination of sulphadoxine and pyrimethamine) or doxycycline may be used for strains resistant to chloroquine alone. In multi-resistant areas, such as South-East Asia, mefloquine, halofantrine or quinine may be used. Generally, these three drugs are not well tolerated compared with the first-choice drugs.

Artemisinin (or quinghaosu), a drug derived from the Chinese medicinal herb, qing hao, or sweet wormwood, is now commonly used for the treatment of drug-resistant malaria. The use of qing hao for the treatment of fevers was recommended in a Chinese handbook for medical emergencies published in AD341, but its use specifically as an antimalarial has only recently been suggested. This drug (and its derivatives, artemeter and artesunate) holds special promise because of its effectiveness against chloroquine-resistant *Plasmodium*, its ease of use (as a suppository), its speed of action and its apparent lack of serious toxicity. Importantly, resistance to it has not been reported. It has been used to great effect in South-East Asia and Latin America. In 2004 the WHO endorsed artemisinin-based combination therapy as first-line treatment where *P. falciparum* is the predominant species. This is the use of artemisinin or one of its derivatives, in combination with another antimalarial drug, to which there is not local resistance.

In addition to chemotherapy, general measures such as physical cooling, antipyretics and fluid management may be necessary. In severe cases, other supportive treatments may be needed, such as blood transfusion (if red cell numbers are drastically reduced) and dialysis for renal failure.

Uncomplicated, benign malaria can be managed on an outpatient basis, but if falciparum is suspected then hospitalisation is usually considered. Severe falciparum is a medical emergency requiring intensive care attention and facilities, and immediate intravenous antimalarial therapy and supportive treatment.

Prevention

Australians and New Zealanders risk acquiring malaria when they travel to regions in the world where malaria is endemic. Currently, protection against malaria is based on avoidance of mosquito bites and on chemoprophylaxis.

Malaria chemoprophylaxis is based on the use of chloroquine where the parasites are sensitive, and

Maloprim (pyrimethamine-dapsone) where resistant. In areas where multiple resistance exists a combination of two of the drugs mefloquine, proguanil and doxycycline is usually prescribed. Up-to-date information on malaria risk and drug susceptibility can be obtained from the World Health Organization <www.who.int/> or Centers for Disease Control <www.cdc.gov/travel/> websites. The most important point, however, is that there is no single drug that is completely effective against all strains and species of malaria parasites. As a result, chemoprophylaxis should be regarded only as an adjunct to the avoidance of exposure to mosquitoes. Fake anti-malarial drugs are sold in pharmacies and shops in SE Asia, so Australian and New Zealand travellers should be advised to obtain preventative medications before departing.

Currently, no effective vaccine is available but intensive research is being undertaken. The overall ineffectiveness of current malaria control programs means that the development of a vaccine is extremely important. Repeated, natural exposure to *P. falciparum* gradually elicits a short-lived immunity to the organism, so the development of an effective vaccine seems feasible.

TOXOPLASMOSIS

Toxoplasmosis is caused by the protozoan *Toxoplasma gondii*, which is a non-motile sporozoan. Cats are an essential part of the life cycle of *T. gondii* (Figure 19.21) because the organism undergoes its sexual phase in the intestine of the cat. Large numbers of oocysts are shed in the faeces of an infected cat. They may then contaminate food or water which can be ingested by other animals and humans. The oocysts contain sporozoites that invade cells to form trophozoites, called tachyzoites. The intracellular parasite reproduces rapidly (*tachys* means speed) and the increased numbers cause the rupture of the host cell, with release of more tachyzoites. As the immune system becomes increasingly effective, the disease enters a chronic phase in which the infected host cell develops a wall to form a tissue cyst. The numerous parasites within such a cyst reproduce very slowly, if at all, and persist for years. Loss of immune function (e.g. in AIDS) allows a reactivation of the infection from such cysts.

Humans generally acquire the infection by ingestion of undercooked meats (e.g. pork, mutton) containing tachyzoites or tissue cysts, although there is a possibility of contracting the disease more directly by contact with cat faeces. In adults, the disease is a rather undefined, mild illness (e.g. low-grade fever, general malaise, myalgia), although occasionally there will be severe effects, especially when the organism attacks nervous tissue. Surveys indicate that 30–40% of the Australian population carries antibodies for this organism; this percentage indicates the high rate of subclinical, unrecognised infections.

The primary danger is in the congenital infection of a foetus. The effects on the foetus can be drastic, including convulsions, severe brain damage, blindness and death. The mother is usually unaware of the disease, as it is being transmitted across the placenta. Studies to determine the

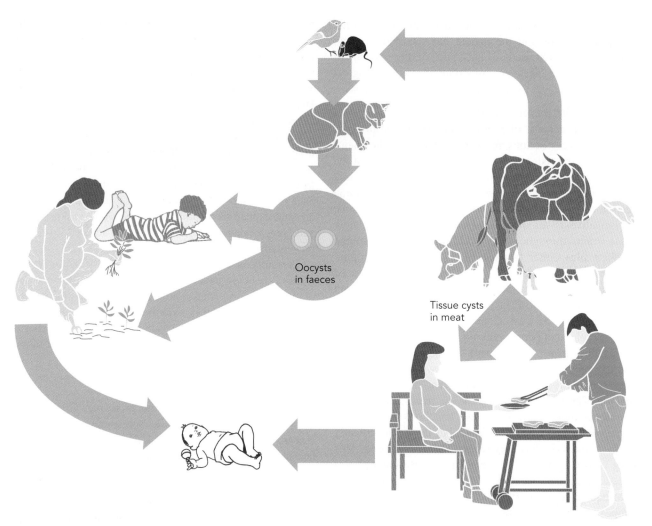

Figure 19.21

Life cycle of *Toxoplasma gondii*
Humans can be infected by cysts of this protozoan from cat faeces or animal meats. Infections in pregnant women can be passed on to the foetus, with severe outcomes.

prevalence of congenital toxoplasmosis are hampered by clinical and technical difficulties, but in Western countries the rate seems to vary from approximately 1 in 500 to 1 in 10 000 births. A large study in Western Australia suggested a prevalence of approximately 1 in 4500 births.[1]

Toxoplasmosis is usually diagnosed in the laboratory by serological tests and/or by PCR testing on body fluids (e.g. CSF, blood, urine) or biopsy material. Pyrimethamine plus sulphadiazine and folinic acid are commonly used to treat toxoplasmosis, but cannot reverse damage in congenital infection.

Systemic helminth infections

SCHISTOSOMIASIS

Schistosomiasis is a debilitating disease caused by a fluke of the genus *Schistosoma*. There are three major species – *S. mansoni*, *S. japonicum* and *S. haematobium*. The species vary with geographical location but the diseases caused by each are similar. More than 200 million people

in the world are thought to be infected, mostly in Asia, Africa, South America and the Caribbean. The disease is not found in Australia, but has been diagnosed in travellers returning from countries where it is endemic.

When water becomes contaminated with *Schistosoma* ova excreted in human wastes, a motile, ciliated larval form of *Schistosoma* (called a miracidium) is released and enters certain species of freshwater snails. The lack of a suitable host snail is a primary reason why schistosomiasis is not transmitted in certain areas of the world (e.g. Australia). Eventually, the pathogen emerges from the snail in an infective form called the cercaria. When the cercaria contact the skin of a person working, washing or swimming in the water, they penetrate the skin (see Figure 19.22) with enzymes which break down its structure. They are then carried by the bloodstream to the liver or urinary bladder. There they mature into an adult form. The male and female mate, producing numerous new eggs, some of which become trapped in tissues.

When egg production begins, symptoms develop,

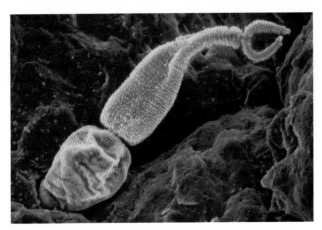

Figure 19.22

***Schistosoma mansoni*, a cause of schistosomiasis**
An electron micrograph showing a cercaria penetrating the skin.

including fever, night sweats, abdominal pain, anorexia, diarrhoea, lethargy, headaches and a non-productive cough. Cell-mediated immune responses occur and produce granulomas like those formed in tuberculosis. The eggs and the immune response to them cause tissue damage in the liver, bladder or intestine. Other eggs excreted into the water continue the cycle.

The adult worm appears to be unaffected by the host's immune system. It apparently coats itself with a layer that mimics the host's tissues.

Laboratory diagnosis consists of microscopic identification of the flukes or their eggs in faecal and urine specimens or serological tests for antibody production.

Praziquantel and oxiaminiquine usually provide effective treatment, although rapid reinfection can occur after completion of treatment. Other forms of control include improved sanitation and elimination of the host snail. Much work has been done towards the development of a vaccine, but it still appears to be some way off.

FILARIASIS

Filariasis can be caused by several different roundworms but most commonly by *Wuchereria bancrofti*. The worms are transmitted to humans by mosquitoes. After entering the tissues, the larvae develop into adult worms which can locate in the lymph glands and ducts of the infected person. Adult worms can be as long as 10 cm and can live in the lymph nodes of a person for years. Microfilariae are forms of the worm that are present in peripheral blood vessels during the night and which retreat to deep vessels, especially those of the lungs, during the day. When a mosquito bites an infected person, it ingests microfilariae that develop into larvae and migrate to the mosquito's mouth parts. When the mosquito bites again, the larvae can infect another person. They enter the blood, develop and reproduce in the lymph glands and ducts, thereby completing the life cycle. Adult worms cause inflammation in lymph ducts, fever and eventual blockage of lymph ducts. Repeated infections over a period of years can lead to **elephantiasis**, a gross enlargement of limbs (Figure 19.23), scrotum or sometimes other body parts, from an accumulation of fluid in the interstitial spaces and an increase in connective tissue.

Filariasis is diagnosed by finding microfilariae in thick blood smears made from blood samples taken at night. Serological tests to detect antibodies are also available, but these do not distinguish active infection from past exposure. There are now rapid tests available for the detection of antigens of the worm in blood. PCR methods have also been developed for detection of worm DNA in blood. The drugs albendazole plus ivermectin are effective in treating the disease. Pressure bandages may be used to force lymph from swollen limbs and, if distortion is not too great, nearly normal size can be regained.

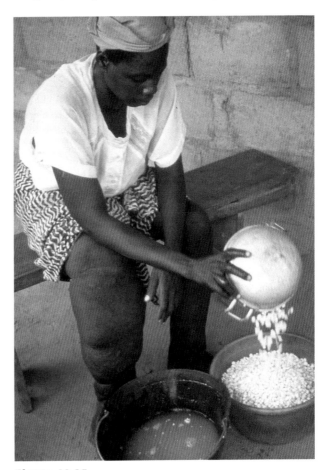

Figure 19.23

Elephantiasis of the leg caused by the roundworm *Wuchereiria bancrofti*

- The circulating blood is normally sterile.
- Infections that spread through the body and reach more than one organ are called systemic infections.
- Bacteraemia refers to the presence of bacteria in the bloodstream.
- Septicaemia is a serious clinical syndrome resulting from bacteria in the bloodstream.

SYSTEMIC BACTERIAL INFECTIONS

- In most cases of septicaemia, the organisms enter the bloodstream from a focus of infection in the body.
- Endotoxic shock is a life-threatening form of septicaemia caused by Gram-negative bacteria.
- The diagnosis of septicaemia is made by blood culture.
- Rheumatic fever is a non-suppurative complication of *Streptococcus pyogenes* sore throat.
- Untreated rheumatic fever can result in deformation and scarring of valves and heart failure, a condition called rheumatic heart disease.
- Infective endocarditis is infection and inflammation of the endocardium. In most cases there is a predisposing heart defect.
- The major pathological feature of infective endocarditis is a growing clump of bacteria, fibrin and platelets, called a vegetation, on the endocardial surface of valves and surrounding structures.
- Osteomyelitis is infection and inflammation of the bone.
- The most common cause of osteomyelitis is *Staphylococcus aureus*.
- Lyme disease is caused by the spirochaete *Borrelia burgdorferi*.
- Lyme disease is transmitted in animals, and to humans, by ticks of the genus *Ixodes*.
- The most common rickettsial infection in Australia is Q fever, caused by *Coxiella burnetii*.
- Scrub typhus (*Orientia tsutsugamushi*) and Queensland tick typhus (*Rickettsia australis*) are the most common arthropodborne rickettsial infections in Australia.
- Leptospirosis is caused by the spirochaete *Leptospira interrogans*. Humans become infected by exposure to meat, water or food contaminated with urine. The bacteria enter through mucous membranes or skin abrasions, reach the bloodstream and are then carried throughout the body.
- Toxic shock syndrome is caused by certain strains of *Staphylococcus aureus* which produce a toxin called toxic shock syndrome toxin-1, or by group A streptococcus.
- Toxic shock syndrome is a potentially life-threatening condition characterised by fever, shock and a red, sunburn-like rash.
- Anthrax is a zoonosis caused by *Bacillus anthracis* and is acquired mainly from sheep, goats and cattle.
- Brucellosis is caused by three species of the genus *Brucella*: *B. melitensis*, *B. abortus* and *B. suis*.
- Transmission of brucellosis from animals to humans occurs by direct contact with infected tissues or animal products, or via dust or aerosols.
- The causative agent of plague is *Yersinia pestis*.
- *Yersinia pestis* infects wild rodents, especially rats, and is transmitted from animal to animal and animal to human by flea bites.

SYSTEMIC VIRAL INFECTIONS

- The cause of AIDS is the human immunodeficiency virus HIV.
- HIV is transmitted by a variety of means, including sexual intercourse, through blood or blood products, from mother to child and as a result of intravenous drug abuse.
- HIV produces disease by chronic infection of cells bearing the CD4 antigen. Helper T lymphocytes (T4 lymphocytes) are the main targets, but antigen-presenting cells are also vulnerable.
- The most common secondary diseases in AIDS patients are *Pneumocystis jiroveci* pneumonia and Kaposi's sarcoma.
- Opportunistic infections are the usual cause of death in patients with AIDS.
- Ross River virus fever is the most important arbovirus infection in australia. it is spread by mosquitoes. The main manifestations are arthritis, with morning joint stiffness, a maculopapular rash, lethargy and flu-like symptoms.
- Dengue fever has a worldwide distribution in tropical areas, and occasionally in the subtropics. Epidemics occasionally occur in Australia.
- The mosquito *Aedes aegypti* is the principal vector of dengue. The disease is characterised by high fever, headache and a rash, often with severe muscle and joint pain.
- A serious form, called dengue haemorrhagic fever, is characterised by high fever, bleeding from the gums, skin and gastrointestinal tract.
- Infectious mononucleosis, or glandular fever, is caused by the Epstein-Barr virus (EBV).
- After an incubation period of 5–6 weeks, EBV causes mild symptoms of fever and headache; fatigue and malaise develop and gradually worsen.
- EBV has been implicated in several malignancies and in chronic fatigue syndrome.
- The majority of cytomegalovirus (CMV) infections produce few symptoms.
- Transplacental transmission of CMV to the foetus leads to spread of the virus to multiple organs and a severe illness.
- CMV is responsible for severe disseminated infections in people with AIDS, cancer patients and organ transplant recipients.
- Fifth disease is a common cause of rash in childhood, caused by parvovirus B19.
- Hand, foot and mouth disease is caused by a number of viruses, particularly coxsackie A16 virus and enterovirus 71. It is characterised by painful oral lesions and a skin rash.
- Yellow fever virus is restricted to parts of South America and

Africa. It is transmitted to humans by the mosquito *Aedes aegypti*.

- Yellow fever is characterised by sudden onset of fever and vomiting, and prostration 3–6 days after infection. Progression to extensive haemorrhagic manifestations and jaundice, leading to coma and death, may occur.
- Haemorrhagic fevers are caused by a number of viruses including the dengue virus, yellow fever virus, Ebola virus and Marburg virus.
- Symptoms of haemorrhagic fevers include fever, malaise, myalgia and widespread haemorrhage, leading to shock and death.
- The incidence of systemic fungal infections has increased because of greater numbers of immunocompromised people.
- Disseminated *Candida* spp. infections occur in transplant patients and patients with neutropenia.
- Disseminated *Aspergillus fumigatus* infections occur in neutropenic patients and people receiving adrenal corticosteroids.
- *Cryptococcus neoformans* is inhaled and causes a lung infection in the immunocompromised, which can spread to other organs including the brain.

SYSTEMIC PROTOZOAL INFECTIONS

- There are 300–500 million cases of malaria in the world each year. The estimated annual death toll from the disease is 2–3 million, mainly children.
- Four species cause human malaria: *Plasmodium falciparum*, *P. vivax*, *P. malariae* and *P. ovale*. Only *P. falciparum* causes significant mortality.

- The malaria protozoa are transmitted to humans by species of *Anopheles* mosquitoes.
- In malaria, a characteristic pattern of recurrent chills followed by fever, drenching sweats, headache, muscular pain and vomiting occurs every 48 or 72 hours, depending on the causative agent.
- Severe falciparum malaria is a medical emergency requiring intensive care attention and facilities, and immediate intravenous antimalarial therapy and supportive treatment.
- Toxoplasmosis is caused by the protozoan *Toxoplasma gondii*.
- *Toxoplasma* oocysts are shed in cat faeces and contaminate food or water.
- In adults, toxoplasmosis is mild and characterised by low-grade fever, general malaise and myalgia. The primary danger is in the congenital infection of a foetus.

SYSTEMIC HELMINTH INFECTIONS

- Schistosomiasis is a debilitating disease caused by a fluke of the genus *Schistosoma*.
- More than 200 million people in the world have schistosomiasis, mostly in Asia, Africa, South America and the Caribbean.
- Filariasis can be caused by several different roundworms, most commonly *Wuchereria bancrofti*. The worms are transmitted to humans by mosquitoes.
- Repeated infections of filariasis over a period of years can lead to elephantiasis, a gross enlargement of limbs, scrotum or sometimes other body parts.

STUDY QUESTIONS

1. Explain the difference between 'bacteraemia' and 'septicaemia'.
2. What is the usual source of organisms causing septicaemia?
3. What predisposing factor exists in the majority of people who develop endocarditis?
4. What is a vegetation in endocarditis?
5. What is the incidence of Lyme disease in Australia?
6. What is toxic shock syndrome and what causes it?
7. What species causes most cases of brucellosis in Australia, and what is the usual source of the organism?
8. What are the three major trends that have emerged in recent years concerning human immunodeficiency virus transmission in Australia?
9. What cell types are targeted by the human immunodeficiency virus?
10. What is the mainstay of treatment for AIDS and how does this drug reduce viral multiplication?
11. Why is it that Ross River virus infection can be acquired almost anywhere in Australia?
12. What is the pathogenesis of dengue haemorrhagic fever?
13. What is chronic fatigue syndrome?
14. What is the most serious form of cytomegalovirus infection?
15. Which species causes the most serious form of malaria and why?

16. What specimen is required for the laboratory diagnosis of malaria?

TEST YOUR UNDERSTANDING

Case History 19.1   Septicaemia
1. Does this patient have septicaemia? If yes, what is the likely cause?
2. What is the likely source of the *Staphylococcus epidermidis*?
3. Why are multiple samples of blood usually collected from a patient for the diagnosis of septicaemia?

Case History 19.2   Osteomyelitis
1. What is the most likely cause of Thomas's osteomyelitis and what is the likely source of the organism?
2. Why is haematogenous osteomyelitis most common in adolescents?

Case History 19.3   Leptospirosis
1. How do humans usually acquire leptospirosis?
2. What is the effective treatment for leptospirosis?

Case History 19.4   Brucellosis
1. Where did the Turkish woman most probably acquire her infection?

2. What important aspect of brucellosis is illustrated by the infection of the laboratory worker?

Case History 19.5   Malaria
1. How is malaria diagnosed in the laboratory?
2. What measures should be taken to prevent getting malaria?
3. Why are antimalarial drugs not always effective in preventing disease?

Further reading

Lew DP & Waldvogel FA 2004, 'Osteomyelitis', *Lancet* 363, p. 369. (Reviews the types, risk factors, pathogenesis, diagnosis and management of osteomyelitis.)

Mackenzie JS, AK Broom, RA Hall et al. 1998, 'Arboviruses in the Australian region, 1990 to 1998', *Communicable Diseases Intelligence* 22(6), p. 93. (This article discusses the major arbovirus infections found in Australia.)

Moorthy VS, MF Good & AVS Hill 2004, 'Malaria vaccine developments', *Lancet* 363, p. 150. (Reviews the pathogenesis of malaria and recent developments in the production of anti-malarial vaccines.)

Moreillon P & Y-A Que 2004, 'Infective endocarditis', *Lancet* 363, p. 139. (Reviews the risk factors, pathogenesis, diagnosis and management of infective endocarditis.)

National Centre in HIV Epidemiology and Clinical Research, *2004 HIV/AIDS, Viral Hepatitis and Sexually Transmissible Infections in Australia, Annual Surveillance Report 2004*, Sydney: NCHECR. (Provides detailed information on the epidemiology of HIV infection. Certain clinical features, such as the median survival time following AIDS, are discussed.)

Remme JHF, P De Raadt & T Godal 1993, 'The burden of tropical diseases', *Medical Journal of Australia* 158, p. 465. (This review article discusses a number of important tropical diseases caused by protozoa and helminths. The burden of malaria and other diseases on the world's population is discussed.)

Scientific American Special Report, 1998, 'Defeating AIDS: what will it take?', *Scientific American*, July, pp. 61–87. (A series of articles by different authors on the epidemiology, pathogenesis, treatment and prevention of HIV infection.)

UNAIDS, 2004, *2004 Report on the Global AIDS Epidemic*, Switzerland: UNAIDS. (Provides a global report of the HIV/AIDS epidemic.)

Whitby M, TA Ruff, AC Street & FJ Fenner 2002, 'Biological agents as weapons 2: anthrax and plague', *Medical Journal of Australia*, 176, p. 605. (Details the epidemiology, clinical features, diagnosis and management of anthrax and plague, and discusses the use of these organisms in bioterrorism.)

Reference

1. Walpole IR, N Hodgen & C Bower 1991, 'Congenital toxoplasmosis: a large survey in Western Australia', *Medical Journal of Australia* 154, p. 720.

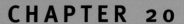

CHAPTER 20

Infections of the Nervous System

[CHAPTER FOCUS]

- **What microorganisms commonly cause infections of the nervous system?**

- **How do microorganisms gain access to the nervous system in order to cause disease?**

- **What are the important clinical aspects of nervous system infections?**

- **How are nervous system infections treated and how may they be prevented?**

Introduction

The central nervous system (CNS) consists of the brain and the spinal cord. The nerves of the peripheral nervous system branch from the CNS. The brain and the spinal cord are surrounded by three layers of membranes or **meninges**, termed the dura mater, arachnoid and pia mater (see Figure 20.1). **Cerebrospinal fluid** (CSF), a clear, lymph-like fluid, circulates in the space between the inner two meninges, called the subarachnoid space, forming a liquid cushion around the CNS organs. This fluid also serves to maintain the chemical balance in the CNS and to nourish the brain. CSF is continuously produced by masses of specialised capillaries (called choroid plexuses) in four ventricles (cavities) within the brain. These capil-laries produce CSF from blood, mainly by active transport and ultrafiltration of substances within the blood plasma. The CSF circulates around the brain and spinal cord and returns to the blood via the arachnoid villi.

Normally, the CSF is produced and drained at a constant rate. However, if its circulation or drainage is blocked (e.g. by tumour or infection), it begins to accumulate and may exert pressure on the brain. This is termed 'hydrocephalus' or 'water on the brain'.

The **blood-brain barrier** comprises the tightly joined endothelial cells of the brain's capillaries (see Figure 20.1). These capillaries are the least permeable in the entire body. The blood-brain barrier protects the brain by ensuring that its internal environment remains stable. The capillaries form a highly selective barrier which allows

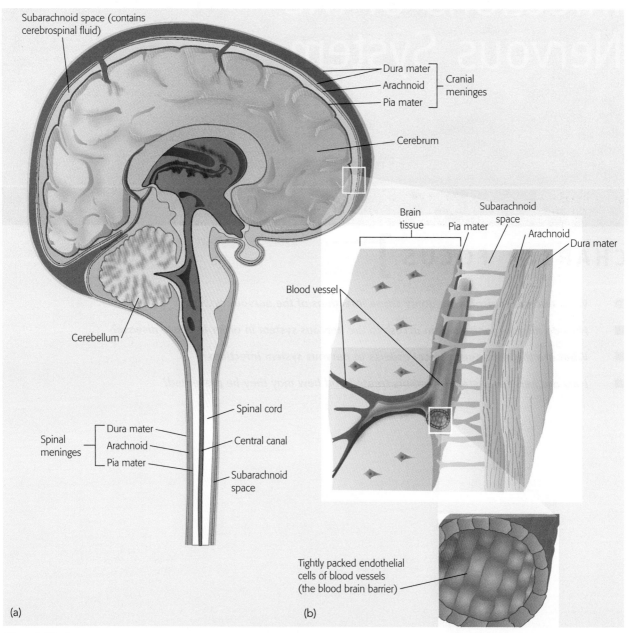

(a) Subarachnoid space (contains cerebrospinal fluid)

Dura mater
Arachnoid
Pia mater
Cranial meninges

Cerebrum

Cerebellum

Dura mater
Arachnoid
Pia mater
Spinal meninges

Spinal cord

Central canal

Subarachnoid space

(b) Brain tissue

Pia mater

Subarachnoid space

Arachnoid

Dura mater

Blood vessel

Tightly packed endothelial cells of blood vessels (the blood brain barrier)

Figure 20.1

(a) The meningeal membranes covering the brain and spinal cord: dura mater, arachnoid and pia mater. (b) The blood-brain barrier – the endothelial cells of the blood vessels of the brain

some substances, such as nutrients (e.g. glucose and essential amino acids), to pass from the circulation to the brain. However, most substances are prevented from entering brain tissue, including wastes (e.g. urea and creatinine) and many drugs (e.g. antibiotics). The blood-brain barrier is less effective in preventing the movement into brain tissue of lipid-soluble substances such as alcohol and certain anaesthetics. Because of their lipid solubility these substances diffuse easily through cell membranes and, therefore, across the blood-brain barrier.

Most antibiotics do not readily cross the blood-brain barrier, although chloramphenicol, a lipid-soluble drug, is able to cross it reasonably well. Injury to the brain may cause a breakdown of the blood-brain barrier due to alteration of the permeability characteristics of the endothelial cells or their tight junctions.

Infections of the central nervous system

Infection of the CNS is a relatively rare occurrence, but when it happens it may have serious consequences, such as permanent neurological damage or death. In most infections, organisms gain access to the CNS from the bloodstream. However, infection may sometimes spread from the ears or sinuses, or via peripheral nerves.

When infection and inflammation of the meninges occurs it is called a **meningitis**. It is most often caused by viruses or bacteria, and occasionally by fungi or protozoa. Infection and inflammation of the brain itself is called **encephalitis** and is almost always caused by viruses. In some circumstances, microorganisms may infect the brain tissue and cause a brain abscess to form. Brain abscesses are mostly caused by bacteria, but sometimes by fungi or protozoa.

BACTERIAL MENINGITIS

Acute bacterial meningitis is a medical emergency requiring urgent and specific treatment. The mortality rate varies with the causative agent, ranging from 5–50%. Up to 30–50% of people who survive bacterial meningitis suffer permanent neurological damage, such as visual or hearing impairment or reduced mental development.

Causative agents, transmission and incidence

The most common causative agents have classically been *Neisseria meningitidis*, *Haemophilus influenzae* and *Streptococcus pneumoniae* but, with the availability of an effective vaccine for *H. influenzae* since 1992, the role of this organism in meningitis has markedly declined. *Escherichia coli* and Group B streptococci (*Streptococcus agalactiae*) are the two most common causes of neonatal meningitis, and *Listeria monocytogenes* affects neonates as well as immunocompromised patients. Patients with CSF shunts or severe head injury, or those who have had neurosurgery may develop meningitis caused by bacteria such as staphylococci, *Propionibacterium* or *Corynebacterium*. *Mycobacterium tuberculosis* is a rare cause of meningitis in Australia.

Meningococcal meningitis. *N. meningitidis*, or the **meningococcus**, is an aerobic Gram-negative diplococcus. It is carried asymptomatically in the nasopharynx by up to 20% of the population. If it spreads from the nasopharynx to the blood, it can reach the meninges and cause disease. Currently, 600–700 cases of invasive meningococcal infection (meningitis and/or septicaemia) are reported in Australia each year, with 40–50 deaths. Yearly notifications have gradually increased over the last decade (see Figure 20.2). Most cases of meningococcal infection occur in the 0–4 years age group, with a smaller peak in the 15–24 years age group. The incidence in Western countries ranges from about 1 to 5 per 100 000 population. Why so many people are colonised and yet so few become infected is not clear, but the possession of antibodies to the organism's capsular antigens seems to be important. This would explain the high incidence in young children, who

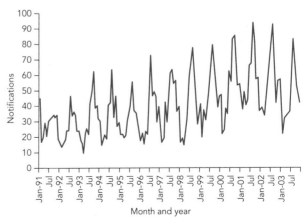

Figure 20.2

Notification rates of meningococcal infection in Australia 1991 to 2003
Source: Communicable Diseases Intelligence, 2005, 29(1), p. 54, © Commonwealth of Australia, reproduced by permission

have lost their maternal-derived antibodies and are yet to produce their own.

Meningococcus serogroups A, B, C, Y and W135 cause the majority of human infections. In Australia, serogroups B and C are the major causes of invasive infections. Meningococcal meningitis is the only type of meningitis that can spread in an epidemic form. This can occur where conditions of overcrowding exist (e.g. military camps) or where person-to-person spread by droplet transmission is enhanced (e.g. dormitories and day-care centres). The last reported epidemic in Australia occurred between 1987 and 1991 in the southern health region of the Northern Territory and the socially linked Anangu Pitjantjatjara Lands of South Australia. In all, 77 cases were diagnosed, with four deaths.

Invasive meningococcal infection usually presents as a meningitis or a septicaemia, or a combination of the two. The meningitis is clinically similar to other forms of acute bacterial meningitis. Meningococcal septicaemia, however, is particularly severe, with a greater mortality (up to 10%) than meningitis. The characteristic feature of meningococcal septicaemia is a haemorrhagic skin rash (see Figure 20.3), although the rash may not be visible on presentation, or be only transiently present. The septicaemic form, sometimes called the Waterhouse-Friderichsen syndrome, can lead to organism invasion of multiple organs, the release of large amounts of endotoxin in the blood, and substantial cytokine release by host cells.

Endotoxin and cytokine release result in disseminated intravascular coagulation (DIC), skin and mucosal haemorrhages, renal failure, bleeding into the brain and adrenal glands and shock, and death is possible within hours.

Meningococcal disease can range from mild or subclinical in some people to rapidly progressive and fatal in others. A rapid diagnosis and immediate commencement of antibiotic therapy are necessary.

Haemophilus meningitis. *Haemophilus influenzae* is an aerobic Gram-negative coccobacillus. There are a number of serological types, but invasive infections are almost always caused by encapsulated type b. The organism is a common inhabitant of the throat of infants and young children, but is found less frequently in adults. Invasion of the meninges is usually preceded by a viral infection of the respiratory tract, the resulting inflammation allowing the organism to invade the bloodstream and then the meninges. In the past, *H. influenzae* type b (Hib) caused about 70% of all cases of childhood bacterial meningitis in Australia, especially in the 0–4 years age group. Prior to 1993 the annual incidence of *H. influenzae* meningitis in Aboriginal children under the age of five was about 150 per 100 000, much higher than the 20–50 per 100 000 in non-Aboriginal children. Up to 5% of cases were fatal, and up to 15% of survivors suffered permanent neurological problems such as deafness or intellectual impairment.

However, in the early 1990s a Hib vaccine became available and there has been a reduction of more than 90% in the incidence of the disease in countries that have included the vaccine in their standard immunisation schedule (see Figure 20.4). The Hib vaccine was introduced in Australia in 1992. There were 29 cases of Hib disease (respiratory or meningeal infection) reported in Australia in 2002.

Pneumococcal meningitis. Pathogenic *Streptococcus pneumoniae* are encapsulated, aerobic, Gram-positive cocci that are carried in the throat of many healthy people. Only rarely does the organism invade the meninges. It causes meningitis mainly in:

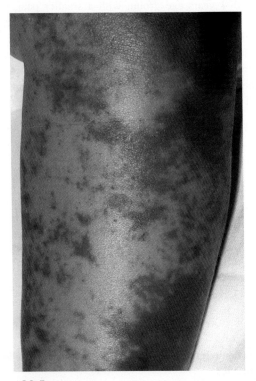

Figure 20.3

Haemorrhagic skin rash of meningococcal septicaemia

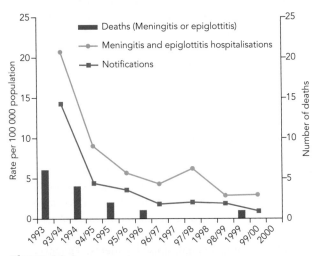

Figure 20.4

Trends in notifications, hospitalisations and death rates of *H. influenzae* infection in Australia 1993–2000
National Health and Medical Research Council 2003, *The Australian Immunisation Handbook*, 8th edn, Australian Government Department of Health and Ageing.

- children under two years of age
- debilitated or splenectomised patients
- head injury victims where there is a skull fracture communicating with the nasopharynx
- the elderly.

About 200 cases of pneumococcal meningitis occur each year in Australia. Children under two years have the highest risk, but the case fatality rate is highest in the elderly (up to 90%).

Acute onset of meningitis may follow otitis media, pneumonia, septicaemia or head injury. Antibodies to capsular polysaccharides opsonise the organism and protect against invasion; however, there are 85 different capsule serotypes. Specific antibodies do provide immunity, but antibodies to one serotype do not protect against the other serotypes.

Neonatal meningitis. Neonatal meningitis can be caused by a wide range of bacteria, but *E. coli* (with capsular type K1) and Group B *Streptococcus* (*Streptococcus agalactiae*) are the most frequent. The strains of *E. coli* and *S. agalactiae* that are pathogenic for the CNS owe their virulence, at least partially, to a polysaccharide capsule. Other causes of neonatal meningitis are shown in Table 20.1.

The incidence of neonatal bacterial meningitis in developed countries, including Australia, is around 2–5 per 10 000 births. Despite appropriate antibiotic therapy and supportive care the mortality rate remains high at approximately 30%, and many of the infants that survive have serious long-term sequelae, including hydrocephalus, cognitive dysfunction, deafness and seizures.

Group B streptococci are part of the genitourinary flora of some women. They have been found to colonise about 20% of women of child-bearing age. A baby born to a colonised mother may itself become colonised in the oral cavity, the rectum or the umbilical stump. A small percentage of colonised infants develop meningitis and/or pneumonia, usually within four weeks but possibly up to

Table 20.1
Bacterial causes of neonatal meningitis

	% CASES
Streptococcus agalactiae	35
Escherichia coli	22
Neisseria meningitidis	6
Coagulase negative staphylococci	5
Listeria monocytogenes	<5
Haemophilus influenzae	<5
Staphylococcus aureus	<5
Enterococcus faecalis	<5
Klebsiella spp.	<5
Citrobacter spp.	<5
Enterobacter spp.	<5
Pseudomonas spp.	<5

CASE HISTORY 20.2
Neonatal meningitis
Baby Sarah was a 3950 gram full-term infant born to a 25-year-old woman. The baby appeared healthy at delivery, but 24 hours later started to show signs of respiratory distress. On examination she was found to be irritable and tachypnoeic. Her axillary temperature was 38.3°C and her pulse 200. The infant had a bulging anterior fontanelle. There was no apparent rash.

Initial CSF findings included: protein 1.15 g/L (normal 0.15–0.45 g/L), glucose 2.1 mmol/L (normal >2.5 mmol/L), many Gram-positive cocci and a few white blood cells.

Comment
In many cases of neonatal meningitis there is no apparent predisposing factor.

three months later. Certain factors are known to place babies at increased risk of these infections, especially:

- prematurity (< 36 weeks)
- prolonged rupture of amniotic membranes
- heavy maternal colonisation
- maternal bacteraemia
- multiple births.

However, many babies have no apparent risk factors. Health-care-associated transmission can occur, especially in crowded nurseries. *E. coli* meningitis in neonates is also often associated with one of the above risk factors, with prematurity and prolonged rupture of membranes being particularly common. Early intestinal colonisation by K1 strains of *E. coli* before the normal flora are established can lead to invasion of the blood and then the CNS.

Listeriosis. **Listeriosis** is caused by *Listeria monocytogenes*, a Gram-positive coccobacillus. This organism causes meningitis mainly in the immunocompromised. It is also an important cause of infection in pregnant women. The infection in pregnant women is usually mild, but the organism can spread to the foetus *in utero* or be transmitted at birth, resulting in severe foetal or neonatal disease. Intrauterine infection can result in abortion, premature labour, intrauterine death or perinatal infection. Perinatal infection is most often manifested as a meningitis.

The organism is found in the intestine of a wide variety of animals and is excreted in their faeces. It is therefore widely distributed in soil, water, sewage and animal feed. Apart from perinatal infections it is predominantly a food-borne pathogen. Foods usually become contaminated in food processing facilities or by contact with soil. Raw foods, such as fruit and vegetables, and uncooked foods of animal origin, such as meat and soft cheeses, are the usual sources of infection. The annual incidence in most Western countries is around 0.2–0.5 per 100 000 population, which amounts to 50–70 cases in Australia. It is usually a mild or often symptomless disease in healthy adults. Mild disease is generally characterised by flu-like symptoms of sore throat, fever, chills and myalgia.

Tuberculous meningitis. *Mycobacterium tuberculosis* is a rare cause of meningitis in Australia. It can occur during active infection or in recrudescent infection (see Chapter 17). From a focus of infection elsewhere, the organism enters the bloodstream and disseminates to the subarachnoid spaces.

The causes, predisposing factors and incidence of bacterial meningitis are summarised in Table 20.2.

Pathogenesis

There are believed to be several critical events in the pathogenesis of many cases of acute haematogenous bacterial meningitis:

1. nasopharyngeal colonisation
2. invasion of the bloodstream and intravascular survival
3. penetration of the blood-brain barrier
4. damage and inflammation of the meninges.

Many of the bacteria that cause meningitis possess surface structures that are thought to enhance mucosal colonisa-

tion. For instance, both *N. meningitidis* and *H. influenzae* possess fimbriae which may facilitate their attachment to the nasopharyngeal mucosa. Polysaccharide capsules are possessed by all the major pathogens and these may also assist them to attach. Immunoglobulin A (IgA), the antibody class found predominantly in mucosal secretions, may inhibit the attachment of bacteria, but many clinical isolates of *N. meningitidis*, *H. influenzae* and *S. pneumoniae* secrete a protease which cleaves and inactivates IgA.

To invade the bloodstream, the bacteria must cross the mucosal epithelium of the nasopharynx. It appears that different pathogens have different methods of invasion. For example, *N. meningitidis* is thought to enter non-ciliated epithelial cells by an endocytic process and pass through the cell in a membrane-bound vacuole. On the other hand, *H. influenzae* invades through separations in the tight junctions of columnar epithelial cells. Once in the bloodstream, the bacteria must then evade the host defence mechanisms there. All the common pathogens (*H. influenzae*, *N. meningitidis*, *S. pneumoniae*, *E. coli* and *S. agalactiae*) are encapsulated, which protects them from phagocytes.

Table 20.2

Bacterial meningitis: causative agents, predisposing factors and incidence

CAUSATIVE ORGANISM	PREDISPOSING FACTORS	INCIDENCE (AUSTRALIA)
Neisseria meningitidis	Young age Close contact Complement deficiencies	2.1 per 100 000 population Most frequent in 0–4 years age group
Haemophilus influenzae	Young age Non-immunised Respiratory tract infection	Low, since vaccine became part of the standard schedule
Streptococcus pneumoniae	Young age Pneumococcal pneumonia Debility Skull fracture Old age	All age groups
Group B streptococcus, *Escherichia coli*	Neonates: • prematurity • prolonged rupture of membranes • heavy maternal colonisation • maternal bacteraemia • multiple births	About 2 per 10 000 births
Listeria monocytogenes	Neonates – maternal infection Immunosuppression, e.g. transplant, cancer	0.25 per 100 000 population
Mycobacterium tuberculosis	Infection elsewhere which spreads to blood	Rare
Staphylococcus *Proprionibacterium* *Corynebacterium*	Entry of skin flora following: • head injury • CSF shunt • neurosurgery	All age groups

---

Pathogenic bacteria are able to pass from the circulation into the CSF by penetrating vulnerable sites of the blood-brain barrier. Bacterial virulence factors such as fimbriae, polysaccharide capsules and endotoxin (lipopolysaccharide) are possibly involved, and the most likely sites of invasion are the choroid plexuses. Once in the CSF, the bacteria have a good chance of survival because humoral defences, particularly immunoglobulin and complement activity, are in very low concentration in this fluid. Even though blood leucocytes enter the CSF during infection, their effectiveness is limited by the lack of antibodies and complement, which normally enhance their activity.

In head-injured patients, organisms may gain direct access to the CNS. The cribriform plate at the anterior part of the base of the skull is in close proximity to the nasal sinuses. This bony plate may be damaged in head injury and organisms found in the nares, particularly *Streptococcus pneumoniae* (the most common cause of meningitis in head-injured patients), may then gain direct access to the CSF.

The tissue dysfunction in bacterial meningitis may be due to focal lesions caused by bacterial growth or toxins. However, there is much evidence to suggest that the intense inflammatory response to the infection has a significant role in producing the neurological problems and death that are so often associated with bacterial meningitis. Studies have indicated that lipopolysaccharides and other bacterial cell wall components play a major role. These are released into the subarachnoid space during natural or antibiotic-induced bacteriolysis and they elicit the local release of cytokines, such as interleukin-1 and tumour necrosis factor, from various cells (e.g. vascular endothelial cells, microglia and astrocytes). These cytokines lead to inflammation and increased blood-brain barrier permeability. The pressure in the subarachnoid space may rise markedly, due to the inflammation, oedema and vascular endothelial injury. Because of the rigid confines of the skull and spinal cord, this pressure spreads to the entire space around the brain and spinal cord. The increased cranial pressure causes a decrease in cerebral blood flow.

The pathophysiologic processes that contribute to the neurologic sequelae of bacterial meningitis are summarised in Figure 20.5.

Clinical features

The clinical presentation of bacterial meningitis is variable and depends on the patient's age, the duration of illness and the causative agent. Headache, fever, altered consciousness, vomiting and nuchal rigidity (neck stiffness) are the most common presenting symptoms. Lethargy, irritability, anorexia and photophobia are also common. These symptoms are often accompanied by upper respiratory symptoms such as a sore throat. In neonates, young infants and the elderly, the symptoms may be more subtle and usually include fever, lethargy, irritability, respiratory distress, lack of interest in food, vomiting and diarrhoea. A rapidly progressing, fulminant form is most often caused by *N. meningitidis* and sometimes *S. pneumoniae*, whereas *H. influenzae* usually has a more insidious onset.

The presence of a haemorrhagic skin rash, associated with septicaemia, is suggestive of *N. meningitidis* infection, although *H. influenzae* can sometimes mimic this. The mortality rate varies from 5–50% depending on a number of factors – including the age of the patient, the causative agent and the duration of illness before commencement of treatment. Up to 10% of survivors experience long-term serious sequelae such as hearing loss, mental retardation and seizures.

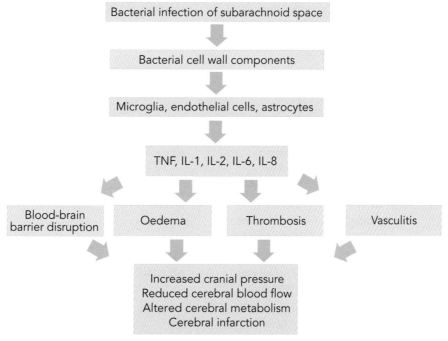

Figure 20.5

Pathophysiology of neurologic dysfunction in bacterial meningitis

Laboratory diagnosis

CSF is the most important specimen for the diagnosis of meningitis. It is usually collected by lumbar puncture but sometimes other methods, such as a ventricular tap, are used. Lumbar puncture may be delayed if there are clinical signs of increased intracranial pressure. If possible, the CSF should be collected into two or three tubes, with 2–5 mL in each. The tubes should be labelled sequentially for different uses in the laboratory. It should be remembered that CSF is a body fluid to which Standard Precautions apply. Laboratory-acquired cases of bacterial meningitis have been reported.

Rapid transport of the specimen to the laboratory is necessary for two important reasons. First, the disease is very serious and thus an accurate diagnosis is needed as soon as possible. Second, most of the common causes are fastidious organisms that may not survive variations in temperature or long transit times. Unlike many other specimens for the microbiology laboratory, CSF specimens should not be refrigerated but maintained at room temperature or at 37°C. Blood cultures should also be collected. Fastidious organisms not isolated from CSF may sometimes be cultured from blood.

Cerebrospinal fluid analysis in the microbiology laboratory usually includes:

- a macroscopic examination
- culture
- a Gram stain
- a cell count
- determination of glucose concentration
- determination of protein concentration.

Preliminary results of all of the above, except culture, should be available within an hour or two after receipt of the CSF specimen in the laboratory. These results may enable bacterial meningitis to be distinguished from other causes of meningitis, as shown in Table 20.3. The differentiation between bacterial causes and viral meningitis may allow for early adjustment to treatment and patient management.

Obvious turbidity in a CSF specimen is suggestive of bacterial infection, and is usually due to the presence of large numbers of white cells and/or bacteria. The differential cell count typically shows polymorphs (polymorphonuclear leucocytes) in acute bacterial meningitis. Bacteria may be detected in a Gram stain if there are greater than

---

Table 20.3

Characteristic changes in cerebrospinal fluid in meningitis

	MACROSCOPIC APPEARANCE	CELLS (x 10⁶/L)	PROTEIN (g/L)	GLUCOSE (mmol/L)	GRAM STAIN
Normal	clear and colourless	0–5	0.15–0.45	≥2.5	
Streptococcus pneumoniae	clear to turbid	elevated, PMN	elevated	reduced	Gram-positive diplococci
Haemophilus influenzae	clear to turbid	elevated, PMN	elevated	reduced	Gram-negative coccobacilli
Neisseria meningitidis	clear to turbid	elevated, PMN	elevated	reduced	Gram-negative diplococci
Escherichia coli	clear to turbid	elevated, PMN	elevated	reduced	Gram-negative rods
Group B streptococci	clear to turbid	elevated, PMN	elevated	reduced	Gram-positive cocci
Listeria monocytogenes	clear to faintly turbid	elevated (mainly lymphocytes)	elevated	reduced	Gram-positive coccobacillus
Mycobacterium tuberculosis	clear to faintly turbid	elevated, lymphocytes (PMN early)	markedly elevated	reduced	negative
Viruses	clear to faintly turbid	elevated, lymphocytes (PMN early)	slightly elevated	normal	negative
Cryptococcus neoformans	clear to faintly turbid	elevated, PMN or lymphocytes	elevated	reduced	yeast cells

PMN = polymorphonuclear leucocytes

10^5 organisms per millilitre of CSF. A negative Gram stain, therefore, does not exclude a bacterial meningitis. A reduction in the CSF glucose level is due to impaired transport of glucose from blood to CSF and its usage by the bacteria and the infiltrating polymorphs. There is usually a significant increase in the protein concentration because of alteration to the blood-brain barrier, resulting in an increased permeability to serum proteins which are normally excluded.

Blood and a nasopharyngeal or throat swab (if meningococcus is suspected) should also be collected for culture.

Antibiotic treatment of meningitis should not be delayed, so specimen collection often follows commencement of therapy. Once therapy is started the ability to isolate bacteria from the CSF is rapidly reduced. The recent development of polymerase chain reaction (PCR) tests on CSF or blood has helped to overcome this problem. Meningococcal DNA can be detected in CSF for up to 72 hours after commencement of antibiotic therapy. Nasopharyngeal swabs may also remain positive for meningococci some time after commencement of antibiotic therapy. Methods for the detection of soluble antigens in CSF, serum or urine have been developed are increasingly being used for rapid diagnosis of the major causes of bacterial meningitis.

If tuberculous meningitis is suspected, a Ziehl-Neelsen stain of centrifuged deposit of CSF is often performed.

Treatment

Prompt treatment of any bacterial meningitis is required. First-line therapy for acute meningitis is most often with benzylpenicillin or amoxycillin plus ceftriaxone or cefotaxime. The third-generation cephalosporins are preferred because (1) they are effective against the three principal causes of bacterial meningitis – *N. meningitidis*, *H. influenzae* and *S. pneumoniae* – and (2) therapeutic levels can be reached in the CSF. It should be remembered that many substances, including antibiotics, do not cross the blood-brain barrier very well. The third-generation cephalosporins are highly potent and seem to enter the CSF in adequate concentration via the leaky capillaries that are characteristic of inflammation.

Therapy may be modified following Gram-stain findings and again once the identity of the organism and its susceptibility pattern is known. Benzylpenicillin is usually the drug of choice for *N. meningitidis* and *S. pneumoniae*, although some resistant strains of *S. pneumoniae* have appeared in recent years. Cephalosporins are usually maintained if *H. influenzae* is identified and found to be susceptible. The treatment of choice for *Listeria* meningitis is ampicillin or penicillin plus cotrimoxazole. Standard anti-tuberculosis drugs (see Chapter 17) are used for tuberculous meningitis.

Because the inflammatory response is at least partially the cause of the injury to the CNS in acute bacterial meningitis, the use of anti-inflammatory agents has been suggested as an adjunct to antibiotic treatment. Experimental and clinical trials have shown that anti-inflammatory agents, such as the corticosteroid, dexamethasone, can diminish the CSF inflammatory response and the subsequent oedema, increased CSF pressure and neurologic sequelae. However, these drugs have minimal or no effectiveness in neonatal infections. Overall, the routine use of anti-inflammatory drugs in acute bacterial meningitis remains controversial and further research on their use is currently being undertaken.

Prevention

There is an increased attack rate of *N. meningitidis* in close contacts of infected individuals, due mainly to higher rates of nasopharyngeal carriage. Antibiotic prophylaxis is therefore recommended in some settings. Household or intimate contacts may be given rifampicin to eliminate carriage and, therefore, the risk of infection. The development of resistance to rifampicin is a concern. Ciprofloxacin may be used as an alternative. To prevent neonatal infection with Group B streptococci, administration of benzylpenicillin to high-risk women during labour has been shown to be effective.

Vaccines are available for the three major causes of bacterial meningitis. Currently, there are two pneumococcal vaccines available in Australia. A 23-valent pneumococcal polysaccharide vaccine is recommended for various high-risk groups, including asplenic individuals (no spleen, anatomical or functional), people over 65 years of age (over 50 years if Aboriginal or Torres Strait Islander), the immunocompromised and patients with CSF leaks. The 7-valent pneumococcal conjugate vaccine is now recommended as part of the standard childhood immunisation schedule at 2, 4 and 6 months. It is also the preferred vaccine for high risk children under 5 years.

A meningococcal serogroup C vaccine has been part of the standard childhood immunisation program since 2003. A tetravalent vaccine for *N. meningitidis* serotypes A, C, Y and W135 is also available. It is recommended for the control of outbreaks, for travellers to high-risk areas (e.g. Nepal and Northern India), for asplenic patients and people with complement deficiencies, and for at-risk laboratory personnel. It is not used for routine mass vaccination mainly because of inconsistent immunogenicity at younger ages. There is no realistic prospect for a serogroup B vaccine in the near future.

Conjugate Hib vaccines to prevent *H. influenzae* infections have been available in Australia since 1992, and part of the standard childhood vaccination schedule since 1993. This provides a dramatic example of the potential success of good vaccines, with Hib infection rates decreasing by more than 90% since introduction of this vaccine (see Figure 20.4). The National Health and Medical Research Council (NHMRC) recommends vaccination of all Australian children at 2 and 4 months, with a booster at 12 months. The vaccine containing PRP-OMP (purified Hib polysaccharide conjugated to meningococcal carrier protein) is recommended.

VIRAL MENINGITIS

Overall, viral meningitis is the most common type of meningitis. Most of these infections are caused by enteroviruses (echoviruses, coxsackie viruses) but other possible causes include the mumps virus and varicella zoster virus. The viruses usually enter the body via the gastrointestinal or respiratory route and, after local multiplication, enter the bloodstream. Viraemia gives the viruses the opportunity to cross the blood-brain barrier and enter the subarachnoid space. As with bacterial meningitis, the incidence of viral meningitis is greatest in infants and young children. The immunocompromised are also at increased risk of viral meningitis.

Viral meningitis is sometimes referred to as **aseptic meningitis**, a general term for any meningitis where microorganisms are not isolated by routine bacteriological culture. Apart from viruses, there are many other causes of aseptic meningitis, including bacteria (not cultured by routine methods), fungi, protozoa and non-infectious causes (e.g. malignancy, autoimmune disease, chemical poisoning).

CASE HISTORY 20.3

Outbreak of viral meningitis

An outbreak of aseptic meningitis due to echovirus 30 occurred in the Wingecarribee Shire during October to November 1994, with 30 cases fitting the clinical case definition. The clinical presentations were fairly typical of viral meningitis. Most patients had fever, headache and meningism. The onset was often short (a few hours) and patients were often debilitated, requiring admission to hospital. Other systemic features of myalgia and arthralgia were also typical.

The mode(s) of transmission in this outbreak remain speculative. There was no obvious geographical clustering. Cases were distributed throughout Wingecarribee Shire, although the majority lived in the Mittagong postal area.

The occurrence of some person-to-person transmission was suggested by the three clinical cases in one family (one confirmed by culture) and a health-care worker who became ill after nursing a case. However, the other cases were not epidemiologically linked to a confirmed case, suggesting other means of transmission.

Although the route of transmission was not established, general measures to stop transmission were implemented when a common water source was excluded on epidemiological grounds. These measures included information on personal, food and domestic hygiene publicised through preschools, schools and the local media. Education of patients and doctors was instituted early.

Source: Communicable Diseases Intelligence 24(5), May 2000, p. 123.

Viral meningitis is generally milder and progresses more slowly than bacterial infections. It is usually manifested by acute onset of headache, mild photophobia, low-grade fever, vomiting, general malaise and minor neck stiffness. This often follows upper respiratory symptoms, gastrointestinal symptoms, or both. Some people with viral meningitis may become tired or sleepy but usually retain full perception and consciousness. Loss of alertness or normal mental status is not typical of viral meningitis but is suggestive of more serious disease, such as bacterial meningitis.

A distinction between viral and bacterial meningitis cannot always be made on clinical grounds. Laboratory examination of CSF in a case of viral meningitis generally shows a moderately increased white cell count with a predominance of mononuclear cells (lymphocytes), although early in infection polymorphs may predominate, mimicking acute bacterial infection. The protein concentration in CSF may be normal or elevated, but is usually lower than in bacterial meningitis. The CSF glucose is usually within normal limits. The characteristic laboratory findings for bacterial and viral infections are compared in Table 20.3.

Diagnosis of viral meningitis can be sometimes achieved by virus isolation, antigen detection or microscopy of CSF. Although virus isolation is successful in some cases, it can take up to 10 days. Antigen detection and microscopy methods generally have a low sensitivity. A definitive diagnosis can be made by the demonstration of a fourfold rise in antibody titre in acute and convalescent sera. However, this can take three weeks or more and is therefore of limited clinical value. Nucleic acid amplification techniques (e.g. PCR) have been developed for some meningitis viruses. They have much higher sensitivity than other diagnostic methods and thus are likely to be further developed and increasingly used.

Therapy for uncomplicated viral meningitis usually involves symptomatic treatment only, although antibacterial drugs are normally given until a non-bacterial cause is confirmed. The great majority of patients recover spontaneously within two weeks, and often within several days. Complications such as chronic fatigue syndrome, chronic muscle weakness and ataxia may occur, but are rare.

FUNGAL INFECTIONS

Very few fungi infect the central nervous system of humans. They include *Coccidioides immitis*, *Histoplasma capsulatum* and *Cryptococcus neoformans*. Except for *Cryptococcus*, these organisms are rarely seen in Australia. Cryptococcal meningitis has become increasingly common in recent years and is most often found in people whose immune system has been compromised in some way.

Cryptococcal meningitis

Before the AIDS epidemic, cryptococcal meningitis was one of those diseases that students were required to learn about but would seldom see. It was associated with exposure to pigeon droppings and occurred in some immunosuppressed people. Today, it is far more familiar. It is now one of the diseases routinely anticipated in patients with AIDS (up to 15% are affected) and is also more common in other people because of the increasing use of corticosteroid therapy and immunosuppressive agents.

Cryptococcus neoformans is a yeast-like fungus with spherical cells. The cells reproduce by budding and have a thick polysaccharide capsule (see Figure 20.6) which is at least partly responsible for its virulence. Serotypes of *C. neoformans* are grouped into three varieties. *C. neoformans* var. *neoformans* and *C. neoformans* var. *grubii* are widely distributed in soil and are commonly found in the droppings of pigeons and other avian species, including chickens, parrots and canaries. These serotypes mostly cause disease in immunocompromised individuals. *C. neoformans* var. *gattii*, on the other hand, has been found to be associated with the bark, flowers and other parts of a number of species of eucalypt and other trees in Australia. It has also been isolated from the dung and under the claws of some Australian native animals (e.g. koalas, possums and echidnas) and these may act as secondary reservoirs. *C. neoformans* var. *gattii* also differs from the other varieties in that it usually affects individuals with no immune impairment.

Infection caused by *C. neoformans* is called cryptococcosis. Humans generally become infected by inhalation of the organism, which then causes a primary infection in the alveoli. In people with normal defences, the disease is often contained within the lungs and is subclinical and regresses spontaneously. However, in immunocompromised people and in a small proportion of infections involving *C. neoformans* var. *gattii*, the organism invades the bloodstream and spreads to other parts of the body, including the brain and meninges. This leads to a subacute or chronic type of meningitis with a slow onset (one or more weeks) that is often fatal if untreated. Complications, such as hydrocephalus, visual disturbances, hearing loss and seizures, may occur.

The typical preliminary CSF findings in cryptococcal meningitis are shown in Table 20.3. If cryptococcal meningitis is suspected, an India ink stain of centrifuged deposit is usually performed. This stain allows the yeast cell and its characteristic large capsule to be seen. Confirmation is by culture of the organism and by a rapid latex agglutination test which can detect cryptococcal antigen in the CSF. The standard treatment is with amphotericin B plus flucytosine, followed by oral fluconazole.

PROTOZOAL INFECTIONS

Few protozoa infect the central nervous system. The notable one in Australia and other Western countries is *Toxoplasma gondii*. Amoebic meningitis caused by *Naegleria fowleri* is a rare disease that occasionally occurs in Australia. The flagellate *Trypanosoma brucei* is the cause of African trypanosomiasis, or sleeping sickness, which affects many thousands of people each year but is restricted mainly to Central and East Africa.

Toxoplasma infection of the CNS

Toxoplasma gondii has for many years been recognised as an important pathogen in congenital infection, but its importance has increased markedly since the AIDS epidemic struck. Cerebral toxoplasmosis is one of the more common neurological complications of HIV infection. The protozoan often produces multiple, well-demarcated lesions throughout the cerebral hemispheres. The clinical manifestations are highly variable and include headache, fever, clumsiness to hemiplegia, seizures, ataxia and cognitive changes. Toxoplasmosis is usually diagnosed in the laboratory by serological methods and/or by PCR testing on body fluids (e.g. CSF, blood, urine) or biopsy material.

Treatment is with pyrimethamine plus sulphadiazine (or clindamycin) plus folinic acid.

ENCEPHALITIS

Encephalitis is almost always caused by viruses, with the herpes simplex virus and various arboviruses (arthropod-borne viruses) being the most common. Different encephalitis-causing arboviruses occur in different parts of the world (see Table 20.4). Each arbovirus type has certain animal reservoirs and is transmitted by a particular arthropod vector. Arbovirus encephalitis in Australia (formerly called Australian encephalitis) is caused by two mosquito-borne flaviviruses – the Murray Valley encephalitis virus and, occasionally, the Kunjin virus. These two viruses infect wild and domestic animals in Australia.

Encephalitis may also occur as a rare complication of certain systemic viral infections (e.g. measles, mumps, cytomegalovirus) or, very rarely, after vaccination with some live attenuated vaccines (e.g. measles, mumps, rubella).

The characteristic manifestations of viral encephalitis represent cerebral dysfunction and include abnormal behaviour, seizures and altered consciousness. Fever, vomiting and nausea are also common. These symptoms reflect necrosis of neurones.

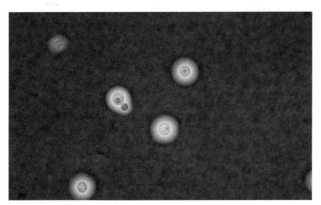

Figure 20.6

India ink stain of *Cryptococcus neoformans* showing the large capsule around the cell

Table 20.4
Arthropod-borne encephalitis viruses

VIRUS	ARTHROPOD VECTOR	GEOGRAPHIC DISTRIBUTION
West Nile encephalitis	Mosquito	Africa, Asia, Europe, USA
Eastern equine encephalitis	Mosquito	USA
St Louis encephalitis	Mosquito	USA, Jamaica
Venezuelan equine encephalitis	Mosquito	USA, South America
Japanese encephalitis	Mosquito	Asia
Louping-ill	Tick	United Kingdom
Russian spring-summer encephalitis	Tick	Europe, Asia
Chandipura virus encephalitis	Sandfly	India
Murray Valley encephalitis	Mosquito	Australia, New Guinea
Kunjin	Mosquito	Australia, New Guinea

Murray Valley encephalitis

Murray Valley encephalitis (MVE) is a severe epidemic-type disease. The MVE virus is considered to be endemic in northern Australia (the Kimberley region of Western Australia and the Top End of the Northern Territory). The MVE virus is believed to have been responsible for severe epidemics in 1917, 1918, 1922 and 1925. It was then known as Australian 'X' disease. The most recent major epidemic occurred in 1974, with a total of 58 cases occurring in all mainland states, resulting in 13 deaths. Epidemics occur mainly during conditions of warm temperature and high rainfall which allow mosquito numbers to increase markedly. The primary hosts of MVE virus are water birds, which maintain infection in mosquitoes. Humans become infected if bitten by an infected mosquito.

Following the 1974 epidemic, a number of sentinel chicken flocks were established by state health authorities. Currently, flocks are maintained in Western Australia, the Northern Territory, New South Wales, Victoria and northern Queensland. The birds in these flocks are regularly tested serologically for antibodies to the MVE and Kunjin viruses, to provide an early warning of any increase in virus activity.

Most infections with MVE virus are subclinical. However, occasionally (about 1 in 1000 infections) the virus crosses the blood-brain barrier and causes damage to the brain tissue. The major presenting symptoms are fever, headache, convulsions or other signs of altered mental state. The case fatality rate can be as high as 40%. Residual neurological impairment, including spastic quadriparesis and facial nerve palsy, can occur in up to 50% of survivors.

MVE is diagnosed by isolation of the virus from a clinical specimen, detection of MVE RNA by PCR in a clinical specimen or by serological evidence: the presence of IgM antibody in serum or CSF, or a fourfold rise in IgG antibody titre. There is no specific therapy for encephalitis caused by arboviruses, making prevention of infection very important. Australian state health departments have contingency plans for disease prevention should virus activity, as indicated by sentinel flocks, be found to be increasing to dangerous levels. Although vaccines have been developed for some other encephalitis arboviruses (e.g. Japanese encephalitis), there is not yet one for MVE.

Japanese encephalitis

Japanese encephalitis is caused by a flavivirus spread by mosquitoes. Its natural hosts are certain wading birds and pigs and it normally spreads to humans when levels are high in local pigs. Japanese encephalitis is a significant problem in some parts of Asia (e.g. India, Sri Lanka, Thailand) and since 1995 has occurred in low incidence in the Torres Strait Islands. In 1998 the first ever case was reported on mainland Australia, on the west coast of Cape York. Since that year no further cases have been identified on mainland Australia.

Most infections are asymptomatic but, when symptomatic, are characterised by headache, fever, convulsions, lowered consciousness and coma, with a high case fatality

---

CASE HISTORY 20.4
Murray Valley encephalitis

A 9-month-old Aboriginal boy from an outstation in the Northern Territory presented to Royal Darwin Hospital, having been ill for a week with fever, diarrhoea, vomiting and lethargy. His conscious state decreased rapidly over 24 hours. Over the next few days he developed a flaccid paralysis of all limbs and signs of brain-stem dysfunction, and required ventilation. Aciclovir was given.

Five weeks after admission his brain-stem functions and respiration had recovered but the limb paralysis persisted. Sera collected on admission and five days later showed a rise in MVE IgG from 1:40 to 1:160.

Comment
Murray Valley encephalitis is considered endemic in some northern areas of Australia and also occurs in epidemic form.

rate (20–50%). There is also a high incidence (up to 50%) of neurological sequelae in those who survive the acute illness. The infection may be diagnosed in the laboratory by isolation of the virus or detection of viral RNA in clinical material, or by serological means. An inactivated vaccine is available for Japanese encephalitis and is currently recommended for travellers spending a month or more in rural areas of Asia or western Papua New Guinea, travellers spending a year or more in Asia (except Singapore), residents of the outer islands of the Torres Strait, and non-residents who will be on the outer islands of the Torres Strait for 30 days or more during the wet season. The Australian Quarantine and Inspection Service maintains herds of sentinel pigs in Torres Strait, Cape York and the Northern Territory to detect Japanese encephalitis virus activity.

Herpes encephalitis

Herpes simplex virus type 1 is most often associated with cold sores. Very rarely, the virus reactivates in the trigeminal ganglia, where it resides latently, and ascends into the brain. The spread of herpes simplex virus type 2 to the brain is even less common, although in neonates both types can cause severe encephalitis. Herpes encephalitis is a very severe disease that causes neurological damage with a high mortality (70% if untreated). Early treatment with aciclovir greatly reduces the mortality and permanent neurological damage. The early diagnosis of herpes encephalitis is therefore important because of the potential for effective treatment.

Diagnosis is usually made by computed tomographic (CT) or magnetic resonance imaging (MRI) scan and EEG. Polymerase chain reaction (PCR) on a CSF specimen provides conclusive evidence but may be falsely negative very early in the course of infection.

OTHER VIRAL CAUSES OF ENCEPHALITIS

A number of other viruses are capable of causing encephalitis in humans. West Nile virus is distributed across Africa, Asia, the US and southern Europe. The natural hosts of the virus are birds, being transmitted between birds and to humans by mosquitoes. Although West Nile virus usually causes a relatively mild illness that only occasionally includes encephalitis, it has been responsible for some large outbreaks of encephalitis in southern Europe and Russia. A significant outbreak occurred in the US in 2002, involving almost 4000 cases and causing over 200 deaths.

The Nipah virus can cause pneumonitis and encephalitis in humans. It has caused outbreaks of encephalitis in Malaysia and Singapore. The natural hosts are bats. Pigs are infected by contact with bat faeces or urine, and then humans are secondarily infected by droplet transmission, initially from infected pigs, and then from infected humans.

Dengue virus occasionally causes encephalitis, although it is more often associated with a systemic infection that doesn't involve the brain. Enterovirus 17, a cause

of hand, foot and mouth disease, is also an occasional cause of encephalitis. Dengue fever and hand, foot and mouth disease are described in Chapter 19.

Other infections involving the nervous system

TETANUS

Tetanus is a rare, but serious, illness caused by the bacterium *Clostridium tetani*, a strictly anaerobic, spore-forming, Gram-positive rod. Tetanus spores are widespread in soil and manure, because the organism is part of the bowel flora of various animals and some humans. The spores are extremely resistant to drying, disinfectants and heat (they are resistant to boiling for 20 minutes) and can survive in soil for years.

Since the development of the tetanus vaccine and its widespread use, tetanus has become a rarity in developed countries. In Australia, fewer than ten cases are notified annually. However, in underdeveloped countries the incidence is much higher and, worldwide, there are more than 50 000 fatalities from tetanus each year. In developed countries, there is often a higher incidence in the elderly because of inadequate past and current immunisation.

Wounds contaminated with faeces or soil can become infected with *C. tetani*. Usually, the spores must be deposited into a deep, necrotic wound where oxygen is lacking, allowing growth of this strict anaerobe to occur. However, many cases of tetanus have occurred following only minor injuries, such as thorns or splinters acquired during gardening. In some developing countries, a high incidence in neonates is associated with the use of

---

CASE HISTORY 20.5

Tetanus

A 58-year-old woman gashed her hand on the branch of a tree while gardening. After examination in the casualty department of her local hospital, her wound was cleaned, she was given an injection of tetanus toxoid and a course of oral flucloxacillin was started.

Six days later she developed a stiffness in her jaw, complained of muscle spasms in her back and had difficulty in swallowing. She was diagnosed as having tetanus, admitted to hospital and given tetanus immunoglobulin. The wound was debrided and cleaned and she was given diazepam to prevent the spasms. This treatment was effective and she was discharged after a week.

Comment

In a non-immune person the most critical part of tetanus treatment is immunoglobulin. This woman would not have developed symptoms of tetanus had this been given initially. Careful taking of her case history should have ascertained whether she was immune or not.

contaminated knives to cut the umbilical cord, or the use of mud to pack the umbilical stump to soothe the infant.

Spores enter a wound and, when bacterial growth and multiplication occur, a potent exotoxin is produced. The non-invasive bacteria remain at the wound site, but the neurotoxin travels along peripheral nerves to the CNS where it blocks the release of transmitters, especially in inhibitory neurones. This causes an overactivity of motor neurones. Sympathetic nerves may also be affected, leading to a similar overactivity in the sympathetic nervous system.

After an incubation period of 4–10 days, muscle rigidity (stiffness) and uncontrolled muscle spasms occur. Uncontrolled contraction of the powerful masseter (jaw) muscles is common, leading to the classic 'lockjaw', or trismus. Contraction of the facial muscles may occur, causing the sneering appearance termed 'risus sardonicus'. Generalised contraction of the muscles of the back, neck, abdomen, arms and legs can give the whole body a stiff, ramrod appearance. In some cases, back muscle contraction may be sufficiently severe to cause the patient's back to arch and even to crush the spinal processes (see Figure 20.7). Death generally results from respiratory failure due to spasm of the respiratory muscles. Variation in blood pressure, tachycardia and sweating may be prominent in the elderly, due to the effects of the toxin on the sympathetic nervous system.

Diagnosis of tetanus is by clinical appraisal since the organism exists only in small numbers and can rarely be isolated. Treatment of tetanus is difficult. Human tetanus immunoglobulin should be given immediately tetanus is suspected. The wound should be thoroughly cleansed and all devitalised tissue removed, and penicillin given to prevent bacterial replication. Muscle relaxants may be used and, in severe cases, ventilatory support may be necessary. Despite treatment, the mortality rate can still be as high as 30%.

Prevention of tetanus involves (1) immunisation and (2) prophylaxis after a tetanus-prone injury is sustained. Tetanus can be effectively prevented if full immunisation is followed. Immunisation is with tetanus toxoid vaccine, a preparation of the toxin that has been treated with formalin, which inactivates its toxicity but retains its antigenicity. It is one of the safest vaccines in current use and is nearly 100% effective. The National Health and Medical Research Council (NHMRC) currently recommends that all people be immunised against tetanus at the ages of 2, 4, 6 months and 4 years, with a booster dose at 15–17 years and again at 50 years.

Certain types of wounds, termed 'tetanus-prone wounds', are likely to favour the growth of tetanus organisms. These include compound fractures, deep penetrating wounds, wounds with extensive tissue damage (e.g. burns) and any wound contaminated with soil, dust or horse manure. For tetanus-prone wounds there are guidelines for the use of tetanus toxoid and tetanus immunoglobulin as prophylactic measures (summarised in Table 20.5).

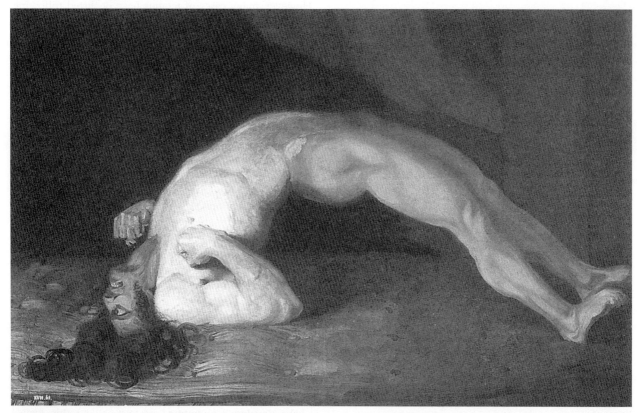

Figure 20.7

A painting of a man dying of the final stages of tetanus
Note the arched back and the sneering appearance of 'risus sardonicus', due to severe muscle spasm of the back and face, respectively.

Table 20.5

National Health and Medical Research Council (NHMRC) guide to tetanus prophylaxis in wound management

HISTORY OF ACTIVE IMMUNISATION	TIME SINCE LAST DOSE	TYPE OF WOUND	TETANUS TOXOID	TETANUS IMMUNOGLOBULIN
Uncertain, or less than three doses		clean, minor wound	Yes	No
		all other wounds	Yes	Yes
Three doses or more	less than 5 years	all wounds	No	No
	5–10 years	clean, minor wound	No	No
		all other wounds	Yes	No
	more than 10 years	all wounds	Yes	No

BOTULISM

Botulism is predominantly a food-borne illness that mainly affects the nervous system, rather than the gastro-intestinal tract. A less common form results from infection of traumatic wounds. Botulism is caused by the anaerobic, spore-forming, Gram-positive rod *Clostridium botulinum*. Generally, the disease is rare in Australia, New Zealand and other developed countries. Since the commencement of notifications in 1992, there have been five cases of infant botulism reported in Australia. Animals, birds and fish are also susceptible to botulism and suffer similar symptoms and outcomes to humans (see Spotlight box, below).

Spores of the organism are widespread in soil and are often found contaminating meat and vegetables. The spores are very resistant to heat, being able to survive boiling for several hours, but are destroyed by standard sterilising processes.

Classically, the disease has been associated with the consumption of canned or preserved foods that have not been adequately sterilised. The foods usually implicated are those preserved at home, when appropriate sterilisation

---

SPOTLIGHT ON
Botulism

During the Easter Thoroughbred Yearling Sales in Sydney in 1994, 42 yearlings were affected by a disease syndrome characterised by variable degrees of flaccid paralysis. Severe respiratory distress signalled the terminal stages of the disease. Thirty-three of the horses died.

It was established that the outbreak was the result of the toxin of *Clostridium botulinum* type C, and was therefore equine botulism. The horse is extremely susceptible to botulinum toxin. The lack of antitoxin in this situation severely handicapped efforts to control the outbreak.

---

procedures have not been followed. The spores germinate inside the can or bottle during storage and the botulinum toxin is released. The ingestion of preformed toxin results in disease. It is absorbed in the intestine and enters the bloodstream. The botulinum toxin then acts on peripheral nerve synapses, blocking the release of acetylcholine, which is the chemical released by neurones to cause muscle cells to contract. The toxin paralyses the muscles in a relaxed state (flaccid paralysis). This neurotoxin is one of the most potent of all natural toxins – 1 µg is sufficient to kill 10 people. It is colourless, tasteless and odourless and thus not noticed when eating contaminated food.

A different form of botulism, called infant botulism, can affect children in the age group of 1–7 months. Unlike the classical form which involves the ingestion of pre-formed toxin in food, infant botulism involves the ingestion of *C. botulinum* cells or spores. Normally, the bacterium itself, and its spores, are unable to compete successfully with the intestinal flora, so their ingestion does not result in disease. But infants are more susceptible because their flora is not fully established. Such cases are often related to the consumption of honey (spores are picked up from flowers and plants by bees) or ingestion of soil.

There are seven different serological types of toxin, which differ in their potency. Types A, B and E are the most common, and A is the most potent.

Symptoms usually begin within 2–3 days of consumption of contaminated food. The disease is characterised by a descending weakness and paralysis. Visual disturbances (e.g. double vision) and dysphagia (pain or difficulty in swallowing) are common early symptoms; as the disease progresses, muscles lower down the body become affected. Muscles in the trunk and limbs are weakened and then paralysed. Eventually, patients may have difficulty breathing and may die from respiratory failure due to dysfunction of respiratory muscles.

Diagnosis is mainly by clinical appraisal and culture and toxin assays of appropriate specimens. Possible specimens, depending on the type of infection, include blood (for serum), gastric contents, faeces, wound tissue and food material. Supportive care (e.g. ventilatory support, intubation of airways, cardiac support) is the most important aspect of patient management. Administration of botulinum antitoxin, which is effective against disease due to toxin types A and E, has been a common aspect of treatment for many years. However, it is produced in horses and has a number of possible, potentially serious side effects, including serum sickness and anaphylaxis, so its use is restricted. Antibiotics are not generally useful, except in wound botulism.

A purified and diluted preparation of neurotoxin A of *C. botulinum*, called Botox, is increasingly being used as a pharmaceutical agent. It has been used with some moderate success in the treatment of disease conditions in which muscles are overactive or in spasm (e.g. in certain eye disorders, some stroke patients, carpel tunnel syndrome). It now also has a very popular cosmetic use – as a beauty treatment. When injected into muscles of the face, it paralyses them and thereby smoothes away wrinkles.

LEPROSY

Leprosy has been known since biblical times. It was a feared disease and, from the 6th century, spread through Europe, leading to the establishment of many isolated leper hospitals and colonies. It is no longer as feared as in the past but remains an important health problem in the world today. The prevalence of leprosy has declined substantially over the last 20 years, largely as a result of the implementation of a multi-drug therapy regime recommended by the World Health Organization in 1981. In 1985 there were an estimated 12 million people with leprosy worldwide. It is believed that this number had been reduced to around 1.3 million cases by 2002. Leprosy was eliminated from 108 countries in that time. However, it is still a problem in certain parts of Asia, Africa and Latin America, with more than half of the world's cases in India.

In Australia, the incidence has been steadily declining since 1944 to a current annual rate of less than 10 notifications per year. Most infections occur in indigenous populations in the Northern Territory and Queensland and in migrants from endemic countries. In New Zealand, fewer than 10 cases per year are generally notified.

Leprosy is caused by the acid-fast bacillus *Mycobacterium leprae*. It has not been possible to culture the organism *in vitro*, so the study of it has been difficult. It has been grown in armadillos, mangabey monkeys and mice for research purposes. The disease appears to be confined to humans, so is always acquired from another person. The organism is present in large numbers in the nasal secretions of infected people and is probably transmitted by nasal droplets followed by uptake through the respiratory mucosa. Skin-to-skin contact is not considered to be an important route. Transmission is enhanced by overcrowding and poor hygiene. The disease has a long incubation period – usually 2–5 years but sometimes

---

CASE HISTORY 20.6

Leprosy

A 23-year-old male, born in North Queensland and of previous good health, presented to his general practitioner with a 12-month history of rash. He had been treated with topical antifungal and corticosteroid creams by other medical practitioners with no effect.

Examination showed numerous, asymmetrically distributed pink-to-brown plaques on the trunk and limbs, some with central healing. Ziehl-Neelson staining of skin biopsies showed numerous acid-fast bacilli. A diagnosis of borderline Hansen's disease was made.

Initially, it appeared that the man had no obvious contact with Hansen's disease. He had lived all his life in North Queensland, had never travelled overseas and denied any contact with people with Hansen's disease.

However, a review of historical data on Hansen's disease in Queensland showed that his grandfather had been incarcerated on Peel Island (the Queensland leprosarium) from 1943 to 1949 and again from 1954 to 1958. It was also noted that in 1982 the grandfather had suffered a clinical relapse. Treatment, including rifampicin, was recommended, but smears were still strongly positive shortly before his death in 1984 at the age of 80.

The current patient was 10 years old when his grandfather died. He had had intermittent, usually short, contact with his grandfather. It was assumed that the grandfather was the source of disease presenting in the grandson 13 years later. The patient was treated with standard multidrug therapy.

Source: Archibald H, PF Fitzpatrick & GH Rée 1999, 'Locally acquired Hansen's disease in North Queensland', *Medical Journal of Australia* 170, p. 72.

---

20 years or more. Infected people may be shedding organisms for years before the onset of symptoms, making control in endemic regions very difficult. Generally, however, and contrary to earlier belief, leprosy is not a highly contagious disease, requiring prolonged and close contact for transmission, such as between children and their infected parents.

M. leprae is an obligate intracellular parasite which resides in histiocytes, endothelial cells, and Schwann cells in peripheral nerves. Its invasion of Schwann cells is the basis for the characteristic nerve damage in the disease. The organism grows extremely slowly, which helps to explain the incubation period of several years or more in human disease. The organism grows best at temperatures below 37°C, and thus has a predilection for cooler parts of the body such as the skin and peripheral structures like the fingers, ears and nose.

After a variable incubation period, the disease can develop with a spectrum of clinical manifestations. In **tuberculoid leprosy**, a strong cell-mediated immune response limits the multiplication of the organism and the disease is confined to patches of skin and certain nerve trunks. This form is characterised by blotchy skin lesions, which may be red or hypopigmented, and areas on the face, trunk and extremities which may have lost sensitivity (e.g. to a pinprick) because of damage to nerves and nerve endings.

Lepromatous leprosy is at the other end of the clinical spectrum and is due to the absence of cellular immunity to the organism. In this form, there is uncontrolled proliferation of the bacteria, which results in extensive skin lesions and nerve involvement. The skin lesions may eventually become very large and nodular in appearance. As the disease progresses, there is loss of eyebrows and a thickening of the nose, ears and cheeks, producing a typical 'leonine' (lion-like) facial appearance. There is progressive destruction of bones in the hands, feet (see Figure 20.8) and nose. With the loss of local sensation, victims suffer frequent physical trauma to extremities which become infected with other organisms, causing further deformity.

Between these two ends of the spectrum, there are intermediate forms referred to as borderline tuberculoid leprosy, borderline leprosy and borderline lepromatous leprosy. The less developed the cell-mediated immune response, the more severe the clinical lesions. The form of disease that an individual develops seems to be at least partly genetically determined.

Diagnosis of leprosy is usually based on clinical grounds – that is, the finding of anaesthetic skin lesions (lesions with a loss of sensation) and thickened peripheral nerves. Laboratory confirmation is provided by the demonstration of acid-fast bacilli in skin smears, obtained by scraping off samples of affected skin with a scalpel blade. The current recommendations of the World Health Organization are that multi-drug therapy should be used for treatment of leprosy. In the less severe forms, rifampicin and dapsone are recommended. In the more severe forms, rifampicin, dapsone and clofazimine are recommended. The rationale for this is that there are many more organisms present in the severe forms and thus a much greater chance of resistant strains emerging.

There is no vaccine for leprosy but the vaccine for tuberculosis (the BCG), which is caused by other mycobacteria, has been reported to provide 20–80% protection against leprosy in different clinical trials. Prophylactic antibiotic therapy may be used for high-risk contacts, but is often unsuccessful.

RABIES AND AUSTRALIAN BAT LYSSAVIRUS INFECTION

Rabies ('rage' or 'madness' in Latin) has been the object of fear and fascination for thousands of years, with written accounts in ancient books of Mesopotamia and Babylon dating back to around 2300 BC. The mere mention of the disease often conjures up visions of a gentle, obedient pet suddenly becoming ferocious and drooling, or a wild, irrational animal emerging from the woods searching for prey, or a human victim dying a horrible death in a state of delirium and rage.

Rabies is an encephalitis caused by a large, enveloped, bullet-shaped virus with single-stranded RNA, belonging to the family Rhabdoviridae. It can infect almost all warm-blooded animals and is primarily a disease of animals. Most human cases are due to dog bites in countries where canine rabies is endemic. In some countries other wild animals, including monkeys, foxes, bats and raccoons, are important sources.

Rabies occurs in most countries of the world and is endemic in much of Africa, Asia, the Americas and Europe. The World Health Organization estimates that over 50 000 people throughout the world die each year from rabies. A number of countries are free of endemic rabies, including Australia, New Zealand, Papua New Guinea, England and Japan, predominantly due to strict quarantine laws and, in some cases, animal vaccination programs. The occasional case of rabies identified in Australia results from infection overseas in endemic countries.

The rabies virus is almost always inoculated by the bite of an infected animal or, rarely, by exposure of mucous membranes or skin lesions to infected saliva or other secretions (e.g. urine). Once in the body, the virus infects local muscle cells where it may lie dormant for a variable period. The virus replicates in the muscle fibres and then travels via peripheral nerves and the spinal cord to the brain where it causes an encephalitis. From there it can spread via nerves to a wide variety of richly innervated sites, such as the salivary glands, respiratory tract, skin and cornea.

The incubation period can vary markedly. The longest well-documented period is about two years, but in most cases it is usually 1–3 months. Clinical illness indicates the arrival of the virus in the CNS. The early symptoms are headache, fever and partial paralysis at the bite site. This is followed by more generalised paralysis, muscle spasms (involving particularly the pharynx and larynx), hydrophobia (fear of water, due to the muscle spasms in the

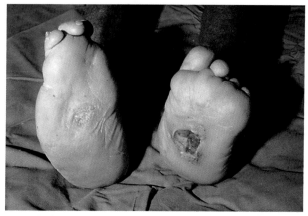

Figure 20.8

Leprosy
In this case a severe destruction of bones in the feet has occurred.

throat and chest that swallowing can induce), hypersalivation, aerophobia (fear of moving air, due to hypersensitivity of the skin), confusion, periods of hyperactivity (running, biting and thrashing about) and hallucinations. After 2–10 days of these acute neurological symptoms, the patient becomes comatose and dies, usually due to heart or respiratory failure. It is almost always fatal once symptoms have developed.

Diagnosis of rabies can be made by detection of viral antigens in skin biopsy specimens using a microscopic immunofluorescence technique, by PCR testing for viral RNA in skin biopsy, saliva or CSF, or by examination of serum or CSF for specific antibodies.

Rabies can be prevented if appropriate prophylactic treatment is given, before symptoms develop, to a person known or suspected of having been exposed to the virus. This treatment is based on:

- prompt and thorough cleaning of the wound with soap and water, followed by application of an antiviral antiseptic (e.g. 70% ethanol or povidone-iodine)
- commencement of rabies vaccination regimen to induce the formation of specific antibodies in the patient
- thorough infiltration of the wound with rabies immunoglobulin to attempt to neutralise viruses before they enter the nervous system.

Such treatment, if administered properly and soon enough, provides protection from disease. Safe, effective vaccines for active immunisation are available, but routine immunisation for Australians is not necessary. However, all workers and travellers who are at high risk of contracting rabies in an endemic area should be immunised, as should health professionals caring for infected patients.

The Australian bat lyssavirus, discovered in 1996, is related to the rabies virus and causes a similar clinical disease. Although it has been found to infect most types of Australian fruit bats (flying foxes) and insectivorous bats, the transfer to humans occurs only rarely (one documented case in 1996 and another in 1998). Rabies vaccine and immunoglobulin also protect against Australian bat lyssavirus infection, so the recommended treatment and preventive measures are similar for both diseases. Rabies immunisation is recommended for any person likely to suffer scratches or bites from bats.

POLIO

Polio (or poliomyelitis) has been known for thousands of years and was once a very common disease. Figure 20.9 shows a typical polio victim recorded on an ancient Egyptian stone slab from the 18th dynasty (1580–1350 BC). Before the availability of vaccines in the mid-1950s, there were more than 20 000 cases of paralytic polio in the United States each year. Since then the incidence has declined to very low numbers. The last notified case of wild-type poliomyelitis in Australia was in 1978, although vaccine-associated cases were reported in 1986 and 1995. Vaccine-associated polio results from the use of the live, attenuated, oral polio vaccine (Sabin vaccine). The vaccine

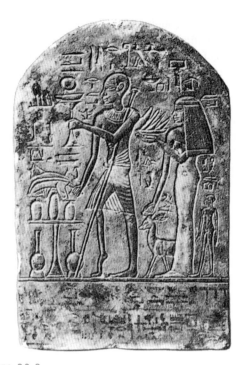

Figure 20.9

A typical polio victim shown on an ancient Egyptian stone slab, circa 1580–1350 BC

viruses become established in the intestine and provide local immunity to wild-type polio viruses. Rarely, in about 1 case per million vaccinated children, the vaccine virus causes disease – called vaccine-associated paralytic poliomyelitis.

In 1988 the WHO initiated a global polio eradication initiative with a view to eradicating the disease from the world. The program has been based on immunisation, surveillance and targeting of high-risk areas. As a result, there has been a progressive fall globally in the reported incidence of polio from an estimated 350 000 cases in 1988 to 2000 cases in 2002. At the same time the number of polio-endemic countries fell from 125 to 7. On 29 October 2000 an independent panel of international public health experts certified the WHO Western Pacific Region, which includes Australia and 36 other countries, as polio-free (see Spotlight box, page 499). This is the second region in the world to be certified. Despite being declared free of polio, it is still essential that population immunity be maintained at a high level as there is always the potential risk of an imported case. Polio is still a significant problem in some developing countries, especially parts of Africa and the Indian subcontinent.

Polio is best known as a cause of paralysis, but the virus produces symptoms in only about 10% of infected people and less than 1% develops the paralytic form. It is caused by the poliovirus, a single-stranded RNA virus, of which there are three distinct serotypes. Humans are the only known reservoir of the virus. It is excreted in the faeces of infected people and is usually transmitted via food, water or hands. It is a fairly stable virus which can remain infectious for long periods outside the body (e.g. in food or

SPOTLIGHT ON
Polio: major milestone reached in global polio eradication

On 29 October 2000 an independent panel of international public health experts certified the World Health Organization Western Pacific Region as polio-free. This Region comprises 37 countries and areas* ranging from tiny islands to the country with the single largest population in the world, the People's Republic of China.

The WHO Western Pacific Region is now the second in the world to be certified polio-free, after the WHO Region of the Americas in 1994.

The Regional Certification Commission on Poliomyelitis Eradication confirmed that no new cases of indigenous polio were detected in the Western Pacific Region in the three years prior to 2000 despite excellent surveillance for the virus – the major benchmark for certification.

Dr Gro Harlem Brundtland, Director-General of the World Health Organization, said from Geneva:

> This is a major milestone in the global effort led by WHO, Rotary International, UNICEF and the Centers for Disease Control to certify the world polio-free by 2005. By certifying that this diverse Region is polio-free, we demonstrate that it is possible to eradicate polio throughout the world. I would like to congratulate the countries involved, donor governments, partner agencies, and in particular the hundreds of thousands of volunteers whose time and effort contributed to this remarkable success.

In polio-free regions, the challenges ahead include maintaining certification-standard surveillance and achieving safe containment of laboratory stocks of the wild poliovirus to prevent inadvertent release. The Western Pacific Region is breaking new ground for the eradication initiative in piloting the Global Action Plan for Laboratory Containment of Wild Poliovirus. The Region will also focus on strengthening routine immunisation programs by systematically building on the lessons learned in polio eradication.

Polio transmission is still likely to occur in up to 20 countries, primarily in West and Central Africa and in the Horn of Africa, as well as in parts of Asia. In these areas, national immunisation days and intensive house-to-house mop-up campaigns are being conducted to interrupt the remaining chains of poliovirus transmission.

*The 37 countries and areas comprising the WHO Western Pacific Region are American Samoa, Australia, Brunei, Darussalam, Cambodia, China, Cook Islands, the Federated States of Micronesia, Fiji, French Polynesia, Guam, Hong Kong (China), Japan, Kiribati, the Lao People's Democratic Republic, Macao (China), Malaysia, Marshall Islands, Mongolia, Nauru, New Caledonia, New Zealand, Niue, Northern Mariana Islands, Palau, Papua New Guinea, the Philippines, Pitcairn Islands, the Republic of Korea, Samoa, Singapore, Solomon Islands, Tokelau, Tonga, Tuvalu, Vanuatu, Vietnam, and Wallis and Futuna.

Adapted from a WHO press release on 29 October 2000.

water). In the early stages of infection, it may also be present in the nose and throat and thus be transmitted by the airborne route.

After initial local multiplication in the intestine or pharynx, the virus reaches the bloodstream. The majority of cases are asymptomatic or have only mild symptoms of headache, sore throat, fever and nausea. One to two per cent of people develop the paralytic form, in which the virus invades the CNS where it infects neurones in the spinal cord and brain. The damage to these cells results in paralysis of the muscles that they innervate. High fever, back or neck pain and muscle spasms are the early symptoms and then several days later a flaccid paralysis occurs. One or more limbs may be affected and some patients also experience difficulties in talking, swallowing or breathing.

Some patients with paralysed respiratory muscles used to be restricted to an 'iron lung' (a predecessor of modern ventilatory equipment) for the rest of their lives. Some paralysis may disappear, but any that persists for several months is usually permanent. One in 200 infections leads to permanent paralysis, usually in the legs (see Figure 20.10).

Laboratory diagnosis of polio involves the isolation and identification of the virus in tissue culture from faeces or a pharyngeal swab. An isolated virus is then tested, by various methods, to determine whether it is a wild-type strain or a vaccine strain.

Post-polio syndrome is a term coined in the 1980s to describe a condition that affects some people who have recovered from paralytic polio many years earlier. The symptoms, which typically appear 30 to 40 years later, are characterised by new and progressive muscle weakness, debilitating fatigue and loss of function, and pain in muscles and joints. A variety of possible causes of post-polio syndrome have been suggested, including degeneration of motor neurones, reactivation of latent virus and immune-mediated response.

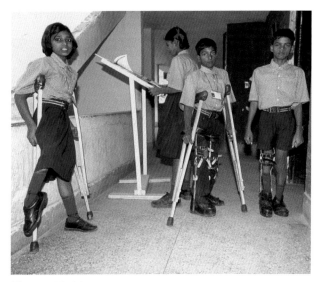

Figure 20.10
Polio victims in India

The first vaccine available for polio was the **Salk vaccine** (IPV – inactivated poliomyelitis vaccine) in 1955. It contains formalin-inactivated viruses and is 70–90% effective. It is administered by intramuscular injection. In the early 1960s, the more effective (nearly 100%) **Sabin vaccine** (OPV – oral poliomyelitis vaccine) was introduced. It contains attenuated, live viruses and is more effective because it induces a strong IgA antibody response at mucosal surfaces where infection first occurs. The OPV has the added advantage of oral administration, as well as providing a longer-lasting immunity if the correct number of doses is given. However, there is still some debate about whether the IPV or the OPV should be used in mass immunisation campaigns, even given the greater efficacy and ease of administration of the latter. The debate is mainly due to the possibility, albeit rare, of vaccine-associated paralytic poliomyelitis. Most cases of vaccine-associated polio occur in young infants (less than four months old) or in the immunocompromised.

The National Health and Medical Research Council in Australia states that IPV or OPV should be used to vaccinate infants from two months of age, but IPV is preferred because of the rare risk of polio associated with OPV. IPV is part of the standard childhood vaccination schedule in Australia and is recommended for use at 2, 4 and 6 months with a further booster dose at 4 years of age.

TRANSMISSIBLE SPONGIFORM ENCEPHALOPATHIES (PRION DISEASES)

Transmissible spongiform encephalopathies (TSEs) are a group of infectious, fatal, neurodegenerative diseases in humans and animals. They are so called because transmission from human to human and animal to human is possible, and the diseases cause damage to the brain tissue that produces microscopic vacuoles, giving it a spongy appearance in histological sections (see Figure 20.11). These diseases are believed to be due to an intracellular accumulation of an abnormal form of a normal cell protein. The infectious protein, PrP, is referred to as a **prion**. The normal cellular isoform of the protein, PrP^c, is

believed to be converted into an abnormal, protease-resistant isoform, referred to as PrP^{res}, in affected brain cells. The normal function of PrP^c. is unknown. After entering a host cell, PrP^{res} appears to act as a template causing conversion of PrP^c to PrP^{res}. The amino acid sequences of PrP^c and PrP^{res} are identical, but their three-dimensional structure is different. How the propagation of PrP^{res} causes damage to brain cells is not known.

Human prion diseases can arise in three distinct ways: sporadic, inherited or acquired. Sporadic disease occurs in very low incidence throughout the world (annual incidence of one per million people). In sporadic diseases the abnormal PrP^{res} protein is spontaneously generated. The inherited disease is the type found in people with a family history of TSE and is due to a mutation in the gene that codes for PrP^c. Acquired prion diseases are caused by the transmission of the infectious agent PrP^{res} during medical or surgical procedures or by consumption of contaminated material.

These infectious agents have a number of unusual properties, including an apparent lack of nucleic acid and a resistance to ultraviolet light, heat and certain chemical agents. For example, infectious prions are not inactivated by boiling, ethylene oxide sterilisation, ethanol, detergents or alcoholic iodine. Even years of storage in formaldehyde does not destroy their infectivity. One of the more remarkable features of all prion diseases is that they do not appear to induce a classical inflammatory response or a specific immune response, normally the hallmarks of infection.

A number of different diseases of animals and humans have been attributed to prions. Scrapie is a prion disease in sheep and goats in which infected animals itch and scrape themselves against fences and posts, often until they bleed. **Bovine spongiform encephalopathy (BSE)**, or **'mad cow disease'**, has possibly affected more than four million cattle in Britain since 1986 and threatened the beef industry there. An infected animal typically loses weight, has a depressed appearance with lowered head and arched back, and suffers increasing difficulty in walking, eventually being unable to stand (see Figure 20.12). The source of the

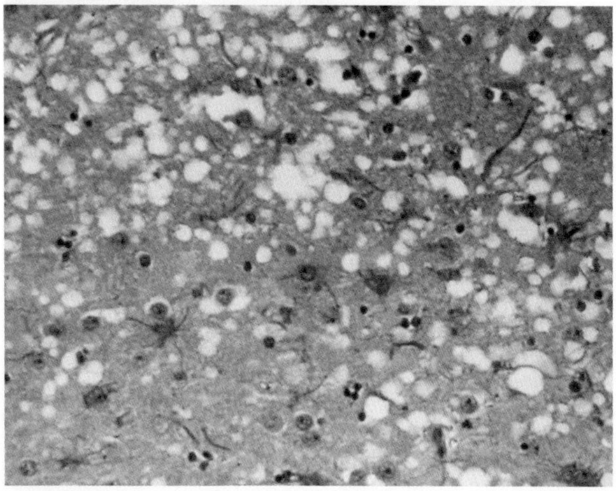

Figure 20.11

A section of brain tissue of a cow with BSE

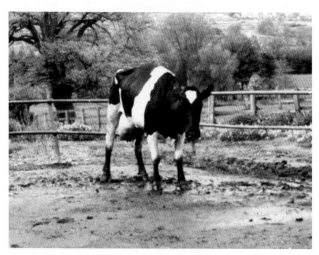

Figure 20.12

Mad cow disease

epidemic is suspected to be cattle feed containing cattle or sheep products (now banned in Britain).

BSE has been reported in much lower incidence in some other countries due to the importation of either cattle feed from the United Kingdom (e.g. France, Portugal, Switzerland) or cattle from the United Kingdom (e.g. Germany, Canada, Italy). Australia and New Zealand are considered to be free of scrapie and BSE.

Creutzfeldt-Jakob disease and variant Creutzfeld-Jakob disease are the most important of the human prion diseases and are discussed in the following sections. The other human prion disease that has been studied extensively is kuru. This disease has been found only in people of the Fore tribes in the highlands of Papua New Guinea. Kuru occurred in about 1 in 10 people in these tribes and was found to be transmitted from person to person by their cannibalistic practices. Their ritual required the consumption of parts of the body of a dead member of the family who, given the incidence of disease, was likely to have died from kuru. No cases of kuru have been seen in those born after 1957, when the practice of cannibalism ceased. D. Carleton Gadjusek, an American scientist, won the Nobel Prize in 1976 for his work on this disease.

Gertsmann-Straussler-Scheinker syndrome is a rare human prion disease with an estimated incidence of less than two cases per 100 million people. This disease, first described by Gertsmann and co-workers in 1928, is mainly an inherited disorder, although studies have shown that it can be transmitted by the injection of brain extracts from affected humans into primates and rodents. Fatal familial insomnia is also an exotic disease of humans attributed to prions.

Creutzfeldt-Jakob disease

Hans Gerhard Creutzfeldt first described a progressive dementing illness in a 22-year-old woman in 1920, and in the following year Alfons Maria Jakob described four similar cases. Worldwide, there is thought to be approximately one new case of Creutzfeldt-Jakob disease (CJD) per 1–2 million people each year.

CJD mainly affects people in the 50–75 years age group. The majority of cases (about 85%) are considered to be of the sporadic type. About 10% of cases appear to be inherited and the remainder are due to transmission of infectious material. Transmission from human to human has been shown to occur through the transfer of infected tissue or body fluids, or via contaminated surgical instruments. Iatrogenic transmission of CJD in treatments involving pituitary hormones and dura mater grafts is most common, but transmission via corneal transplants and neurosurgical equipment has also been reported. The use of pituitary-derived growth hormone and gonadotrophin, collected and pooled from cadaveric pituitary glands in the 1980s, was responsible for more than 140 cases of CJD in the United States, the United Kingdom, France, New Zealand and Australia. There is no evidence that CJD is transmissible by blood or blood products, although it is

theoretically possible. There are concerns that the variant form of CJD could be transmitted in this way (see next section).

There is no evidence to suggest that CJD is transmitted during normal social contact or sexual contact, or from mother to foetus. There is no direct evidence to support the hypothesis of transmission of CJD via food.

A number of reports of CJD in health-care workers (including neurosurgeons, doctors, dentists, nurses and histopathology technicians) suggest the possibility of workplace infection, although precise evidence of this has not been demonstrated in most of these cases.

From iatrogenic infections it has been established that, when the agent is introduced into or near the brain, the incubation period is in the order of months, but in peripheral transmission the incubation period is usually years or even decades. The dominant features of CJD are muscle weakness and dementia. Early symptoms may include loss of balance and muscle coordination, slurred speech, failing vision and myoclonic (quick, jerky) movements of the extremities or head. The symptoms become progressively more severe, leading to dementia and a variety of other neurological disturbances such as dysphasia, spasticity and seizures in a period of only months. Myoclonic jerking movements are the most frequent physical sign. The patient eventually becomes comatose. The disease is uniformly fatal, usually in less than a year from the onset of symptoms.

A definitive diagnosis of CJD can only be made at autopsy with the demonstration of spongy neuropathological changes and the demonstration of PrP^{res} deposits in brain tissue. A presumptive diagnosis, before death, can be made on clinical grounds, together with EEG and MRI scans and examination of CSF for non-specific markers of neuronal injury.

Because prions are unusually resistant to heat and many chemical disinfectants, specific methods for sterilisation and disinfection are followed when contamination with these agents is suspected. Recommendations from the Australian Government Department of Health and Ageing, in *Infection Control Guidelines*, 2004, are:

- incineration of disposable instruments and clinical waste
- autoclaving of instruments for reuse for 18 minutes at 134°C
- immersion of heat-sensitive instruments in 2% sodium hypochlorite solution or 1 molar NaOH for 1 hour
- disinfection of surfaces with 5% sodium hypochlorite or 1M NaOH, allowed to stand for 1 hour.

There is no proven treatment for CJD and no vaccine.

Variant Creutzfeld-Jakob disease

Variant Creutzfeld-Jakob disease (vCJD) was first described in the United Kingdom in 1996, associated with the consumption of meat from cattle with mad cow disease (bovine spongiform encephalopathy – BSE). By November 2002, around 139 people had been diagnosed with vCJD across Europe, of which 129 were reported in Britain.

The BSE epidemic began in the UK in 1986 and is thought to have originated from the similar disease in sheep known as scrapie. It is postulated that the disease crossed the species barrier as a result of the practice of using sheep carcasses to produce protein-rich supplements for cattle feed. The height of the epidemic was in 1993, when 1000 new cases per month were being identified. In the next two to three years the epidemic was largely brought under control by the banning of feed containing cattle or sheep products and by the slaughter of 200 000 diseased cattle and 4.5 million asymptomatic cattle (due to the anticipated long incubation period). BSE had by then had a crippling effect on the British livestock industry and other industries reliant on bovine-derived products (e.g. gelatin and pharmaceutical industries). BSE had also spread to other European countries, presumably due to their importation of live animals or livestock food supplements from the UK.

Variant CJD is a clinical syndrome that is somewhat different to classical CJD:

- vCJD occurs in much younger people than is seen in the classical form
- vCJD tends to have a longer duration of illness than classical CJD (median of 4.5 months compared to 14 months)
- the histological changes in the brain tissue are more common in vCJD.

As for all TSEs, the disease is invariably fatal.

Evidence is emerging that vCJD may be transmitted by blood transfusion. Also, experimental studies have shown that it is possible to transmit BSE by blood between sheep. As a result, a number of countries, including Australia, have banned blood donation from anyone who visited Britain for a cumulative period of six months or more between 1980 and 1996.

The diagnosis of vCJD is similar to that of classic CJD, although the clinical criteria for a presumptive diagnosis are somewhat different.

SUMMARY

- The brain and the spinal cord are surrounded by three membranes, or meninges.
- Cerebrospinal fluid (CSF) circulates in the space between the two inner meninges.
- The blood-brain barrier consists of the tightly joined endothelial cells of the brain's capillaries, and allows only certain substances to pass from the circulation to the brain.
- Meningitis is an infection and inflammation of the meninges, most often caused by viruses or bacteria.
- Encephalitis is an infection and inflammation of the brain itself and is almost always caused by viruses.

BACTERIAL MENINGITIS

- The most common causative agents of acute bacterial meningitis are *Neisseria meningitidis* and *Streptococcus pneumoniae*.
- *Haemophilus influenza* was a major cause until an effective vaccine against it became available in 1992.
- Most cases of meningococcal meningitis (*N. meningitidis*) occur in the 0–4 years age group.
- A serious form of meningococcal infection is meningococcal septicaemia.
- Pneumococcal meningitis (*Streptococcus pneumoniae*) usually follows septicaemia or head injury.
- Neonatal meningitis is caused mainly by *E. coli* (with capsular type K1) or *Streptococcus agalactiae*.
- *Listeria monocytogenes* mainly causes meningitis in neonates or immunocompromised people.
- *Mycobacterium tuberculosis* can cause meningitis by entering the bloodstream and disseminating to the meninges.

- The tissue dysfunction in bacterial meningitis results from focal lesions due to bacterial growth or toxins, and the host inflammatory response.
- Headache, fever, altered consciousness, vomiting and nuchal rigidity (neck stiffness) are the most common presenting symptoms of bacterial meningitis.
- The mortality rate in bacterial meningitis varies from 5–50%. Up to 10% of those who survive bacterial meningitis experience serious long-term sequelae.
- CSF is the most important specimen for the diagnosis of meningitis. Blood cultures should also be collected.
- Prompt treatment of any bacterial meningitis is required.
- First-line therapy for acute meningitis is most often with benzylpenicillin or amoxicillin plus cefotaxime or ceftriaxone.
- Vaccines are available for some causes of bacterial meningitis.

VIRAL MENINGITIS

- The major causes of viral meningitis are enteroviruses.
- The incidence of viral meningitis is greatest in infants and young children.
- The immunocompromised are at increased risk of viral meningitis.
- Viral meningitis is generally milder and progresses more slowly than bacterial infections.
- A definitive diagnosis of viral meningitis is usually made by culture of CSF or the demonstration of a fourfold rise in antibody titre in acute and convalescent sera.
- Therapy for viral meningitis usually involves symptomatic treatment only.

FUNGAL INFECTIONS

- Fungal meningitis is rare in Australia, except for cryptococcal meningitis.
- Humans generally become infected with *Cryptococcus neoformans* by inhalation of the organism, after which it causes a primary lung infection. The organism may then invade the bloodstream and spread to other parts of the body, including the brain and meninges.
- Cryptococcal meningitis is confirmed by culture of the organism and by a rapid latex agglutination test which can detect cryptococcal antigen in CSF.

PROTOZOAL INFECTIONS

- Few protozoa infect the central nervous system. The notable one is *Toxoplasma gondii* which causes toxoplasmosis.
- Cerebral toxoplasmosis is one of the more common neurological complications of HIV infection.
- Diagnosis of toxoplasmosis is based on serological methods or PCR testing on body fluids.
- Treatment of cerebral toxoplasmosis is with pyrimethamine, sulphadiazine and folinic acid in combination.

ENCEPHALITIS

- Encephalitis is almost always caused by viruses; herpes simplex virus and arboviruses are the most common.
- Viral encephalitis is characterised by cerebral dysfunction, including abnormal behaviour, seizures and altered consciousness.
- Murray Valley encephalitis (MVE) is a severe, epidemic-type disease found mostly in the northern parts of Australia. It is mainly caused by the mosquito-borne MVE virus.
- Most infections with the MVE are subclinical, but occasionally the virus crosses the blood-brain barrier and causes damage to the brain tissue.
- Australian encephalitis is diagnosed by isolation of the virus, detection of viral RNA or serological evidence.
- Japanese encephalitis is caused by a flavivirus spread by mosquitoes. It is a significant problem in some parts of Asia.
- There is no specific therapy for encephalitis caused by arboviruses.
- Herpes encephalitis is a very severe disease that causes neurological damage and has a high mortality rate. Early treatment with aciclovir greatly reduces the mortality and permanent neurological damage.
- Other viral causes of encephalitis include the West Nile virus, Nipah virus, dengue virus and enterovirus 71.

TETANUS

- Tetanus is a rare, but serious, illness caused by the bacterium *Clostridium tetani*.
- Tetanus spores are widespread in soil and manure.
- Tetanus spores usually cause infection when deposited into a deep, necrotic wound where oxygen is lacking.
- The tetanus toxin travels from the wound to the CNS where it blocks the release of transmitters, resulting in an overactivity of motor neurones. Death generally results from respiratory failure.
- Diagnosis of tetanus is by clinical appraisal.
- Human tetanus immune globulin should be given immediately tetanus is suspected; the wound should be thoroughly cleansed and penicillin given.
- Prevention of tetanus involves immunisation and prophylaxis after a tetanus-prone injury is sustained.

BOTULISM

- Botulism is a form of food poisoning which affects the nervous system; it is caused by *Clostridium botulinum*.
- Spores of *C. botulinum* are widespread in soil and are often found contaminating meat and vegetables.
- Infant botulism is generally related to consumption of honey or ingestion of soil.
- The botulinum toxin acts on peripheral nerve synapses, blocking the release of acetylcholine and causing a flaccid paralysis of the muscles. Patients may have difficulty breathing and may die from respiratory failure.
- Diagnosis of botulism is mainly by clinical appraisal, culture and toxin assays.
- Supportive ventilatory and cardiac care is the most important aspect of patient management.

LEPROSY

- Leprosy is caused by the acid-fast bacillus *Mycobacterium leprae*.
- Leprosy is not a highly contagious disease, requiring prolonged close contact for transmission.
- Invasion of Schwann cells by the organism is the basis for the characteristic nerve damage in leprosy.
- Diagnosis of leprosy is based on clinical grounds and a microscopic examination of skin scrapings.
- Multi-drug therapy should be used in the treatment of leprosy.

RABIES

- Most cases of rabies in developing countries are due to dog bites.
- Countries that have been declared free of rabies include Australia, England, Japan, Sweden and Norway.
- Rabies virus replicates in muscle fibres and then travels to the brain, where it causes an encephalitis.
- The symptoms of rabies are generalised paralysis, muscle spasms, hydrophobia, hypersalivation, aerophobia, confusion, periods of hyperactivity and hallucinations. Eventually, the patient becomes comatose and dies, usually due to heart or respiratory failure.
- Diagnosis of rabies is based on detection of viral antigens or RNA in skin biopsy specimens, or by detection of specific antibodies.
- All workers and travellers at high risk of contracting rabies in an endemic area should be immunised, as should health professionals caring for infected patients.
- The Australian bat lyssavirus is related to the rabies virus and causes a similar clinical disease.

POLIO

- Polio (or poliomyelitis) is caused by the polio virus.
- Effective vaccines were developed in the mid-1950s and the incidence in developed countries declined to very low numbers.
- Polio is best known as a cause of paralysis, but the virus produces symptoms in only about 10% of infected people.
- Laboratory diagnosis of polio involves the isolation of the virus from faeces or a pharyngeal swab.
- Post-polio syndrome is a condition affecting some people who had recovered from paralytic polio many years earlier.
- In Australia, the inactivated polio vaccine (IPV) is preferred for mass immunisation.

TRANSMISSIBLE SPONGIFORM ENCEPHALOPATHIES (PRION DISEASES)

- Prions are transmissible agents that cause a number of fatal, neurodegenerative diseases in humans and animals.
- The prion diseases are believed to be due to an accumulation of an abnormal form of a cell protein in brain cells, called PrP (prion protein).

- Human prion diseases can occur sporadically, can be inherited or can be transmitted.
- Prions appear to lack nucleic acid and have an unusual resistance to ultraviolet light, heat and certain chemical agents.
- Creutzfeldt-Jakob disease (CJD) and variant CJD are the most important of the human prion diseases.
- Iatrogenic transmission of CJD through corneal transplants, stereotactic equipment, pituitary hormones and dura mater grafts has been reported.
- Early symptoms of CJD may include loss of balance and muscle coordination, slurred speech, failing vision and myoclonic (quick, jerky) movements of the extremities or head, leading to dementia.
- Variant Creutzfeldt-Jakob disease (vCJD) is associated with consumption of meat from cattle with mad cow disease (BSE).
- The characteristics and course of vCJD are different from those of CJD.
- Definitive diagnosis of CJD and vCJD can only be made at autopsy. A presumptive diagnosis before death is based on clinical grounds and non-specific tests.
- There is no treatment for CJD or vCJD and no vaccine.

STUDY QUESTIONS

1. What is the blood-brain barrier?
2. Define the terms 'meningitis' and 'encephalitis'.
3. What are the three most common causes of bacterial meningitis, and how do these organisms reach the meninges?
4. What are the two most common causes of neonatal meningitis, and how do these organisms reach the meninges?
5. What are the critical events in the pathogenesis of acute bacterial meningitis?
6. What are the major clinical features of acute bacterial meningitis?
7. What specimens should be collected from a patient suspected of having meningitis?
8. What preliminary results from the laboratory would be suggestive of a bacterial meningitis?
9. How can meningitis due to *Haemophilus influenzae* be prevented?
10. What is aseptic meningitis?
11. What are the most common causes of viral meningitis?
12. What is the most common cause of fungal meningitis in Australia, and what are the common predisposing factors?
13. What protozoan most commonly causes infection of the central nervous system in Australia, and what are the common predisposing factors?
14. What are the causes of Australian encephalitis and how is this disease transmitted?
15. What factors usually predispose to the development of a brain abscess?
16. What is the causative agent of tetanus and where is this organism commonly found?
17. Describe the pathogenesis of tetanus.
18. How does the treatment of tetanus differ from its prevention?

19. Name the causative agent of botulism and describe the pathogenesis of the disease.
20. Name the causative agent of leprosy and describe how the disease is transmitted.
21. Differentiate between tuberculoid leprosy and lepromatous leprosy.
22. What is rabies?
23. Why is rabies rare in Australia?
24. Describe the pathogenesis of paralytic poliomyelitis.
25. Why is polio a rare disease in Australia?
26. What is a spongiform encephalopathy? Give two examples.
27. What is the cause of Creutzfeldt-Jakob disease and how is it transmitted?
28. What is a prion?

TEST YOUR UNDERSTANDING

Case History 20.1   Meningococcal infection

1. What would be the typical observations in a Gram stain of CSF from a person with meningococcal meningitis?
2. How is meningococcal infection spread from person to person?
3. How can the spread of meningococcal infection be prevented?

Case History 20.2   Neonatal meningitis

1. What is the most likely cause and source of this infection?
2. What evidence is there to suggest that this is a bacterial infection?
3. What problems are associated with antimicrobial drug treatment of bacterial meningitis?

Case History 20.3   Outbreak of viral meningitis

1. What are the likely predisposing factors of viral meningitis in this case?
2. What laboratory findings support the diagnosis of viral meningitis?
3. How does the prognosis for viral meningitis compare with that for bacterial meningitis?

Case History 20.4   Murray Valley encephalitis

1. Why was aciclovir given to the child in this case?
2. Why is this referred to as an arbovirus infection?
3. What evidence confirmed this as a case of Murray Valley encephalitis? Explain.

Case History 20.5   Tetanus

1. Why did this woman develop tetanus?
2. What part of the treatment do you think was most responsible for the prevention of serious disease?
3. What is the major pathogenic mechanism of *Clostridium tetani*, and how does this relate to how tetanus is treated?

Case History 20.6   Leprosy

1. What does this case demonstrate about the incubation period of leprosy?
2. Why does therapy for leprosy involve administration of multiple drugs?

Further reading

Britton WJ & DNJ Lockwood 2004, 'Leprosy', *Lancet*, 363, pp. 1209–19. (Reviews the epidemiology, pathogenesis, clinical features, management and prevention of leprosy.)

Collins SJ, VA Lawson & CL Masters 2004, 'Transmissible spongiform encephalopathies', *Lancet*, 363, pp. 51–61. (Reviews the pathogenesis of prion diseases in humans.)

Halstead LS 1998, 'Post-polio syndrome', *Scientific American*, April, p. 36. (Gives a general overview of the pathogenesis of polio and post-polio syndrome.)

Kennedy PGE 2004, 'Viral encephalitis: causes, differential diagnosis, and management', *Journal of Neurology, Neurosurgery and Psychiatry*, 75, pp. 10–15. (Reviews the causes, differential diagnosis and management of viral encephalitis.)

Montoya JG & O Liesenfeld 2004, 'Toxoplasmosis', *Lancet*, 363, pp. 1965–76. (Reviews the epidemiology, pathogenesis, pathology, clinical features, diagnosis, management and prevention of toxoplasmosis.)

National Health & Medical Research Council 2003, *The Australian Immunisation Handbook*, 8th edn, Australian Government Department of Health and Ageing. (This book gives useful information on vaccine-preventable diseases and details the current recommendations and contraindications of the available vaccines.)

Prusiner SB 2001, 'Shattuck lecture – neurodegenerative diseases and prions', *New England Journal of Medicine*, 344(20), pp. 1516–26. (Reviews the pathogenesis of prion diseases with comparisons to other neurodegenerative diseases, such as Alzheimer's disease.)

Saez-Llorens X & GH McCracken 2003, 'Bacterial meningitis in children', *Lancet*, 361, pp. 2139–48. (Reviews the epidemiology, pathogenesis, clinical features, diagnosis, management and prevention of bacterial meningitis.)

Thorley BR, KA Brussen, V Stambos & H Kelly 2003, 'Annual report of the Australian National Poliovirus Reference Laboratory, 2002', *Communicable Diseases Intelligence*, 27(3), pp. 352–6. (Details current surveillance methods and incidence of poliovirus in Australia.)

Tuomanen E 1993, 'Breaching the blood-brain barrier', *Scientific American*, February, 56. (Provides a description of the blood-brain barrier and how bacteria may affect its integrity.)

Warrell MJ & DA Warrell 2004, 'Rabies and other lyssavirus diseases', *Lancet*, 363, pp. 959–69. (Reviews the incidence, pathogenesis, clinical features, management and prevention of lyssavirus infections.)

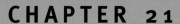

CHAPTER 21

Infections of the Urinary and Reproductive Systems

[CHAPTER FOCUS]

- *What microorganisms cause urinary tract infections?*

- *How do urinary tract infections develop and what forms of infection occur?*

- *What are the major types of infections that involve the reproductive system?*

- *How can sexually transmissible diseases be prevented?*

Introduction

In this chapter we examine the infectious diseases of the urinary tract and reproductive system. The urinary tract is one of the more common sites of infection, especially in females, and is frequently the site of hospital-acquired infection. The reproductive (genital) system has a close anatomical relationship with the urinary tract and is also a common site of infection. Many infections of the genital tract are acquired during sexual activity and are therefore called **sexually transmissible infections** (STIs). STIs are a major public health problem throughout the world.

Normal flora of the urinary and reproductive systems

The anatomy of the male and female genitourinary tracts and the sites that have a normal microbial flora are shown in Figure 21.1. In a healthy person, the upper urethra, the urinary bladder and the organs of the upper urinary tract are sterile. In contrast, the lower urethra has a normal flora that usually includes *Staphylococcus epidermidis*, *Enterococcus faecalis*, corynebacteria, species of *Neisseria* and *Bacteroides*, and members of the *Enterobacteriaceae*, such as *Escherichia coli* and *Proteus*.

The upper regions of the urinary tract are normally kept free of microorganisms by a variety of defence mechanisms. One of the more critical of these is the normal flow of urine that washes over the surface of the urethral epithelium, flushing away microorganisms. The lower urethra is also cleansed by this mechanism, but recolonisation there occurs quickly.

In the genital tract of males, normal flora organisms are found only in the anterior urethra, that is, near the external opening. In contrast, the genital tract of females, in particular the vagina, has a very complex normal flora. This microbial population is significantly influenced by sex hormones and is thus different in neonates, pre-pubertal girls and pre- and post-menopausal women. Its composition also varies during the menstrual cycle.

In adult females, the major residents of the vagina are the lactobacilli. These bacteria assist in maintaining the acidic pH of the normal vagina (around pH 4.4 to 4.6) by breaking down the glycogen in vaginal secretions with the formation of lactic acid. Only microorganisms capable of growth and multiplication at this pH are found in the normal flora. In addition to the lactobacilli, these include enterococci, corynebacteria, a variety of anaerobic bacteria and the yeast *Candida albicans*. In healthy females, protection against infection of the genital and urinary tracts is afforded by the low pH and the normal flora of the vagina. In situations where the pH and/or the normal flora are modified (e.g. with broad spectrum antibiotic therapy or use of spermicides), infection often ensues.

Urinary tract infections

Urinary tract infections occur much more frequently in females. Approximately 10–20% of women experience a urinary tract infection (UTI) at some time in their life. In contrast, less than 5% of males under 60 years of age suffer an episode of urinary tract infection, although the incidence of UTI increases markedly above that age in association with an increased incidence of prostatic hypertrophy (causing urinary obstruction). UTIs represent 30–40% of all hospital-acquired infections, and are often related to urinary catheterisation. Although the majority of infections are short-lived, recurrences are possible, and severe infections can result in renal damage.

CAUSATIVE ORGANISMS

The vast majority of infections are caused by microorganisms that ascend the urethra and thereby reach the bladder and sometimes the kidneys. Occasionally, in patients with septicaemia, organisms spread from the bloodstream to the kidneys to cause infection.

Ascending infections are most often caused by the enteric bacterium, *E. coli*. Other common causes include *Staphylococcus aureus*, coagulase negative staphylococci (*Staphylococcus epidermidis*, *Staphylococcus saprophyti-*

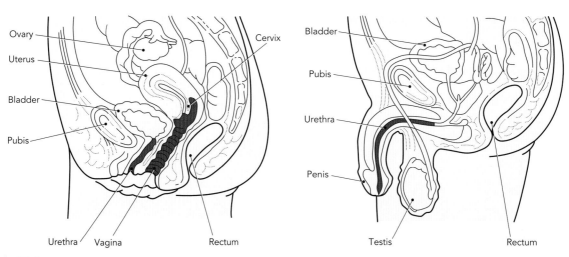

Figure 21.1

The male and female genitourinary tracts, showing the areas where normal flora reside (*coloured red*)

cus), *Enterococcus faecalis*, *Pseudomonas*, and *Enterobacteriaceae* such as *Proteus*, *Klebsiella* and *Enterobacter*. These organisms are derived mainly from the patient's own gastrointestinal tract. *E. coli* is the most common cause of both community-acquired and hospital-acquired UTI, but organisms such as *Proteus mirabilis*, *Staphylococcus aureus*, *Enterococcus faecalis* and *Pseudomonas aeruginosa* have a more prominent role in hospital infections than in community-acquired infections (see Table 21.1). Hospital-acquired organisms are often multiply resistant to antibiotics and therefore difficult to treat.

Strictly anaerobic bacteria, and viruses, fungi (other than *Candida albicans*), protozoa and helminths are rare causes of UTI. *Leptospira interrogans* is a bacterium which can infect the kidneys of certain mammals, including humans, and it may also spread to other organs (see Chapter 19). A number of sexually transmitted organisms cause urethritis (inflammation of the urethra). These are discussed in a later section on reproductive system infections.

PATHOGENESIS OF URINARY TRACT INFECTIONS

Host factors predisposing to infection

The much higher incidence of urinary tract infection in women is attributed to the proximity of the anus to the urethral opening and the shortness of the female urethra compared with that of males. The proximity of the anal and urethral orifices favours the colonisation of the lower urethra with gastrointestinal flora. The short urethra means that bacteria have less distance to travel to reach the bladder and establish infection (see Figure 21.2). Good personal hygiene is important in preventing the transfer of organisms from the anus to the vagina and periurethral areas. Sexual intercourse can facilitate the movement of organisms into and up the urethra, especially in females, explaining the higher frequency of UTI in the sexually active compared with the celibate woman.

Because the flushing of microorganisms from the urethra during the normal passage of urine is an important defence mechanism, any factor that prevents normal urine

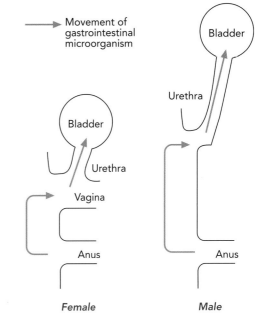

Figure 21.2

Susceptibility of females to urinary tract infections
Females are more susceptible than males because of the proximity of the anus to the urethra and the shorter urethra.

flow or complete bladder emptying makes the individual more susceptible to UTI. Pregnancy, renal calculi and tumours are common causes of urinary obstruction and are therefore predisposing factors of urinary tract infection. And, as stated earlier, there is a marked increase in the incidence of UTI in men above the age of 60 due to urinary obstruction caused by hypertrophy of the prostate. Loss of neurological control of the bladder leading to incomplete emptying, such as can occur in paraplegia, also makes the individual more prone to UTI. Retained urine in the bladder provides a reservoir for microbial persistence.

Urinary catheterisation

The high incidence of urinary tract infection in hospitalised people is partly due to the use of indwelling urinary catheters. Up to 25% of catheterised patients develop a bacteriuria. During insertion of the catheter, bacteria already in the urethra may be carried into the bladder or, if proper

Table 21.1
Common causes of urinary tract infection

CAUSE	PERCENTAGE OF CASES	
	COMMUNITY-ACQUIRED	HOSPITAL-ACQUIRED
• *E. coli*	80	40
• Other organisms including:		
Proteus mirabilis		
Klebsiella		
Enterobacter		
Pseudomonas aeruginosa	20	60
Coagulase negative staphylococci		
Staphylococcus aureus		
Candida albicans		

aseptic technique is not used, organisms from the hospital environment or on the hands of a staff member may be introduced. Generally, the longer a catheter is in place the greater the risk of infection, because the catheter provides several potential sites of entry for microorganisms.

The catheter also prevents the normal flushing of the urethra with urine, and bacteria are able to move upwards between the outside of the catheter and the surface of the urethra. The longer a catheter is in place, the more its outer surface becomes encrusted with mineral deposits beneath which large numbers of bacteria are able to reside. There the bacteria are protected from host defences and antibiotics.

Bacterial virulence factors

Since *E. coli* is the most common cause of UTI, the bulk of the research into virulence factors of urinary pathogens has centred on this organism. Only certain strains of *E. coli* are able to cause UTI, and this has been attributed mainly to their possession of pili. These are filamentous protein structures (see Chapter 4) that allow bacteria to attach to surfaces – in this case to the urethral and bladder epithelium. Non-piliated strains of *E. coli* that cause UTI are thought to have other adhesins that allow them to stick to epithelium. Adhesins have also been identified in other urinary tract pathogens.

Other virulence factors of urinary pathogens include the capsular polysaccharide (K) antigens of *E. coli*, which help it to evade being phagocytosed by tissue macrophages. *Proteus* and some strains of *E. coli* have an enzyme called *urease* and are thought to survive well on the outer surface of catheters by encrusting themselves with minerals released from the breakdown of urea, thereby protecting themselves as described in the previous section.

SITES AND CLINICAL FEATURES OF URINARY TRACT INFECTIONS

Most UTIs are initiated by microorganisms ascending the urinary tract. Infection may initially be in the urethra, resulting in an inflammation of that site, called **urethritis**. As the organisms ascend the tract, subsequent infection of the bladder may occur. The bladder tissue becomes inflamed, and the patient is said to have **cystitis**. In some cases, the organisms may travel further up the urinary tract and infect the kidney(s), resulting in inflammation of one or both kidneys, which is called **pyelonephritis**. It is also possible for individuals to have large numbers of bacteria in their urine without displaying any symptoms. This is termed an **asymptomatic bacteriuria**.

Asymptomatic bacteriuria

As there are no symptoms present, asymptomatic bacteriuria is usually detected during routine screening of a person. It is thought to represent multiplication of bacteria in the bladder urine without involvement of tissues, although in some cases a limited degree of tissue infection may be present. In most cases, treatment is unnecessary because infection never occurs. However, in pregnant women, young children and people about to undergo instrumentation of the urinary tract there is a significant risk of renal infection. In such cases treatment is warranted.

Cystitis

Acute infections of the bladder are usually characterised by symptoms of:

- **dysuria** – difficult or painful (burning) urination
- **urgency** – an urgent need to urinate
- **frequency** – the need to urinate more frequently than usual.

In addition, the urine is cloudy due to the presence of large numbers of leucocytes (**pyuria**) in response to infection, and may occasionally contain blood (**haematuria**) because of tissue damage.

Infections of the bladder recur in some people, with the possibility of scarring and permanent damage to the urinary tract. Such recurrences may be caused by the same or different organisms.

Pyelonephritis

Infection of the kidney(s) can result from movement of bacteria upwards from the bladder, or occasionally from the bloodstream. The clinical presentation of pyelonephritis is similar to that of cystitis although, in pyelonephritis, fever and haematuria are more common. Flank pain and tenderness in the kidney region may also be present. Pyelonephritis is a serious condition because there is a potential for serious kidney damage. If the pyelonephritis becomes chronic, permanent damage and loss of kidney function may occur.

LABORATORY DIAGNOSIS

The appropriate methods for collection and transport of urine specimens for diagnosis of UTIs are described in Chapter 15. The specimen most commonly collected is a 'clean-catch' or mid-stream specimen of urine (MSU). Urine may be collected by other methods, depending on the circumstances – for example, suprapubic aspiration of urine from young children, a specimen from an indwelling urinary catheter, or a specimen collected during cystoscopy.

An amount of 2–50 mL should be collected into a sterile, plastic, wide-mouth container. Because urine is a good growth medium and quantitative bacterial counts are required (see below), the specimen should be transported to the laboratory without delay. The specimen may be refrigerated if a delay is unavoidable or if another specimen cannot be collected at a more appropriate time.

Usually, patients are started on antibiotic therapy before the results of the laboratory tests are available. Wherever possible, it is important that the urine specimen is collected before antibiotic therapy is initiated, so that an accurate laboratory diagnosis is obtained (see Chapter 15).

In the laboratory the urine specimen is examined microscopically and cultured. A microscopic examination of urine allows the presence of white cells, red cells, epithelial cells, casts and bacteria to be determined. The presence of any one of these does not necessarily indicate infection, but all of them, together with culture results, are used to build a clinical picture from which a diagnosis can be made. Most patients with symptomatic infection have pyuria (a raised polymorphonuclear cell count in urine), but pyuria without infection is common.

The clinical significance of these microscopic elements is summarised in Table 21.2.

Since the lower urethra is usually colonised by bacteria, even properly collected MSU specimens may be contaminated with (non-infecting) periurethral organisms. Since some species of bacteria that colonise the lower urethra are also potential urinary pathogens, the *number* of bacteria in a urine sample is more important than their mere presence. Therefore, infection is assessed and distinguished from contamination by quantitative culture methods.

Significant bacteriuria is usually defined as a count of 10^8/L in a properly collected MSU. However, it should be recognised that, in certain situations, fewer than this number may represent infection. Less than 10^8/L can be significant in:

- infections caused by Gram-positive bacteria, fungi, or slow-growing or fastidious organisms
- catheter specimens
- specimens collected during cystoscopy
- specimens collected by suprapubic aspiration
- specimens from patients already receiving antibiotic therapy
- specimens from patients with high urine output (causing dilution of the bacteria).

A number of laboratory findings indicate improper specimen collection. One or more of the following in a specimen of urine casts doubt on its quality:

- greater than normal numbers of epithelial cells
- culture of more than one type of bacterium (since most UTIs are caused by a single organism)
- the presence of organisms without white cells (in some cases)
- the presence of Gram-positive rods (i.e. lactobacilli from vaginal flora).

There are also several rapid methods in use for detecting bacteriuria including filtration, bioluminescence and photometric techniques.

TREATMENT AND MANAGEMENT

The choice of antimicrobial therapy should be based on culture and sensitivity results. This is particularly important in health-care-associated infections or recurrent infections, both of which may be caused by antibiotic-resistant organisms. In catheterised patients, management includes the removal or replacement of the catheter, since it is likely to be acting as a source of infection. Supportive measures such as the raising of the pH of the urine with urinary alkalinisers (to slow bacterial growth) and high fluid intake (to help to flush out organisms) may also be instituted.

Because of the seriousness of pyelonephritis, more aggressive therapy (e.g. intravenous rather than oral antibiotics) for a longer period (e.g. 10 days) is often warranted. Unfortunately, pyelonephritis is not always distinguished from cystitis by either clinical or laboratory findings.

PREVENTION

The incidence of community-acquired UTI in women may be reduced by such measures as promotion of good personal hygiene, adequate fluid intake and regular

---

Table 21.2

The clinical significance of urinary elements found during microscopic examination of urine

ELEMENT	POSSIBLE CLINICAL SIGNIFICANCE
White cells (>4 per hpf* or >10^8/L)	• bacterial infection • acute glomerulonephritis • bladder tumour • drug therapy • strenuous exercise
Red cells (>2 per hpf)	• infection of the kidney or bladder • renal trauma • renal calculi • malaria • endocarditis • carcinoma of the urinary tract
Epithelial cells (>10 per hpf)	• poor specimen collection (i.e. not a mid-stream urine) • inflammatory conditions of upper urinary tract
Casts (more than occasional)	• infection • many other types of renal disease

* high power field

emptying of the bladder. In women with recurrent UTIs, voiding urine after intercourse may reduce the frequency of infection. In hospitals, prevention is based on similar principles plus avoidance of catheterisation wherever possible and proper catheter care.

Suggested guidelines for catheter care are listed in Table 21.3.

Infections of the reproductive system

Most diseases of the reproductive (genital) system are transmitted during sexual activity and are thus referred to as **sexually transmissible infections** (STIs). They were formerly called venereal diseases, after Venus, the Roman goddess of love. It is important to recognise that a number of STIs can also be transmitted by other body fluids, especially blood and blood products (e.g. the human immunodeficiency virus (HIV) and the hepatitis B and C viruses), which is why the term 'sexually transmissible infection' is used.

Table 21.4 lists the common STIs and syndromes and their causative agents. Notice that some syndromes (e.g. urethritis, pelvic inflammatory disease) can be caused by a number of different organisms. This can make the diagnosis and treatment of infection much more difficult. All these syndromes are discussed in this chapter, except for AIDS (see Chapter 19) and hepatitis (see Chapter 18), because these two infections predominantly involve body systems other than the genital tract.

Although many of the genital infections are preventable if appropriate precautions (e.g. use of condoms) are taken, and many are readily cured with antimicrobial treatment,

Table 21.4

Sexually transmissible infections and their causative agents

SYNDROME	CAUSATIVE AGENTS
• Gonorrhoea	Neisseria gonorrhoeae
• Syphilis	Treponema pallidum
• Urethritis	Neisseria gonorrhoeae
	Chlamydia trachomatis
	Mycoplasma genitalium
	Ureaplasma urealyticum
	Herpes simplex virus
• Vaginitis	Trichomonas vaginalis
	Candida albicans
• Cervicitis	Neisseria gonorrhoeae
	Chlamydia trachomatis
	Herpes simplex virus
• Genital warts and carcinoma	Human papilloma viruses
• Genital ulcer disease	Herpes simplex virus
	Treponema pallidum
	Haemophilus ducreyi
	Chlamydia trachomatis L1, L2, L3
	Calymmatobacterium granulomatis
• Pelvic inflammatory disease	Neisseria gonorrhoeae
	Chlamydia trachomatis
	Mycoplasma hominis
	Vaginal normal flora
• AIDS	Human immunodeficiency viruses 1 and 2
• Hepatitis	Hepatitis A,B,C,D viruses

Table 21.3

Procedures for the prevention of catheter-associated urinary tract infection

- Avoid catheterisation of a patient where possible.
- Catheter and associated equipment must be sterile before use.
- Wash hands thoroughly before and after inserting a catheter or other manipulation of the catheter.
- The external meatal opening should be cleansed prior to insertion of the catheter.
- The catheter must be inserted using good aseptic technique.
- The catheter should be inserted in such a way as to cause minimal damage to mucosal surfaces.
- A closed drainage system should be used wherever possible.
- The catheter tubing should not be allowed to come loose from the collecting bag.
- The collecting bag must not be allowed to fill to the level of the inlet tube.
- Keep duration of catheterisation to a minimum.
- Use intermittent rather than continuous catheterisation where possible.

they still represent a major health problem in both developed and developing countries throughout the world. The World Health Organization (WHO) estimates that worldwide there are over 340 million new cases of STI each year. Reasons commonly given for the continuing high incidence of STIs include:

- increased sexual activity at a younger age
- frequent partner change
- the production of few or no symptoms by some pathogens
- the social stigma of these diseases and the non-seeking of medical advice and/or notification of sexual partners
- the sexual freedom resulting from contraception
- ignorance
- the failure to use barrier preventive measures (e.g. condoms)
- the lack of effective vaccines for most STIs.

The numbers of cases of STIs reported by health authorities generally represent only a fraction of the actual cases, because many are not diagnosed. As you will see, in some STIs a large percentage of infected people may be asymptomatic. Furthermore, many symptomatic people do not seek medical advice, because of the social stigma associated with sexually transmissible infections.

STIs are also of major health importance because **genital ulcer disease** (e.g. syphilis, herpes, chancroid) increases the risk of transmission of the human immunodeficiency virus (HIV), especially in heterosexuals. Genital ulcers provide a direct site of entry for the HIV. There is also evidence that HIV transmission is enhanced in the presence of certain STIs (see section on syphilis, for example).

GONORRHOEA

Causative organism and incidence

Gonorrhoea is an infection caused by the bacterium *Neisseria gonorrhoeae*, sometimes called the 'gonococcus'. It is named after Albert Neisser who first described it in 1879. The disease was somewhat misnamed as gonorrhoea (after the ancient Greek *gonos* meaning 'seed', and *rhoia* meaning 'flow') because the male urethral discharge was mistaken for semen. The bacterium is a Gram-negative round or oval-shaped diplococcus with flattened sides (see Figure 21.3), so that it often has the appearance of a pair of coffee beans.

Gonorrhoea is a major global disease with estimates of around 60 million cases annually. In developed countries the majority of male cases occurs in the male homosexual community. Currently, in Australia, 5000–7000 notifications of gonococcal infection are received per year by the National Notifiable Diseases Surveillance System, with the greatest rates of infection in Queensland, the Northern Territory and Western Australia. The vast majority of infections occur in indigenous Australians (see Figure 21.4). This includes gonorrhoea and other forms of gonococcal infection (e.g. eye infections), but the vast majority are genital infections. There has been a gradual, increasing trend of gonococcal infection over the past decade.

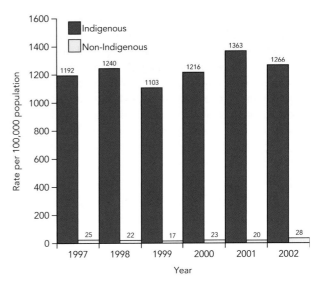

Figure 21.4

Notifications of gonococcal infection in Northern Territory, South Australia and Western Australia (combined) 1997–2002, by indigenous status
Source: *Communicable Diseases Intelligence* 2004, 28(1): 42, © Commonwealth of Australia, reproduced by permission

Transmission

N. gonorrhoeae is fairly sensitive to drying and survives for only a short time on dry surfaces. It can, however, survive for several hours in pus. Given its inability to survive well outside the body, it is usually transmitted by direct person-to-person contact. It is a disease only of humans.

The efficiency of transmission appears to be gender-dependent. It is thought that an infected male will transmit the infection 60% of the time to non-infected contacts, whereas a female will transmit it only 30% of the time. This difference seems to be related to the high organism load in semen. There are several high-risk transmission factors, the most important being multiple sexual partners and disregard of safe sex practices. Pharyngeal and rectal infections have become more common in both homosexuals and heterosexuals because of more varied sexual practices.

N. gonorrhoeae can also be transmitted vertically from an infected mother to baby at birth. This usually results in an eye infection called **ophthalmia neonatorum** (see Chapter 16). While this infection has been controlled in many Western countries through the use of antibiotics or silver nitrate eye-drops, it remains a major problem in developing countries.

Pathogenesis

Once the gonococci are introduced into the vagina, or the urethra of males, they attach by way of pili to the mucosal cells. This attachment prevents them from being washed away by the flow of urine or secretions. The bacteria multiply rapidly and spread up to the cervix in females or up the urethra in males. Survival of the bacteria is aided by their production of an IgA protease which inactivates IgA antibodies found in mucous secretions.

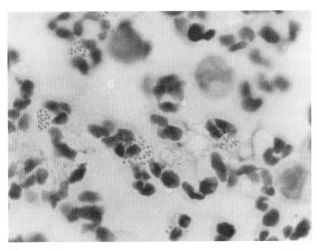

Figure 21.3

Neisseria gonorrhoea
Gram stain of the gonococcus in pus cells (polymorphonuclear leucocytes).

The bacteria invade the epithelial cells lining the cervix and urethra and multiply within them. Inside these cells they are protected from phagocytes and antibodies. Eventually, they are discharged from the basement membrane of the epithelial cells into the subepithelial connective tissue. There they cause local damage and elicit an inflammatory response. Occasionally, they invade blood vessels and then spread to other parts of the body, such as joints. Persistent infections cause chronic inflammation and fibrosis of the tissues.

Clinical features

Symptoms usually develop within a week (often in 1–2 days) of infection. In men gonococcal infection is usually characterised by a urethral discharge (see Figure 21.5) and **dysuria** (pain on passing urine). The infection may be very mild or asymptomatic in up to 50% of cases. A small percentage of untreated cases can develop an **epididymitis** (infection and inflammation of the epididymis).

Up to 50% of infected women also have very mild symptoms or are completely asymptomatic. Symptomatic infection is usually characterised by a cervico-vaginal discharge and cervical oedema. Abnormal menses, dyspareunia (painful intercourse) and dysuria (due to urethral infection) are also common.

The asymptomatic nature of infection in many women is important for two main reasons. First, they are an important, unrecognised source of infection. Second, in up to 30% of untreated women the infection spreads further up the genital tract to cause inflammation in the fallopian tubes (**salpingitis**) and sometimes the ovaries (**oophoritis**), or in the whole of the peritoneal cavity (**peritonitis**). Inflammation in one or more of these sites is called **pelvic inflammatory disease** (PID).

Persistent infection, especially in the fallopian tubes, can cause scarring and blockage of the tubes, leading to infertility or ectopic (tubal) pregnancy, as well as increased susceptibility to recurrent attacks of PID. Pelvic inflammatory disease is not only caused by *N. gonorrhoeae*. Other organisms, especially *Chlamydia trachomatis*, can also cause it, alone, or in coexistence with

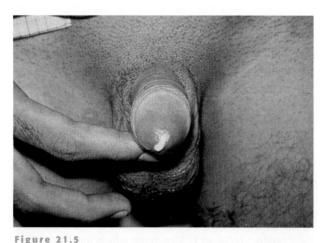

Figure 21.5

A purulent urethral discharge in a male with gonorrhoea

the gonococcus. PID is dealt with more fully on page 523.

Anorectal infection is often asymptomatic, but otherwise can be characterised by rectal pain, discharge, constipation and tenesmus (painful defecation). Gonococcal pharyngitis, acquired during oral sex, is clinically indistinguishable from any other bacterial pharyngitis, but is also usually asymptomatic. Disseminated gonococcal infection can occur but is rare. Usually, joint symptoms (tenosynovitis or arthritis), a skin rash and fever are the major manifestations. A meningitis or endocarditis is also possible.

Diagnosis

Diagnosis has classically been based on microscopy and culture of an appropriate specimen. In men, this is a urethral swab. In women, a cervical swab is usually collected and, additionally (not alternatively), a sample of vaginal discharge if purulent. A rapid, presumptive diagnosis can be made by microscopic examination of a Gram stain if intracellular Gram-negative diplococci are seen. Microscopy is only generally appropriate for urethral and cervical specimens. It should be remembered that the organism is sensitive to drying and extremes of temperature, so the specimen should be inoculated directly onto culture media at the bedside or transported immediately to the laboratory in transport medium containing activated charcoal (to neutralise toxic substances), and must not be refrigerated. A pharyngeal or rectal swab may also be collected for culture if appropriate.

Polymerase chain reaction (PCR) tests for gonorrhoea (and *Chlamydia trachomatis* – see later section) are now commercially available and have the major advantage of being suitable for use on urine. Gonococci and *Chlamydia* are found in urine because these organisms often colonise the urethra. Urine is a less invasive specimen than the swabs above, and urine PCR tests for gonorrhoea and *Chlamydia* infections have made possible mass screening programs in high-risk populations.

The major disadvantage of the use of the PCR test for diagnosis is that this methodology does not provide antibiotic sensitivity information. Given the variability in antibiotic sensitivity of different strains of gonococci, sensitivity results may be important. So culture of a swab specimen should also be performed, if possible. Dual testing, by culture and PCR, increases the likelihood of detecting the microbe in an infected person.

All patients found to have an STI should be evaluated for other STIs. As noted earlier, *Chlamydia* co-infection is common in a person with gonorrhoea. In addition, all patients should be evaluated for syphilis, HIV infection and hepatitis B.

Treatment and prevention

Since the early 1980s there has been a marked and disturbing increase in the incidence of antibiotic resistance in *N. gonorrhoeae*. Pencillins have been one of the standard treatments for gonorrhoea, but a high proportion of infections are now caused by penicillin-resistant strains.

Increasing resistance to the quinolone antibiotics (e.g. ciprofloxacin) and to tetracyclines has also been observed. Although resistance to later-generation cephalosporins (e.g. ceftriaxone) and spectinomycin is currently rare, there is concern that the gonococcus may gradually develop resistance to these drugs as well, with their increasing use. As a result of concerns over resistance the World Health Organization established the Gonococcal Antimicrobial Surveillance Programme (GASP) to monitor susceptibility and resistance patterns of the gonococcus in different regions of the world.

Currently, treatment is usually with ceftriaxone, although penicillins and quinolones are still appropriate for use in regions where resistance is low. The advantage of the latter groups of antibiotics is that they can be administered orally. Follow-up cultures 4–7 days after treatment is strongly recommended to confirm effectiveness of treatment. Since many patients have a coexistent infection with *Chlamydia trachomatis*, treatment should also include an effective anti-chlamydial drug, usually azithromycin.

Prevention of gonorrhoea is based on the use of condoms and the tracing and presumptive treatment of patient contacts. Despite extensive effort, no vaccine is currently available.

SYPHILIS

Causative organism and incidence

Syphilis is an STI that has been recognised for centuries and still remains a global health problem, especially in parts of Africa and Asia. Recent major increases in incidence in the former Soviet Union and other eastern European countries have been observed. It is caused by the spirochaete *Treponema pallidum*, a thin, coiled and highly motile organism with fastidious growth requirements. Between 1000 and 2000 cases of syphilis are notified in Australia per year. The highest incidences occur in some Aboriginal populations (see Figure 21.6).

Transmission

Transmission of syphilis requires close, personal contact. The organism survives poorly outside the body because it is very sensitive to drying, heat (as low as 42°C) and disinfectants. The organism is present in the skin or mucous membrane lesions of an infected person and enters the body of a sexual contact through the mucous membranes or through abrasions (even minute) in the skin. An infected woman may also transmit the organism to her foetus *in utero*, especially after the first trimester, often resulting in congenital malformations.

Pathogenesis and clinical features

The treponemes typically multiply slowly and so there is an average incubation period of three weeks before symptoms develop. Classically, the course of infection is divided into three stages, but only some patients experience all stages.

1. **Primary syphilis** is characterised by the development of a papular lesion at the site of infection, usually on the

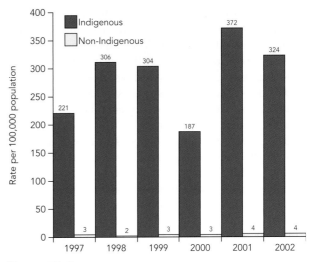

Figure 21.6

Notifications of syphilis in Northern Territory, South Australia and Western Australia (combined) 1997–2002, by indigenous status

Source: Communicable Diseases Intelligence 2004, 28(1): 44, © Commonwealth of Australia, reproduced by permission

genitals, but sometimes on the rectum, lip or hand. In males, there is usually a lesion on the penis which is seen, but in females the primary lesion usually occurs on the cervix and therefore often goes unnoticed. The papular lesion breaks down to form a painless, hard-based ulcer called a **chancre** (see Figure 21.7). The papule and ulcer contain large numbers of organisms and are highly infectious. Also, inguinal lymph nodes may be enlarged. In 2–6 weeks the lesion heals spontaneously, to the relief of those who have not sought medical advice. Unfortunately, this is often only a temporary respite.

2. In approximately 50% of untreated cases, **secondary syphilis** develops 2–10 weeks later. From the time of initial infection, the treponemes begin to spread from the site of entry to local lymph nodes and then to the bloodstream. The secondary stage involves the multiplication of bacteria and the production of lesions, especially in skin and mucous membranes. It is charac-

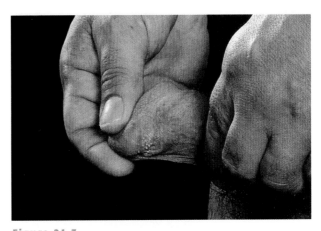

Figure 21.7

The chancre of primary syphilis on penis

terised by the appearance of a red, maculopapular rash anywhere on the skin, anogenital region, mouth, throat or cervix (see Figure 21.8). The rash may even occur on the palms or soles of the feet. This may be accompanied by malaise and mild fever. These lesions are highly infectious. The symptoms again subside spontaneously after a few weeks, followed by a prolonged asymptomatic period of 3 to 30 years.

3. After this latent period, signs of disease reappear in about 30% of untreated cases. This is called **tertiary** (or late) **syphilis**. Renewed multiplication, dissemination and a cell-mediated hypersensitivity response of the immune system combine to form lesions in various organs. Soft, granulomatous lesions (**gummas**) may form in the skin, bones, liver or other organs. If lesions form in the central nervous system, **neurosyphilis** is the result. Degenerative changes may lead to mental illness, paresis (weakness or partial paralysis), or *tabes dorsalis* (poor muscle coordination and unstable gait). The paresis plus gradual loss of higher integrative functions in tertiary syphilis is sometimes referred to as 'general paralysis of the insane'.

In **cardiovascular syphilis** aortic aneurysm and blood vessel and valve damage may occur, leading to heart failure. The treponemes are rarely found in the lesions of tertiary syphilis because the symptoms appear to be due mainly to a hypersensitivity reaction to the microbes.

The pathogenesis and clinical features of syphilis are summarised in Table 21.5.

Congenital infection occurs when the organism crosses the placenta. In many cases the infection may not become apparent for many months after birth, but in some it may cause miscarriage, stillbirth or severe symptoms at birth, including hepatosplenomegaly, prolonged jaundice, thrombocytopaenia and failure to thrive. Possible congenital abnormalities include mental retardation, blindness, deafness, bone disease and, later, facial and tooth deformities.

As noted earlier, diseases such as syphilis, in which genital ulcers are produced, have the added problem of increasing the risk of HIV (human immunodeficiency virus) transmission and acquisition. Not only do the ulcers provide a site of entry for the HIV, but there is evidence that activated CD4 lymphocytes are attracted to the site of infection. These lymphocytes are the key target of the HIV. In addition, HIV infection can increase the likelihood of clinical progress of syphilis.

Diagnosis

Treponema pallidum cannot be readily grown in the laboratory. Therefore, the laboratory diagnosis of syphilis hinges on microscopic and serologic methods. The quickest and most direct method is microscopy. The primary and secondary lesions of syphilis usually contain large numbers of organisms. The bacteria may be readily seen in exudate from the lesions when examined by dark-ground microscopy (see Figure 2.8, page 26) or in a UV microscope after treating the specimen with fluorescein-labelled anti-treponemal antibodies. The exudate must be sent to the laboratory immediately after collection. The exudate is highly infectious and must be handled with care.

In the absence of lesions, serology is the mainstay of diagnosis. The serological tests used are of two types: the non-specific (non-treponemal) tests and the specific (anti-treponemal antibody) tests. The non-specific tests do not detect antibodies to treponemal antigens, but rather detect an antibody-like substance called *reagin*. The antigen used in these assays is cardiolipin, an extract from normal mammalian tissue. The two non-specific tests in common use are the VDRL (Venereal Diseases Research Laboratory) and the RPR (Rapid Plasma Reagin). False positive results are possible with these non-specific methods, so a positive result is confirmed using a specific test, such as the fluorescent treponemal antibody absorption test (FTA-ABS), the *Treponema pallidum* particle agglutination test (TPPA) or enzyme linked immunosorbent assay (ELISA). Unless seroconversion is demonstrated, these serological methods do not distinguish between past and current infection.

Treatment

Penicillin is very active against *Treponema pallidum* and is the drug of choice. A single intramuscular injection of benzathine penicillin remains active in the body for two weeks and is usually effective for syphilis of less than two years duration. For older infections, three intramuscular injections at weekly intervals, or daily injections of procaine penicillin for three weeks are the usual regimes. If the patient is allergic to penicillin, oral doxycycline may be used.

Prevention

Prevention is based on the practice of safe sex, and contact tracing and screening. Prevention of secondary and tertiary disease depends on early diagnosis and treatment. Congenital infection is preventable if women are screened (by serology) early in pregnancy and treated. Re-screening in the third trimester is warranted in high-incidence regions. In the US syphilis screening is performed on all blood donors and as part of routine pre-marital checks.

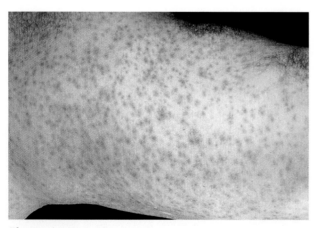

Figure 21.8

Secondary syphilis showing a papular rash

Table 21.5

Pathogenesis and clinical features of syphilis

STAGE OF DISEASE	PATHOGENESIS	SIGNS AND SYMPTOMS
Incubation period (2–10 weeks)	Multiplication at site of entry	
Primary syphilis (lasting 2–6 weeks)	Spread to regional lymph nodes and bloodstream	• primary chancre • enlarged inguinal nodes
Asymptomatic period (2–10 weeks)		
Secondary syphilis (2–6 weeks)	Multiplication in extra-genital sites	• maculopapular rash anywhere on skin or mucous membranes • malaise and mild fever
Asymptomatic period (3–30 years)	Organisms dormant in liver, spleen and central nervous system	

Tertiary syphilis	Renewed multiplication and invasion plus a cell-mediated hypersensitivity response	• gummas in skin, bone, liver
		• cardiovascular syphilis:
		  – aortic lesions
		  – heart failure
		• neurosyphilis:
		  – general paresis of insane
		  – tabes dorsalis

SPOTLIGHT ON

Syphilis screening program: a success story

Syphilis rates in the Kimberley region of far northern Western Australia are among the highest in the nation. As a result a structured program of periodic syphilis screening, based on a regional population register of Aboriginal Kimberley residents, was established in 1986. It aimed to reduce the incidence of syphilis by detecting and treating prevalent cases.

The program offered annual syphilis serology (SS) testing to all Aboriginal Kimberley residents aged 15–40 years, and testing every second year to those aged below 40 years. In addition, syphilis testing was also recommended for all patients presenting with sexually transmitted infection (STI) symptoms, and named contacts of STI cases, and as part of routine antenatal screening. In 1996, following evaluation of the program and discussions with the Kimberley Aboriginal Services Council, the target group was modified to include all Kimberley residents aged 15–25 years.

In addition, rather than being centrally managed using a regional population register, the responsibility for initiating SS testing in first-time patients and for recalling patients for repeat testing was devolved to local health services.

Aboriginal people comprise one-half of the resident population of about 30 000 people scattered across the Kimberley, an area of more than 420 000 square kilometres. There are six major towns (with populations ranging from 2000 to 10 000) and more than 200 discrete Aboriginal communities ranging in size from just a few families to over 500 people. Health care is provided predominantly by government and community controlled organisations. Each of the major towns has a hospital and one or more primary-care services. Remote-area clinics staffed by nurses and Aboriginal health workers are present in fewer than 20 Aboriginal communities.

Syphilis represents an STI-control success story in the Kimberley. The syphilis incidence rate has decreased 10-fold since the mid-1980s and the proportion of cases transmitted locally is decreasing.

In January 2000, the periodic syphilis screening program was discontinued. The effect of this policy change will be closely monitored using indicators to ensure that, should the decision not to screen prove to have been misjudged, any increase in syphilis incidence is detected early and managed appropriately.

Source: DB Mak & CDJ Holman 2000, 'A decision to end a periodic syphilis screening program in the Kimberley region', *Communicable Diseases Intelligence*, 24(12): 386.

CHLAMYDIAL INFECTIONS

Causative organisms and incidence

Chlamydia are very small bacteria that are obligate intra-cellular parasites. Four species are currently recognised, but only *Chlamydia trachomatis* infects the genital tract. This species can be subdivided into different serotypes (serovars) which are associated with different infections:

- serotypes A, B and C cause an eye infection called trachoma (see Chapter 16)
- serotypes D to K cause genital and associated infections
- serotypes L1, L2 and L3 cause a specific genital infection called lymphogranuloma venereum.

Genital chlamydial infections caused by serotypes D to K have a high incidence in many countries and are currently the most prevalent of the bacterial STIs. The Centers for Disease Control in the United States estimates that around three million Americans are infected by *Chlamydia* each year. In Australia, *Chlamydia* infection has the highest incidence of any notifiable disease, with more than 24 000 cases notified in 2002. The number of notifications has increased fourfold over the last decade, although some of this increase is due to increased surveillance, more sensitive screening tests, and public awareness campaigns. Notifications include all types of chlamydial infection although the majority are genital infections. The real incidence is probably many times that number because many cases are asymptomatic.

Most infections occur in the 15–24 years age group, with a predominance in females (see Figure 21.9). Geographically, highest rates of notification come from the Aboriginal populations in northern Queensland, Western Australia and the Northern Territory (see Figure 21.10). The large number of people who are infected asymptomatically and who shed the organism in their genital secretions makes transmission very easy.

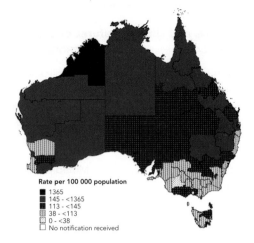

Rate per 100 000 population
- 1365
- 145 - <1365
- 113 - <145
- 38 - <113
- 0 - <38
- No notification received

Figure 21.10

Notification rates of *Chlamydia* infection in Australia, 2003, by statistical division of residence
Source: Communicable Diseases Intelligence 2005, 29(1): 32, © Commonwealth of Australia, reproduced by permission

Lymphogranuloma venereum (LGV) is a serious disease found in restricted regions of the world, particularly tropical and subtropical Africa, Asia and South America. It is rare in developed countries. It is a notifiable disease in only some Australian states. Fewer than five cases a year are notified and they are generally acquired overseas.

Pathogenesis and clinical features

Serotypes D to K probably enter through minute abrasions in the mucosal surface. The organisms grow in columnar and transitional epithelial cells and the clinical disease is then determined by the site of infection. Infection of the cervix leads to **cervicitis**, which produces no or mild symptoms in 50% of women. Symptomatic women may experience slight vaginal discharge or intermenstrual bleeding. The absence of symptoms means that many women are not treated and are thus at risk of the infection spreading to the fallopian tubes, resulting in **pelvic inflammatory disease** (see page 523). Infection can be spread from mother to baby at birth causing an eye infection – opthalmia neonatorum.

Urethral infection (**urethritis**) in men is also often asymptomatic, with only about 50% experiencing a mucoid urethral discharge. The asymptomatic person may remain infectious for months and unknowingly transmit the infection to sexual partners.

In LGV, a primary lesion develops at the site of organism inoculation (usually on the genitals, but occasionally in the oral cavity or rectum) within two weeks of infection. The lesion heals rapidly, but draining lymph nodes become infected. Typically, inguinal buboes form, which gradually enlarge. Abscesses may form in the nodes and eventually suppurate and discharge through the skin. The organisms may spread via the lymphatics to the rectum (proctitis) and other tissues (e.g. pneumonitis, meningo-encephalitis, hepatitis).

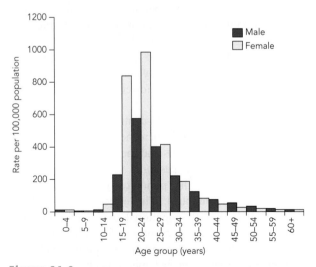

Figure 21.9

Notification rates of *Chlamydia* infection in Australia, 2003, by age group and sex
Source: Communicable Diseases Intelligence 2005, 29(1): 32, © Commonwealth of Australia, reproduced by permission

Diagnosis

Chlamydial infections cannot be reliably distinguished from infections caused by other organisms by clinical examination alone, so laboratory testing is essential. Culture is the gold standard, but is slow and requires specialised techniques because the organism can be grown only in cell culture (it is an obligate intracellular parasite). For culture, a cervical or urethral swab is usually collected (by scraping the site with a swab in order to obtain infected cells) as well as discharge. The difficulties associated with culture means that other diagnostic methods are often used. Antigen detection methods (e.g. ELISAs) are commonly used. Nucleic acid amplification tests (e.g. polymerase chain reaction, ligase chain reaction) are available, although their cost is currently a limiting factor. They have superior sensitivity over culture and antigen detection methods, especially for asymptomatic infections. They also have the major advantage of being suitable for use with less invasive specimens – first-catch urine specimens and vulval or vaginal swabs.

In LGV, bubo pus or tissue biopsy are the common specimens. Swabs, scrapings and small amounts of tissue should be transported in an appropriate transport medium.

Treatment

Treatment is usually with azithromycin, which can be given as a single oral dose, or doxycycline for one week. Sexual contacts should also be treated whether or not they are symptomatic, because of the ease of spread and the potential seriousness of fallopian tube infection. Because concurrent chlamydial and gonococcal infections are common, patients receiving treatment for gonorrhoea should also receive treatment for *Chlamydia*.

MYCOPLASMA GENITALIUM

Mycoplasma genitalium is difficult to culture, so most data on its role in genital infections is based on PCR and serological tests. Our knowledge of the pathogenesis of this organism is rudimentary, but its capacity to cause urethritis in men is accepted. Its role in infection in females is less certain. There is some evidence that this organism may cause cervicitis and pelvic inflammatory disease. However, most men and women from whom *M. genitalium* alone is isolated are asymptomatic. Diagnosis of infection is currently based on PCR testing of a urethral swab from men or a cervical swab from women.

GENITAL HERPES

Causative agents and incidence

There are two major types of herpes simplex virus: herpes simplex virus type 1 (HSV-1) and herpes simplex type 2 (HSV-2). Both types have been found to cause genital and oral (cold sores) herpes, but type 2 predominates in the genital region while type 1 is the more common cause of oral infection.

Infection with at least one of the herpes viruses seems to occur in most people, although mainly asymptomatically. Up to 75% of adults have antibodies to HSV-1 and up to 50% have antibodies to HSV-2. Approximately 15% of women attending public antenatal clinics are found to be seropositive for HSV-2, and the prevalence is much higher in homosexual men, sex workers and people attending STI clinics.

The Centers for Disease Control in Atlanta estimates that 50 million adults in the United States have recurrent genital herpes. National notifications are not compiled in Australia.

Pathogenesis and clinical features

HSV-2 is readily inactivated by drying at room temperature. Therefore, transmission is essentially by direct contact with infected secretions or mucosal surfaces. The virus appears able to invade intact mucosal surfaces, but infects skin only through breaks or abrasions.

Initial infection may be completely asymptomatic or so mild that it is unrecognised. As many as 50–70% of genital herpes infections may fall into this category. The majority of people with antibodies to HSV-2 do not have a history of clinical genital herpes. If symptomatic, the primary lesions usually occur on the penis, anus, vulva, cervix or vagina 3–14 days after exposure. The classic lesions are usually small, grouped vesicles filled with a clear fluid and surrounded by an area of inflammation (see Figure 21.11). In a primary infection, groups of lesions often appear on more than one site. The vesicles break down after several days to form painful, shallow ulcers. If the lesions occur over a large area of the genitalia, walking, or even the wearing of clothing, can be painful.

Local lymph nodes are usually swollen and the patient may be lethargic and feverish. Neurologic signs (headache, stiff neck, photophobia) occur in some primary infections, reflecting a viral meningitis. In males, a

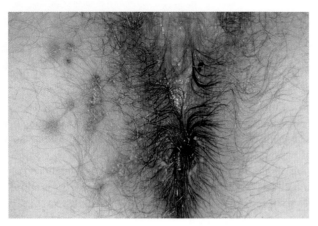

Figure 21.11
Vesicles of genital herpes

urethritis with a watery discharge may occur. Herpes pharyngitis can occur after oral sexual contact.

The primary lesions usually heal within two weeks, but by that time the virus has travelled along the local sensory nerve to the sensory root ganglion where it lies dormant. Virus persistence there lasts for a lifetime. The virus can reactivate and travel back down the nerve, exit the cell and be shed asymptomatically, or spread to, and infect, mucocutaneous epithelial cells, causing cell destruction and new lesions.

There is considerable variation in the frequency of recurrent symptomatic attacks. In some people recurrence is rare; less than 50% of infected people have a recurrence within one year. Others may have many recurrent attacks in a year. The lesions in recurrent attacks are usually fewer in number, involve only one site and resolve sooner than the primary lesions.

Recurrent infection may or may not be symptomatic, but an asymptomatic person can be shedding the virus. Shedding always occurs when lesions are present and days of asymptomatic shedding occur around these symptomatic episodes. Studies indicate that a large proportion of infections are transmitted from asymptomatic people.

Latency, reactivation and recurrent infections are typical of herpes viruses. HSV-1 undergoes a similar cycle in sensory nerves and cutaneous tissue in causing recurrent cold sores. The mechanisms involved in the establishment of latency or in the reactivation of herpes viruses are not well understood, except that reactivation can occur apparently spontaneously or in response to certain stimuli such as physical or emotional stress, ultraviolet light and fever.

HSV-2 can also be transmitted from a symptomatic or asymptomatic mother to her baby during pregnancy, at birth or postnatally. The great majority of neonatal infections are acquired at birth, especially if the mother is suffering from primary infection at that time. The virus can invade the skin, eyes, CNS and visceral organs. Many cases of neonatal infection are fatal; in a large proportion of non-fatal infections, mental retardation and defective sight and hearing are typical outcomes.

Similar to *Treponema pallidum* (see section on syphilis), HSV-2 infection has the important effect of increasing the risk of HIV acquisition. Both organisms have this effect by providing a lesion for direct entry of the HIV, as well as by causing an influx of activated CD4 lymphocytes, the target of the HIV, to the site of infection.

Diagnosis

The diagnosis of genital herpes is sometimes possible by clinical appearance, but it cannot always be distinguished from other types of genital ulcer. Furthermore, many cases are asymptomatic. The virus can be cultured from vesicle fluid or ulcer swabs, and this is the definitive diagnostic approach. Fluid in vesicles should be aspirated with a syringe, or the vesicles should be opened with a small gauge needle and the base of the lesion rubbed with a cotton swab. The swab should be placed in viral transport medium. If transport to the laboratory is delayed, specimens should be refrigerated.

The major disadvantages of culture are that it requires specialised laboratory techniques, and so may not be available, and it takes five days or more. PCR is the assay with the greatest sensitivity for detecting HSV in genital lesions and can provide a result within 24 hours, but only some laboratories currently offer this test. As a result, antibody detection (e.g. by ELISA or Western Blot) is still commonly used to diagnose HSV infection. However, these serological methods do not reliably distinguish between past and current infection.

Treatment

There is currently no fully effective cure for genital herpes. Treatment with aciclovir, valaciclovir or famciclovir reduces the duration of symptoms and virus shedding in clinical and subclinical cases, but does not eliminate latent infection. A continuous, low dose of one of these drugs may be used for a limited time in people with frequent recurrences, and this may be effective in reducing the frequency and severity of recurrences and in reducing subclinical shedding. Strains of herpes simplex virus resistant to aciclovir and famciclovir have been found on rare occasions.

Prevention

Prevention of transmission of genital herpes is based on the general use of safe sex practices. Infected people should be advised to have total abstinence from sex when symptomatic because they may shed the virus from any part of the genital region. Therefore, the use of a condom does not guarantee protection against HSV infection when one partner is symptomatic.

If a pregnant woman is symptomatic near term, caesarean delivery is indicated and will often prevent neonatal infection if performed before rupture of the membranes. This does not always prevent infection of the baby, however, since *in utero* and postnatal transmission are possible. Current HSV vaccines have limited efficacy, especially in women.

GENITAL WARTS

Causative agents and transmission

More than 100 different types of human papillomaviruses (HPV) that infect the skin and mucous membranes have been identified. At least a third of these are associated with anogenital infections. Infection normally occurs through mucous membranes or traumatised skin, although vertical and oral transmission are also possible. PCR and serological studies have shown that papillomavirus infection is very common. However, the exact prevalence in Australia is not known because it is not a notifiable disease.

Clinical features

Genital warts (**condyloma acuminatum**) appear as pinkish-brown masses, usually in clusters, on the penis, scrotum, vulva, cervix or perineal or perianal regions (see Figure 21.12). They can appear at any time from 1 to 8 months or more after infection and then resolve spontaneously within 1–2 years. Warts in the vulva can become very large and extend into the vagina.

The majority of infections are subclinical. Why some people develop warts after infection and others remain asymptomatic is not known. The importance of asymptomatically infected people is that they represent a large, unidentified reservoir of the virus. Furthermore, in a symptomatic person, areas of genital skin where warts are not present are possibly also infected.

One of the major concerns of genital warts is the epidemiological association of certain virus types with carcinoma. Certain types of HPV (e.g. types 16, 18, 31 and 45) have been strongly implicated in the development of vulval, cervical and anal cancer in women. There is also thought to be an association between certain virus types and anal and penile carcinoma in men. There is a relatively low incidence of cancer compared to the incidence of infection, suggesting that other factors may be important for cancer development, particularly smoking and immunosuppression (e.g. from HIV infection).

Diagnosis

Diagnosis of infection is based mainly on clinical examination; histological examination of a biopsy specimen can be used in cases of clinical uncertainty. Human papillomaviruses cannot be cultured, but the virus can be identified by DNA or RNA typing of specimens containing infected cells. Cervical infection is often initially indicated by the presence of abnormal cells in a Pap smear (see Spotlight box, page 98) and then confirmed by colposcopy. The application of 3–5% acetic acid can be used to demonstrate subclinical infection of the vulva, cervix, penis and anus. Infected tissue shows as areas of whitening (called acetowhite lesions), but acetowhitening is not specific for HPV infection.

PCR has recently been used in some epidemiological studies but the role of this method in diagnosis is uncertain.

Treatment

As for warts in other areas of the body, treatment involves removal of the warts, most often with podophyllotoxin (a plant extract) or imiquimod cream, both of which can be applied by patient self-treatment. Other possible treatments include freezing with liquid nitrogen or dry ice, laser therapy or surgical excision.

Early identification and treatment of abnormal cervical cells may prevent the formation of cancerous lesions. Treatment of warts, however, is not always successful. Removal of warts may remove one focus of infection, but viruses may persist in nearby, apparently normal tissue and later cause a local recurrence.

Prevention

Papillomaviruses may exist on most areas of genital skin of an infected person even where no obvious warts are present. Thus, condom usage may reduce transmission but it does not offer complete protection. A major advance in prevention of genital warts and their sequelae is the development of vaccines against some of the viruses. Success has been reported with a vaccine against HPV type 16, and currently clinical trials of vaccines against multiple types are being undertaken.

DONOVANOSIS

Also called **granuloma inguinale**, donovanosis is caused by the encapsulated Gram-negative rod *Calymmatobacterium granulomatis* (also called *Klebsiella granulomatis*). It is rare in temperate climates but common in tropical and subtropical regions such as the Caribbean, New Guinea and India, and is endemic in Aboriginal populations in central and northern Australia. Fewer than 50 cases are reported annually, with the majority occurring in the Northern Territory.

The infection is characterised by nodules, usually on the genitalia, which erode to form granulomatous ulcers. As the disease progresses, the ulcers may spread peripherally, involving more and more tissue. In some cases, extragenital lesions may occur; these are thought to be due to auto-inoculation. The epidemiology of the disease is unclear. The role of sexual transmission is controversial since sexual contacts are often not infected.

Diagnosis of the disease is based on clinical appearance and microscopic examination of a stained smear of a

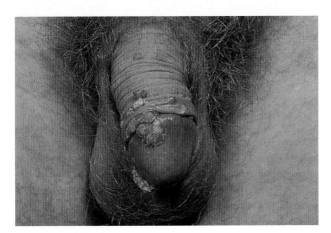

Figure 21.12
Genital warts on the penis

biopsy or scraping from the lesion. Stained organisms are typically found inside large mononuclear cells. PCR, if available, is highly sensitive and can also provide a diagnosis. Treatment is usually with azithromycin.

CHANCROID

Chancroid is an STI caused by a small Gram-negative rod, *Haemophilus ducreyi*. It is most frequently seen in Africa, the Caribbean and South-East Asia. Although notifiable in almost all Australian States and Territories, fewer than ten cases, on average, are reported each year. The disease is manifested by soft, painful genital ulcers 3–5 days after infection (see Figure 21.13). Local lymphadenitis becomes apparent after several days. The lymph nodes gradually enlarge to such an extent that eventually they may break through the skin, discharging pus. Extragenital lesions, such as on the tongue and lip, may also be seen. The lesions are highly infectious.

The organism is difficult to culture in the laboratory and can take up to nine days. However, culture remains the definitive diagnostic method. A Gram stain of an aspirate from the ulcer margin or enlarged lymph node shows short Gram-negative rods inside or outside polymorphonuclear leucocytes. Co-infection with other sexually transmissible organisms is common, so assessment for other STIs is warranted. Multiplex PCR methodology allows the simultaneous detection of *T. pallidum*, herpes simplex virus and *H. ducreyi*. The organism is becoming increasingly resistant but is still sensitive to a number of drugs, including erythromycin and ciprofloxacin.

VAGINITIS

Vaginitis is characterised by a vaginal discharge with an inflamed vaginal mucosa. It is most commonly caused by the yeast *Candida albicans* or the protozoan *Trichomonas vaginalis*.

Candida albicans is a normal inhabitant of the vagina but in certain circumstances (e.g. during antibiotic usage, immunosuppression, pregnancy, diabetes) its numbers increase sufficiently to cause a vaginitis. It typically causes an intensely irritating (itchy) infection with a yellow, cheesy discharge.

Trichomonas vaginalis is a flagellated protozoan (see Figure 21.14) that is a recognised cause of STI. Not only does this organism have a role in causing vaginitis, but it is now recognised as a factor promoting HIV transmission, as a cause of low weight or premature birth and as a factor that can predispose women to pelvic inflammatory disease. In up to 50% of women the infection may be asymptomatic.

When symptomatic there is a vaginal discharge that can be thin and scanty to profuse and thick. The classic symptom of a profuse, frothy yellow/greenish discharge occurs in only 10–30% of women. Urethritis is the most common outcome of infection in men.

The laboratory diagnosis of vaginitis can often be made by direct microscopic examination and culture of discharge. In a microscopic examination yeast cells may be seen in *Candida* infection, or motile trophozoites in *Trichomonas* infection. In *Candida* infections, culture is a more sensitive diagnostic tool than microscopy, and should especially be performed in recurrent infections.

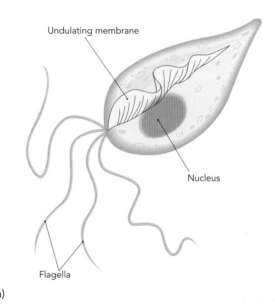

Undulating membrane

Nucleus

Flagella

(a)

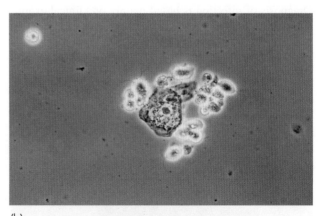

(b)

Figure 21.14

***Trichomonas vaginalis*, the protozoan that causes trichomoniasis**

(a) Schematic drawing of the organism; (b) phase contrast wet mount of *Trichomonas* in vaginal discharge.

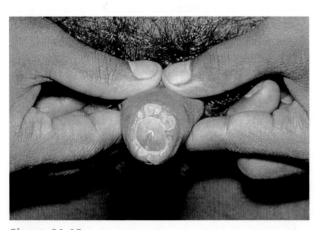

Figure 21.13

Chancroid lesion on the penis

Rapid PCR tests have been developed for *Trichomonas*, but they are not commercially available at present.

Oral or topical metronidazole is effective against *Trichomonas* and allows repopulation of the vagina with lactobacilli. *Candida* is treated with a topical antifungal (e.g. nystatin, clotrimazole) or an oral antifungal like ketoconazole. Sexual partners should be treated if *Trichomonas* is found to be the cause.

NON-SPECIFIC URETHRITIS

Non-specific urethritis (NSU) is inflammation of the urethra not caused by *Neisseria gonorrhoeae* or *Chlamydia trachomatis*. The organisms most often associated with NSU are *Mycoplasma genitalium*, *Trichomonas vaginalis*, herpes simplex virus and *Ureaplasma urealyticum*. However, in many cases a causative agent is not identified. Symptoms are similar to gonorrhoea, but are usually milder. They may include a watery to milky discharge, stinging or burning during urination and itching, tingling or irritation inside the penis.

Once *N. gonorrhoea* and *C. trachomatis* have been excluded, specific tests for the other possible causes, as described earlier in this chapter, may be undertaken. *Ureaplasma urealyticum* infection can be diagnosed by culture of discharge. NSU is often treated empirically with doxycycline or azithromycin. If this treatment is ineffective in preventing recurrent episodes of urethritis, *T. vaginalis* or herpes simplex virus are likely causes.

PELVIC INFLAMMATORY DISEASE

Pelvic inflammatory disease (PID) is defined as the clinical syndrome associated with infection of the pelvic organs, particularly the uterus, fallopian tubes and ovaries, and sometimes the whole of the peritoneal cavity. The most important sites of infection are the fallopian tubes (**salpingitis**), because this can lead to ectopic pregnancy or sterility. It is estimated that as many as one million new cases of PID occur each year in the United States and that many thousands of women have been rendered sterile as a result.

Causative agents, pathogenesis and clinical features

PID may be uni- or poly-microbial. Most infections are caused by *Neisseria gonorrhoeae*, *Chlamydia trachomatis*, or both. Polymicrobial infection can occur with one or both of these organisms in conjunction with the causative agents of bacterial vaginosis. Bacterial vaginosis is common in women with PID. It is thought that *N. gonorrhoeae* and *C. trachomatis* set up infection by initially damaging the upper genital tract, and then vaginal flora (anaerobes and facultative anaerobes) ascend the tract and gradually take over. *Mycoplasma genitalium* is also recognised as a potential cause of PID.

The symptoms associated with PID are extremely variable. Most cases of PID are asymptomatic, and only come to light during investigations for infertility. When symptomatic, the most common symptom is a dull and constant lower abdominal pain. Also, patients often have cervical

---

> **CASE HISTORY 21.3**
> ### Pelvic inflammatory disease
> A 21-year-old woman attended the casualty department of her local hospital complaining of the gradual onset of severe pain in the lower part of her abdomen. Over the last few hours she had also begun to feel feverish and nauseated. Prior to this she had noticed no other symptoms.
>
> A pelvic examination revealed a yellowish discharge from the cervical os. A cervical swab was taken and a Gram stain showed intracellular Gram-negative diplococci. Culture results the next day confirmed infection with *Neisseria gonorrhoeae*. She stated that her two sexual partners did not have any signs of infection.
>
> *Comment*
> This woman had an asymptomatic gonorrhoeal infection until the organism reached the upper parts of her genital tract. *Neisseria gonorrhoeae* is a common cause of pelvic inflammatory disease but a number of other organisms can also cause PID.

motion tenderness (pain when the cervix is moved from side to side). Other manifestations include abnormal vaginal discharge, intermenstrual bleeding, fever and postcoital bleeding.

Persistent infection can lead to fibrosis and scarring of the fallopian tubes, which can block the passage of the ovum from the ovary to the uterus. This can result in sterility or the implantation of the fertilised egg in the uterine tube rather than in the uterus (called an 'ectopic' or 'tubal' pregnancy).

Diagnosis and treatment

The diagnosis is usually made clinically on the findings of abnormal discharge or bleeding, together with lower abdominal tenderness, cervical motion tenderness and adnexal tenderness. Laparoscopy is considered the gold standard method for diagnosis of PID, but is not always performed because it is invasive, not cost-effective and does not identify all cases.

Treatment of PID usually involves the use of a combination of antibiotics because of the possibility of polymicrobial infection. Several different treatment regimens exist – a typical one is metronidazole, doxycycline and ceftriaxone or ciprofloxacin. Male partners should be assessed for both gonorrhoea and chlamydial infection.

PREVENTION OF STIs

Since the AIDS pandemic began, the practice of 'safe sex' has become the plea of governments and health departments throughout the world. In the past, safe sex meant protection from unintended pregnancy, but today it refers mainly to protection from the human immunodeficiency virus (HIV) and other sexually transmissible infections. Vaccines have been heralded as the ultimate solution to the global epidemic of STIs but, despite intensive research, the only successful vaccines developed to date for STIs are for hepatitis B and possibly some papillomaviruses. Prevention is therefore based on the following approaches.

Avoidance of high-risk encounters

Avoidance of high-risk encounters is clearly the best method for prevention of STIs. A high-risk encounter is unprotected, penetrative sex (without a condom) with:

- multiple partners, or with someone who has multiple partners
- someone who uses intravenous drugs
- someone other than a monogamous partner
- a prostitute.

A safe encounter is sex with a faithful, uninfected partner.

Since HIV and some other sexually transmissible infections can be transmitted by blood, the sharing of needles and syringes in drug usage is also risky behaviour. A major reason for the high incidence of STIs throughout the world is that many infections are asymptomatic and risk of infection is not always obvious.

Barrier contraceptive devices

Barrier contraceptive devices, specifically condoms, are the best alternative to abstinence or safe sex with one partner. The success of the condom is directly related to its consistent usage and structural integrity. In experimental studies, intact latex condoms have been found to be impervious to bacteria and viruses. However, if the device fails (breakage, leakage or slipping off) during use, its effectiveness will clearly be reduced.

Condoms are only partially effective for protection against those diseases in which the organisms may infect all parts of the genital skin – that is, herpes simplex infections and genital warts. 'Natural' condoms made from animal membranes are less effective because they are more easily broken; also, they are not impervious to smaller particles, like viruses. Other devices, such as the 'female condom' (a sheath or pouch), can also potentially eliminate direct contact with genital secretions.

Spermicides

Spermicides are agents that have been developed for contraceptive purposes. They do this by interfering with sperm viability. Nonoxynol-9 is the most frequently used and best studied compound. It is a detergent that disrupts the membranes of sperm and also microorganisms. *In vitro* studies have demonstrated that most spermicides have potent antimicrobial and antiviral activity, but the clinical effectiveness of these substances has not yet been established. In addition, there is some concern that the detergent action of spermicides may cause vaginal irritation, which may enhance HIV transmission.

Contact tracing

The tracing of sexual contacts of people with STIs, and their screening and treatment, is a vital part of any prevention program. Unfortunately, this is not always possible or is not performed adequately.

SUMMARY

- The urinary tract is one of the more common sites of infection and is frequently the site of hospital-acquired infection.
- In a healthy person, the upper urethra, the urinary bladder and the organs of the upper urinary tract are sterile.
- Protection against infection of the genital and urinary tracts in females is afforded by the low pH and the normal flora of the vagina.

URINARY TRACT INFECTIONS

- Urinary tract infections occur much more frequently in females than in males.
- UTIs represent 30–40% of all hospital-acquired infections.
- The vast majority of urinary tract infections are caused by microorganisms ascending the urethra and reaching the bladder.
- Ascending infections are most often caused by the enteric bacterium, *E. coli.*
- The flushing of microorganisms from the urethra during the normal passage of urine is an important defence mechanism.
- The high incidence of UTI in hospitalised people is partly due to the use of indwelling urinary catheters.
- A catheter provides several potential sites of entry and colonisation for microorganisms and prevents the normal flushing of the urethra with urine.

- Asymptomatic bacteriuria represents multiplication of bacteria in the bladder urine, without involvement of tissues, although in some cases infection is present.
- Cystitis is an acute infection of the bladder, usually characterised by symptoms of dysuria, urgency and frequency.
- Pyelonephritis is an infection of the kidney(s).
- The specimen most commonly collected for the diagnosis of UTIs is a clean-catch or mid-stream specimen of urine (MSU).
- Significant bacteriuria is usually defined as a count of 10^8/L in a properly collected MSU.
- The incidence of community-acquired UTI in women may be reduced by promotion of good personal hygiene, adequate fluid intake and regular emptying of the bladder.
- In hospitals, prevention of UTIs is based on similar principles plus avoidance of catheterisation wherever possible.

INFECTIONS OF THE REPRODUCTIVE SYSTEM

- Most diseases of the reproductive (genital) system are transmitted during sexual activity and are referred to as sexually transmissible infections (STIs).
- There is a strong association between the organisms that cause genital ulcer disease (e.g. syphilis, herpes, chancroid) and transmission of the human immunodeficiency virus (HIV).

Gonorrhoea

- Gonorrhoea is caused by the bacterium *Neisseria gonorrhoeae* (the 'gonococcus').
- The gonococcus is usually transmitted by direct person-to-person contact.
- The gonococcus can be transmitted vertically from an infected mother to baby at birth.
- In men, gonococcal infection is usually characterised by a urethral discharge and dysuria.
- Up to 50% of infected women have very mild symptoms or are completely asymptomatic; symptomatic infection is usually characterised by a cervico-vaginal discharge and cervical oedema.
- In untreated women, the infection may spread further up the genital tract to cause pelvic inflammatory disease (PID).
- Diagnosis is based on microscopy and culture of an appropriate specimen: in men, a urethral swab or urethral discharge; in women, a cervical swab. Urine PCR tests are now available.
- All patients with gonococcal infection should be evaluated for other STIs.
- Treatment is with an appropriate antibiotic; resistance to some drugs exists.

Syphilis

- Syphilis is caused by the spirochaete *Treponema pallidum*.
- Transmission of syphilis requires close personal contact.
- An infected woman may transmit the organism to her foetus *in utero*, resulting in congenital malformations.
- Primary syphilis is characterised by the development of a papular lesion at the site of infection. The papular lesion breaks down to form a painless, hard-based ulcer called a chancre.
- The secondary stage of syphilis is characterised by the appearance of a red, maculopapular rash anywhere on the skin, anogenital region, mouth, throat or cervix.
- In about 30% of untreated cases, the disease progresses to tertiary syphilis and granulomatous lesions (gummas) form in various organs.
- The primary and secondary lesions of syphilis usually contain large numbers of organisms, which are readily seen microscopically in exudate from the lesions.
- In the absence of lesions, serology is the mainstay of diagnosis.
- Penicillin is very active against *Treponema pallidum* and is the drug of choice.
- Prevention is based on the practice of safe sex, and contact tracing and screening.

Chlamydial infections

- Genital infections caused by serotypes D to K of *Chlamydia trachomatis* are the most prevalent of all STIs.
- Serotypes L1, L2 and L3 of *C. trachomatis* cause lymphogranuloma venereum (LGV).
- Infection in the urethra is termed chlamydial urethritis; infection of the cervix leads to cervicitis.
- Many infections are asymptomatic or have only mild symptoms.

- In LGV, a primary lesion develops at the site of organism inoculation. Inguinal buboes form, which gradually enlarge.
- Treatment is usually with azithromycin.

Mycoplasma genitalium

- *Mycoplasma genitalium* causes urethritis in males; its role in causing infection in females is less certain.

Genital herpes

- Herpes simplex virus type 1 (HSV-1) and herpes simplex type 2 (HSV-2) cause genital and oral (cold sores) herpes, but type 2 predominates in the genital region.
- Initial infection may be completely asymptomatic or so mild that it is unrecognised.
- The primary lesions usually occur on the penis, anus, vulva, cervix or vagina. They are usually small, grouped vesicles filled with a clear fluid and surrounded by an area of inflammation; they break down after several days to form painful, shallow ulcers.
- The virus travels up the local sensory nerve to the sensory root ganglion where it lies dormant; virus persistence there lasts for a lifetime.
- The virus can reactivate and travel back down the nerve where it causes a recurrent attack.
- The virus can be cultured from vesicle fluid or ulcer swabs. PCR is sometimes used for diagnosis.
- Treatment with aciclovir, valaciclovir or famciclovir reduces the duration of symptoms and virus shedding.
- Prevention of genital herpes is based on safe sex practices, and total abstinence when symptomatic.

Genital warts

- At least 30 different types of human papillomaviruses (HPV) are associated with anogenital infections.
- Infection normally occurs through mucous membranes or traumatised skin.
- Genital warts (condyloma acuminatum) appear as pinkish-brown masses, usually in clusters, on the penis, vulva, cervix or perineal or perianal regions.
- Subclinical infection is extremely common.
- A major concern with genital warts is the association of certain virus types with cervical cancer.
- Diagnosis of infection is based on clinical examination.
- Treatment involves removal of warts with podophyllotoxin or imiquimod, freezing with liquid nitrogen or dry ice, or surgical excision. Treatment is not always successful.

Donovanosis

- Donovanosis (granuloma inguinale) is caused by the Gram-negative rod *Calymmatobacterium granulomatis*.
- The infection is characterised by nodules, usually on the genitalia, which erode to form granulomatous ulcers.
- Diagnosis of the disease involves microscopic examination of a stained smear from the lesion.
- Treatment is with azithromycin.

Chancroid

- Chancroid is an STI caused by the small Gram-negative rod *Haemophilus ducreyi*.

- The disease is manifested by soft, painful genital ulcers. The lymph nodes gradually enlarge and eventually break through the skin, discharging pus.
- Culture is the definitive diagnostic method.
- The organism is sensitive to a number of drugs.

Vaginitis
- Vaginitis is characterised by a vaginal discharge and inflammation of the vaginal mucosa.
- Vaginitis is most commonly caused by the yeast *Candida albicans* or the protozoan *Trichomonas vaginalis*.
- The laboratory diagnosis of vaginitis can often be made by direct microscopic examination of discharge.

Non-specific urethritis
- Non-specific urethritis (NSU) is any inflammation of the urethra not caused by *Neisseria gonorrhoeae* or *Chlamydia trachomatis*.
- Symptoms include a watery discharge and dysuria, but many infections are asymptomatic.

Pelvic inflammatory disease
- Pelvic inflammatory disease (PID) is usually asymptomatic. It is associated with infection of the pelvic organs, particularly the uterus, fallopian tubes, ovaries and peritoneal cavity.
- Most infections are caused by *Neisseria gonorrhoeae*, *Chlamydia trachomatis*, or both.
- The symptoms are extremely variable; the most common is a dull and constant lower abdominal pain.
- Persistent infection can lead to fibrosis and scarring of the fallopian tubes which can result in sterility or ectopic (tubal) pregnancy.
- The diagnosis is usually made on clinical grounds.
- Treatment of PID usually involves a combination of antibiotics.

Prevention of STIs
- Avoidance of high-risk encounters is the best method of preventing STIs.
- Barrier contraceptive devices, specifically condoms, are the best alternative to abstinence or safe sex with one partner.
- Tracing the sexual contacts of people with STIs, and their screening and treatment, is vital.

STUDY QUESTIONS

1. Which parts of the urinary and reproductive systems of humans have a normal microbial flora?
2. Why are females generally more susceptible to urinary tract infections than males?
3. From where do urinary tract pathogens usually originate?
4. How does normal urine flow protect the urinary tract from infection?
5. Why do urinary catheters increase the risk of urinary tract infection?
6. Define the terms 'pyelonephritis', 'cystitis' and 'asymptomatic bacteriuria'.
7. Why should urine for microbiological analysis be transported to the laboratory promptly?
8. What is significant bacteriuria?
9. What laboratory results indicate that a urine specimen is of poor quality?
10. Why are sexually transmissible infections considered to be a major health problem?
11. How is gonorrhoea usually transmitted?
12. Why is asymptomatic gonorrhoeal infection in women so important?
13. What specimen(s) should be collected from a woman suspected of having gonorrhoea?
14. What are the differences between primary and secondary syphilis?
15. What are the two main methods for diagnosing syphilis in the laboratory, and what specimens are needed for each?
16. What types of genital infections does *Chlamydia trachomatis* cause?
17. What is the most common cause of genital herpes?
18. How does the genital herpes virus cause recurrent infections?
19. What are the common causes of genital warts?
20. What important sequela is associated with genital warts in women?
21. How are genital warts treated?
22. What is donovanosis?
23. What are the common causes of vaginitis?
24. What is non-specific urethritis and what are the common causes?
25. What is pelvic inflammatory disease and what are the possible serious sequelae of this disease?
26. How is pelvic inflammatory disease diagnosed?
27. List the ways by which sexually transmissible infections can be prevented.

TEST YOUR UNDERSTANDING

Case History 21.1   Urinary tract infection
1. What do the urinalysis results indicate?
2. Why are the numbers of organisms in urine quantitated?

Case History 21.2   Urethritis
1. Assuming Mr K did have gonorrhoea, what are the possible reasons for the incomplete effectiveness of the treatment?
2. What should have Mr K been treated with?

Case History 21.3   Pelvic inflammatory disease
1. What organs might be involved in this infection?
2. Are any serious complications associated with this infection?
3. Should the woman's asymptomatic sexual partners be notified and treated?

Further reading

Bowden FJ, SN Tabrizi, SM Garland & CK Fairley 2002, 'Sexually transmitted infections: new diagnostic approaches and treatments', *Medical Journal of Australia* 176: 551. (A review of the diagnosis and treatment of common STIs.

Bowen S 2003, 'How to treat sexually transmitted infections', Parts 1 & 2, *Australian Doctor* 17 and 23 January. (Reviews the diagnosis and management of common sexually transmitted diseases.) <www.australiandoctor.com.au>

Donovan B 2004, 'Sexually transmissible infections other than HIV', *Lancet* 363: 545. (A general review of the epidemiology, diagnosis and management of STIs.)

Jensen JS 2004, '*Mycoplasma genitalium*: the aetiological agent of urethritis and other sexually transmitted diseases', *Journal of the European Academy of Dermatology and Venereology* 18: 1. (A review of the role of *Mycoplasma genitalium* in genital infections.)

Lee N (ed.) 1990, Laboratory diagnosis of urinary tract infection, *Clinical Microbiology Update Program*, University of New South Wales. (A detailed description of laboratory methods used in urinalysis and the interpretation of results.)

Lehker MW & JF Alderete 2000, 'Biology of trichomonosis', *Current Opinion in Infectious Diseases* 13(1): 37. (A review article detailing the clinical aspects, diagnosis and treatment of *Trichomonas vaginalis* infections.)

National Centre in HIV Epidemiology and Clinical Research 2004, *Annual Surveillance Report*: *HIV/AIDS, Viral Hepatitis and Sexually Transmissible Infections in Australia*.

National Health & Medical Research Council 2003, *The Australian Immunisation Handbook*, 8th edn, Australian Government Department of Health and Ageing. (This book gives useful information on vaccine-preventable diseases and details current recommendations and contraindications of available vaccines.)

Glossary

abscess A sac of pus walled off by a layer of fibrin.

acetyl CoA An activated compound which is an important intermediate in carbohydrate metabolism and is also able to enter other metabolic pathways.

acid-fast bacilli Bacteria belonging to the genus *Mycobacterium*, which are identifiable in an acid-fast stain.

acid-fast stain A differential stain used to identify bacteria that belong to the genus *Mycobacterium*. Also called a **Ziehl-Neelsen stain**.

acquired immune system A functional system consisting of a variety of cells and organs that protect the body against pathogens which evade the non-specific defences; it also protects against future attack by the pathogen. Also called **adaptive immune system**, **specific immune system** or **specific defences**.

acquired immunodeficiency syndrome (AIDS) A disease caused by the human immunodeficiency virus which impairs the ability of the body to produce a specific immune response.

activation energy The amount of energy required for a reaction to occur.

active immunisation The use of a vaccine to prevent a specific disease in a person.

active immunity The development of antibodies or other specific defences by the acquired immune system in response to microorganisms or other foreign substances which enter the body.

active site The area of an enzyme which binds specifically to its substrate.

active transport The movement of substances across a membrane against a concentration gradient.

acute bronchitis An inflammation of the tracheobronchial tree.

acute diarrhoea A sudden disruption in bowel habits in which normally formed stools are replaced by more frequent, liquefied movements.

acute glomerulonephritis Inflammation of the kidneys due to the deposition of immune complexes in the glomeruli.

acute inflammatory response A non-specific defence that is the body's response to tissue injury, characterised by redness, heat, swelling and pain.

acute otitis media Acute infection and inflammation of the middle ear.

adaptive immune system See **acquired immune system**.

adenine A purine base that pairs with thymine in DNA and uracil in RNA.

adenosine triphosphate (ATP) A small molecule which is important for the storage of energy released during metabolism.

adherence The attachment of microorganisms to host tissues or other surfaces.

adhesins The substances or structures on the surfaces of microorganisms that enable them to attach to cell surfaces.

aerial hyphae Long filaments of fungal cells that grow above the mycelium and bear spores.

aerobe, obligate An organism that can only grow in the presence of oxygen.

aerobic respiration The process whereby cells gain energy from the breakdown of organic molecules, using the electron transport chain, with oxygen as the final electron acceptor.

aetiology The study of the cause and origin of a disease.

aflatoxin A carcinogenic toxin produced by *Aspergillus flavus*.

agammaglobulinaemia A primary immunodeficiency disease characterised by a lack of antibodies.

agar A polysaccharide derived from seaweed and used as a solidifying agent for bacterial culture media.

agar plate A solid medium contained in a petri dish for growing bacteria or fungi.

agglutination The clumping of the particles due to their cross-linking by specific antibodies.

AIDS See **acquired immunodeficiency syndrome**.

airborne transmission The spread of infectious microorganisms through the air, usually over distances greater than one metre from the infected host.

algae A group of photosynthetic eucaryotic organisms.

algal bloom An overgrowth of algae seen on waterways.

allergen An antigen that evokes an allergic response.

allergy See **immediate hypersensitivity**.

alternate pathway A pathway for the activation of the complement system initiated by polysaccharides present on the surface of certain microorganisms.

Ames test A bacterial test used to identify potential carcinogens.

aminoglycosides A group of antibiotics containing amino sugars.

amoeba A single-celled protozoan (eucaryotic organism) that moves by extending pseudopods.

amoebic dysentery A severe form of inflammatory diarrhoea caused by *Entamoeba histolytica*.

anabolism The synthesis of complex organic molecules from simple components in living cells.

anaerobe, obligate An organism that can only grow in the absence of oxygen.

analogue A compound that has a structure similar to the substrate for an enzyme and that can be bound by the enzyme.

anaphylactic shock A potentially life-threatening disorder resulting from a generalised allergic reaction throughout the body.

anaphylatoxins Substances which bind to mast cells, basophils and platelets, triggering the release of histamine and other inflammatory mediators.

anaphylaxis A systemic allergic reaction which occurs when an allergen enters the blood and circulates through the body.

Animalia A kingdom in the Linnaean classification system, containing multicellular eucaryotic organisms that do not have cell walls.

anthrax A zoonosis caused by *Bacillus anthracis* that is characterised by cutaneous, respiratory or intestinal disease.

antibacterial agent A compound that can kill bacteria or inhibit their growth.

antibiotic A chemical substance produced naturally by a microorganism that can kill or inhibit another microorganism.

antibiotic-associated colitis A serious gastrointestinal disease which can sometimes follow antibiotic therapy, caused by the establishment of *Clostridium difficile* in the intestine.

antibody A protein found in blood and other body fluids that is secreted by plasma cells in response to an antigen, and which is capable of binding specifically with that antigen. Also called **immunoglobulin**.

antibody titre The amount of antibody in a person's blood or other body fluid.

antifungal agent A compound that can kill or inhibit fungi.

antigen A foreign substance which, when introduced into the body, activates the acquired immune system and induces an immune response. Also called **immunogen**.

antigen-antibody complex See **immune complex**.

antigen-binding fragments (Fab) The end of the antibody molecule comprising the two arms responsible for binding of antigen.

antigen-binding sites The sites on an antibody molecule where binding to antigen occurs.

antigen-presenting cell A macrophage or other cell that engulfs an antigen and then presents fragments of it to lymphocytes to activate them.

antigenic Capable of inducing an immune response.

antigenic determinant The small part of the whole antigen molecule to which antibodies or activated lymphocytes bind.

antigenic drift A term used for repeated, minor mutations in the genes that code for the antigen of a microorganism.

antigenic shift A major antigenic change in a virus due to a recombination of genes when two different strains of a virus infect the same cell.

antigenic variation A phenomenon in which certain microorganisms are able to repeatedly or progressively change their cell surface antigens, enabling them to evade the immune system.

antihistamine A drug used to alleviate the redness and swelling prominent in some allergic conditions like hay fever and hives.

antimicrobial agent Any compound that kills or inhibits microorganisms. It may be synthetic or naturally occurring.

antiprotozoal agent A compound that can kill or inhibit protozoa.

antipyretic A drug used to reduce fever.

antiseptic A chemical agent used on skin or living tissue to kill or remove microorganisms without damaging the tissue.

antiserum A fluid derived from blood which contains antibodies.

antitoxin An antibody preparation derived from the serum of immune humans or animals which neutralises a microbial toxin.

antiviral agent A compound that can inactivate viruses.

apoptosis A process of programmed cell death in which a cell begins to kill itself.

APSGN—acute post-streptococcal glomerulonephritis A serious inflammation of the kidneys after a streptococcal infection elsewhere in the body.

arbovirus A virus which is transmitted to humans by biting arthropods (e.g. insects and ticks).

Archaea One of the three bacterial domain classifications, containing ancient bacteria such as thermophiles and halophiles.

archaebacteria Procaryotic organisms (bacteria) of ancient origin that lack peptidoglycan in their cell walls.

arthropod vector A member of the phylum Arthropoda (spiders, mites, ticks and insects) that carries an infectious agent from one host to another.

artificial active immunity Immunity produced in response to a vaccination.

artificially acquired active immunity Active immunity produced following vaccination.

artificially acquired passive immunity Immunity due to the injection of preformed antibodies derived from another person.

ascariasis A gastrointestinal disease caused by the roundworm *Ascaris lumbricoides*.

aschelminth A roundworm.

asepsis The absence of disease-producing microorganisms.

aseptic meningitis A general term used for any meningitis where microorganisms are not isolated by routine bacteriological culture, especially viral meningitis.

aseptic technique Procedures used to minimise the transfer of microorganisms.

asexual reproduction Reproduction that does not involve cells of different mating strains.

asymptomatic bacteriuria A condition in which a person has large numbers of bacteria in the urine without displaying any symptoms.

athlete's foot A fungal infection of the skin of the foot. Also called *tinea pedis*.

attenuation Any process that substantially reduces or eliminates the disease-producing ability of a microorganism, while still keeping it alive.

atypical pneumonia Pneumonia characterised by diffuse, patchy lesions in the lung, an insidious onset and a non-productive cough.

autoantibody An antibody produced against one's own tissue.

autoimmune disease Tissue damage and disease due to the presence of auto-antibodies.

autoclave Equipment used for sterilisation by steam under pressure.

autotroph An organism that uses carbon dioxide from the air as its principal carbon source.

B cell See **B lymphocyte**.

B lymphocyte A cell which is a major component of the humoral immune system, giving rise to antibody-secreting plasma cells when stimulated by antigen.

bacillary dysentery Diarrhoea caused by *Shigella* spp. Also called **shigellosis**.

bacillus (pl: bacilli) A rod-shaped bacterium.

bacteraemia The presence of bacteria in the bloodstream.

bacteria Microorganisms that have a procaryotic cell structure.

bactericidal Able to kill bacteria.

bacteriophage A virus that infects bacteria.

bacteriostatic Able to inhibit bacterial growth.

Bairnsdale ulcer A cutaneous ulcer caused by *Mycobacterium ulcerans*.

basal body A structure that connects flagella to the cell wall and membrane of a bacterium.

basophil A white blood cell which contains granules of histamine and other inflammatory mediators.

BCG vaccine (Bacillus of Calmette and Guerin), a live attenuated strain of *Mycobacterium bovis* used to provide immunity to tuberculosis.

benign malaria A type of malaria in which there is a pattern of intermittent illness and well-being, caused by *Plasmodium vivax*, *P. ovale* and *P. malariae*.

beta-lactamase An enzyme produced by bacteria that are resistant to antibiotics such as penicillin and cephalosporin and contain a ß-lactam ring.

beta-lactams Compound containing a five-membered beta-lactam ring.

binary fission The process of reproduction that involves splitting into two identical daughter cells.

biofilm A multilayer community of bacteria held together on a surface by polysaccharide secretions of some of the bacteria.

biogenesis The idea that living cells can arise only from pre-existing living cells.

biological transmission The method of transmission of a pathogen that involves replication in an insect vector.

biotechnology The industrial use of living cells to produce biological materials.

bioterrorism The fear created by the threat of biological warfare.

biotin A sulfur-containing vitamin.

blepharitis Infection and inflammation of the eyelid margin.

blepharoconjunctivitis Infection and inflammation of the eyelid.

blood agar A nutrient agar culture medium to which defibrinated horse or sheep blood is added.

blood-brain barrier The tightly joined endothelial cells of the brain's capillaries that prevent the passage of most substances and thus help to ensure that the brain's environment remains stable.

blood culture A culture of a blood sample performed in the investigation of a patient with fever or other manifestations of systemic infection.

blue-green algae See **Cyanobacteria**.

boil A large, pus-filled nodule that develops when the deeper areas of a hair follicle become infected by *Staphylococcus aureus*. Also called a **furuncle**.

booster vaccination A second or subsequent dose of a vaccine given to produce large numbers of memory cells and antibody levels in blood that remain high for many years.

botulism A disease of the nervous system caused by a neurotoxin of *Clostridium botulinum*, acquired by consumption of contaminated food.

bovine spongiform encephalopathy A prion disease of cattle that can be transmitted to humans to cause variant Creutzfeld-Jakob disease.

bright-field microscopy A type of compound light microscopy in which the specimen is fully illuminated with light.

broad spectrum antimicrobial agent A chemical which is active against a number of different microorganisms.

bronchiolitis Infection and inflammation of the bronchioles.

bronchopneumonia A diffuse, patchy inflammation of the lungs, with numerous, small discrete foci of consolidation occurring throughout the lungs. Caused by viruses and some bacteria.

brucellosis A systemic zoonosis caused by the bacteria *Brucella melitensis*, *B. abortus* and *B. suis*. Also called **undulant fever** or **Malta fever**.

Bruton's agammaglobulinaemia A primary immunodeficiency caused by incomplete maturation of B lymphocytes.

bubo An enlarged lymph node due to inflammation.

bubonic plague A systemic infection caused by the bacterium *Yersinia pestis*, characterised by large, tender buboes, most frequently in the armpit or groin.

bulla A large blister containing clear fluid, more than 0.5 cm in diameter.

campylobacteriosis A gastrointestinal infection caused by Campylobacter.

candidaemia A systemic infection caused by *Candida albicans*.

candidiasis An infection caused by the yeast *Candida albicans*. Also called **moniliasis** or **thrush**.

CAPD—continuous ambulatory peritoneal dialysis A procedure whereby a patient is able to undergo dialysis without being confined to bed.

capsid The protein coat surrounding the viral nucleic acid.

capsomere One of the protein units that make up the viral capsid.

capsule A protective outer layer present in some bacteria and composed of polysaccharide; also called **glycocalyx** or **slime layer**.

carbapenem A group of ß-lactam compounds with a broad spectrum of antibacterial activity.

carbuncle A large abscess or multiple abscesses in adjacent areas of skin caused by *Staphylococcus aureus*.

carcinogen A substance that can cause cancer.

cardiovascular syphilis A form of tertiary syphilis in which aortic aneurysm and blood vessel and valve damage may occur.

caries Tooth decay.

carrier A person who harbours and continuously sheds a pathogen without showing any symptoms of disease.

catabolism The process of breakdown of complex molecules in living cells with release of energy.

catalase An enzyme produced by some bacteria, which breaks down hydrogen peroxide.

catalyst A substance that lowers the activation energy of a reaction.

category-specific isolation precautions A method of infection control in which diseases are assigned to categories and the body substances that are considered infective within each category are specified.

CD4 cell See **helper T cell**.

CD8 cell See **cytotoxic T cell**.

cell culture Animal or plant cells grown in the laboratory.

cell-mediated hypersensitivity See **delayed type hypersensitivity**.

cell-mediated immunity An immune response in which T lymphocytes act directly against target cells, release chemicals that enhance inflammation, or activate other defence cells to cause destruction of the target cells. Also called **cellular immunity**.

cell membrane See **cytoplasmic membrane**.

cell wall The outer layer of bacteria and most algal, plant and fungal cells. It provides shape and structural support for the cell.

cellular immunity See **cell-mediated immunity**.

cellulitis An infection of subcutaneous tissue.

centrioles A pair of cylindrical structures which take part in eucaryotic cell division.

cephalosporins A group of ß-lactam antibiotic compounds, derived from the fungus Cephalosporium, that inhibit the synthesis of peptidoglycan.

cercariae The free-swimming larval form of flukes (e.g. Schistosoma) which are released into the water from the intermediate snail host.

cerebrospinal fluid The fluid that circulates in the space between the inner two meningeal membranes of the brain and spinal cord.

cervicitis Infection and inflammation of the cervix.

cestode Tapeworm.

chancre A painless, hard-based ulcer found in the primary stage of syphilis.

chancroid A sexually transmissible disease caused by *Haemophilus ducreyi*, characterised by soft, painful genital ulcers.

chemically defined medium A culture medium in which the amount of each pure chemical compound is known.

chemokine A cytokine that is responsible for the attraction, migration or homing of a certain cell in the body.

chemostat Equipment used to control the chemical composition of the culture medium during microbial growth. Can be used for the continuous culture of microorganisms.

chemotaxis The attraction of phagocytes to sites of damaged tissue or microbial invasion by chemicals released at the site.

chemotherapy The treatment of an illness or infection with a chemical substance.

chickenpox A highly infectious disease characterised by skin lesions caused by the varicella zoster virus.

chlamydiae Very small bacteria which have a complex life cycle and can only reproduce inside a living cell.

chloramines Organic chlorine compounds used in water purification.

chloramphenicol A broad spectrum antibiotic which inhibits protein synthesis.

chlorophyll The pigment in algae and green plants that absorbs energy from the sun for photosynthesis.

chloroplast The organelle in green plants that is the site of photosynthesis.

cholera An acute and profuse diarrhoeal disease caused by *Vibrio cholerae*.

chromosome A structure containing DNA and carrying hereditary information.

chronic fatigue syndrome (CFS) A condition in which excessive fatigue and general malaise are chronic complaints, often following an initial viral-like illness.

chronic hepatitis The persistence of hepatitis virus antigens in the bloodstream for at least six months.

chronic infection An infection that persists in the body and is accompanied by continuous shedding of the pathogen.

chronic inflammation A type of inflammation in which large numbers of lymphocytes and macrophages are involved, occurring if the acute inflammatory response is unsuccessful in clearing organisms or foreign material from the tissue.

chronic mucocutaneous candidiasis A chronic infection caused by *Candida*, usually seen in immunodeficient patients.

chronic suppurative otitis media (CSOM) A severe, chronic form of middle ear infection.

ciguatera A toxin produced by certain species of marine algae that can cause poisoning if it enters the food chain.

cirrhosis A disease of the liver characterised by reduced liver function and an increase in connective tissue.

classical pathway A pathway for the activation of complement proteins initiated by antigen-antibody complexes.

clean technique Procedures designed to minimise the spread of infection.

clonal selection A theory proposed to explain the activation of a specific clone of lymphocytes by antigen, giving rise to a larger population of cells with the same specificity.

clone A population of cells all derived from the same parent cell.

coagulase An enzyme produced by pathogenic staphylococci that coagulates fibrinogen to form a deposit of fibrin around the bacterial cells.

coccobacilli Small rod-shaped bacteria which resemble cocci.

coccus (pl: cocci) A spherical bacterium.

codon A specific sequence of three nucleotide bases, responsible for the binding of a particular amino acid.

coenzyme An organic molecule associated with an enzyme and required for enzyme activity.

cofactor A non-protein component of an enzyme that is required for enzyme activity.

collagenase A microbial enzyme that breaks down tissue collagen.

colonisation The process in which microorganisms live and reproduce on the human body without causing disease.

colony-forming units The number of individual bacterial colonies visible on an agar plate. Each colony may have arisen from one or more cells.

colony stimulating factor A cytokine that stimulates certain cells to divide and differentiate.

commensalism A symbiotic association between two organisms in which one benefits without harming the other.

common vehicle transmission Transmission of a pathogen to a number of people from a common source such as food or water.

communicable disease A disease which is transmitted from one host to another.

community-acquired infection An infection acquired in the community, not in a health-care facility.

community strain A strain of microorganism that originates in the community, not from a hospital. A community strain of a microorganism is usually sensitive to antimicrobial drugs.

complement A complex system of proteins circulating in the blood in an inactive state; they are involved in body defences when activated.

complement fixation The activation of complement proteins and fixation to a receptor on antibody molecules in antigen-antibody complexes.

complete antigen A foreign substance that stimulates specific lymphocytes, inducing them to produce an immune response.

complex medium A culture medium in which the exact chemical composition of each of the nutrients is not defined.

compound light microscope A microscope with more than one lens, which uses visible light as the illumination source.

condyloma acuminatum Genital warts, appearing as pinkish-brown masses on the penis, vulva, cervix or perineal or perianal regions.

congenital infection An infection of the foetus that occurs *in utero*.

congenital rubella syndrome A potentially severe rubella infection in the foetus due to the virus crossing the placenta from the mother's circulation.

conidia (conidiospores) Asexual fungal spores that develop on aerial hyphae.

conjugate vaccine A vaccine prepared by combining the desired antigen with another protein.

conjugation The transfer of genetic material from one bacterium to another by means of sex pili.

conjunctivitis Infection and inflammation of the conjunctiva of the eye.

contact inhibition A property of cells that regulates growth.

contact transmission Spread of a pathogen from one host to another by contact.

contagious Easily spread from one person to another.

contamination The unwanted presence of microorganisms.

continuous cell line A cell culture consisting of cells that can be propagated over many generations.

continuous culture The process of growing and harvesting microorganisms in such a way that optimal growth conditions are maintained.

coryza See **rhinitis**.

Creutzfeldt-Jakob disease (CJD) A disease caused by a prion, characterised by fatal degeneration of brain tissue.

cristae Folds of the inner membrane of mitochondria.

crossing over An event in meiosis in which part of the DNA from one chromosome is exchanged with the DNA from another.

cross-resistance Situation where an organism that has developed a mechanism of resistance to one drug will also be resistant to related drugs.

croup Inflammation of the larynx and trachea, characterised by stridor, hoarseness and a resonant cough.

crust The dried exudate from an erosion or ulcer.

cryptococcosis Lung or meningeal infection caused by *Cryptococcus neoformans*.

cryptosporidiosis Intestinal infection caused by *Cryptosporidium parvum*.

crystallisable fragment (Fc) The tail part of an antibody molecule where complement fixation and phagocyte adherence occurs.

culture A growth of microbes in/on a culture medium.

culture medium A preparation of nutrient material for the growth of microorganisms.

cutaneous mycoses Fungal infections which affect the epidermal layers of the skin.

cyanobacteria A group of photosynthetic bacteria, formerly called blue-green algae.

cyst (i) A sac with a defined wall containing fluid or other material, e.g. hydatid cyst; (ii) a form of some protozoa and helminths in which the cell is surrounded by a protective layer.

cystitis Infection and inflammation of the urinary bladder.

cytokine A soluble factor released by cells which regulates the activity of other cells involved in body defences.

cytolysis The destruction of cells by damage of their cell membranes.

cytopathic effects The microscopically observable changes to a cell caused by virus infection of the cell.

cytoplasm The contents of cells inside the plasma membrane (excluding the nucleus).

cytoplasmic membrane The membrane containing the cytoplasm of the cell. Also called **plasma membrane**.

cytosine A pyrimidine base that pairs with guanine in RNA and DNA.

cytotoxic hypersensitivity Destruction of body cells by the binding of antibodies to antigens on the surface of a cell, followed by complement activation and cell lysis. Also called **type II hypersensitivity**.

cytotoxic T cell A type of T lymphocyte which directly kills infected cells that display microbial antigens on their surface.

dark-field microscopy A type of compound light microscopy using a special condenser so that objects in the specimen appear bright against a black background.

debridement Removal of necrotic tissue from a wound.

decline phase The phase of an illness when the acute symptoms have subsided.

decontamination The process of removal of undesirable substances or pathogens from an object or area by cleaning or disinfecting.

defensin A small peptide in the body that has killing activity against a broad range of microorganisms.

definitive host The organism that harbours the adult sexually mature form of a parasite.

degranulation The release of granules containing histamine and other inflammatory chemicals by mast cells and basophils in allergic reactions.

delayed type hypersensitivity Hypersensitivity reactions that are mediated by T cells and take a day or more to appear after the introduction of antigen. Also called **cell-mediated hypersensitivity** or **type IV hypersensitivity**.

delayed type hypersensitivity T cells T cells responsible for delayed type hypersensitivity reactions. When stimulated by antigen, they secrete lymphokines which activate macrophages and cause inflammatory reactions.

dendritic cells A group of bone marrow derived cells found in skin and lymphoid tissues that play an important role in antigen presentation to lymphocytes.

dengue fever A systemic infection caused by the dengue virus and transmitted by mosquitoes.

dengue haemorrhagic fever A serious form of dengue fever characterised by bleeding from the gums, skin and gastro-intestinal tract.

deoxyribose A pentose sugar which is part of the DNA molecule.

dermatomycosis A fungal skin infection.

dermatophytes Fungi that grow on skin.

dermis The inner layer of the skin.

diapedesis The process by which neutrophils move out of the bloodstream and into the tissue space in inflammation.

diarrhoea A disruption in bowel habits characterised by more frequent passing of loose, watery stools.

differential medium A microbial growth medium that allows the differentiation of one microorganism from another.

dimorphism The ability of an organism to grow in two different forms under different environmental conditions.

diphtheria An acute infection of the upper respiratory tract caused by toxin-producing strains of *Corynebacterium diphtheriae*. The toxin can subsequently cause heart, kidney and nervous tissue disease.

diplococci Spherical bacteria that occur in pairs.

diploid cell A cell that has two sets of chromosomes.

disaccharide A carbohydrate molecule composed of two sugar units.

disease A harmful alteration to the physiological or metabolic state of a host.

disease-specific isolation precautions A set of procedures to be followed to prevent the transmission of a specific disease.

disinfectant A chemical substance normally used for the disinfection of inanimate objects.

disinfection The destruction, removal or reduction in numbers of harmful microorganisms to an acceptable level.

disseminated infection An infection which spreads throughout the body.

disseminated intravascular coagulation The non-specific activation of blood coagulation mechanisms by endotoxin, resulting in the blockage of small vessels by thrombi in a variety of organs.

DNA (deoxyribonucleic acid) The molecule which carries genetic information.

domains Part of the classification system for living organisms.

donovanosis A genital ulcer disease caused by *Calymmato-bacterium granulomatis*. Also called **granuloma inguinale**.

dot blot method A method of analysing DNA.

droplet transmission The spread of infectious agents in small liquid droplets through the air.

dry heat sterilisation A method of sterilisation using dry heat at 160°C for 60 minutes.

dysentery A severe diarrhoea characterised by blood and pus in the stools.

dysuria Difficult or painful passing of urine.

ecology The study of the relationship between organisms and their environment.

ecosystem The living and non-living components of a particular environment.

ectoparasite A parasite that lives on the surface of another organism.

electron micrograph A photograph of a specimen taken with an electron microscope.

electron microscope A microscope that uses electrons to produce an image of the specimen.

electron transport chain A chain of specialised compounds that can pass electrons along the chain to a final electron acceptor (molecular oxygen), releasing energy as ATP.

elephantiasis A gross enlargement of limbs, scrotum or other body parts caused by repeated infection by the worm *Wuchereria bancrofti*.

ELISA A method of detection of antibodies in blood. From Enzyme Linked Immunosorbent Assay.

Embden-Meyerhof pathway See **glycolysis**.

empyema Infection of the pleural space.

encephalitis Infection and inflammation of the brain.

endemic disease A disease which is always present in a given population.

endocarditis Inflammation of the internal membrane lining of the heart.

endocytosis The process by which phagocytes take up foreign material.

endogenous infection An infection caused by microorganisms from the patient's own body.

endogenous pyrogen A fever-producing substance derived from body cells.

endophthalmitis An infection and inflammation of the fluid behind the cornea.

endoplasmic reticulum A network of membranes in eucaryotic cells connecting the nuclear membrane to the plasma membrane and providing sites for ribosomal attachment.

endospore A resistant structure with a thick coat, formed within some Gram-positive bacterial cells.

endotoxic shock A severe, life-threatening form of septicaemia caused by the release of large amounts of endotoxin from Gram-negative bacteria.

endotoxin A lipopolysacccharide which occurs as part of the cell wall of most Gram-negative bacteria and is released when the cell dies. May produce toxic effects in the human host.

endotracheal intubation The insertion of a tube into the trachea to open the airway.

enriched medium A microbial growth medium that contains special growth factors for fastidious organisms.

enteritis Inflammation of the intestine.

Enterobacteriaceae A group of facultatively anaerobic Gram-negative bacteria, many of which are found in the human intestine.

enterotoxin An exotoxin that acts specifically on the intestine.

enzyme A protein molecule that acts as a biological catalyst.

eosinophil A blood cell present in large numbers in allergic reactions.

epidemic A sudden rapid rise in the incidence of a disease in a particular population or area.

epidemic keratoconjunctivitis An infection of the conjunctiva and cornea caused by adenoviruses.

epidemic polyarthritis A systemic infection caused by the Ross River virus and spread by mosquitoes.

epidemiology The study of the occurrence, spread and control of disease.

epidermis The outer layer of the skin.

epididymitis Infection and inflammation of the epididymis.

epiglottitis Infection and inflammation of the epiglottis.

epitope The small part of a whole antigen molecule that is the immunogenic component; the site of binding of antibodies or activated lymphocytes.

erosion A superficial, circumscribed loss of epidermis, which heals without scarring.

erysipelas A bacterial skin infection, often on the face, that typically appears as a bright red, swollen lesion with a sharply demarcated edge.

erythema Reddened skin, usually due to inflammation.

erythema migrans A unique skin lesion with a bulls-eye appearance which occurs in the early stage of Lyme disease.

eschar The thick crust or scab that forms over a burn.

essential nutrients Substances that are essential for growth.

etiology See **aetiology**.

eubacteria All procaryotes (bacteria) containing peptidoglycan cell walls. Also called **true bacteria**.

Eucarya One of the domains used for classification of living organisms.

eucaryotic Describes organisms that have their DNA enclosed in a nucleus and contain other membrane-bound organelles. Includes animals, plants and fungi.

evidence-based practice The use of research evidence to support changes in clinical procedures.

excoriation An area of skin denuded of epidermis by scratching.

exfoliatin An exotoxin possessed by some strains of *Staphylococcus aureus* that causes layers of cells in the epidermis to separate and sheets of skin to be shed (scalded skin syndrome).

exogenous infection An infection caused by microorganisms from a source external to the patient.

exogenous pyrogen A fever-producing substance derived from outside the body, often components of bacteria, and especially lipopolysaccharides.

exotoxin A toxin secreted by a bacterium into its environment.

exponential growth Growth of a bacterial culture characterised by a doubling of cell numbers in each time period.

exudate An accumulation of plasma fluid and proteins in a tissue during inflammation.

F plasmid Extrachromosomal DNA found in F+ donor cells capable of conjugation.

facilitated diffusion The movement of substances across a membrane from a region of high concentration to a region of lower concentration using carrier proteins.

facultative anaerobes Organisms which can grow in the presence or absence of oxygen.

faecal-oral transmission The mode of transmission of pathogens that enter the body via the gastrointestinal tract and are excreted in faeces.

falciparum malaria The most severe form of malaria, caused by *Plasmodium falciparum*.

false negative A negative test result in a person who actually has the disease.

false positive A positive test result in a person who does not have the disease.

fastidious microorganism A microorganism that requires special growth factors.

fatty acid Long chain aliphatic compound containing a terminal carboxyl group.

fermentation The enzymic breakdown of pyruvate in the absence of oxygen.

fever (pyrexia) Abnormally high body temperature, representing severe or systemic infection and/or inflammation.

fibroblast A cell which gives rise to collagen and connective tissue.

fifth disease A common infection of children characterised by a rash on the cheeks, caused by parvovirus B19.

filamentous fungi Fungi consisting of thin filaments or hyphae which form a mat called a mycelium.

filariasis A systemic infection caused by several different roundworms; most commonly by *Wuchereria bancrofti*.

filtration A method for separation of solids from liquids or gases by passage through special filters which retain the solids. Used to remove bacteria from solutions and air.

fimbriae Hair-like appendages on bacteria, used for attachment to surfaces.

five-kingdom classification A system of classification proposed by Whittaker, in which all living organisms are grouped into one of five kingdoms: Procaryota, Protista, Fungi, Plantae and Animalia.

flagella Long thin appendages that are found on some organisms and that enable them to move.

flatworms A primitive group of worms, the main parasitic ones being flukes and tapeworms.

fluid mosaic model The model proposed for the structure of the cell membrane, consisting of proteins embedded in a phospholipid bilayer.

flukes Flatworms with complex life cycles.

fluorescence microscopy The use of ultraviolet light in a microscope to visualise objects that fluoresce.

folliculitis Infection of a hair follicle, usually caused by *Staphylococcus aureus*. Also called a **pimple** or **pustule**.

fomite Any inanimate object that can be involved in the spread of infection.

food biosecurity The prevention of the intentional contamination of food and water with hazardous agents, including pathogens and toxins.

food intoxication A gastrointestinal disease caused by the presence of preformed toxins (microbial or non-microbial) in food.

food poisoning A gastrointestinal disease related to the consumption of food, including microbial and non-microbial causes. Also called **food-borne illness**.

food-borne illness See **food poisoning**.

frame-shift mutation A mutation involving the deletion or insertion of one or more bases, resulting in a change in the codon and the insertion of a different amino acid into the protein.

free radical A very reactive particle containing an unpaired electron.

frequency The need to urinate more frequently than usual.

fulminant hepatitis A clinical syndrome in which there is severe impairment or necrosis of liver cells, often resulting in liver failure and death.

fulminating disease A sudden very severe disease, often with a fatal outcome.

fungaemia The presence of fungi in the bloodstream.

fungi Eucaryotic organisms with cell walls that are not capable of photosynthesis.

furuncle See **boil**.

fusidic acid A bacteriostatic agent that inhibits protein synthesis.

gammaglobulin (i) An antibody preparation extracted from the pooled serum of large numbers of blood donors; (ii) the fraction of blood proteins that contains antibodies.

gangrenous infection An infection of the soft tissue below the dermis.

gastritis Inflammation of the internal lining of the stomach.

gastroenteritis Inflammation of the gastrointestinal tract, including the stomach and intestine.

gastrointestinal infection A disease of the gastrointestinal tract caused by the establishment and multiplication of microorganisms in the gastrointestinal tract.

gene A linear segment of DNA which codes for a particular hereditary characteristic.

generalised transduction The transfer of genetic material from one bacterial cell to another by a lytic phage genital ulcer disease.

generation time The time taken for a bacterial cell to reproduce itself.

genetic engineering Manipulation of the genetic material of an organism in order to alter the characteristics of the organism in a particular way.

genetic recombination Formation of DNA involving the reciprocal exchange of homologous (paired) segments of DNA at any place on the chromosome.

genital ulcer disease Any infection characterised by ulceration of the genital region.

genus Part of the binomial classification system above the level of species, e.g. *Staphylococcus* in *Staphylococcus aureus*.

germ theory of disease The principle proposed by Koch that microorganisms can cause disease.

German measles See **rubella**.

germicide A substance that kills microorganisms (germs).

Ghon complex The characteristic finding in tuberculosis of tubercles (small granulomas) in the lung plus enlarged lymph nodes.

giardiasis A gastrointestinal infection caused by the protozoan *Giardia intestinalis*.

gingivitis A periodontal disease involving inflammation or infection of the gums.

glandular fever A systemic infection caused by the Epstein-Barr virus. Also called **infectious mononucleosis**.

glomerular haematuria The presence of blood in the urine due to inflammation or infection of the glomeruli of the kidneys.

glomerulonephritis Inflammation of the glomeruli of the kidneys.

glycerol An organic alcohol containing three carbon atoms. It combines with fatty acids to form triglycerides.

glycocalyx A structure consisting of polysaccharides found outside the cell wall of some bacteria. Also called **capsule** or **slime layer**.

glycogen A branched polysaccharide containing glucose units which acts as a carbon storage molecule.

glycolysis The anaerobic metabolic pathway in which glucose is converted to pyruvate.

Golgi complex A membranous organelle in eucaryotic cells involved in the secretion of proteins.

gonorrhoea A sexually transmissible disease caused by the bacterium *Neisseria gonorrhoeae*.

Gram-negative Describes a bacterium which stains red with the Gram stain.

Gram-positive Describes a bacterium which retains the blue colour of the Gram stain.

Gram stain A standard procedure for staining bacteria which divides almost all bacteria into two groups, and serves as the first step in classifying and identifying them.

granuloma A lesion associated with chronic inflammation that typically consists of a mass of different types of cells arranged in fairly discrete layers, and completely walled off by collagen.

granuloma inguinale See **donovanosis**.

guanine A purine nucleotide base that pairs with cytosine in RNA and DNA.

gumma A soft, granulomatous lesion in the skin, bones, liver or other organs, characteristic of tertiary syphilis.

gut-associated lymphoid tissue (GALT) Clusters of lymphoid cells lining the mucosal surface of the intestinal tract.

haemagglutination Aggregation (agglutination) of red blood cells.

haematuria The presence of blood in urine.

haemoflagellates A flagellated protozoan usually found in the bloodstream of its host.

haemolysin A toxin that breaks down red cells.

haemolytic uraemic syndrome (HUS) A possible complication of some infections caused by toxigenic strains of *E. coli*, characterised by haemolytic anaemia, uraemia, thrombo-cytopaenia and renal failure.

haemorrhagic fever A disease characterised by fever, malaise, myalgia, prostration, multisystem involvement and widespread haemorrhage, and caused by a number of different viruses.

half-life The time taken for half of a substance to be used or destroyed.

hapten A small molecule that cannot initiate an immune response on its own, but which reacts with antibodies or activated T cells produced against it.

heavy (H) chain The longer polypeptide chain of an antibody molecule.

helminths Worms.

helper T cell A regulatory T lymphocyte that plays a central role in the immune response.

hepatitis Injury and inflammation of the liver.

hepatitis A Hepatitis caused by the hepatitis A virus.

hepatitis B Hepatitis caused by the hepatitis B virus.

hepatitis C Hepatitis caused by the hepatitis C virus.

hepatitis D Hepatitis caused by the hepatitis D virus.

hepatitis E Hepatitis caused by the hepatitis E virus.

hepatocellular carcinoma Cancer of the liver.

herd immunity The principle that individuals who are immune to an infectious disease will not be carriers of the organism, reducing the reservoir of that microbe in the community, and therefore the number of susceptible people who will encounter it.

herpes encephalitis Infection of the brain caused by the herpes virus, especially serious in neonates.

heterotroph An organism which requires an organic source of carbon for energy.

hexachloraphene Human parvovirus.

hexose A sugar molecule containing six carbon atoms.

Hfr strain A bacterial strain which exhibits a high frequency of recombination due to the insertion of an F+ plasmid into the chromosomal DNA.

histamine A substance present in many body cell types, especially mast cells, basophils and platelets, that causes vasodilation and increased capillary permeability.

histones Proteins associated with DNA in eucaryotic chromosomes.

hookworm A type of roundworm which enters the body by burrowing through the skin and travels via the bloodstream and attaches to the lungs and intestines.

horizontal transmission Transmission of a disease from one person to another, usually by physical contact.

hospital strain A strain of microorganism that originates in hospitals. This organism is likely to be resistant to some antimicrobial drugs.

hospital-acquired infection An infection acquired in a hospital. Also called a **nosocomial infection**.

human leucocyte antigen A major histocompatibility (MHC) protein that is found on the surface of leucocytes.

humoral immune response An immune response to foreign antigen characterised by the activation of B lymphocytes and the production of specific antibodies against the antigen.

humoral immunity Immunity provided by antibodies present in the body's fluids.

hyaluronidase An enzyme produced by some bacteria which breaks down the hyaluronic acid of connective tissue.

hydatid disease A disease characterised by the production of fluid-filled sacs in the body, containing developing forms of the tapeworm *Echinococcus granulosis*.

hydrophilic Water loving.

hydrophobic Water hating; does not mix with water.

hypersensitivity An over-reaction of the immune system to an antigen which it has previously encountered.

hypertonic A solution with a higher concentration of dissolved substances than is present in a cell.

hyphae Long filaments of cells found in fungi.

hypotonic A solution with a lower concentration of dissolved substances than is present in a cell.

iatrogenic infection An infection resulting from a medical procedure or treatment.

IgA A class of antibody molecules found mainly in mucosal secretions and breast milk.

IgD A class of antibody molecules found on the surface of B lymphocytes.

IgE The class of antibody molecules responsible for allergic reactions.

IgG The major class of antibody molecules in blood, and the class which crosses the placenta from mother to foetus.

IgM The class of antibody molecules in blood that are produced early in response to infection and that are indicative of recent infection.

imidazoles A group of antifungal drugs that inhibit sterol synthesis.

immediate hypersensitivity A hypersensitive reaction that occurs within minutes to hours after a sensitised person comes in contact with a foreign antigen. Also called **allergy** or **type I hypersensitvity**.

immune complex An antibody molecule bound specifically to its antigen.

immune complex hypersensitivity A hypersensitive reaction that results when antigen-antibody complexes are not cleared quickly from the body, instead being deposited in tissues. Also called **type III hypersensitivity**.

immune response The specific response to the presence of a microorganism or foreign substance in the body.

immune surveillance The mechanisms of the immune system that enable it to seek out and destroy tumour cells.

immune system The system of specific and non-specific defences the body has to eliminate foreign microorganisms and substances, and to provide long-term immunity to them.

immunisation The exposure of a person to material that is antigenic but not pathogenic to make them immune to a certain microorganism. Also called **vaccination**.

immunity The capacity of the immune system to successfully defend the body against a potentially infectious agent.

immunocompromised Having a defect in one or more of the key components of the immune system (lymphocytes, phagocytes or complement).

immunodeficiency A condition in which the production or function of one of the key components of the immune system (lymphocytes, phagocytes or complement) is abnormal.

immunodeficiency disease A disease which causes immuno-deficiency.

immunofluorescence A method of diagnosis involving labelling with fluorescent antibodies.

immunogen See **antigen**.

immunogenic Capable of inducing an immune response.

immunoglobulin See **antibody**.

immunological memory The property of the immune system which enables it to react more rapidly and vigorously on subsequent exposures to the same antigen.

immunology The study of the body's immune system.

immunosuppression A depletion or reduction of the immune defences of the host.

impetigo A highly infectious skin infection caused by staphylococci, streptococci, or both.

in vitro Outside a living organism; in the laboratory.

in vivo In a living organism.

incidence rate The proportion of a population that contracts a disease within a given time period.

inclusions Small deposits found inside cells, e.g. storage granules.

incubation period The period of time which elapses between exposure to a pathogen and the appearance of disease symptoms.

index case The first case of a disease in an epidemic.

inducer A substance which stimulates the expression a gene.

inducible enzyme An enzyme which is synthesised under the influence of an inducer.

induration A raised red area on the skin resulting from tuberculin sensitivity.

infection The growth of pathogenic microorganisms in the body.

infectious disease A disease which is caused by a pathogenic microorganism or its products.

infectious mononucleosis See **glandular fever**.

infective dose The number of microorganisms which must gain entry to the body in order to establish an infection.

infective endocarditis An inflammation of the endocardium caused by a microorganism.

inflammation The body's response to tissue injury, characterised by redness, swelling, heat and pain.

inflammatory diarrhoea Diarrhoea characterised by stools containing blood, mucus and pus.

influenza A respiratory infection caused by influenza A and B viruses.

innate immunity See **non-specific immunity**.

integrase An enzyme that integrates viral DNA into the host cell genome. The human immunodeficiency virus (HIV) has an integrase.

interferon (IFN) (i) A protein secreted by virus-infected cells which helps neighbouring cells to resist infection; (ii) a lymphokine secreted by activated T lymphocytes.

interleukin A cytokine that acts as a chemical messenger between leukocytes.

interleukin-1 (IL-1) A cytokine released by macrophages and other cells that stimulates activated T cells.

interleukin-2 (IL-2) A cytokine that encourages activated T cells to proliferate and differentiate.

intermediate host The host which harbours the immature or larval form of a parasite.

intoxication A disease due to a microbial toxin.

invasive phase The stage in a disease when the pathogen is invading the host and causing severe symptoms.

iodophor An antiseptic preparation containing iodine and an organic compound.

ischaemia Loss of blood supply to a tissue.

isomers Organic compounds with the same chemical formula but different molecular structures.

isotonic A solution containing the same concentration of dissolved substances as is found in a cell.

keratin A tough protein found in skin, nails and hair that is resistant to most weak acids, bases, and bacterial enzymes and toxins.

keratinase A microbial enzyme that degrades keratin.

keratitis Infection and inflammation of the cornea.

keratoconjunctivitis Infection and inflammation of the conjunctiva and cornea.

kinases A group of enzymes produced by certain bacteria that enable them to dissolve fibrin clots.

kinins Small peptides present in blood and other body fluids in an inactive form which, when activated, cause vasodilation, increased vascular permeability and pain.

Koch's Postulates A set of criteria proposed by Robert Koch, which should be met in order to determine whether an organism is responsible for causing a particular disease.

Koplik's spots Found in measles, they are areas of white necrosis on a reddened mucosa in the mouth.

Krebs cycle See **TCA cycle**.

kuru A human prion disease which has been found in people of the Fore tribes in Papua New Guinea.

lactoferrin A substance, present in a number of body secretions, that inhibits the growth of some microorganisms by binding the growth factor iron.

lag phase The period of bacterial growth during which bacteria are exposed to fresh medium but do not increase in number.

laryngitis Infection and inflammation of the larynx.

laryngotracheitis Infection and inflammation of the larynx and trachea.

latent Refers to the presence of a pathogen in the body without replicating.

latent viral infection An infection in which the virus remains dormant in the host for long periods without replicating or producing disease symptoms.

legionellosis See **Legionnaires' disease**.

Legionnaires' disease A pneumonia caused by *Legionella pneumophila* or other species of Legionella. Also called legionellosis.

leishmaniasis Also called kala azar, a disease transmitted by sandflies, resulting in visceral or skin lesions, caused by species of *Leishmania*.

lepromatous leprosy A form of leprosy in which there is uncontrolled proliferation of the bacterium resulting in extensive skin lesions and nerve involvement.

leprosy An infection of skin and nerves caused by *Mycobacterium leprae*.

leptospirosis A systemic bacterial infection caused by *Leptospira interrogans*.

lesion An area of damaged tissue.

leukocidin A toxin that kills phagocytic leukocytes (neutrophils and macrophages).

leukocyte A white blood cell.

leukocytosis A significant increase in the number of white cells in blood.

leukopenia A decrease below normal numbers of white cells in the blood.

leukotriene A mediator of inflammation synthesised from arachidonic acid, derived from mast cell membranes.

ligand A carbohydrate-specific binding protein involved in adherence.

ligase chain reaction A combined nucleic acid probe and amplification technique for diagnosis of some microbial diseases.

light (L) chain The shorter polypeptide chain of an antibody molecule.

light microscopy The use of a microscope which uses white light to visualise the specimen.

lincosamides A group of antibacterial agents which inhibit protein syntheis.

lipase An enzyme which breaks down fats into glycerol and the component fatty acids.

lipid A An endotoxin which occurs as part of the cell wall of Gram-negative bacteria.

lipopolysaccharide A kind of molecule composed of lipid and polysaccharide units. The lipopolysaccharides which occur as part of the wall of Gram-negative bacteria are called **endotoxins**.

lipoproteins Molecules composed of lipid and protein units.

listeriosis A systemic bacterial infection caused by *Listeria monocytogenes*.

lobar pneumonia An infection and consolidation of the lung confined to certain lobes.

localised infection An infection which is confined to one area of the body.

log phase The period of bacterial growth when the bacteria are dividing at their maximum rate and cell numbers are increasing exponentially.

logarithmic growth Growth of a bacterial culture during which there is a doubling of cell numbers in each specified time interval.

Lyme disease A systemic infection caused by the spirochaete *Borrelia burgdorferi*.

lymph nodes Small, bean-shaped organs occurring throughout the lymphatic system and important in immune responses.

lymphadenopathy A swelling of the lymph nodes.

lymphocyte A white blood cell that plays a critical role in immune responses.

lymphogranuloma venereum A sexually transmissible disease caused by *Chlamydia trachomatis*.

lymphokines Cytokines secreted by activated helper T cells.

lyophilisation Removal of water under controlled conditions.

lysis The rupture of a cell due to osmotic pressure or viral infection.

lysogeny A state in which phage DNA is incorporated into the DNA of the bacterial cell that it has infected, but does not replicate or cause cell lysis.

lysosomes Organelles that contain digestive enzymes; particularly prominent in phagocytes.

lysozyme An enzyme found in body secretions that breaks down the cell wall of many bacteria.

lytic cycle Infection of a cell by a virus resulting in lysis (destruction) of the host cell.

macrolides A group of bacteriostatic antibiotics which affect protein synthesis; used as an alternative for people who are allergic to penicillin.

macrophage A large phagocytic cell found in most tissues and organs of the body.

macule A circumscribed, flat area of altered skin colour.

mad cow disease See **bovine spongiform encephalopathy**.

major histocompatibility complex (MHC) The gene complex which codes for proteins that are used as recognition molecules by lymphocytes. The proteins are important antigens in transplant rejection.

malaise A general feeling of being unwell.

malaria A systemic infection caused by protozoa of the genus *Plasmodium*.

Malta fever See **brucellosis**.

Mantoux skin test A skin test for immunity to tuberculosis. Also called the **tuberculin skin test**.

margination The process by which neutrophils stick to the inner walls of the capillaries prior to their movement through the capillary wall and into the tissues.

mast cell A cell found throughout the body that contains histamine and other inflammatory mediators.

measles A systemic disease characterised by a skin rash caused by the rubeola virus. Also called **rubeola**.

measles encephalitis A rare complication of measles infection in which the virus persists in brain tissue.

mechanical transmission The transmission of an infectious agent on the outside of an insect's body or on a person's hands.

mediators of inflammation The chemicals that are responsible for the physiological events that occur in inflammation.

medical asepsis Procedures that limit the number, growth and spread of microorganisms by practices such as good hygiene, handwashing and disinfection.

meiosis The process in reproduction that leads to a halving of the number of chromosomes in a eucaryotic cell, from diploid to haploid.

melioidosis An infection caused by the bacterium *Burkholderia pseudomallei*. Usually a pneumonia, but the organism can form abscesses in many body organs.

membrane attack complex The components of the complement system that damage membranes of cells, resulting in their lysis.

memory cell A lymphocyte that persists in the body for months to years and provides long-term immunity.

meninges The three membranes that surround the brain and the spinal cord.

meningitis Infection and inflammation of the meninges.

meningococcaemia The presence of *Neisseria meningitidis* in the bloodstream.

meningococcal meningitis Meningitis caused by *Neisseria meningitidis*.

meningococcus Another name for *Neisseria meningitidis*.

merozoite A form of the malarial parasite found in the liver or infected blood cells.

merozoites A stage in the life cycle of the malaria parasite. Merozoites are released from the liver into the bloodstream and produce the typical symptoms of malaria at regular intervals.

mesophile An organism which grows in the temperature range between about 10°C and 50°C.

messenger RNA (mRNA) The type of RNA that carries the genetic message from DNA to the ribosome where it acts as a template to direct the incorporation of the correct amino acids into protein.

metabolic pathway A sequence of enzymically directed reactions in which the product of one reaction serves as the substrate for the next reaction.

metabolism The sum of all the chemical reactions which occur in a living cell.

methicillin-resistant *Staphylococcus aureus* (MRSA) A strain of *Staphylococcus aureus* that is resistant to methicillin and usually a number of other antimicrobial drugs.

metronidazole A widely used antiprotozoal drug.

microbiota Normal microorganisms present on the human body.

microfilaria A microscopic roundworm larva which may ultimately block the lymph capillaries and cause elephantiasis.

microflora See **normal flora**.

mid-stream specimen of urine (MSU) A specimen of urine that is collected after the first few millilitres is allowed to pass.

miliary tuberculosis A serious form of tuberculosis in which the bacterium spreads throughout the body.

minimum inhibitory concentration (MIC) The lowest concentration of an antimicrobial agent which will prevent the growth of a particular microorganism.

mitochondria Membrane-rich organelles found in eucaryotic cells; the site of oxidative phosphorylation reactions which produce ATP.

mitosis The process by which eucaryotic nuclei divide, maintaining the same number of chromosomes.

MMR vaccine A vaccine to protect against measles, mumps and rubella.

molluscum contagiosum A skin infection caused by viruses of the pox group.

Monera See **Procaryota**.

moniliasis See **candidiasis**.

monocyte A phagocytic blood cell that is the precursor of the tissue macrophage.

monosaccharide A simple carbohydrate consisting of a single sugar unit containing five or six carbon atoms.

morbidity (i) The incidence of disease in the total population; (ii) the state of being diseased.

morphology The external appearance.

mortality The number of deaths that result from a particular disease.

motile Describes microorganisms that are able to move by the use of appendages such as cilia and flagella.

mucinase An enzyme produced by some bacteria which digests a component of mucus, enhancing their ability to colonise mucous membranes.

mucociliary escalator The ciliated epithelium of the upper respiratory tract which moves mucus and anything trapped in it upwards away from the lungs.

mucocutaneous Relating to the mucous membranes and the epithelium.

multi-resistant *Staphylococcus aureus* (MRSA) A strain of *Staphylococcus aureus* that is resistant to a number of antimicrobial drugs. These strains are responsible for many infections in hospitals.

mutagen An agent which can cause a mutation.

mutation A permanent change in the structure of DNA.

mutualism A symbiotic relationship between two organisms in which both organisms benefit.

mycelium A mass of fungal hyphae which intertwine forming a mat.

mycoplasmas Very small bacteria which lack a cell wall.

mycosis A fungal infection.

naive lymphocyte A mature lymphocyte that has not encountered its specific antigen.

naked virus A virus that is not surrounded by an envelope.

narrow spectrum antimicrobial agent A drug which is active against a limited number of microorganisms.

narrow spectrum drug An antimicrobial agent which is active against only a few species of organisms.

natural immunity See **non-specific immunity**.

natural killer (NK) cells A group of non-specific lymphoid cells that destroy cancer cells and virus-infected cells.

naturally acquired active immunity Immunity that develops after an infection.

naturally acquired passive immunity Immunity due to the natural transfer of antibodies, e.g. immunity acquired by the foetus via transplacental transfer of antibodies.

necrosis Tissue death.

necrotising fasciitis Infection and inflammation in the soft tissue below the dermis (the superficial fascia).

necrotising infection Infection of the soft tissue below the dermis.

nematode A roundworm.

neoplasia The alteration of cellular DNA in such a way that the cell multiplies uncontrollably.

nephrotoxicity Able to cause damage to the kidneys.

neurosyphilis A form of tertiary syphilis in which lesions form in the central nervous system.

neurotoxin An exotoxin which acts predominantly on nervous tissue.

neutralisation A process in which antibodies bind to and block specific attachment sites on viruses or bacterial exotoxins.

neutropenia A decrease in the number of neutrophils in the blood.

neutrophil The most abundant type of white blood cell. It is highly phagocytic and actively motile. Also called a **polymorphonuclear leukocyte (PMN)**, **polymorph** or **pus cell**.

neutrophilia A significant increase in the number of neutrophils in blood. It is a characteristic sign of severe bacterial infection.

nitrogen fixation The ability of some microorganisms to use nitrogen from the air to grow.

nodule A circumscribed, elevated area of skin, larger than 1 cm in diameter.

non-communicable diseases Diseases which are not usually spread from person to person.

non-inflammatory diarrhoea A diarrhoea characterised by watery stools without blood, mucus or pus.

non-polar Describes a substance which does not carry any positive or negative charge on its molecules.

non-specific defences Defences that offer general protection against all potentially harmful agents. These defences include the skin and mucous membranes, cellular defences, inflammation, antimicrobial proteins and fever.

non-specific immunity Immunity provided by the non-specific defences to prevent the entry of pathogens into the body, or to immediately destroy them if they do manage to enter. Also called **innate immunity** and **natural immunity**.

non-specific urethritis Any infection of the urethra not caused by *Neisseria gonorrhoeae* or *Chlamydia trachomatis*.

nonsense codon A codon that does not code for an amino acid.

normal flora The microorganisms that inhabit the human body without causing disease.

normal immunoglobulin An immunoglobulin preparation containing a mixture of antibodies that is extracted from the serum of large numbers of blood donors.

nosocomial infection An infection that is acquired in a hospital or other health-care facility.

nuclear membrane The membrane enclosing the nucleus.

nucleocapsid Refers to the protein-nucleic acid complex of the virus.

nucleoli Areas in the nucleus of a eucaryotic cell where ribosomal RNA is formed.

nucleoside A compound consisting of a purine or pyrimidine base joined to a pentose sugar molecule.

nucleotide A nucleoside joined to one or more phosphate groups.

nucleus An organelle in eucaryotic cells where chromosomes are located.

obligate aerobe See **aerobe, obligate**.

obligate anaerobe See **anaerobe, obligate**.

oedema Swelling of a tissue due to an accumulation of fluid.

oncogenic Cancer-causing.

oophoritis Inflammation of the ovaries.

ophthalmia neonatorum An eye infection in neonates caused by *Neisseria gonorrhoeae*, acquired from the mother during passage through the birth canal.

opportunistic infections Infections caused by organisms that do not usually cause disease, but can become pathogenic under certain conditions, such as depression of the immune system.

opsonin A serum protein (antibody or complement) that enhances phagocyte activity.

opsonisation The enhancement of phagocyte activity with opsonins.

organelle A structure bounded by a membrane and found within eucaryotic cells.

organic Describes a compound containing carbon.

ornithosis See **psittacosis**.

osmosis The movement of water from an area of high water concentration to an area of low concentration across a selectively permeable membrane.

osmotic pressure The pressure required to prevent the movement of water by osmosis.

osteomyelitis Infection and inflammation of a bone.

otitis media Infection and inflammation of the middle ear.

ototoxicity Able to cause damage to the ears or hearing.

oxidation The loss of electrons from a molecule.

oxidative phosphorylation The process whereby the energy of electrons from oxidation reactions is coupled to the synthesis of ATP.

pandemic An epidemic that spreads worldwide.

papule A circumscribed, elevated area of skin, less than 1 cm in diameter.

parasitaemia The presence of protozoa or helminths in the blood.

parasite An organism that derives its nutrients from another living organism (the host).

parasitism A symbiotic relationship in which one organism benefits while the other, the host, is harmed.

paronychia An infection of the finger or toe nail.

passive immunisation Immunisation involving the transfer of preformed antibodies to an individual.

passive immunity The immunity resulting from the transfer of pre-made antibodies or immune cells from an immune person to a non-immune person.

pasteurisation A method of mild heat treatment developed by Pasteur to destroy microorganisms responsible for food spoilage and some pathogens.

pathogen An organism that is able to produce disease.

pathogen associated molecular patterns Molecules found on microorganisms, but not on human cells.

pathogenicity The ability of a microorganism to cause disease.

pediculosis A lice infestation usually involving the scalp, pubic area or trunk.

pelvic inflammatory disease A clinical syndrome due to infection of the pelvic organs, particularly the uterus, fallopian tubes, ovaries or the whole peritoneal cavity, which may lead to scarring and blockage of the fallopian tubes.

penicillin The first antibiotic to be discovered; one of a group of bacteriocidal compounds which inhibit cell wall synthesis.

pentose A sugar molecule containing five carbon atoms.

peptide A chain of amino acids joined by peptide bonds.

peptidoglycan A major structural component of bacterial cell walls.

perforins Protein molecules which are inserted into the plasma membrane of a target cell bringing about its death.

perinatal infection An infection acquired at birth.

peritonitis Infection and inflammation of the peritoneal cavity.

pertussis A potentially severe infection of the respiratory tract caused by *Bordetella pertussis*. Also called **whooping cough**.

petechia A small flat haemorrhage.

phage See **bacteriophage**.

phage typing A method of identification of different strains of bacteria by determining their susceptibility to infection by specific bacteriophage.

phagocyte A cell that actively ingests and digests foreign material in the body.

phagolysosome A structure in a phagocyte derived from the fusion of a phagosome with lysosomes and in which lysosomal enzymes break down foreign material.

phagosome A phagocytic vacuole which contains ingested foreign material formed within the cytoplasm of a phagocyte.

pharyngitis Infection and inflammation of the oropharynx.

pharyngoconjunctival fever A syndrome of sore throat and conjunctival infection caused by adenoviruses.

phospholipid A compound consisting of glycerol, two fatty acids, phosphate and various bases.

phospholipid bilayer A double layer of phospholipid molecules which form the basic structure (matrix) of cell membranes.

photosynthesis The process occurring in green plants in which energy from the sun is used to synthesise carbohydrate (glucose) from carbon dioxide and water.

pili Appendages on a bacterial cell some of which are used to transfer DNA during conjugation and some of which are for attachment to surfaces.

pinworm A tiny roundworm that lives in the human intestine. Also called threadworm.

pityriasis versicolor A skin infection caused by the yeast *Malassezia furfur*. Also called **tinea versicolor**.

plague An infection of lymph nodes and other organs caused by the bacterium *Yersinia pestis*.

Plantae Plants, one of the original Linnaean classifications.

plaque A coating of microorganisms and organic matter on tooth enamel.

plasma The fluid part of blood without the cells and platelets.

plasma cell The cell responsible for synthesis and secretion of antibodies in humoral immunity.

plasma membrane See **cytoplasmic membrane**.

plasmid A small piece of cyclic DNA found in some bacteria which replicates independently of the chromosomal DNA.

plate count A method of determining the number of bacteria in a sample.

platyhelminthes Flatworms.

pleomorphic Occurring in more than one form.

pleural effusion The entry of an inflammatory exudate into the space between the lung tissue and pleural membranes.

pleurisy Inflammation of the pleural membranes.

pneumonia Infection and inflammation of the lung(s).

pneumonic plague Infection of the lungs by the plague bacterium, *Yersinia pestis*.

point mutation The substitution of one base for another in DNA, causing mutation.

polar Refers to a molecule which carries a positive or negative charge.

polio (poliomyelitis) A systemic infection caused by the polio virus in which infection of the central nervous system may occur and may result in paralysis.

polyenes A group of antifungal compounds which interfere with sterol synthesis.

polymerase chain reaction A technique used to copy a specific nucleotide sequence contained within a sample of DNA, thus increasing the quantity of DNA to detectable levels.

polymorph See **neutrophil**.

polymorphonuclear leukocyte (PMN) See **neutrophil**.

polypeptide A long chain of amino acids, joined by peptide bonds.

polyribosome A ribosome complex where a number of ribosomes are bound along a strand of mRNA.

polysaccharide A polymer of sugar units.

Pontiac fever A mild form of *Legionella* infection, characterised by myalgia, fever, malaise and headache.

portal of entry The point of entry of a pathogen into the body.

portal of exit The point at which a pathogen exits from the body.

post-operative infection Any infection that occurs as a result of surgery.

post-polio syndrome A syndrome in which symptoms of muscular weakness occur late in life in people who have recovered from childhood polio.

post-streptococcal glomerulonephritis Infection of the glomeruli of the kidneys, following a streptococcal infection elsewhere in the body.

PPD (purified protein derivative) The antigen used in the Mantoux skin test for immunity to tuberculosis.

precipitation The cross-linking of soluble antigens by antibody to form large complexes which precipitate out of solution.

prevalence rate The proportion of people with a particular disease at a given point in time.

primary cell line Animal cells extracted from live tissue which are grown in tissue culture in the laboratory.

primary immune response The response of the acquired immune system the first time it is exposed to a particular antigen.

primary immunodeficiency Abnormal production or function of phagocytes, lymphocytes or complement due to a genetic or developmental defect.

primary infection An acute infection which is the cause of the initial illness.

primary lymphoid organs The thymus and the bone marrow which are the sites of lymphocyte maturation.

primary metabolite A compound produced during the active growth phase of a microorganism.

primary syphilis The first stage of syphilis infection characterised by the development of a papular lesion at the site of infection.

prion An infectious protein agent that causes fatal, neuro-degenerative diseases in humans or animals.

probe A small fragment of DNA containing a nucleotide sequence which is specific to the particular organism being looked at.

Procaryota The classification kingdom which contains all the bacteria. Also called **Monera**.

procaryotic Having characteristics of the procaryotes, including a lack of subcellular organelles.

prodromal period The period in the course of a disease when non-specific symptoms are present before the onset of specific signs or symptoms.

proglottid Segment of a tapeworm.

prophage Bacteriophage DNA which has been integrated into the bacterial host DNA.

prophylactic antibiotic An antibiotic administered in order to prevent the occurrence of an infection.

prophylaxis The administration of a drug to prevent a disease.

prostaglandins A group of biologically active substances, some of which are mediators of inflammation.

prosthetic group A molecule bound to an enzyme that is necessary for enzyme activity.

protease An enzyme that breaks down proteins. The human immunodeficiency virus (HIV) has a protease that is crucial in the formation of new virus particles.

protective asepsis Infection control procedures designed to prevent the transmission of an infection to or from a patient.

proteinuria The presence of protein in the urine.

Protista The biological kingdom comprising unicellular eucaryotic organisms.

protoplast A bacterium without its cell wall, enclosed by the cell membrane.

protozoa Single-celled eucaryotic organisms belonging to the kingdom Protista.

pseudopod 'False foot'—an extension of the cell membrane allowing the cytoplasm to flow into it.

psittacosis A pneumonia caused by *Chlamydia psittaci*, usually acquired from birds. Also called **ornithosis**.

psychrophile An organism which grows best in cool temperatures ($15°$ to $20°C$).

puerperal fever An acute streptococcal infection of the uterus and surrounding area, associated with childbirth, also known as childbed fever.

pulse field gel electrophoresis A technique for analysis of DNA composition.

PUO—pyrexia of unknown origin The presence of a fever without any obvious infection.

pure culture A culture consisting of only one species of organism.

purpura Numerous petechiae; small flat haemorrhages on the skin.

pus A thick, creamy-coloured fluid comprising a mixture of dead or dying neutrophils, tissue debris and remaining pathogens.

pus cell See **neutrophil**.

pustule See **folliculitis**.

pyelonephritis Inflammation of one or both kidneys.

pyogenic Pus forming.

pyrexia Fever.

pyrogen A substance which produces fever.

pyruvic acid A compound containing three carbon atoms, the main product of the metabolism of glucose via the glycolytic pathway.

pyuria The presence of large numbers of leucocytes (pus) in urine.

Q fever A pneumonia caused by the bacterium *Coxiella burnetii*.

quinine An antimicrobial drug extracted from the bark of the chinchona tree.

quinolones A group of antibacterials which interfere with DNA synthesis.

rabies An infection of the central nervous system caused by the rabies virus.

recombinant DNA DNA formed from two different species.

regeneration The restoration of a tissue's orginal structure and function after damage by the replacement of cells by mitosis.

repression The process whereby a repressor molecule prevents the synthesis of a protein.

repressor A protein that interferes with the expression of a gene.

reservoir of infection A site where microorganisms persist and which acts as a continual source of infectious agents.

resident flora See **normal flora**.

resistance The ability of the body to prevent the occurrence of an infection.

resistance factors (R) Genes which bestow antimicrobial resistance on bacteria, usually carried on plasmids.

respiration In metabolism, the aerobic breakdown of carbohydrates with release of energy.

restriction endonucleases Enzymes derived from bacteria which are able to cut double-stranded DNA at specific sites on the DNA molecule. Used in genetic engineering.

Restriction Fragment Length Polymorphisms (RFLPs) Fragments of DNA produced by digestion with restriction endonucleases and used to characterise the DNA by electrophoresis.

retinitis Inflammation of the retina.

retroviruses A class of single-stranded RNA viruses which replicate by first synthesising DNA from RNA.

reverse barrier nursing See **protective asepsis**.

reverse transcriptase A viral enzyme that transcribes RNA into DNA.

Reye's syndrome A sometimes fatal disease occasionally seen in children after a viral infection which was treated with aspirin.

rheumatic fever A non-infectious complication of *Streptococcus pyogenes* sore throat in which immune damage to heart and other tissues occurs.

rheumatic heart disease Scarring and deformation of the heart valves due to rheumatic fever.

rheumatoid arthritis A combination autoimmune disease and immune-complex hypersensitivity which causes chronic inflammation and joint damage.

rheumatoid factor An anti-IgG antibody found in the blood of people with rheumatoid arthritis.

rhinitis Infection and inflammation of the nasal passages. Also called **coryza**.

ribose A pentose sugar which occurs in ribonucleic acid.

ribosomes Particles containing RNA and protein found in the cytoplasm and acting as the site of protein synthesis.

rickettsiae Small intracellular bacteria.

rifampicin An antibiotic which inhibits RNA synthesis, used to treat TB.

ringworm A skin infection caused by several different fungi. Also called **tinea**.

RNA (ribonucleic acid) Nucleic acid which takes part in protein synthesis.

rubella A systemic disease characterised by a skin rash and caused by the rubella virus. Also called **German measles**.

rubeola See **measles**.

Sabin vaccine The oral poliomyelitis vaccine containing an attenuated virus.

Salk vaccine The inactivated poliomyelitis vaccine administered by intramuscular injection.

salmonellosis A mainly gastrointestinal infection caused by species of Salmonella.

salpingitis Inflammation of the fallopian tubes.

sanitisation Thorough cleaning of an object to remove most microorganisms.

SARS Severe acute respiratory syndrome; a type of pneumonia caused by a coronavirus.

scabies A skin infestation caused by the mite *Sarcoptes scabiei* var. *hominis*.

scalded skin syndrome A skin disorder caused by strains of *Staphylococcus aureus* which produce the exfoliatin toxin.

scale An abnormal accumulation of keratin in skin.

scanning electron microscope An electron microscope that provides a three-dimensional image of a specimen at very high magnifications.

scar tissue replacement Replacement of damaged tissue with scar tissue, which does not have the physiological functions of the original tissue.

scarlet fever An erythematous skin rash caused by some strains of *Streptococcus pyogenes* which produce an erythrogenic toxin.

schistosomiasis A debilitating systemic disease caused by flukes of the genus Schistosoma.

schizogony The process of multiple fission in which one cell divides many times to produce multiple daughter cells.

scolex The head of a tapeworm.

secondary immune response The immune response resulting from exposure to the same antigen for the second time. The response is faster, stronger and longer lasting than a primary response.

secondary immunodeficiency Immunodeficiency resulting from damage or suppression of otherwise normal components of the immune system by infection, cancer, malnutrition, drugs or other therapies.

secondary infection An infection that occurs following a primary infection, when the patient is in a weakened state.

secondary lymphoid organs The collection of lymphoid organs and tissues that are the sites in the body where immune reactions occur.

secondary metabolites Products of microbial metabolism, usually accumulating in the stationary phase.

secondary syphilis The secondary stage of syphilis characterised by a skin rash or lesions on mucous membranes.

selective medium A microbial culture medium that allows some organisms to grow but not others.

selective toxicity The ability of an antimicrobial agent to inactivate or destroy a microorganism without harming the host cell.

semi-permeable membrane The membrane surrounding most living cells that controls the passage of substances in and out of the cell. Also called selectively permeable membrane.

sepsis Poisoning due to infection by microorganisms.

septic shock A life-threatening disorder due to the presence of large amounts of endotoxin in the body.

septicaemia A serious clinical syndrome resulting from the presence of bacteria in the bloodstream.

serial dilution A method used to dilute a sample so that the number of bacteria present can be counted accurately.

seroconversion The development of antibodies to an antigen in a person's blood.

serology The detection of antibodies or antigens in a sample of blood or other body fluid.

seroprevalence The prevalence of a disease in the community as determined by the number of people who are carrying antibodies to the disease at any one time.

serotypes Different antigenic strains of a microorganism.

serum The liquid part of blood after the cells and clotting factors have been removed.

sex pilus See **pili**.

sexually transmissible infection An infection acquired during sexual activity.

shigellosis See **bacillary dysentery**.

shingles A disease caused by the reactivation of the varicella zoster (chickenpox) virus characterised by painful, vesicular lesions on the skin.

significant bacteriuria A bacterial count of 108/L or more in a properly collected mid-stream specimen of urine.

signs of disease Measurable changes which can be observed in the patient.

sinusitis Inflammation of the sinus cavities.

slime layer See **glycocalyx**.

smallpox A serious systemic disease that has been eradicated from the world.

source of infection The individual or object from which an infection is acquired.

southern blot A technique for DNA analysis.

specialised transduction The accidental inclusion of a piece of chromosomal DNA adjacent to a prophage when the prophage is transferred to another cell.

species A group of organisms with similar properties; the second name in bacterial classification.

specific defences See **acquired immune system**.

specific immunoglobulin (SIG) An antibody preparation obtained from the serum of people who are convalescing from a particular infection and have a large amount of a specific antibody.

specific immune system See **acquired immune system**.

spermine An antibacterial substance found in semen.

spirillum A spiral-shaped bacterium.

spirochaete A spiral-shaped bacterium with an axial filament.

spongiform encephalopathy A prion disease producing microscopic vacuoles in the brain, giving it a spongy appearance.

spontaneous generation The theory that life can arise spontaneously from non-living matter.

sporadic disease Occasional or random outbreak of disease.

sporangiophore An aerial hypha which carries a sporangium.

sporangium A sac containing spores.

spore An asexual reproductive structure formed by fungi and actinomycetes. See also **endospore**.

spore coat The thick protective layer formed around a bacterial endospore.

sporozoan A kind of non-motile protozoan.

sporozoite A trophozoite of malaria which occurs in the salivary glands of mosquitoes.

sputum A specimen from the lungs produced from a deep cough.

staining The application of a stain or dye to microorganisms prior to examination under a microscope.

staphylococci A genus of Gram-positive bacteria characterised by small round cocci which occur in clusters.

staphylokinase An enzyme produced by *Staphylococcus aureus* which breaks down fibrin clots.

starch A carbohydrate polymer consisting of branched chains of glucose units.

stationary phase A stage in growth of a bacterial culture when the number of new cells being produced equals the number of cells which die.

stereospecificity The way in which the spatial configuration (shape) of a molecule determines its ability to bind to another molecule.

stereoisomers Two molecules which have the same chemical structure, but differ in shape; mirror images of each other.

sterile technique Methods used to ensure that an object or area is free of all microorganisms.

sterilisation The complete destruction or removal of all microorganisms including viruses and endospores.

sterility The complete absence of any microorganisms.

streak plate method The method by which microorganisms are isolated as separate colonies on an agar plate.

streptococci A genus of Gram-positive bacteria which occur as chains of cocci.

streptokinase An enzyme produced by some streptococci which breaks down fibrin and which is used therapeutically as a thrombolytic agent.

subacute sclerosing panencephalitis (SSPE) A rare and serious complication of measles due to viral persistence in brain tissue.

subclinical infection An infection which does not produce any recognisable signs or symptoms, but elicits an immune response.

subcutaneous infection An infection involving tissue beneath the skin.

substrate The molecule which an enzyme reacts with.

subunit vaccine A vaccine based on a part of a microorganism.

sulfa drug Synthetic drug containing sulphur.

sulphonamides A group of bacteriostatic agents which interfere with folic acid synthesis.

superantigens Substances produced by some microbes that activate large numbers of T cells, resulting in a massive release of cytokines and tissue injury.

superficial mycosis A fungal infection located on the skin or hair shaft.

superinfection An overgrowth of a resistant microbial species, usually after a period of antimicrobial therapy.

superoxide The free radical O_2^-.

superoxide dismutase An enzyme that destroys the free radical O_2^-.

surgical asepsis The procedures followed to maintain sterility.

surgical site infection A post-operative infection involving the operative field.

surveillance The collection of data on all aspects of the occurrence and spread of a disease.

susceptibility The lack of resistance or a vulnerability to an infection.

symbiosis Two different organisms living together.

symptoms of disease Changes felt and reported by the patient as a result of disease.

syncytia A multi-nucleate mass of fused body cells.

syndrome A group of signs and symptoms which are characteristic of a particular disease.

synergism A situation where the effect of two drugs working together is greater than the action of the drugs working alone.

syphilis A sexually transmissible disease caused by the spirochaete *Treponema pallidum*.

systemic candidiasis See **candidaemia**.

systemic disease A disease which affects the whole body.

systemic infection An infection in which microorganisms enter the bloodstream and are disseminated through the body.

systemic inflammatory response An immune response to an infection that enters the bloodstream and circulates through the body.

systemic mycosis A fungal infection which occurs in deep tissue or involves various organs in the body.

T4 cell A T lymphocyte that possesses the CD4 receptor on its surface; it displays helper activity. Also called a **helper T cell**.

T8 cell A T lymphocyte that possesses the CD8 receptor on its surface; it may display cytotoxic or suppressor activity. Those with cytotoxic activity are called **cytotoxic T cells**.

T cell See **T lymphocyte**.

T dependent antigen An antigen which requires the involvement of T cells in order for activation of B cells to occur.

T lymphocyte A type of lymphocyte which matures in the thymus gland. Responsible for cell-mediated immunity and regulation of immune responses.

tapeworm A segmented flatworm, the adult stage of which lives in the intestine.

TCA—tricarboxylic acid cycle A pathway in carbohydrate metabolism whereby pyruvic acid is converted to carbon dioxide and water with the release of large amounts of energy stored as ATP.

teichoic acid A polysaccharide which occurs in the walls of Gram-positive bacteria.

temperate phage A bacteriophage which exists in a lysogenic state in the host cell.

template A pattern for the replication of a certain structure, as in DNA or RNA.

teratogen A substance causing abnormalities to the foetus *in utero*.

tertiary syphilis The third stage of syphilis infection in which bacterial multiplication and dissemination and a cell-mediated hypersensitivity response of the immune system combine to form lesions in various organs.

tetanus A disease characterised by severe muscle spasm caused by the exotoxin of *Clostridium tetani*.

tetracyclines A group of bacteriostatic drugs which inhibit protein synthesis.

therapeutic index Ratio of the effective dose of a drug to the dose that will be lethal for the host (patient).

thermal death point The lowest temperature at which all the microorganisms present will be killed in a given time.

thermophile An organism which grows well at high temperatures (50° to 60°C).

threadworm See **pinworm**.

thrush A superficial infection of mucous membranes characterised by milky-white patches of inflammation.

thymine A pyrimidine base in DNA which pairs with adenine.

thymine dimer A compound produced by the formation of bonds between adjacent thymine molecules in DNA chains exposed to UV radiation.

thymus An organ found in the upper thoracic region beneath the sternum. Immature lymphocytes develop into mature T cells under the influence of thymic hormones.

tincture of iodine A solution of iodine in alcohol.

tinea See **ringworm**.

tinea capitis Tinea of the scalp.

tinea corporis Tinea of the body (trunk).

tinea cruris Tinea of the groin.

tinea pedis See **athlete's foot**.

tinea unguium Tinea of the nails.

tinea versicolor See **pityriasis versicolor**.

tissue tropism The ability of a virus to attach to specific receptor molecules on the cell surface.

titre A measure of the amount of specific antibody in blood or other body fluid. The reciprocal of the greatest dilution of the fluid that shows a positive reaction in an antibody-antigen reaction.

tolerance A non-responsiveness of the immune system to a given antigen.

toll-like receptor A type of non-specific receptor for a foreign particle or microorganism found on the surface of phagocytes and certain other cell types. It recognises molecules called pathogen associated molecular patterns.

tonsillitis Infection and inflammation of the tonsils.

toxaemia The presence of toxins in the bloodstream.

toxic shock syndrome A systemic disease caused by certain strains of *Staphylococcus aureus* that produce the toxic shock syndrome toxin.

toxin A substance produced by microorganisms that interferes with the normal functioning of host cells or tissues.

toxoid A bacterial exotoxin that has been modified to remove its toxicity while still retaining its ability to elicit an immune response.

toxoplasmosis A systemic infection caused by the protozoan *Toxoplasma gondii*.

TPN—total parenteral nutrition A procedure whereby all nutrition and drugs are administered via a central catheter.

tracheitis Infection and inflammmation of the trachea.

trachoma An eye infection which can lead to blindness, caused by *Chlamydia trachomatis*.

transcription The process of synthesis of messenger RNA using DNA as a template.

transduction Transfer of DNA from one bacterial cell to another by a bacteriophage.

transfer RNA A small RNA molecule responsible for transferring the correct amino acid to the growing peptide chain in protein synthesis.

transformation The process in which naked DNA passes from one bacterial cell to another resulting in a change in the properties of the recipient cell.

transient flora Microorganisms which are found on the human body for only a short time and do not cause disease.

translation The formation of a polypeptide on a messenger RNA template.

transmissible spongiform encaphalopathy A group of progressive, fatal, neurodegenerative diseases (e.g. Creutzfeld-Jacob disease) caused by prions.

transmission electron microscope An electron microscope used to study the internal structures of cells at high magnification.

transport medium A liquid or semi-liquid medium into which some specimens are placed to prevent them from drying and to maintain microorganism viability.

transport proteins Proteins located in the cell membrane and responsible for the transport of substances into and out of the cell.

transposon A fragment of cellular DNA in which genes for resistance to a number of different antimicrobials are located beside each other and so can be transferred to other cells during conjugation.

traveller's diarrhoea The acute diarrhoea that frequently occurs in people visiting a foreign country. Often caused by *E. coli*.

trematodes See **flukes**.

trichinosis A disease caused by the nematode *Trichinella spiralis* which is acquired by eating poorly cooked meat (mainly pork).

trichomoniasis An infection caused by *Trichomonas vaginalis*.

triple antigen vaccine (DTP) A vaccine used to immunise against diphtheria, pertussis and tetanus.

trophozoite A vegetative form of a protozoan.

true bacteria The largest group of bacteria in the three-domain classification scheme.

trypanosomes A group of flagellated protozoa.

tubercle A granuloma lesion characteristic of tuberculosis infection.

tuberculin A protein of the *Mycobacterium* cell used in the Mantoux skin test.

tuberculin skin test See **Mantoux skin test**.

tuberculoid leprosy The form of leprosy in which a strong cell-mediated immune response limits the multiplication of the organism and the disease is confined to patches of skin and certain nerve trunks.

tuberculosis An infection of the lungs or other organs caused by species of *Mycobacteria*.

tumour-associated antigen A chemical grouping, recognised as foreign by the immune system, found on the surface of tumour cells.

tumour necrosis factor (TNF) A cytokine which kills virus-infected cells as well as being important in inflammation and lymphocyte proliferation.

turbidity Cloudiness of a liquid.

type I hypersensitivity See **immediate hypersensitivity**.

type II hypersensitivity See **cytotoxic hypersensitivity**.

type III hypersensitivity See **immune complex hypersensitivity**.

type IV hypersensitivity See **delayed type hypersensitivity**.

ulcer An area of tissue loss, varying in depth. An ulcer may involve skin only, or may extend more deeply into subcutaneous tissue.

ultraviolet radiation Low-energy short-wavelength radiation which can disrupt chemical bonds, e.g. in DNA, causing mutation or cell death.

undulant fever See **brucellosis**.

Universal Precautions A set of infection control procedures designed to prevent transmission of blood-borne pathogens.

urethritis Infection and inflammation of the urethra.

urgency The urgent need to urinate; symptomatic of urinary tract infection.

vaccination See **immunisation**.

vaccine A preparation containing one or more antigens that is used to immunise a person against a specific disease.

vacuole A membrane-bound structure in the cytoplasm of cells, usually containing gas or storage molecules.

vaginal candiasis An infection of the vagina due to *Candida albicans*.

vaginitis Inflammation of the vagina.

variant Creutzfeldt-Jakob disease A prion disease acquired by consumption of contaminated beef from a cow with mad cow disease.

varicella Chickenpox.

vasoconstriction A decrease in the diameter of blood vessels.

vasodilation Dilation of blood vessels.

vegetation A clump of bacteria, fibrin and platelets on the endocardium, characteristic of infective endocarditis.

vegetative cells Actively growing cells.

vertical transmission Transmission of an infection from mother to foetus *in utero*.

vesicle A small blister containing clear fluid, less than 0.5 cm in diameter.

vibrio A small curved (comma-shaped) bacterium.

viraemia The presence of viruses in the blood.

viral attachment proteins Proteins on the surface of the virus which attach to specific receptors on the surface of the target cell.

viral genome The genetic material of a virus.

virion An entire mature virus particle, occurring outside a host cell and consisting of nucleic acid, protein capsid and sometimes an envelope.

viroid An infectious particle consisting only of circular RNA and lacking a capsid.

virulence The degree of pathogenicity of an organism.

virulence factors The factors which contribute to an organism's ability to cause disease.

virus A tiny infectious particle consisting of nucleic acid and a protein coat.

virustatic Able to inhibit viral replication.

volutin Granules of polyphosphate in bacterial cells.

wart A benign mass of tissue on the skin or mucous membrane caused by a papilloma virus.

water-borne transmission Transmission of an infectious agent in contaminated water.

Weil's disease See **leptospirosis**.

wet preparation A suspension of microorganisms in a drop of fluid for microscopic examination.

wheal A raised, often itchy erythematous lesion.

whooping cough See **pertussis**.

X-linked agammaglobulinaemia A primary immunodeficiency disease caused by incomplete maturation of B lymphocytes.

yeast A unicellular fungus.

yellow fever A systemic infection caused by the yellow fever virus and transmitted by mosquitoes.

Ziehl-Neelsen stain See **acid-fast stain**.

zone of inhibition A clear area corresponding to inhibition of bacterial growth which appears on an agar plate around an antimicrobial disk.

zoonosis An infection of animals that can be transmitted to humans.

zoster Shingles.

Credits

All references are to figures.

Page xv author photo Dr Bishop, by Andrew Taylor
Page xv author photo Dr Lee, by John Wong

1.3	The Granger Collection
1.4	Walter and Eliza Hall Institute
1.5	Professor Peter Doherty
1.6	UNAIDS Report, XV International Conference, Bangkok, 2004, <www.unaids.org>
2.5(a), (b)	Dr A Smithyman, Cellabs, Sydney
2.5(c)	Professor Adrian Lee, Department of Microbiology, University of New South Wales
2.8	Dr Gary Lee
2.9	Photograph courtesy of Dr A Smithyman, Cellabs, Sydney
2.10	J O'Rourke, School of Microbiology and Immunology, University of New South Wales
2.11	Phillips Scientific and Industrial Electronics
2.12	Photolibrary
2.13	David Ellis, Adelaide Women and Children's Hospital
2.15	G Jayachandran, Faculty of Health Sciences, University of Sydney
2.16	Professor Richard Lumb
2.17	G Jayachandran, Faculty of Health Sciences, University of Sydney
3.17	Dr Penny Bishop
3.18	David Sheumack & Marianne Muir, Hanitro, PL
4.2(a)	Centers for Disease Control
4.2(b)	Dr Gary Lee
4.3	Centers for Disease Control
4.4(b)	Dr Penny Bishop
4.5	Gautham P Jayachandran, Faculty of Health Sciences, University of Sydney
4.6	B2201250: Photolibrary/Dr Stannard UCT/ SPL
4.9(b)	Photographic Library of Australia Pty Ltd, North Sydney
4.14	G Jayachandran, Faculty of Health Sciences, University of Sydney
4.15	G Jayachandran, Faculty of Health Sciences, University of Sydney
4.24	Photographic Library of Australia Pty Ltd, North Sydney
4.27	Dr Penny Bishop
5.4	Dr Penny Bishop
5.7	Centers for Disease Control
5.8	Photograph courtesy of Dr A Smithyman, Cellabs, Sydney
5.9	Department of Infectious Diseases, University of Sydney
6.1	David Ellis/Kaminski's Library of Medical Mycology
6.2	SPL-00002505-001: Photolibrary/J. Forsdyke/ Gene Cox/SPL
6.4	David Muir, Royal North Shore Hospital, Sydney
6.5	Audio Visual Services, Royal Prince Alfred Hospital, Sydney
6.6	David Ellis/Kaminski's Library of Medical Mycology
6.7	David Ellis/Kaminski's Library of Medical Mycology
6.8	David Ellis/Kaminski's Library of Medical Mycology
6.9	David Ellis/Kaminski's Library of Medical Mycology
6.10	Dr Gayle Fischer
6.11	Photograph courtesy of Dr A Smithyman, Cellabs
6.12	Professor Tania Sorrell/ David Ellis/Kaminski's Library of Medical Mycology
6.13	David Ellis/Kaminski's Library of Medical Mycology
6.14	David Ellis/Kaminski's Library of Medical Mycology
6.16	Professor Andrew Thompson, Murdoch University/Dr A Smithyman, Cellabs, Sydney
6.17	Stephen Neville, Department of Microbiology, Southwestern Area Pathology Service, Liverpool, NSW
6.20	Stephen Neville, Department of Microbiology, Southwestern Area Pathology Service, Liverpool, NSW
6.21	Centers for Disease Control
7.1(a)	eyeofscience, Germany, www.eyeofscience.com
7.1(b)	SPL-00038560-001: Photolibrary/Southhampton General Hospital/SPL
7.3	Centers for Disease Control
7.4–7.10	Medical Illustrations Department, Princess Margaret Hospital for Children, Perth, WA
7.9(c)	Centers for Disease Control
8.1(a)	CSIRO scienceimage.csiro.au
8.1(b)	Dr Raina Plowright
8.4	Christine Bishop
9.3	Boehringer-Ingelheim Pty Ltd
9.25	The Granger Collection
9.36(a)	SPL-00027411-001: Photolibrary/Andrew Syred/ SPL
9.36(b)	B786710: Photolibrary/Eye of Science/SPL
10.3	Bb2348: Photolibrary/SciMAT/Photo Researchers

Index